SPRIGG'S ESSENTIALS OF
Polysomnography
A Training Guide and Reference for Sleep Technicians

Lisa M. Endee, MPH, RRT-SDS, RPSGT, RST

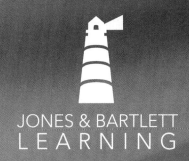

JONES & BARTLETT
LEARNING

World Headquarters
Jones & Bartlett Learning
5 Wall Street
Burlington, MA 01803
978-443-5000
info@jblearning.com
www.jblearning.com

Jones & Bartlett Learning books and products are available through most bookstores and online booksellers. To contact Jones & Bartlett Learning directly, call 800-832-0034, fax 978-443-8000, or visit our website, www.jblearning.com.

Substantial discounts on bulk quantities of Jones & Bartlett Learning publications are available to corporations, professional associations, and other qualified organizations. For details and specific discount information, contact the special sales department at Jones & Bartlett Learning via the above contact information or send an email to specialsales@jblearning.com.

Production Credits

VP, Product Management: Amanda Martin
Director of Product Management: Cathy L. Esperti
Product Specialist: Rachael Souza
Project Specialist: Rachel DiMaggio
Project Specialist, Navigate: Rachel DiMaggio
Digital Project Specialist: Angela Dooley
Director of Marketing: Andrea DeFronzo
Marketing Manager: Michael Sullivan
VP, Manufacturing and Inventory Control: Therese Connell

Composition and Project Management: Exela Technologies
Cover Design: Scott Moden
Text Design: Scott Moden
Media Development Editor: Troy Liston
Rights Specialist: Rebecca Damon
Cover Image (Title Page, Part Opener, Chapter Opener): © Agsandrew/ Shutterstock
Printing and Binding: LSC Communications
Cover Printing: LSC Communications

Library of Congress Cataloging-in-Publication Data

Names: Endee, Lisa, author. | Spriggs, William H. Essentials of polysomnography.
Title: Sprigg's essentials of polysomnography: a training guide and reference for sleep technicians / Lisa Endee.
Other titles: Essentials of polysomnography
Description: Third edition. | Burlington, MA: Jones & Bartlett Learning, [2021] | Preceded by: Essentials of polysomnography: a training guide and reference for sleep technicians / by William H. Spriggs. Second edition. 2015. | Includes bibliographical references and index.
Identifiers: LCCN 2019031300 | ISBN 9781284172218 (paperback)
Subjects: MESH: Polysomnography—methods | Sleep Wake Disorders—diagnosis | Allied Health Personnel | Sleep Medicine Specialty–organization & administration | Sleep—physiology
Classification: LCC RC547 | NLM WM 188 | DDC 616.8/498075—dc23 LC record available at https://lccn.loc.gov/2019031300

6048

Printed in the United States of America
24 23 22 21 20   10 9 8 7 6 5 4 3 2 1

Brief Contents

© Agsandrew/Shutterstock

Contents

Preface

Essentials of Polysomnography, third edition, is a full-color text designed specifically for sleep technicians and professionals. The new comprehensive all-in-one package and compact design makes it the ideal choice for training new sleep technicians, as well as students interested in studying polysomnography, physicians, sleep lab managers, durable medical equipment reps, and sleep lab front office staff members. It is also a great reference and study tool to help prepare for the RPSGT and CPSGT certification exams.

What's New in This Edition?

This third edition of *Essentials of Polysomnography* includes the following:

- **NEW** Chapter 17, "Medications and Sleep," contains content on commonly prescribed sleep aids and the effect of drugs on sleep efficiency and architecture.
- **NEW** Chapter 18, "Other Therapeutic Modalities," is dedicated to the various therapeutic options for the treatment of sleep disorders.

- **NEW and UPDATED content** that reflects the latest American Academy of Sleep Medicine scoring rules and sleep-disorder nosology and is correlated to the most recent Registered Polysomnographic Technologist exam blueprint, which was released in 2018.
- **EXPANDED** content on the far-reaching consequences of sleep deprivation, various risk factors for sleep disorders, components of the sleep consultation and physical assessment examination, clinical practice guidelines for PAP titration, home sleep testing and reporting, pediatric sleep testing and scoring, and emergency preparedness and maintaining patient safety in the sleep-testing environment.
- **NEW** case studies have been integrated within the chapters to facilitate the application of content and to foster critical thinking.
- In **all-in-one packaging**, a pocket guide and flash cards are included in the back of the book and are perforated for easy use.

How to Use This Book

Key Features

Each chapter of the book begins with a list of Learning Objectives to help you focus on the most important concepts in that chapter.

Each chapter contains tables that highlight important information, such as **Table 17-3**, Medication Classes Associated with Insomnia.

This text is highly illustrated with diagrams and photos demonstrating a variety of concepts such as **Figure 8-27**, An Example of Muscle Artifact in the C4 Channel.

Several chapters conclude with a Case Study to help the reader review and put into practice what they have learned.

Table 17-3
Medication Classes Associated with Insomnia

Anti-epileptics
Beta blockers
Bronchodilators
Decongestants
Diuretics
Steroids
Selective serotonin reuptake inhibitors (SSRIs)
Stimulants

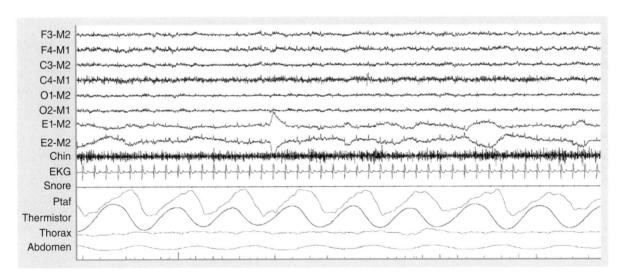

FIGURE 8-27 An example of muscle artifact in the C4 channel.
Courtesy of Polysomnographic Technology Program, Stony Brook University School of Health Technology and Management.

The appendixes at the end of the text outline complex topics such as patient hookup, identifying artifacts, and interpreting electrocardiograms.

A posttest and posttest answer key allow students to test themselves on the content of the text.

Removable flashcards as well as a pocket guide are included for students to study from.

Case Study Example

A 21-year-old women reports to the sleep disorders center complaining of severe excessive daytime sleepiness that has progressively gotten worse over the last 5 years. She reports difficulty staying awake in her college classes and episodes of "sleep attacks" daily.

Think about what other questions or information you would like to collect from this patient to narrow down which sleep disorders are relevant.

Physical exam reveals a patient with a BMI of 21 and a neck size and oral anatomy within normal limits. No nasal congestion or deviation is observable. The patient's sleep diary demonstrates a regular and sufficient nighttime sleep routine, and a subjective sleep assessment reveals moderate daytime sleepiness. On further questioning, the patient describes vivid lifelike dreams at sleep onset and times when she wakes up but feels like she cannot move.

These features are consistent with which sleep disorder or disorders?

This patient reports chronic EDS, episodes of sleep paralysis, and hypnogogic hallucinations. These clinical features are highly suggestive of narcolepsy. Alternatively, hypersomnia is also possible. The patient's history does not indicate a high risk for sleep-related breathing disorder, but it cannot be ruled out at this time.

What type of testing is indicated?

To confirm a diagnosis of narcolepsy, an overnight sleep study followed by a multiple sleep latency test is indicated. In this case, testing revealed an overnight sleep study within normal limits with the exception of short sleep onset and REM latencies. There were no abnormal respiratory events observed. The MSLT revealed three SOREMPs and a mean sleep latency of 5 minutes.

What Is the Most Likely Final Diagnosis?

The overnight testing ruled out the presence of sleep-related breathing disorders. The presence of SOREMPs on the MSLT also rules out hypersomnia. Instead, the MSLT findings support the diagnosis of narcolepsy type II because the patient does not report cataplectic episodes.

Instructor and Student Resources

Qualified instructors will receive a full suite of instructor resources, including the following.

For the Instructor

- A comprehensive chapter-by-chapter PowerPoint deck
- A test bank with questions on a chapter-by-chapter basis as well as a midterm and a final exam

For the Students

- The pocket guide from the previous edition has now been updated and added to the end matter of the text as appendixes that are perforated for easy removal
- A full suite of flash cards to be used as a study tool
- A comprehensive practice exam available online to help students prepare for the RPSGT and CPSGT certification exams
- Case studies online as writeable PDFs
- An interactive eBook is available for all students who purchase the text

About the Author

Lisa Mastropietro Endee, MPH, RRT-SDS, RPSGT, RST

Lisa Endee is Clinical Associate Professor of polysomnographic technology and respiratory care at Stony Brook University in the School of Health Technology and Management. She possesses nearly 20 years of experience in adult and pediatric sleep diagnostics and therapeutics. Lisa's academic background includes the completion of a Bachelor of Science degree from Fordham University in 1996, a Bachelor of Science degree in Respiratory Care from the State University of New York at Stony Brook in 1999, and a Master of Public Health degree from the State University of New York at Stony Brook in 2018. She received her Registered Respiratory Therapist (RRT) credential in 1999, Registered Polysomnographic Technologist (RPSGT) in 2000, and Sleep Disorders Testing and Therapeutic Intervention credential (RRT-SDS) in 2012.

Lisa's career in polysomnography includes experience in both clinical and academic settings. She entered the profession as an entry-level therapist, gaining proficiency in sleep diagnostic testing, therapeutics, and patient education. Lisa quickly advanced to a lead position, where she was responsible for scoring sleep studies, generating reports, and working closely with sleep physicians on study interpretation, therapy recommendations, and the many aspects of clinical sleep medicine. In 2005, Lisa advanced to Clinical Coordinator at Good Samaritan Hospital's Sleep Apnea Center in West Islip, New York. In this role, she expanded the adult Sleep Apnea Center, led the facility toward success in obtaining American Academy of Sleep Medicine Accreditation, coordinated the establishment of a satellite Pediatric Sleep Disorders Center, and managed all of the clinical operations and staff at both facilities. In addition, Lisa was actively involved in policy development and various departmental and hospital-level quality-assurance and performance-improvement initiatives.

After providing more than 10 years of service as a clinical instructor, Lisa transitioned to academia in 2012. In her current role as Clinical Associate Professor, her responsibilities include clinical instruction of students on all aspects of sleep diagnostics, interpretation, and therapeutics. Lisa has been an item writer for the National Board for Respiratory Care's sleep specialty exam and has coauthored several articles for the American Association of Respiratory Care's Sleep Section and the *Journal of Respiratory Care*. In addition, she has served on numerous committees for the Board of Registered Polysomnographic Technologists and the American Association of Sleep Technologists.

Lisa's professional areas of interest include patient and public education in the areas of sleep wellness and health. She has led various community-based research projects targeting the prevention of drowsy driving. Through grant funding, she has spearheaded the development of a unique, educational website—stopdrowsdriving.org—and the launch of a social media campaign to prevent drowsy driving and reduce incidence of crashes and injuries. She has also served as the Principal Investigator of a research project that led to the development of a data-driven curriculum targeting drowsy driving prevention among young adults. This curriculum is currently being expanded across colleges and universities in New York state.

Acknowledgments

Many thanks to William H. Spriggs for his authorship of the previous two editions of this textbook and to his colleagues at Sleep Healers Labs who assisted in providing many of the figures and images that have been maintained in this edition. Sleep study images in this updated edition were gathered from studies provided to Stony Brook University School of Health Technology and Management's Polysomnographic Technology Program by Dr. Kala Sury.

Reviewers

Jacqueline Compton, RPSGT, RST, CSE, CCSH, M.Ed.
Instructor
Highline College
St Louis, MO

Kelly Cummins, MSOM, RPSGT, CCSH, RRT
Program Chair Polysomnography Technology/
Instructor Respiratory Care
Southeast Community College
Lincoln, NE

Douglas E. Masini, RRT-ACCS, FCCP, FAARC
Chair Diagnostic and Therapeutic Sciences
Armstrong State University
Savannah, GA

Michell Oki, SDS, RPSGT, RRT, NPS, ACCS, RPFT
Associate Professor
Weber State University
Ogden, UT

Christine Robinson, RRT, RPSGT
Polysomnographic Technology Program Director
Baker College
Flint, MI

Dr. Mark G. Ryland, AuD, RPSGT, R RP/EEG T, RNCST,
CNCT, FASET
Associate Professor of Neurodiagnostics Technology
and Polysomnography
Cuyahoga Community College
Pharma, OH

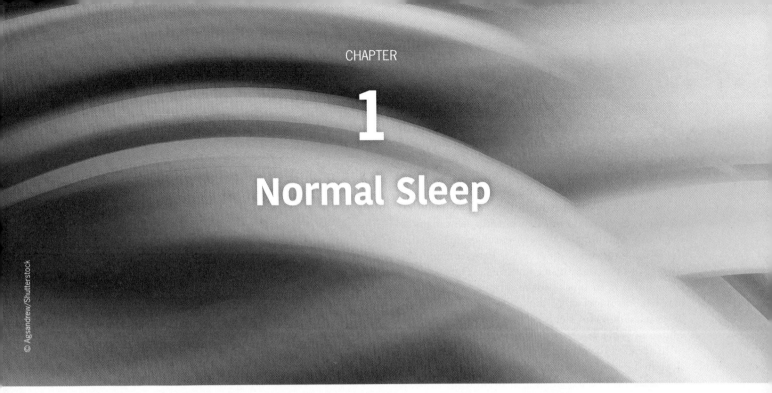

CHAPTER

1

Normal Sleep

© Agsandrew/Shutterstock

CHAPTER OUTLINE

LEARNING OBJECTIVES

1. Understand the importance of sleep.
2. Discover differences between the sleep of humans and that of other animals.
3. Understand why the human body and mind need sleep.
4. Discuss common mediators of sleep deprivation.
5. Describe some of the consequences of sleep deprivation on health and well-being.
6. Learn more about the circadian rhythm and its effects on our daily lives.
7. Understand normal sleep patterns.
8. Discuss the significance of changes in sleep patterns from the norm.
9. Learn how the normal aging process affects sleep.
10. Understand how pregnancy can affect sleep.

KEY TERMS

sleep
sleep deprivation
sleep hygiene
chronic sleep deprivation
sleep debt
circadian rhythm
rapid eye movement (REM)
thermoregulation
thalamus
reticular activating
   system (RAS)
suprachiasmatic
   nucleus (SCN)
dopamine
acetylcholine
noradrenaline
histamine
glutamate
sleep state
nonrapid eye movement
   (NREM)
stage R

phasic REM
tonic REM
stage N1
stage N2
sleep spindles
stage N3
sleep architecture
stage W
wake after sleep
   onset (WASO)
sleep efficiency
histogram
hypnogram
sleep latency
sleep onset
excessive daytime
   sleepiness (EDS)
first night effect
total wake time
rebound sleep
stage R latency
stage R onset

The Need for Sleep

Like it needs food, water, and oxygen, the human body needs sleep to survive. **Sleep** is defined as "a natural and periodic state of rest during which consciousness of the world is suspended."[1] Sleep is a state during which the body and mind are allowed to rest and become restored.

The sleep of hundreds of different species of mammals has been researched extensively. This research has provided us with further information about human evolution and our relationship as humans to these other mammals. Most research on mammalian sleep has determined that there is variation among species of mammals in sleep need (see **Figure 1-1**), some only requiring as little as 3 hours while others may need as many as 19 hours every 24-hour period. The varied need for sleep in several species is represented in **Table 1-1**.[2]

In addition to varying sleep lengths, some mammals sleep in different ways than others. For example, dolphins sleep with only half of their brain while the other half is still awake. This allows them to continue swimming and watching for predators while sleeping.

In humans, sleep is critical for growth and repair, learning, memory consolidation, safety, and optimal health. Human sleep need changes across the life span (see **Figure 1-2**). Infants and children have an increased sleep need to ensure proper growth, development, and learning. The National Sleep Foundation recommends that adults obtain between 7 and 9 hours of sleep each night.[3] However, 35% of American adults report getting fewer than 7 hours of sleep in a 24-hour period.[4] Despite the importance of sleep, only 10% of Americans prioritize it over other aspects of their health and wellness.[5]

When an individual does not obtain the duration, consistency, or type of sleep necessary, **sleep deprivation**, a condition that has various deleterious effects on function and overall health, results. The prevalence of insufficient sleep varies among U.S. states, with geographic hot spots of sleep deprivation along the East Coast, the southeastern United States, Alaska, and Hawaii.[6] Common mediators of sleep deprivation

Table 1-1
Mammalian Sleep

Species	Sleep/Day (Hours)	Stage R/Day (Hours)
Armadillo	17.0	3.0
Baboon	9.5	1.0
Bat	19.0	3.0
Cat	12.5	3.0
Dolphin	10.0	minimal to absent
Echidna	8.5	temperature dependent
Elephant	4.0	minimal & only when lying down
Ferret	14.5	6.0
Giraffe	4.5	0.5
Guinea pig	9.5	1.5
Hamster	14.0	3.0
Horse	3.0	0.5
Human	8.0	2.0
Koala	14.5	has never been observed in the wild
Mole	8.5	2.0
Opossum	18.0	5.0
Platypus	14.0	7.0
Rat	13.0	2.5
Seal	6.0	1.5

include social and environmental factors. Our modern busy lifestyle is undoubtedly one of the main causes for America's lack of sleep. Before the invention of the light bulb in 1879, the average American slept 10 hours per night. Now that number is just under 7 hours.[7]

Balancing work and family responsibilities with obtaining sufficient sleep has proved to be particularly difficult for the working class population in the modern era, especially among women. Research has shown that women's sleep is likely to be curtailed, interrupted, or both, by responding to the needs of family members. In addition, in struggling to meet their occupational and familial obligations while fatigued and sleepy, they tend to stress their bodies in ways that can contribute further to sleep debt.[8]

In addition, shift work, primary sleep disorders, and poor **sleep hygiene** are often the cause of chronic

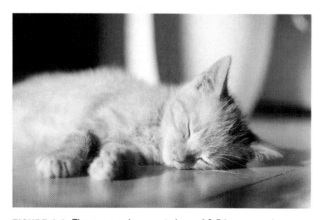

FIGURE 1-1 The average housecat sleeps 12.5 hours per day.
© Dalibor Valek/Shutterstock.

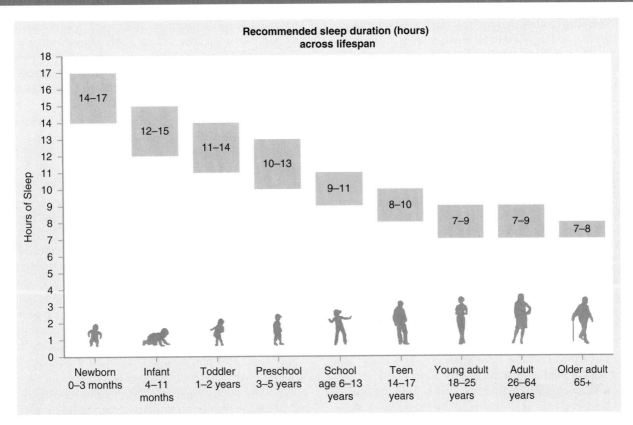

FIGURE 1-2 Sleep needs across the life span.

sleep issues. *Sleep hygiene* refers to the practice of good habits surrounding the sleep–wake routine that promote increased quantity and quality of sleep. Sleep hygiene includes the recommendation for a regular sleep routine, obtaining sufficient sleep on a nightly basis, and avoiding poor habits that can impact sleep such as using digital devices in the hour before bed.[9] Digital media has become an important cause of sleep deprivation in teenagers and young and middle-aged adults. Ninety percent of Americans report using a technological device in the hour before bed. The more interactive the device, the more likely difficulties falling asleep and unrefreshing sleep were reported.[10] For a list of the recommendations for proper sleep hygiene, see **Table 1-2**.

Chronic sleep deprivation, or a consistent lack of necessary sleep over an extended period of time, can have drastic and sometimes deadly effects. As a person consistently fails to receive adequate sleep, **sleep debt** increases. *Sleep debt* refers to the amount of sleep a person has lost over a period of time compared with what he or she should receive. If an individual requires 8 hours of sleep every night but obtains only 6 hours, then he or she has accumulated a sleep debt of 2 hours in just one night. If this pattern continues for four nights, he or she will have accumulated 8 hours of sleep debt.

Table 1-2
Sleep Hygiene

Do	Avoid
Establish a regular, relaxing, bedtime routine	Staying in bed awake for more than 20 minutes Brighter areas; if you cannot sleep, move to another dimly lit or dark location until you are sleepy
Go to bed the same time each night	Stimulants (caffeine, nicotine, etc.) close to bedtime
Wake up the same time each morning	Use of digital devices (smartphones, computers, laptops, video games) at least 1 hour before bed
Exercise daily	Strenuous exercise too close to bedtime
Ensure adequate daily exposure to natural light	Heavy, rich, fatty or spicy foods before bed
Limit daytime naps to 30 minutes	Long daytime naps, which can interfere with the normal sleep routine
Create a comfortable, cool, and dark sleep environment	Watching TV, doing homework, reading in bed

Sleep deprivation has far-reaching consequences. According to Dr. William Dement, increased sleep debt is directly correlated with increased adverse effects, including daytime sleepiness, poor performance, lack of concentration, and multiple health problems.[11] Adults who sleep fewer than 7 hours per night are more likely to report chronic health conditions, including increased risk for heart attack, coronary artery disease, hypertension, stroke, diabetes, depression, and cancer.[12] Short sleep duration in children is associated with a significantly increased risk of obesity.[13] Other potential results of increased sleep deprivation include decreased memory, poor decision making, irritability, morning headaches, lack of motivation, and increased risk of injury.

Some of the most visible effects of sleep deprivation today are seen in traffic accidents. In 2013, 72,000 crashes, 44,000 injuries, and 800 deaths were attributed to drowsy driving.[14] The National Highway Traffic Safety Administration reports that 2.5% of fatal motor vehicle crashes and 2.0% of all crashes with nonfatal injuries involve drowsy driving every year.[15] These statistics are believed to be greatly underestimated because driving while drowsy leaves behind limited physical evidence at the scene of the crash. Modeling studies and published reports have estimated that between 15% and 33% of fatal crashes may involve drowsy drivers.[16,17] Thirty-two percent of adults report having driven drowsy at least once per month during the past year.[18] Crashes attributed to drowsiness behind the wheel result in billions of dollars in lost property and productivity a year. Sleep deprivation plays an important role in risk. Individuals who sleep fewer than 6 hours per night are more likely to report falling asleep at the wheel.[14]

Truck drivers are a high-risk population for sleep deprivation and crashes. In Salina, Kansas, in May 2005, a truck driver fell asleep at the wheel and crashed into an SUV, killing a mother and son and injuring two other vehicle occupants. In October 2007, the truck driver was sentenced to 6 months in prison for two counts of vehicular homicide. Many states now recognize the gravity of drowsy driving. In August 2003, New Jersey became the first state to criminalize a drowsy driving crash that leads to a fatal accident. Penalties can be as high as 10 years in prison and $100,000 in fines. In some states, drowsy driving can draw penalties as serious as driving while intoxicated.

Work-related accidents and loss of productivity resulting from sleep deprivation also plague our world. Twenty-nine percent of adults report that they have fallen asleep or became extremely sleepy while at work. Almost 20% report being late, leaving early, or not going in to work because of sleepiness.[19] This has resulted in an estimated $50 billion in lost productivity in the United States. Among the most costly and devastating

known work-related accidents that were believed to be attributed to sleep deprivation are the Three Mile Island nuclear meltdown in 1979; the gas leak in Bhopal, India, in 1984; the *Challenger* space shuttle disaster in 1986; the Chernobyl nuclear accident in 1986; and the *Exxon Valdez* oil spill in 1989.

Three Mile Island's Unit 2 nuclear power plant near Middleton, Pennsylvania, was the site of the most serious U.S. nuclear plant accident in history. The accident started around 4 A.M. on March 28, 1979, when a cooler malfunctioned. It is believed that poor judgment by sleep-deprived workers led to the meltdown. Luckily, no known injuries or health problems occurred because of this event.

On December 3, 1984, a storage tank of a pesticide ingredient in Bhopal, India, overheated, releasing large amounts of deadly gas. This accident also occurred in the early morning hours when workers were drowsy and inattentive. As a result, 15,000 people died and approximately 600,000 people were injured.[20]

In early 1986, the United States was celebrating the "space race" as it prepared to send the first school-teacher, Christa McAuliffe, along with a crew of six other astronauts, into space. The mission was highly publicized as the country anxiously gathered to watch the launch. The shuttle had several problems, and crews worked around the clock for days leading up to the launch to make the shuttle ready for its anticipated launch time. The managers who approved the launch reportedly slept little the night before. On January 28, 1986, the *Challenger* space shuttle exploded just over a minute after liftoff, killing the entire crew (see **Figure 1-3**). This tragic event was also thought to be attributed to poor judgments made by a sleep-deprived crew.

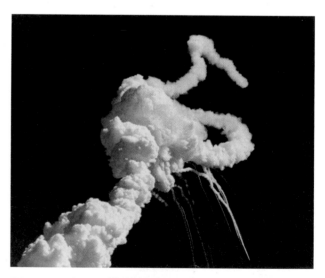

FIGURE 1-3 January 28, 1986: The space shuttle *Challenger* explodes shortly after liftoff. Many experts believe sleep deprivation may have played a role in the events leading up to this disaster.
Courtesy of NASA.

Later the same year in Ukraine, Reactor 4 at Chernobyl was to be shut down and tested at 1 A.M. Several of the safety features were turned off by the sleepy crew, leading to a large steam explosion and fire. This caused at least 5% of the radioactive core to be released into the surrounding area. Twenty-eight people in the area died within 4 months from radioactive or thermal burns, and at least 75 deaths since that time are believed to have been caused by the exposure.[21]

On March 23, 1989, the Exxon oil tanker *Valdez* struck a large reef while maneuvering through a remote Alaskan coastline. Reports claim the crew was poorly rested, and many believe this to be one of the primary causes of the crash. The tanker spilled approximately 11 million gallons of oil, although exact amounts are difficult to determine. Hundreds of thousands of animals died instantly, and many more have died since. Massive lawsuits and large-scale economic and environmental consequences resulted.

Obtaining an adequate quantity and quality of sleep affords significant benefits to health, safety, and overall well-being. Specifically, individuals who are free of sleep disorders, practice good sleep hygiene, and get the recommended amount of sleep tend to be happier, have greater levels of energy and motivation and, ultimately, live longer than those who do not obtain adequate sleep.[22]

The Human Circadian Rhythm

To understand human sleep, we must first discuss the human **circadian rhythm**. A circadian rhythm is a daily cycle of biological activity influenced by variations in the environment, such as the alteration of day and night.[23] A circadian rhythm can include sleeping and waking in animals, tissue growth and differentiation in certain fungi, or the opening and closing of certain flowers. In humans, circadian rhythm includes not only the 24-hour sleep–wake cycle, but also varying levels of alertness during wakefulness.

While we are awake, our circadian rhythm oscillates approximately every 90 minutes. People often note higher levels of alertness during the morning hours and a lower energy level after lunch in the early afternoon hours. Although this often varies according to the amount and quality of sleep a person obtains, daily activities and exercise, and the types of food eaten, it is also affected by an internal biological clock. Extensive research has shown that several factors can affect the circadian rhythm, including the following:

- *Light:* Light is considered to be the most dominant factor affecting the human circadian cycle. Evidence of this can be seen in humans' tendency to be awake during the day and asleep at night. Further evidence is seen in studies involving bright light therapy to treat insomnia and certain circadian rhythm disorders.

- *Temperature:* Temperature has been shown to be another factor affecting circadian rhythm. Slightly increasing room temperature may cause a person to be drowsy, whereas decreasing the temperature may increase alertness for short periods of time. As a person enters **rapid eye movement (REM)** sleep, the core body temperature becomes unstable and drops.
- **Thermoregulation:** The body's ability to regulate its own temperature decreases during REM.
- *Food:* A lunch composed of fatty, greasy foods is often followed by periods of drowsiness, whereas eating healthier foods can encourage higher levels of alertness.
- *Drugs:* Stimulants, depressants, and other drugs can have profound effects on the circadian rhythm. Some of these effects may be short-term and others long-term. Certain drugs such as melatonin can aid in the quality of sleep by decreasing the amount of time needed to initiate sleep and decreasing the amount of wake time after sleep onset. For more information on how different types of drugs affect our sleep, see Chapter 17.
- *Activity:* Research has shown that exercise can increase our alertness and help us sleep better at night. However, sleep hygiene techniques instruct us to avoid strenuous exercise shortly before bedtime because this can have a negative impact on our ability to initiate sleep.

Although countless factors can influence our circadian rhythms both when awake and when asleep, those listed are among the most influential and common.

Human Sleep

To understand normal human sleep, we must first discuss the functions of certain structures in the brain as they relate to sleep.

Brain Structures Related to Sleep

The brain is made up of the brain stem, the diencephalons, the cerebrum, and the cerebellum. The brain stem consists of the pons, the midbrain, and the medulla oblongata. The diencephalons are made up of the hypothalamus, the thalamus, the epithalamus, and the pineal gland.

Many structures of the brain affect alertness, wakefulness, and sleepiness. The primary structures of the brain involved in the circadian rhythm and the sleep–wake process are as follows (see **Figure 1-4**).[24]

Thalamus
Medulla oblongata
Hypothalamus
Pons
Midbrain
Spinal cord

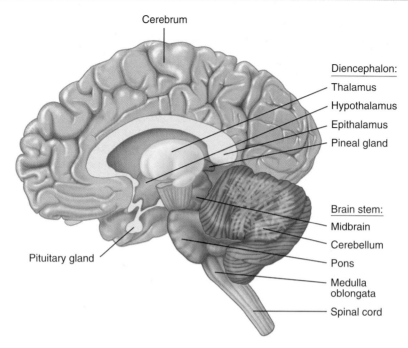

FIGURE 1-4 The human brain.

Raphe nuclei
Basal forebrain
Hippocampus
Suprachiasmatic nuclei
Reticular formation neurons

The **thalamus** constitutes the main part of the dien-cephalons and is known to have multiple functions. Among other things, it is responsible for sending spe-cific sensory data from the body to different areas of the brain, especially the cerebral cortex. As data between the thalamus and the cortex become blocked, aware-ness of external stimuli decreases, and consciousness is lost. This sensory blockage is caused by a deactivation of the **reticular activating system (RAS)**. The RAS con-sists of several neurons in the reticular formation and is believed to be the center of arousal and motivation. Deactivation of the RAS leads to decreased alertness and develops spindle activity in the thalamus seen in stage N2 (for more information on N2 and other stages of sleep, please see the "States and Stages of Sleep" section in this chapter). Reticular formation neurons stimulate other neurons through the thalamus to the cortex, which develops the cerebral activation that leads to wakefulness.

The **suprachiasmatic nucleus (SCN)** is a bilateral area of the brain located in the hypothalamus. It is strongly affected by light and is responsible for controlling the circadian rhythm. The SCN is often referred to as the pacemaker for the circadian rhythm.

The primary chemicals involved in the circadian rhythm and the sleep–wake process include dopa-mine, acetylcholine, noradrenaline, histamine, and glutamate. The primary responsibility of **dopamine** is the arousal of the cortex, movement, and responsive-ness. **Acetylcholine** activates the cortex. Acetylcholine levels are highest during wakefulness and rapid eye movement sleep (stage R). **Noradrenaline** primarily maintains and enhances the activation of the cerebral cortex. **Histamine** also activates the cortex. **Glutamate** includes excitatory amino acids that progress to the cortex, forebrain, and brainstem. Glutamate is primarily responsible for central activation of the cortex.

States and Stages of Sleep

Sleep is divided into two main **sleep states**: REM and **non-rapid eye movement (NREM)**. Just as there are vary-ing levels of wakefulness and alertness in the circadian rhythm, there are also different levels or stages of sleep. Rather than being considered a state of unconscious-ness, sleep is considered a state of altered or decreased consciousness.

Stage R, or REM sleep, is characterized by the pres-ence of rapid eye movements during sleep. **Phasic REM** refers to periods of stage R in which the eyes move back and forth in rapid motions. **Tonic REM** refers to the occurrence of stage R without rapid eye move-ments. Saw-toothed electroencephalogram (EEG) waves, a characteristic waveform often seen in stage R, are mostly seen during phasic REM. The areas of the brain mostly responsible for causing stage R include the hippocampus, the pons, and the medulla oblon-gata. Other characteristics of stage R include muscle atonia; a low-voltage, mixed-frequency EEG pattern; a decrease in core body temperature; altered respiratory patterns; and penile erections in males. Stage R appears to be associated with memory, cognition, and feelings of restorative sleep.

NREM is divided into three stages: N1, N2, and N3. **Stage N1** is considered a transitional stage of sleep, which has characteristics of both wake and sleep. During stage N1, a subject may occasionally be able to hear and respond to external stimuli. Often a person may awaken from a brief period of N1 unaware that he or she was asleep. **Stage N2** is a slightly deeper stage of sleep in which **sleep spindles** first occur. Sleep spindles are unique EEG waveforms that indicate a blockage of external stimuli such as sounds. Therefore, in N2 we become significantly less aware of our surroundings than when we are in N1. **Stage N3**, formally called *delta sleep*, is considered to be the deepest stage of sleep because of the lack of responsiveness during this stage. N3 is typically the most difficult stage from which to awaken an individual. The primary structures in the brain playing roles in NREM sleep are the raphe nuclei, the forebrain, the thalamus, and the hypothalamus.

Periods of REM and NREM oscillate throughout the night in approximately 90-minute cycles, continuing the 90-minute circadian rhythm seen during wakefulness.

Sleep Architecture

Sleep architecture refers to the patterns of sleep stages through which we progress during our sleep period. In this section we will discuss the norms and averages of sleep patterns across normal, healthy adults. Changes to normal sleep architecture occur as a result of several different factors, including age, internal and external stimuli, medical conditions, and psychological conditions. To discuss sleep architecture, we must further detail each sleep stage.

Stage W (Wake)

During wake (**stage W**), muscle activity and cognitive responsiveness are high, and levels of alertness vary according to many different factors. Wakefulness comprises two-thirds of the 24-hour cycle in humans, or approximately 16 hours per day. EEGs can be difficult to read during wakefulness because of frequent movement and muscle activity. However, EEGs during stage Wake are typically high frequency with mixed voltages. When resting awake with the eyes closed, alpha waves are present in the occipital regions of the brain, electromyogram (EMG) amplitudes are high, the eyes roll slowly, and airflow varies according to the activity levels. The average latency to sleep in normal, healthy adults is 10–20 minutes.

Wake after sleep onset (WASO) is the amount of wake time in minutes during the attempted sleeping period, after sleep onset has been achieved. WASO is often characterized by lower activity levels than wake periods during daytime hours. The average person is asleep at least 90% of the sleep period (from sleep onset to the final awakening). In other words, WASO should constitute less than 10% of the sleep period. The percentage of the night that a person spends asleep is called **sleep efficiency**. Sleep efficiency is calculated by dividing the total sleep time by the total time in bed. A sleep efficiency greater than 90% is considered normal and optimal.

Stage N1

Stage N1 makes up approximately 5–10% of the sleep period. A person in stage N1 can sometimes detect and even respond to external stimuli, T. When in stage N1, the EEGs present a relatively low voltage pattern with mixed-frequency waves in the frontocentral regions of the brain, EMG amplitudes remain high, the eyes continue to roll slowly, and airflow tends to become more regular. Most people enter sleep through stage N1, which is why it is often called a *transitional* stage. A person in stage N1 is often unaware that he or she is asleep.

Stage N2

Stage N2 characteristics include a relatively low voltage mixed-frequency EEG pattern, a moderate-level EMG amplitude, and the absence of eye movements. In addition, the EEGs during stage N2 include sleep spindles and K-complexes that originate in the central areas of the brain. Stage N2 makes up approximately 45–50% of the total sleep period in normal, healthy young adults. It is during stage N2 that the senses begin to be blocked from external stimuli.

Stage N3

In stage N3, the EEG is characterized by a moderate amount of low-frequency, high-amplitude activity accompanied by a low amplitude EMG. Stage N3 is considered to be an extremely deep stage of sleep because subjects are difficult to awaken out of this stage; awakening from stage N3 often results in grogginess and disorientation. Stage N3 makes up approximately 20–25% of the sleep period in normal, healthy young adults, and is predominant during the first third of the night. Stage N3 tends to decrease dramatically with age. The human growth hormone is released during stage N3, making stage N3 a restorative sleep for the body.

Stage R

Stage R is characterized by low-voltage mixed-frequency EEG pattern, rapid eye movements (REMs), and an EMG amplitude that is lowest relative to the other stages. Periods of tonic REM are also common in which no rapid eye movements are seen. Stage R is often referred to as a *paradoxical* sleep because the brain activity resembles the activity during wakefulness, but the muscles are paralyzed. Muscle tone is at its lowest point of the circadian rhythm during stage R. Like stage N3, stage R makes up approximately 20–25% of the sleep period in normal, healthy young adults. This tends to decrease with many different sleep disorders. The patterns of stage R are the opposite of those in stage N3. Stage R periods are typically shorter in the beginning of the sleep period and become longer as the sleep period progresses. Whereas stage N3 is restorative for the body, stage R is restorative for the mind. Research suggests that memory is diminished when stage R is deprived. The average latency to stage R is 90–120 minutes.

Typical Progression of Sleep

Figure 1-5 shows a typical sleep **histogram** (or **hypnogram**) for a normal, healthy young adult. A histogram is a chart or graph showing sleep architecture throughout the night, and it often includes other channels such as muscle tone, abnormal events, or oxygen level. Figure 1-5 shows a typical progression of sleep stages throughout the night for a normal, healthy young adult. Notice that the periods of stage N3 are longest during the first third of the night and gradually decrease in length as the night progresses. Conversely, periods of stage R tend to be brief at the beginning of the night and progressively become longer. Each sleep cycle is approximately 90 minutes in length, although this can certainly vary. Occasional unexplained awakenings are considered normal during the night and may be evidence of an evolutionary defense mechanism. Sleep is typically entered through stage N1, and periods of this stage are usually brief.

There are various internal and external factors that can result in changes to the normal sleep cycle and pattern. The normal aging process can have a significant impact on sleep patterns.

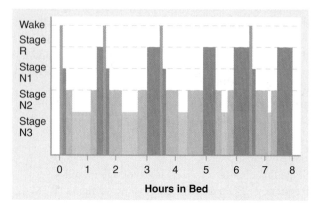

FIGURE 1-5 Sleep staging histogram for a normal, healthy young adult.

Sleep and Aging

As humans age, there are various impacts on sleep. First, there is evidence suggesting that with age comes a decreased need for sleep: For example, infants may need more than 12 hours of sleep per 24-hour period, whereas adolescents need 8–10 hours, young adults need 7–8 hours of sleep on average, and older adults may need less than 7 hours of sleep per night on average. Although this is true in general, individual differences are typically greater than age differences as a whole.

Sleep efficiency is also impacted with age. Specifically, the number of EEG arousals and awakenings per hour of sleep, also known as the *arousal index*, tends to increase as adults age. The increased prevalence of arousals may result from several factors including stress, medications, medical conditions, pain, respiratory events, limb movements, psychological conditions, or sensitivity to the environment. Therefore, although older adults may spend more time in bed, time spent sleeping tends to decrease. Although young adults typically enjoy more than 90% sleep efficiency, many older adults experience sleep efficiencies between 70% and 80%.

Sleep architecture is also affected by age. Specifically, stage N3 sleep decreases significantly with age. Where infants have high percentages of slow wave sleep, many older adults may achieve little of it during the night. This phenomenon may be the result of decreasing EEG amplitude with age. As stage N3 is lost, the percentage of total sleep time spent in stages N1 and N2 increases (see **Figure 1-6**). The changes in sleep architecture and reduction in sleep quality experienced by adults as they age often results in the common complaint of insomnia. Unfortunately, many will attempt to use over-the-counter or prescription medications, herbal remedies, or alcohol to help them sleep. Among adults aged 65–80 years, 31% report using sleep medications at least three times a week, 29% report using them for 1–3 years, and 62% report using them for more than 3 years.[25]

As we age, the prevalence of sleep disorders tends to increase. For some disorders, risk factors increase with age—for example, REM behavior disorder and obstructive sleep apnea. Sleep problems can also arise because of the increasing presence of other medical conditions that occur with age. For example, arthritis can cause an individual to have difficulty initiating or maintaining sleep. Certain psychological factors that may increase with age—including fear, guilt, and anxiety—may also affect the ability to initiate or maintain sleep. Stressors such as financial stress, marital stress, family pressures, or job changes can also greatly affect a person's ability to sleep. As a result of reduced quality sleep and the increased risk for sleep disorders, older adults have an increased risk of the deleterious consequences of sleep deprivation, especially depression, cognitive defects, injuries, and falls.

Sleep Parameter	Effect of Aging
Sleep Latency	Remains fairly consistent across lifespan (in the absence of underlying sleep disorders) until older age when it tends to increase
WASO	Increases steadily after age 35 years due to increases in age-related sleep fragmentation
REM	Remains fairly consistent as a percentage of total sleep time with the exception of infancy, where is makes up approximately 50% of TST
SWS	A significant decrease occurs in the second decade of life, followed by a slower decline with advancing age
Stage 2	Remains fairly consistent as a percentage of total sleep time with increases occurring with advancing age as SWS declines
Stage 1	Remains fairly consistent as a percentage of total sleep time with increases occurring with advancing age as SWS declines

FIGURE 1-6 Impact of age on sleep architecture.

Table created by Lisa M. Endee; based on Citation: Ohayon MM, Carskadon MA, Guilleminault C, Vitiello MV (2004). Meta-analysis of quantitative sleep parameters from childhood to old age in healthy individuals: developing normative sleep values across the human lifespan. Sleep 2004;27(7):1255–73.

Changes to Normal Sleep Architecture

The sleep-staging histogram presented previously is an example of the sleep architecture of a typical healthy young adult. There can be small variations in sleep architecture among individuals. However, significant changes in an individual's sleep architecture, either in percentage of time spent in each stage or in cycling through the various sleep stages, often indicates an underlying issue. **Figure 1-7** provides an example of an abnormal sleep histogram. Following are a few important factors to pay attention to.

Sleep Latency

Sleep latency is the amount of time, in minutes, it takes a person to fall asleep. The measurement of sleep latency on a *polysomnogram*, or sleep study, begins at "lights out," when the lights are turned off and the patient attempts to fall asleep; the measurement ends at **sleep onset**, or the first 30-second epoch of sleep on a polysomnogram, which is usually stage N1. A sleep latency of 10–20 minutes is considered normal. A decreased sleep latency may indicate **excessive daytime sleepiness (EDS)**. A person who is excessively sleepy will usually fall asleep quicker than a person who is not sleepy. This excessive daytime sleepiness may be caused by many reasons but can often indicate that a person's sleep is being interrupted by upper airway obstruction or periodic limb movements. A decreased sleep latency may indicate that a person has difficulty staying awake and therefore may be dangerous behind the wheel of a motor vehicle. A sleep latency longer than 20 minutes may indicate that a person is

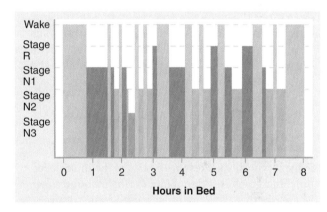

FIGURE 1-7 Abnormal sleep histogram.

having difficulty initiating sleep. This could be the result of a **first night effect** while being tested, problems with insomnia, or getting too much sleep the previous night. First night effect refers to the stresses and other factors that a patient feels during the first night of testing in a sleep lab, which may affect his or her ability to initiate and maintain sleep.

Sleep Efficiency

As mentioned previously, normal sleep efficiency for a healthy young adult is 90% or higher. A decreased sleep efficiency, by definition, indicates increased **total wake time**. Increased total wake time may indicate a disruption during sleep from any number of factors, including leg movements, apnea, pain, insomnia, and so on. Increased sleep efficiency may be indicative of **rebound sleep**. Rebound sleep is often observed in patients with obstructive sleep apnea sleeping with positive airway pressure (PAP) therapy for the first time. Rebound sleep can also lead to increases in stages N3 and R.

Total Stage N1 Time

A healthy adult should spend approximately 5–10% of the night in stage N1 sleep. Because stage N1 is a transitional stage, an increase in stage N1 often indicates increased wakefulness or disruptions to sleep, such as those already cited. A decrease in stage N1 often indicates decreased disruptions to sleep.

Total Stage N2 Time

Stage N2 makes up approximately 45–50% of the total sleep time. Increases or decreases in stage N2 are usually associated with increases or decreases in stage N3 or stage R sleep, which may be better indicators of significant problems during sleep.

Total Stage N3 Time

Stage N3 makes up approximately 20–25% of the total sleep time. This naturally decreases with age and is often absent in older adults. Decreases to stage N3 in young adults may indicate a disruption to sleep, perhaps caused by too much sleep during the night before testing or anxiety resulting from first night effect. Stage N3 may be increased because of rebound sleep or from certain medications such as sedatives or alcohol.

Total Stage R Time

Stage R typically makes up 20–25% of the total sleep time. Increases are often found during rebound sleep. Decreases to stage R are often caused by disruptive sleep, often the result of apneas, periodic limb movements, pain, or external factors.

Stage R Latency

Stage R latency is defined as the amount of time, in minutes, from sleep onset to **stage R onset**. Stage R onset is the first 30-second epoch of Stage R. The normal latency to stage R is 90–120 minutes. A decreased stage R latency may indicate EDS or rebound sleep. An increased stage R latency may indicate problems with insomnia, disruptive sleep, or too much sleep the previous night.

Stage R Periods

The length of individual periods of stage R can provide insight into the causes of abnormal sleep architecture. Although a patient's total stage R time in a night may be consistent with the norm, he or she may start the night with short stage R periods and end the night with excessively long stage R periods. This is often seen during a PAP titration when the pressures at the beginning of the night may not be sufficient to allow

the patient to remain in stage R, but the increased air pressure at the end of the night may allow the patient to experience a long stage R rebound. Circling back to the abnormal sleep histogram shown in Figure 1-7, note the increase in sleep latency, total wake time, and time spent in stage N1 sleep as well as the decrease in stage N3 and stage R as compared to the normal histogram shown in Figure 1-5.

Pregnancy and Sleep

Pregnancy can cause significant changes in a woman's body, many of which can affect sleep. Weight gain is one of the most important changes that can affect sleep during pregnancy. Additional weight caused by pregnancy, specifically in the abdominal and thoracic areas, can greatly increase the likelihood of obstructive respiratory events, including apneas, hypopneas, and snoring.[26] The comorbidities of obstructive sleep apnea syndrome—such as morning headaches, decreased stage R, increased EEG arousals and awakenings, increased limb movements, increased blood pressure, and many others—often increase in frequency and severity during pregnancy. Obstructive sleep apnea during pregnancy can also lead to excessive daytime sleepiness, fatigue, drowsiness, falling asleep unintentionally, decreased sleep efficiency, and an increased desire to take naps.

It is also common for pregnancy-related morning sickness to interrupt sleep. As mentioned previously in this chapter, periods of stage R are longest in the early morning hours. If morning sickness associated with pregnancy occurs early enough, it can disrupt the amount of stage R sleep a pregnant woman obtains.

Pain and discomfort related to pregnancy can also profoundly affect the amount and quality of sleep obtained. Particularly in the third trimester of pregnancy, discomfort increases, often causing the subject to experience increased difficulty initiating sleep, increased sleep latencies, increased awakenings after sleep onset, and decreased sleep efficiency.

Leg movements, both periodic limb movements in sleep (PLMS) and the occurrence of restless legs syndrome (RLS), are increased during pregnancy, possibly related to hormonal changes.[26] The occurrence of RLS can increase sleep latency, and PLMS can increase nocturnal awakenings and EEG arousals and decrease sleep efficiency.

The National Sleep Foundation's 2007 "Sleep in America" poll focused on sleep in women. A large section of the report focused on the sleep of pregnant women. The poll showed that although 82% of women reported sleeping well before they were pregnant, only 60% reported sleeping well during pregnancy.[27] This dropped to 54% in women during the third trimester of pregnancy. Among the top factors reported to have the largest negative effects on sleep in pregnant women were getting up to go to the bathroom, pain, dreams, heartburn, nasal congestion, and leg cramps.

Chapter Summary

Sleep is one of the most important functions the human body performs. This is especially evident when the body is deprived of sleep. Sleep deprivation can have profoundly negative effects, including daytime sleepiness, poor performance, lack of concentration, memory loss, and multiple health problems. *Sleep debt* refers to the amount of sleep we have lost over a period of time compared with what we should have received. In addition to countless automobile and work-related accidents, many large-scale disasters may be related to sleep deprivation. Some of these include the Three Mile Island nuclear meltdown in 1979; the gas leak in Bhopal, India, in 1984; the *Challenger* space shuttle disaster in 1986; the Chernobyl nuclear accident in 1986; and the *Exxon Valdez* oil spill in 1989. Although the exact events leading to these disasters may never be fully known, it is believed that sleep deprivation may have played important roles in each.

The circadian rhythm affects not only our alertness during the daytime but also our sleep patterns at night. Many factors can affect our circadian rhythm, including light, temperature, food, drugs, and activity levels.

Many different parts of the brain affect our circadian rhythm and our sleep. The main parts of the brain involved in sleep include the thalamus, medulla oblongata, hypothalamus, pons, midbrain, spinal cord, raphe nuclei, basal forebrain, hippocampus, suprachiasmatic nuclei, and reticular formation neurons.

Mammalian sleep can vary greatly among species. Among the most interesting is the dolphin, which can sleep with half of its brain at a time, allowing it to stay alert at all times and avoid predators.

Human sleep architecture consists of stages W, N1, N2, N3, and R (rapid eye movement) sleep. Stage N1 is a transitional stage from wake to sleep and constitutes approximately 5–10% of the total sleep time. Stage N2 is characterized by sleep spindles and K-complexes in the EEGs and makes up approximately 45–50% of the total sleep time. Stage N3 is the stage in which the body's tissues and muscles are restored and makes up approximately 20–25% of the night. Stage R is characterized by rapid eye movements and a decreased amplitude in the chin EMG and constitutes approximately 20–25% of the night. Deprivation from stage R has been shown to lead to memory loss and a lack of concentration. Normal sleep architecture shows a decrease in stage N3 as the night progresses and longer periods of stage R.

Many changes to our sleep come naturally with age. Among the most significant are a decrease or even complete loss of stage N3, a decreased sleep efficiency, and increased complaints of insomnia. Pregnancy can also greatly affect sleep in women. Additional weight from pregnancy can increase the likelihood of obstructive sleep apnea and primary snoring, and certain hormonal changes may play a role in the increase of leg movements during pregnancy. Other factors such as pain, discomfort, and increased urination can also negatively impact the sleep of pregnant women.

Chapter 1 Questions

Please consider the following questions as they relate to the material in this chapter.

1. What is sleep debt? How can an increased sleep debt impact our daily lives?
2. How is our cycle of alertness during the day related to our sleep patterns at night?
3. How does human sleep differ from the sleep of other animals?
4. What are the stages of sleep, and how are they normally distributed during the night?
5. How does the normal aging process affect our sleep?
6. What is the significance of a decreased sleep latency? A decreased sleep efficiency?
7. How can pregnancy affect sleep?

Footnotes

1. Princeton University (2010). About WordNet. WordNet. Princeton University.
2. Kryger, M. H., Roth, T., & Dement, W. C. (2017). *Principles and practice of sleep medicine.* Philadelphia: Elsevier.
3. Hirshkowitz, M., Whiton, K., Albert, S. M., et al. (2015). National Sleep Foundation's sleep time duration recommendations: Methodology and results summary. *Sleep Health, 1*(1), 40–43. doi:10.1016/j.sleh.2014.12.010
4. Liu, Y., Wheaton, A. G., Chapman, D. P., Cunningham, T. J., Lu, H., & Croft, J. B. (2016). Prevalence of healthy sleep duration among adults—United States, 2014. *MMWR. Morbidity and Mortality Weekly Report, 65*(6), 137–141. doi:10.15585/mmwr.mm6506a1
5. National Sleep Foundation (2018). Sleep in America poll: Sleep prioritization and personal effectiveness. *Sleep Health.* doi.org/10.1016/j.sleh.2018.02.007
6. Centers for Disease Control and Prevention (CDC). (2017). Short sleep duration among U.S. adults. Accessed on November 8, 2017, from https://www.cdc.gov/sleep/data_statistics.html
7. National Sleep Foundation (2002). Sleep in America poll: Adult sleep habits. *Sleep Health.* doi:10.1016/j.sleh.2015.04.001
8. Maume, D. J., Sebastian, R. A., & Bardo, A. R. (2010). Gender, work-family responsibilities, and sleep. *Gender & Society, 24*(6), 746–768.
9. National Sleep Foundation (2018). Sleep hygiene. Accessed on November 8, 2017, from https://www.sleepfoundation.org/articles/sleep-hygiene
10. Gradisar, M., Wolfson, A. R., Harvey, A. G., Hale, L., Rosenberg, R., & Czeisler, C. A. (2013). The sleep and technology use of Americans: Findings from the National Sleep Foundation's 2011 Sleep in America poll. *Journal of Clinical Sleep Medicine.* doi:10.5664/jcsm.3272
11. Dement, W. C., & Vaughan, C. C. (2000). *The promise of sleep: A pioneer in sleep medicine explores the vital connection between health, happiness and a good night's sleep.* New York: Dell.
12. CDC. (2017). Short sleep duration among US adults. Accessed November 8, 2017, from https://www.cdc.gov/sleep/data_statistics.html

13. Wu, Y., Gong, Q., Zou, Z., Li, H., & Zhang, X. (2017). Short sleep duration and obesity among children: A systematic review and meta-analysis of prospective studies. *Obesity Research & Clinical Practice, 11*(2), 140–150. doi:10.1016/j.orcp.2016.05.005

14. CDC. (2017). Drowsy driving. Accessed on November 8, 2017, from https://www.cdc.gov/features/dsdrowsydriving/index.html

15. National Highway Traffic Safety Administration. (2011). Traffic safety facts crash stats: Drowsy driving. Washington, DC: US Department of Transportation, National Highway Traffic Safety Administration.

16. CDC. (2013). Drowsy driving—19 states and the District of Columbia, 2009–2010. *Morbidity and Mortality Weekly Report (MMWR), 61*(51–52), 1033.

17. Wheaton, A. G., Shults, R. A., Chapman, D. P., Ford, E. S., & Croft, J. B. (2014). Drowsy driving and risk behaviors—10 states and Puerto Rico, 2011–2012. *Morbidity and Mortality Weekly Report (MMWR), 63*(26), 557.

18. National Sleep Foundation. (2018). Sleep in America poll: Sleep prioritization and personal effectiveness. *Sleep Health.* doi.org/10.1016/j.sleh.2018.02.007

19. National Sleep Foundation. (2008). Sleep in America poll: Sleep, performance, and the workplace. Accessed on November 8, 2017, from https://www.sleepfoundation.org/professionals/sleep-america-polls/2008-sleep-performance-and-workplace

20. Long, T. (2008, December 2). Dec. 3, 1984: Bhopal, "Worst industrial accident in history." Retrieved from http://www.wired.com/science/discoveries/news/2008/12/dayintech_1203

21. United States Nuclear Regulatory Commission. (2013). Backgrounder on Chernobyl nuclear power plant accident. Accessed at http://www.nrc.gov/reading-rm/doc-collections/fact-sheets/chernobyl-bg.html

22. Dement, W. C., & Vaughan, C. C. (2000). *The promise of sleep: A pioneer in sleep medicine explores the vital connection between health, happiness and a good night's sleep.* New York: Dell.

23. *American Heritage Science Dictionary.* Circadian rhythm. Accessed from https://ahdictionary.com/word/search.html?q=circadian+rhythm

24. Mattice, C., Brooks, R., & Lee-Chiong, T. (2012). *Fundamentals of sleep technology.* Wolters Kluwer Lippincott Williams & Wilkins.

25. University of Michigan. (2017). National poll on healthy aging: Trouble sleeping? Don't assume it's a normal part of aging. Retrieved from https://www.healthyagingpoll.org/report/trouble-sleeping-dont-assume-its-normal-part-aging

26. National Sleep Foundation. (2019). Pregnancy and sleep. Accessed from https://www.sleepfoundation.org/articles/pregnancy-and-sleep

27. National Sleep Foundation. (2007). Sleep in America poll: Women and sleep. Accessed from https://www.sleepfoundation.org/professionals/sleep-america-polls/2007-women-and-sleep

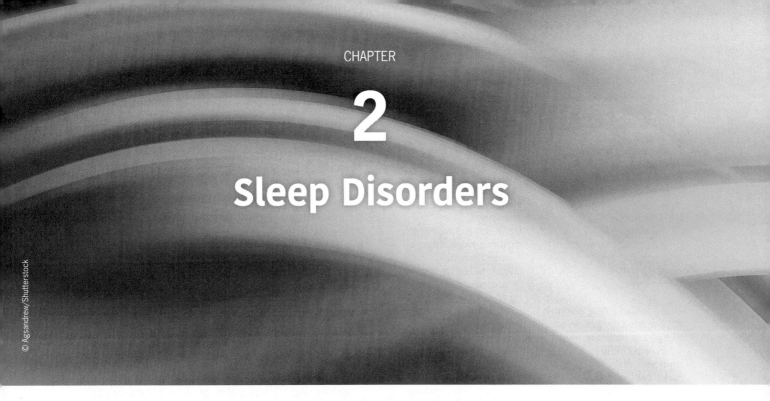

2

Sleep Disorders

© Agsandrew/Shutterstock

CHAPTER OUTLINE

LEARNING OBJECTIVES

1. Discuss a brief history of sleep disorders.
2. Learn the classification of sleep disorders as outlined by the AASM.
3. Describe the features and symptoms of each disorder.
4. Discuss the social and personal impact of specific disorders.

KEY TERMS

Pickwickian syndrome
Association of Sleep
  Disorders Centers
  (ASDC)
*International Classification
  of Sleep Disorders* (ICSD)
insomnia
chronic insomnia disorder
psychophysiological
  insomnia
idiopathic insomnia
paradoxical insomnia
sleep diary
sleep log
sleep hygiene
limit-setting disorder

behavioral insomnia
  of childhood
short-term insomnia
  disorder
group therapy
light therapy
sleep restriction
self-control techniques
biofeedback
sleep-related breathing
  disorders
obstructive sleep
  apnea (OSA)
obstructive apnea
hypopnea
oxygen desaturation

EEG arousal
paradoxical breathing
micrognathia
retrognathia
apnea–hypopnea
  index (AHI)
respiratory disturbance
  index (RDI)
respiratory effort–related
  arousal (RERA)
upper-airway resistance
  syndrome
excessive daytime
  sleepiness (EDS)
sudden infant death
  syndrome
central sleep apnea (CSA)
central apnea
continuous positive airway
  pressure (CPAP)
hypercapnia
hypocapnia
Cheyne–Stokes breathing
high-altitude periodic
  breathing
primary central
  sleep apnea
primary sleep apnea
  of infancy
treatment-emergent
  central sleep apnea
complex sleep apnea
obesity hypoventilation
  syndrome (OHS)
congenital central
  alveolar hypoventilation
  syndrome (CCHS)
late-onset central
  hypoventilation with
  hypothalamic dysfunction

alveolar hypoventilation
idiopathic central alveolar
  hypoventilation
snoring
primary snoring
sleep-related groaning
catathrenia
CPAP therapy
positional therapy
tonsillectomy
adenoidectomy
bi-level therapy
multiple sleep latency
  test (MSLT)
maintenance of
  wakefulness test
narcolepsy
cataplexy
sleep paralysis
hypnagogic hallucinations
narcolepsy tetrad
automatic behavior
microsleep
narcolepsy type I
hypnagogic
hypnopompic
sleep-onset REM
  period (SOREMP)
narcolepsy type II
idiopathic hypersomnia
recurrent hypersomnia
periodic hypersomnolence
Kleine-Levin syndrome
hypersomnia
insufficient sleep
  syndrome
circadian rhythm
circadian rhythm sleep–
  wake disorder (CRSWD)
actigraphy

delayed sleep–wake phase disorder
advanced sleep–wake phase disorder
irregular sleep–wake rhythm disorder
free-running circadian rhythm
non–24-hour sleep–wake rhythm disorder
shift work disorder
jet lag disorder
parasomnia
confusional arousal
sleepwalking
somnambulism
sleep terror
night terror
sleep-related eating disorder
REM-related parasomnias
REM sleep behavior disorder (RBD)
isomorphism
recurrent isolated sleep paralysis
nightmare
posttraumatic stress disorder (PTSD)
exploding head syndrome
sleep-related hallucinations
nocturnal enuresis
bedwetting
sleep enuresis
sleep talking

somniloquy
sleep-related movement disorders
restless legs syndrome (RLS)
periodic limb movement disorder (PLMD)
periodic limb movements in sleep
PLM index
sleep-related leg cramps
bruxism
sleep-related bruxism
rhythmic masticatory muscle activity
sleep-related rhythmic movement disorder
body rocking
head banging
myoclonus
benign sleep myoclonus of infancy
propriospinal myoclonus at sleep onset
excessive fragmentary myoclonus (EFM)
hypnagogic foot tremor
alternating leg muscle activation
sleep start
hypnic jerk
environmental sleep disorder

History of Sleep Disorders

Since the beginning of time, humans have been fascinated with sleep. Many early writings discuss sleep and sleep disorders in a variety of ways. In 1836, Charles Dickens published a series of papers called the "Posthumous Papers of the Pickwick Club."[1] In these writings, he describes a boy named Joe who was overweight and extremely tired, and who snored heavily. A drawing of the boy shows an obese young man with a short, fat neck. From this, the term **Pickwickian syndrome** was coined; although it is not used today, the symptoms have many similarities with the sleep disorder called *obesity hypoventilation syndrome.*

Pioneering sleep researchers in the 1950s and 1960s such as Nathaniel Kleitman, William Dement, and others identified different stages of sleep and were able to recognize specific patterns of these stages throughout the night. Along with the development of new technologies designed to read and record physiological activities, this gave way to the development of the field of sleep disorders. In 1961, the Sleep Research Society began informally with such sleep pioneers as Doctors William Dement, Allan Rechtschaffen, Nathaniel Kleitman, Michel Jouvet, and Eugene Aserinsky. In 1968, Rechtschaffen and Dr. Anthony Kales produced *A Manual of Standardized Technology Techniques and Scoring Systems for Sleep Stages of Human Patients,*[2]

which defined scoring techniques for sleep studies for the next 40 years.

In 1970, Dement started the first sleep-disorders lab, which provided all-night evaluations of patients with sleep complaints; within 5 years there were four more sleep centers in business. In 1975, the **Association of Sleep Disorders Centers (ASDC)** was developed, which is now known as the American Academy of Sleep Medicine (AASM). Its sleep center accreditation went into effect 2 years later in 1977. By the early 1990s, several professional sleep societies had developed, including the ASDC, Clinical Sleep Society, Association of Professional Sleep Societies, American Board of Sleep Medicine, and National Sleep Foundation. The American Academy of Sleep Medicine was known as the Clinical Sleep Society from 1984 to 1986 and the American Sleep Disorders Association from 1987 to 1998; in 1999 it became the American Academy of Sleep Medicine.

In 1990, the AASM developed the first edition of the *International Classification of Sleep Disorders* (ICSD), which categorized and described all known sleep disorders. A second edition of the ICSD was published in 2005 (ICSD-2), and the third edition was published in 2014 (ICSD-3). The information in this chapter reflects the updated definitions and classifications of sleep disorders found in the third edition.

Classification of Sleep Disorders

The following pages categorize sleep disorders as outlined in the third edition of the ICSD[3]:

1. Insomnia
   a. Chronic insomnia disorder
   b. Short-term insomnia disorder
   c. Other insomnia disorders
   d. Isolated symptoms and normal variants

2. Sleep-related breathing disorders
   a. Obstructive sleep apnea disorders
      i. Obstructive sleep apnea, adult
      ii. Obstructive sleep apnea, pediatric
   b. Central sleep apnea syndrome
      i. Central sleep apnea with Cheyne–Stokes breathing
      ii. Central sleep apnea due to a medical disorder without Cheyne–Stokes breathing
      iii. Central sleep apnea due to high-altitude periodic breathing
      iv. Central sleep apnea due to a medication or substance
      v. Primary central sleep apnea
      vi. Primary central sleep apnea of infancy
      vii. Primary central sleep apnea of prematurity
      viii. Treatment-emergent central sleep apnea

c. Sleep-related hypoventilation disorders
   i. Obesity hypoventilation syndrome
   ii. Congenital central alveolar hypoventilation syndrome
   iii. Late-onset central hypoventilation with hypothalamic dysfunction
   iv. Idiopathic central alveolar hypoventilation
   v. Sleep-related hypoventilation due to a medication or substance
   vi. Sleep-related hypoventilation due to a medical disorder
d. Sleep-related hypoxemia disorder
e. Isolated symptoms and normal variants
   i. Snoring
   ii. Catathrenia

3. Central disorders of hypersomnolence
   a. Narcolepsy type I
   b. Narcolepsy type II
   c. Idiopathic hypersomnia
   d. Kleine-Levin syndrome
   e. Hypersomnia due to a medical disorder
   f. Hypersomnia due to a medication or substance
   g. Hypersomnia associated with a psychiatric disorder
   h. Insufficient sleep syndrome

4. Circadian rhythm sleep–wake disorders
   a. Delayed sleep–wake phase disorder
   b. Advanced sleep–wake phase disorder
   c. Irregular sleep–wake rhythm
   d. Non–24-hour sleep–wake rhythm disorder
   e. Shift work disorder
   f. Jet lag disorder
   g. Circadian rhythm sleep–wake disorder not otherwise specified

5. Parasomnias
   a. NREM-related parasomnias
      i. Disorders of arousal from NREM sleep
      ii. Confusional arousals
      iii. Sleepwalking
      iv. Sleep terrors
      v. Sleep-related eating disorder
   b. REM-related parasomnias
      i. REM sleep behavior disorder
      ii. Recurrent isolated sleep paralysis
      iii. Nightmare disorder
   c. Other parasomnias
      i. Exploding head syndrome
      ii. Sleep-related hallucinations
      iii. Sleep enuresis
      iv. Parasomnia due to a medical disorder
      v. Parasomnia due to a medication or substance
      vi. Parasomnia, unspecified

d. Isolated symptoms and normal variants
   i. Sleep talking

6. Sleep-related movement disorders
   a. Restless legs syndrome
   b. Periodic limb movement disorder
   c. Sleep-related leg cramps
   d. Sleep-related bruxism
   e. Sleep-related rhythmic movement disorder
   f. Benign sleep myoclonus of infancy
   g. Propriospinal myoclonus at sleep onset
   h. Sleep-related movement disorder due to a medical disorder
   i. Sleep-related movement disorder due to a medication or substance
   j. Sleep-related movement disorder, unspecified
   k. Isolated symptoms and normal variants

Insomnia

Insomnia can be defined as a complaint of a lack of sleep or of nonrestorative sleep and can occur in all age groups. The ICSD-3 defines insomnia as "persistent difficulty with sleep initiation, duration, consolidation, or quality that occurs despite adequate opportunity and circumstances for sleep, and results in some form of daytime impairment."[3] Daytime impairments may include daytime sleepiness, reduced motivation, impaired memory or concentration, irritability, behavioral issues such as aggression, and proneness toward errors. The ICSD-2 identified several different types of insomnia. The ICSD-3 consolidates these types and groups them into the categories of chronic and short-term insomnia.

Chronic Insomnia Disorder

Chronic insomnia disorder is associated with sleep disturbances and daytime symptoms as previously described that occur at least three times a week for at least 3 months. There are several clinical subtypes defined and described below.

Psychophysiological Insomnia

Psychophysiological insomnia is caused by excessive focus and anxiety about sleep, learned sleep-prevention habits, and a heightened level of arousal. The subject typically has no difficulty falling asleep when sleep is not planned or when outside of their usual sleep setting, but sleep onset is difficult to achieve at the normal bedtime and during planned naps.

Idiopathic Insomnia

Perhaps the most detrimental and debilitating form of insomnia is **idiopathic insomnia**. Idiopathic insomnia, also termed *lifelong insomnia*, is first identified at infancy or early childhood and persists throughout the patient's life. There appears to be no external cause for this insomnia, although genetic and congenital aberrations are suspected.

Paradoxical Insomnia

Formerly termed *sleep state misperception*, **paradoxical insomnia** consists of the subject's complaint of insomnia without any actual evidence of insomnia. Many times in the sleep lab, a patient will report that he or she remained awake all night, even though the technician was able to determine by viewing the electroencephalograms (EEGs) that sleep was achieved. In some cases, the patient may have had a normal sleep efficiency, but still insists he or she did not sleep at all. This type of comment should always be included in the technician's notes because the patient may have paradoxical insomnia. A useful tool for both the clinician and patient when facing paradoxical insomnia is a **sleep diary** or a **sleep log**, which is a self-report of sleep habits over a period of time. Sleep diaries usually last at least 5 days and sometimes as long as a month. **Figure 2-1** shows a sample sleep diary.

A sleep diary can help patients see abnormalities in their own sleep habits, such as irregular or inconsistent bedtimes or daytime naps that may affect their sleep schedules at night. Clinicians can use a patient's sleep diary to point out some of these inconsistencies or poor sleep habits. They can also use the sleep study report to demonstrate to the patient the discrepancy between actual sleep and perceived sleep.

Inadequate Sleep Hygiene

The term **sleep hygiene** refers to habits that are healthy for one's sleep. Therefore, inadequate sleep hygiene is a set of habits or practices that are detrimental to a person's sleep or may cause a person to sleep poorly. Sleep hygiene techniques are practices that everyone should follow to fall asleep more easily and stay asleep longer. Often a clinician finds that a person's insomnia may be the result of bad habits. In this case, it is beneficial to educate patients about proper and beneficial sleep habits (see Figure 1-2). Following these habits can greatly improve one's ability to fall asleep and stay asleep.

Day	Date	Time in Bed	Time Out of Bed	Total Time in Bed	Time Asleep	Awake Time	Total Sleep Time	Estimated Sleep Efficiency	Notes
1									
2									
3									
4									
5									
6									
7									
8									
9									
10									
11									
12									
13									
14									
15									
16									
17									
18									
19									
20									
21									

Time in Bed: The final time of day the subject got in bed to go to sleep.
Time Out of Bed: The time of day the subject got out of bed for the last time in the morning.
Total Time in Bed: The total time in minutes the subject spent in bed during the night. This equals the Time Out of Bed minus the Time in Bed.
Time Asleep: The estimated time of day the subject fell asleep for the first time.
Awake Time: The estimated time of day the subject awoke for the last time in the morning.
Total Sleep Time (TST): The estimated total amount of time the subject actually slept.
Estimated Sleep Efficiency: This is calculated by dividing the TST by the Total Time in Bed. A sleep efficiency >90% is considered normal.

FIGURE 2-1 Sleep diary.

Behavioral Insomnia of Childhood

Also called **limit-setting disorder**, **behavioral insomnia of childhood** is comparable to inadequate sleep hygiene for children or infants. In addition to the sleep hygiene practices listed in the previous section, parents should consider other sleep hygiene practices that are specific for children such as not putting toys or other distractions in the crib, allowing the child to fall asleep alone rather than in a parent's arms, or preventing the infant from becoming dependent on a bottle to initiate sleep. Although some of these actions may be appropriate at certain developmental stages in infancy or early childhood, their persistence into older childhood increases the likelihood of the child having difficulty initiating and maintaining sleep. A normal, healthy bedtime routine for a child is recommended, such as reading for a short period of time.

Insomnia Due to a Mental Disorder

As its name implies, this insomnia is caused by a diagnosed mental illness and persists for at least 1 month. Common mental illnesses contributing to insomnia include depression and anxiety disorders. Clinicians are faced with the challenge of determining whether the mental illness is causing the insomnia or if another type of insomnia is causing the mental illness. For example, a patient suffering from a chronic insomnia can experience depression as a result of the inability to sleep. Alternately, a person who is depressed will often experience insomnia as a symptom.

Insomnia Due to a Medical Condition

Various medical conditions have the potential to cause symptoms of insomnia, either short-term or long-term. Some of the most common and persistent insomnia-causing medical conditions include those associated with pain or discomfort. These are more common in the elderly but can occur at any age.

Insomnia Due to a Drug or Substance

Another form of insomnia is secondary to substance abuse or substance withdrawal. These substances most often include alcohol, hypnotic drugs, sedatives, stimulants, and opiates. Most drugs have the ability to alter or create a disturbance in sleep in one form or another. These disturbances can vary greatly, depending on the type of drug used and the amount, duration, and regularity of its use, as well as individual factors. Alcohol can have many effects on sleep, including a reduced sleep latency, reduced wakefulness, and reduced rapid eye movement (REM) sleep and increased slow-wave sleep during the first third of the night. During the latter portions of the night, alcohol can increase the number of arousals and produce sleep fragmentation. It can also increase the likelihood of nightmares because of a REM rebound. The use of alcohol, sedatives, and pain medications can increase the likelihood of sleep disturbances resulting from obstructive respiratory events. These drugs relax the muscles, which can lead to the likelihood of obstructions in the upper airway.

Prescription and illegal drugs alike can cause sleep problems, including insomnia. Medications with insomnia as a side effect include, but are not limited to, the following:

- Beta blockers
- Corticosteroids
- Adrenocorticotropic hormones
- Monoamine oxidase inhibitors
- Diphenylhydantoin
- Calcium blockers
- Alpha methyldopa
- Bronchodilators
- Stimulating tricyclics
- Stimulants
- Thyroid hormones
- Oral contraceptives
- Antimetabolites
- Decongestants
- Thiazides

Short-Term Insomnia Disorder

Also called *adjustment insomnia* or *acute insomnia*, **short-term insomnia disorder** is extremely common, especially in today's busy, high-stress culture. Almost everyone experiences difficulty initiating or maintaining sleep for a night or two at some point in life. Adjustment insomnia is often associated with a specific stressor that can include work, school, or marital stress; excitement; anticipation; financial hardship; illness; and the death of a loved one or a natural disaster. The diagnosis of short-term insomnia is used when the disturbance has been present for less than 3 months. Although adjustment insomnia is common, it also typically corrects itself when the stressor is relieved. If a college student experiences adjustment insomnia because of stress from upcoming final exams, for example, the insomnia will likely be corrected when final exams are completed.

Other Insomnia Disorder

This diagnosis is used sparingly for individuals who experience difficulty initiating or maintaining sleep but do not meet the full criteria for chronic or short-term insomnia.

Isolated Symptoms and Normal Variants

Individuals who routinely allot time in bed in excess of their sleep need and those who routinely obtain less than 6 hours of sleep per night without daytime impairments (short sleepers) fall into this category.

Insomnia Treatment Options

Insomnia can occur as a primary condition or secondary to another issue. When insomnia is the primary condition, or the primary condition is unknown, the clinician must seek to resolve the insomnia independently. Various therapeutic options are available to help patients treat their insomnia, including **group therapy**, **light therapy**, sleep hygiene, **sleep restriction**, **self-control techniques**, and **biofeedback**. Group therapy is useful by allowing the patient to explore possible underlying psychological causes for the insomnia and hear the causes of other people's insomnias. Light therapy can help adjust the circadian rhythm and help the patient initiate sleep at the appropriate time. Biofeedback mechanisms train the patient to control certain physiological parameters such as muscle tension, skin temperature, and EEG recordings to gain control over their insomnia. These techniques have been shown to be effective in patients who are especially tense or stressed. Self-control techniques are more psychological in nature than biofeedback mechanisms, but the underlying purpose is the same: to allow the patient to gain control over his or her ability to initiate and maintain sleep. These are helpful for patients who feel that their lives are out of control because of any number of reasons. Sleep restriction is another useful tool for treating chronic insomnia, especially for older patients. This is particularly useful for people who tend to stay in bed for longer and longer periods of time per night. Many people with chronic insomnia may stay in bed for 10 hours per night but only sleep 6 hours. For these patients, the clinician may decide to treat the insomnia by restricting the amount of time the patient is in bed per night. This is another case in which a sleep diary may be useful.

When insomnia develops as a result of another medical or psychological condition, treatment often focuses on the primary condition. For example, a woman experiencing insomnia as a result of painful arthritis will likely be able to sleep better if her pain is reduced by medications.

Sleep-Related Breathing Disorders

Sleep-related breathing disorders are divided into those of central origin and those caused by an obstruction. Central breathing disorders are characterized by a lack of respiratory effort caused by either a central nervous disorder or a cardiac dysfunction.[3] Obstructive respiratory events are caused by partial or complete collapse of the upper airway.

Obstructive Sleep Apnea, Adult

Obstructive sleep apnea (OSA) is one of the most common sleep disorders. Although both common and dangerous, it is relatively easily diagnosed and treated. OSA is characterized by the presence of repeated obstructive apneas and hypopneas. **Obstructive apneas** are respiratory events classified by a complete cessation (defined as a decrease in amplitude of at least 90%) of airflow and continued respiratory effort. A **hypopnea** is a respiratory event characterized by a reduction in airflow by 30% to 90% in amplitude that is associated with a 3% **oxygen desaturation** (a decrease in the amount of hemoglobin saturated by oxygen) or a brief (3 seconds or longer) shift in EEG frequency called an **EEG arousal**. In adults, both apneic and hypopneic events must last at least 10 seconds in duration. Often these events are associated with body jerks, limb movements, **paradoxical breathing** (chest and abdominal effort asynchrony), and snoring.

Symptoms of OSA include snoring, gasping or choking during sleep, witnessed pauses in breathing by the bedpartner, restless sleep, sweating, waking with the bed in disarray, and morning headaches.

Risk factors for OSA include obesity, advanced age, being male, smoking, and having a crowded upper airway. Crowding of the airway can result from various factors, including enlarged tonsils, adenoids, or tongue; nasal obstruction; high arched (narrow) palate; **micrognathia** (having a small jaw) or **retrognathia** (having a recessed jaw); craniofacial abnormalities; and large neck size. An older male patient who is obese and has a large neck is at particularly high risk for OSA.

Diagnostic criteria for OSA call for an **apnea–hypopnea index (AHI)** of at least a total of five apneas and hypopneas per hour of sleep with complaints of daytime sleepiness as well as gasping, choking, or snoring or a **respiratory disturbance index (RDI)** of at least 15 in the absence of these complaints. AHI is calculated by dividing the total apneas and hypopneas by the total sleep time in hours. RDI is calculated by dividing the total apneas, hypopneas, and **respiratory effort–related arousals (RERAs)** by the total sleep time in hours. A RERA is an EEG arousal that is associated with a marked decrease in airflow and continued or increasing respiratory effort. **Upper-airway resistance syndrome** is characterized by frequent RERAs during sleep and results in symptoms similar to those of OSA.

Figure 2-2 illustrates an obstructive apnea. The airflow is absent despite the persistence of respiratory effort. An airway obstruction exists when the chest and abdomen expand and contract but no air flows through the nose or mouth.

Figure 2-3 illustrates a hypopnea, also an obstructive respiratory event. Like obstructive apneas, effort persists; however, airflow is not completely absent but rather decreased.

Figure 2-4 shows an obstructive apnea. The respiratory effort decreases slightly but persists despite the cessation of airflow. At the end of the event, the patient kicks their legs and has an EEG arousal.

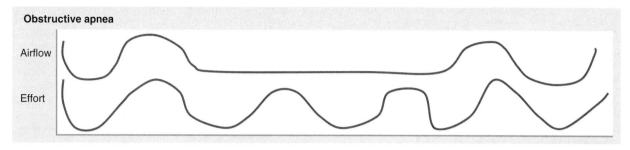

FIGURE 2-2 An obstructive apnea.

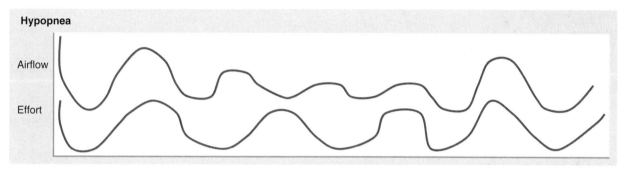

FIGURE 2-3 A hypopnea.

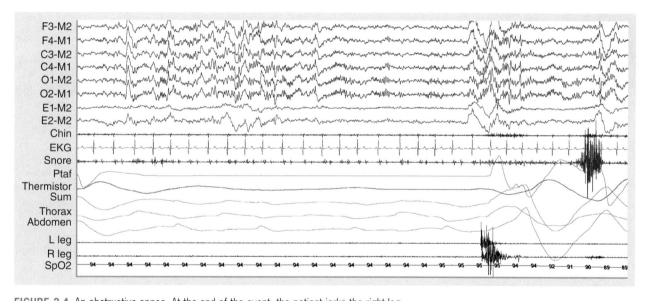

FIGURE 2-4 An obstructive apnea. At the end of the event, the patient jerks the right leg.

Figure by Lisa M. Endee; produced from a sleep study provided to Stony Brook University School of Health Technology and Management's Polysomnographic Technology Program by Dr. Kala Sury.

The sample in **Figure 2-5** shows another obstructive apnea with an associated EEG arousal and limb movements.

The sample in **Figure 2-6** shows an obstructive apnea during REM sleep. **Figure 2-7** also shows an obstructive apnea.

The epoch or designated time period in **Figure 2-8** shows a subtle hypopnea. The decrease in airflow would be extremely difficult to see using just a thermistor.

OSA has been highly associated with cardiovascular risk factors and increased mortality. OSA-associated intermittent hypoxia and sleep fragmentation result in sympathetic activation, oxidative stress, and systemic inflammation; left untreated, they increase the risk of hypertension, coronary artery disease, atrial fibrillation, heart failure, and stroke.[4]

OSA has also been linked to many other serious health consequences, including insulin resistance

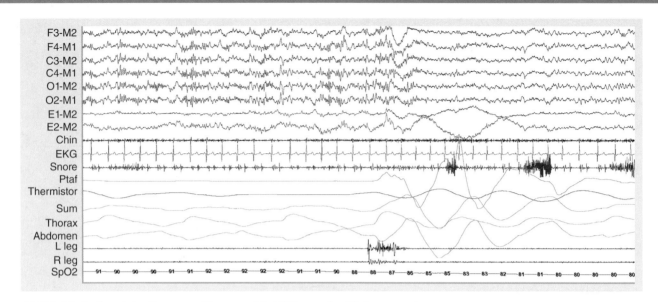

FIGURE 2-5 Another obstructive apnea with an associated EEG arousal and limb movements.

Figure by Lisa M. Endee; produced from a sleep study provided to Stony Brook University School of Health Technology and Management's Polysomnographic Technology Program by Dr. Kala Sury.

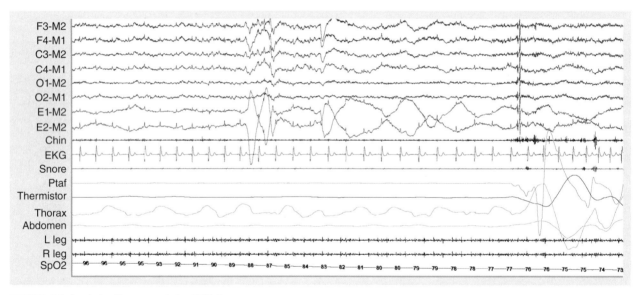

FIGURE 2-6 An obstructive apnea during REM sleep.

Figure by Lisa M. Endee; produced from a sleep study provided to Stony Brook University School of Health Technology and Management's Polysomnographic Technology Program by Dr. Kala Sury.

and metabolic syndromes. Further, control of many comorbidities such as hypertension, asthma, chronic obstructive pulmonary disease, and diabetes will be quite difficult if there is an underlying sleep disorder. Finally, there are various cognitive and psychosocial detriments associated with OSA. These include **excessive daytime sleepiness (EDS)**, lack of motivation, memory loss, lack of concentration, social withdrawal, depression, and increased risk of occupational errors, accidents, and drowsy driving.

Obstructive Sleep Apnea, Pediatric

Like OSA in adults, pediatric OSA is characterized by obstructive apneas and hypopneas. The events are also often associated with snoring, labored, or paradoxical breathing, as well as morning headaches, oxygen desaturation, and hypercapnia. The main difference between pediatric and adult OSA is in the duration of the respiratory events. Although events in adults must be at least 10 seconds long, obstructive apneic and hypopneic events in children are scored using a two-breath duration criteria.

OSA has been shown to be more prevalent in infants and children who are obese, and those with Down syndrome or other craniofacial abnormalities. Even mild cases of pediatric OSA can have lasting and severe effects. OSA in infants and children can impact both physical and mental growth, and it is believed to

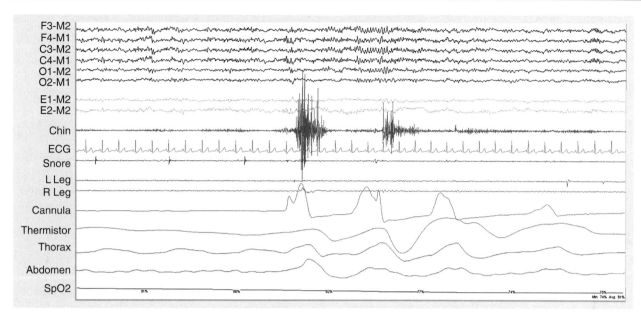

FIGURE 2-7 An obstructive apnea.

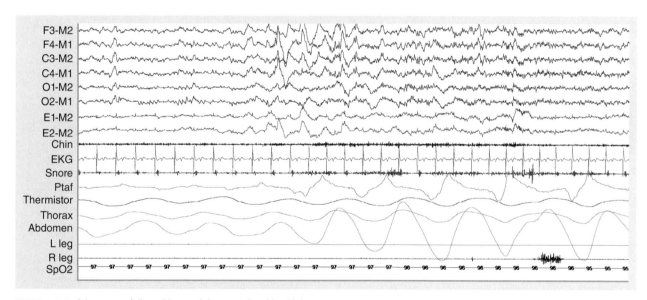

FIGURE 2-8 A hypopnea followed by a subtle arousal and leg kick.

Figure by Lisa M. Endee; produced from a sleep study provided to Stony Brook University School of Health Technology and Management's Polysomnographic Technology Program by Dr. Kala Sury.

be associated with **sudden infant death syndrome**, an occurrence in which an infant dies during sleep seemingly without warning. Diagnostic criteria for pediatric OSA require an average of only one obstructive apnea or hypopnea per hour of sleep.

Central Sleep Apnea Syndromes

Currently, there are eight different central sleep apnea syndromes. **Central sleep apnea (CSA) is** characterized by cessation of airflow with a concurrent cessation of respiratory effort. **Central apneas** are often seen in older patients, those with congestive heart failure, neurological conditions, or on opioid medications, as well as in patients using **continuous positive airway pressure (CPAP)** for the first time or those with high CPAP pressures.

The normal drive to breathe is prompted by the levels of carbon dioxide (CO_2) in our bodies. Normal CO_2 levels range from 35 mm to 45 mm Hg. When CO_2 levels are high (**hypercapnia**), feedback loops relay a message to the brain to prompt breathing, and CO_2 levels are reduced at exhalation. Conversely, low CO_2 levels (**hypocapnia**) decrease the drive to breathe. CSA is thought to result from an unstable ventilatory control, especially during sleep–wake transitions, and low CO_2 levels that are more likely to drop below the apnea threshold. Patients with resting partial pressure carbon dioxide ($PaCO_2$) levels less than 40 mm Hg are more likely to have CSA.

Diagnostic features of CSA include an average of at least five central apneas per hour during sleep. Occasional central apneas are also common at sleep onset. **Figure 2-9** illustrates a typical central apnea. The airflow ceases at the same time as the respiratory effort and resumes as the breathing effort resumes.

The sample epoch in **Figure 2-10** shows a central apnea. The airflow drops as a result of the lack of respiratory effort. When the patient attempts to breathe at the end of the apnea, he is able to do so without any difficulty because there is no obstruction present.

The sample epoch in **Figure 2-11** shows another central apnea, approximately 15 seconds long. Notice in these samples that there is almost no oxygen desaturation, as is common in central events.

Figure 2-12 is another example of a central apnea, this one during REM and lasting at least 20 seconds.

Central Sleep Apnea with Cheyne–Stokes Breathing

Cheyne–Stokes breathing is characterized by a pattern of central apnea or hypopnea alternating with a distinct waning and waxing breathing pattern. This pattern is typically seen during nonrapid eye movement (NREM) sleep and is corrected during REM. Most patients with Cheyne–Stokes breathing are males over age 60. The diagnostic criteria for Cheyne–Stokes breathing is five or more central apneas or hypopneas per hour of sleep, greater than 50% of the total respiratory events being central in origin, and a crescendo–decrescendo pattern.

Central Sleep Apnea Due to a Medical Disorder without Cheyne–Stokes Breathing

Medical conditions such as degenerative brain stem lesions have been known to cause central respiratory events. In this case, the central respiratory events occur as a secondary disorder. In this disorder, five or more central apneas or hypopneas per hour of sleep, greater than 50% of the total respiratory events being central in

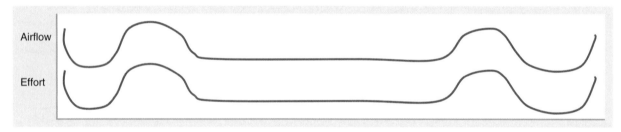

FIGURE 2-9 A typical central apnea.

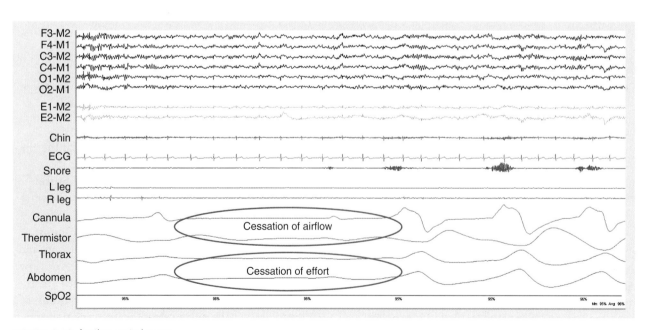

FIGURE 2-10 Another central apnea.

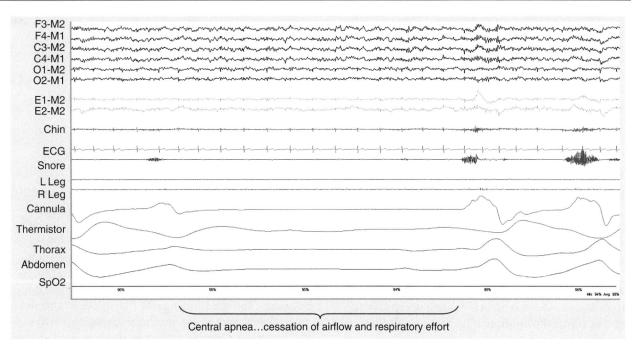

FIGURE 2-11 A 15-second-long central apnea.

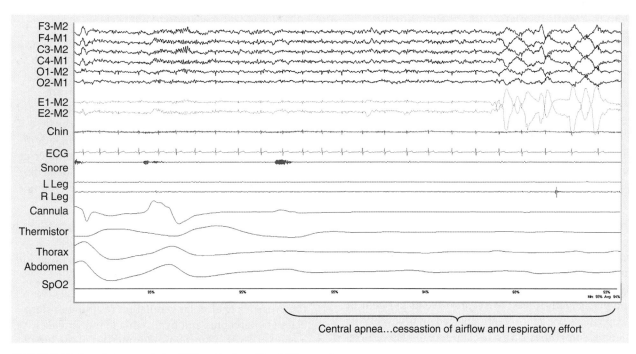

FIGURE 2-12 A central apnea during REM and lasting at least 20 seconds.

origin, and *the absence of* a crescendo–decrescendo pattern is diagnostic.

Central Sleep Apnea Due to High-Altitude Periodic Breathing

High-altitude periodic breathing disorder is characterized by central apneas and hypopneas occurring during a recent ascent to at least 4,000 meters (approximately 12,000 feet). The events occur at least five times per hour of sleep. The occurrence of central events during an altitude adjustment such as this is considered a normal response, and the condition tends to correct itself when the subject returns to lower altitudes.

Central Sleep Apnea Due to a Medication or Substance

Certain drugs, including methadone and hydrocodone, have been known to occasionally cause central respiratory events. In this case, the disorder is secondary in nature.

Primary Central Sleep Apnea

Primary central sleep apnea is idiopathic and cannot be explained by the use of a medication, substance, or the presence of a medical illness. Diagnostic criteria include five or more central apneas or hypopneas per hour of sleep, greater than 50% of the total respiratory events being central in origin, and *the absence of* a crescendo–decrescendo pattern.

Primary Central Sleep Apnea of Infancy

This life-threatening disorder occurs in infants who are at least 37 weeks conceptional age, and is characterized by prolonged central apnea, lasting at least 20 seconds (or a periodic breathing pattern at least 5% of the sleep time), desaturation, and apnea or cyanosis noted by an observer. **Primary central sleep apnea of infancy** is usually attributed to a developmental issue or secondary to another medical condition. It is extremely dangerous for newborns and should be diagnosed and treated as quickly as possible.

Primary Central Sleep Apnea of Prematurity

Central sleep apnea is common in premature infants and sometimes requires ventilator support. The diagnostic criteria for primary central sleep apnea of prematurity includes being a conceptional age of less than 37 weeks and either recurrent central apneas of at least 20 seconds in duration or periodic breathing for at least 5% of the duration of sleep study monitoring. The condition usually improves with maturation of the ventilatory control centers.

Treatment-Emergent Central Sleep Apnea

Treatment-emergent central sleep apnea, often referred to as **complex sleep apnea**, is diagnosed after the patient has been diagnosed with OSA and has had a subsequent PAP titration. After resolution of obstructive events during the titration, central events emerge and persist with at least five central events per hour of sleep. These patients are often placed on bi-level PAP therapy, sometimes with a backup rate to help resolve the central events.

Sleep-Related Hypoventilation Disorders

Sleep-related hypoventilation disorders have the common feature of abnormally elevated arterial PCO_2 (>45 mmHg), or hypercapnia, during sleep.

Obesity Hypoventilation Syndrome

Also referred to as hypercapnic sleep apnea, **obesity hypoventilation syndrome (OHS)** is characterized by hypoventilation during sleep in obese individuals. Diagnostic criteria for this disorder include a $PaCO_2$ greater than 45 mm Hg during wakefulness, a body mass index (BMI) (measured by kg/m²) greater than 30, and the absence of a medical disorder or medication that may cause hypoventilation. Overnight sleep testing on patients with OHS often reveals worsening of hypoventilation during sleep, especially during REM, and the presence of obstructive sleep apnea.

Congenital Central Alveolar Hypoventilation Syndrome

Congenital central alveolar hypoventilation syndrome (CCHS) is a rare disorder characterized by the failure of automatic central control of breathing attributed to a genetic mutation in the PHOX2B gene. Patients with CCHS experience sleep-related hypoventilation, hypercapnia, and oxygen desaturation. Hypoventilation may also be present during wakefulness but is typically worse during sleep. The condition usually first appears at birth but may present later in life in some individuals. The disorder persists for life and often requires lifelong treatment with ventilatory support.

Late-Onset Central Hypoventilation with Hypothalamic Dysfunction

Patients with **late-onset central hypoventilation with hypothalamic dysfunction** are typically healthy until approximately age two, when they develop severe obesity and central hypoventilation. Diagnostic criteria include the absence of symptoms during the first few years of life, sleep-related hypoventilation, lack of PHOX2B gene mutation, obesity, and either endocrine dysfunction, neural tumor, or severe psychosocial disturbance. Patients with this disorder will often require ventilatory support during sleep.

Idiopathic Central Alveolar Hypoventilation

Formerly called **alveolar hypoventilation** or central alveolar hypoventilation, **idiopathic central alveolar hypoventilation** is defined in the ICSD-3 as "the presence of alveolar ventilation resulting in sleep-related hypercapnia and hypoxemia in individuals with presumed normal mechanical properties of the lung and respiratory pump."[3] Diagnostic criteria for this disorder include the presence of sleep-related hypoventilation that cannot be attributed to impairments in respiration, obesity, medication use, or another medical disorder. The disorder usually presents in adolescence and is gradually progressive.

Sleep-Related Hypoventilation Due to a Medication or Substance

This disorder is characterized by hypoventilation during sleep that can be attributed to a medication or other substance that is known to reduce ventilatory drive.

Sleep-Related Hypoventilation Due to a Medical Disorder

This disorder is characterized by hypoventilation during sleep that can be attributed to an underlying medical disorder, including airway disease, muscular and neurological disorders, and disorders affecting the chest wall, not including obesity.

Sleep-related Hypoxemia Disorder

This diagnosis is applied when significant oxygen desaturation during sleep is present to levels at or below 88% in adults and at or below 90% in children. In this disorder, the hypoxemia is not associated with hypoventilation or primarily attributed to obstructive or central sleep apneic–hypopneic events. Often, primary lung disease is an underlying factor of this disorder.

Isolated Symptoms and Normal Variants

This subcategory includes sleep-related symptoms that may be benign in some patients but can be indicative of the presence of an underlying sleep disorder. Often the symptoms warrant further testing to rule out a primary sleep disorder.

Snoring

Snoring is an audible vibration of the upper airway during sleep. It is most often associated with inspiration but can occur during the expiration as well. Snoring is caused by turbulent airflow moving through the airway. The intensity can vary from mild to loud and can cause the person to wake up or disrupt a bedpartner or others in adjacent rooms. Snoring often leads to dry mouth or irritated tissues in the throat. If snoring is not associated with symptoms, it is referred to as **primary snoring**. However, snoring is one of the most common symptoms of obstructive sleep apnea. Therefore, the occurrence of daytime sleepiness, fatigue, insomnia, frequent arousals, gasping, choking, or witnessed pauses in breathing or if the patient has been diagnosed with hypertension, cognitive dysfunction, coronary artery disease, stroke, congestive heart failure, atrial fibrillation, or type 2 diabetes warrants further evaluation through sleep testing.

Catathrenia

Sleep-related groaning, or **catathrenia**, consists of repeated groaning during exhalation, mainly in REM sleep. Typically the patient is not affected by this disorder, but the bed partner's sleep is often disrupted as a result. This disorder is rare but appears to be more common in males than in females.

Sleep-Related Breathing Disorders Treatment Options

The most effective and common treatment option for OSA is **CPAP therapy**. This mode of treatment uses air pressure to act as a split to maintain the patency of the airway, effectively eliminating apnea, hypopnea, flow limitation, and snoring. Alternative treatment options include dental appliances, **positional therapy**, and various surgical procedures. The effectiveness of many of these treatments varies greatly according to the severity and other characteristics of the patient.

In infants and children with large tonsils or adenoids, the most appropriate first-line OSA treatment would be a **tonsillectomy** or **adenoidectomy**. CPAP is occasionally prescribed but should be used with careful consideration. Treatment of central apnea and hypoventilation disorders includes using **bi-level therapy** and other modes of ventilatory support. These therapies will be discussed in more detail in subsequent chapters.

Central Disorders of Hypersomnolence

The ICSD-3 refers to this group of sleep disorders as those in which "the primary complaint is daytime sleepiness not caused by disturbed nocturnal sleep or misaligned circadian rhythms."[3] Sleepiness can often be classified by questionnaires such as the Epworth Sleepiness Scale or the Stanford Sleepiness Scale or by tests such as the **multiple sleep latency test (MSLT)** or the **maintenance of wakefulness test**.

Narcolepsy Type I

The term **narcolepsy** is derived from the Greek words *narke*, meaning numbness or stupor, and *lepsis*, meaning attack. As the name suggests, narcolepsy is a disorder characterized by sleep attacks. Narcolepsy is primarily caused by a physiological or pathological abnormality. Although the severity and symptoms of narcolepsy may vary greatly between individuals, the disorder includes a variety of symptoms, which may include EDS, **cataplexy**, and other REM sleep phenomena such as **sleep paralysis** and **hypnagogic hallucinations**. These four characteristics constitute the **narcolepsy tetrad**. Few narcoleptic patients suffer from all of the listed symptoms, but many suffer from more than one. Frequent and often irresistible napping is also a common symptom of narcolepsy. Another common symptom of narcolepsy seen in approximately 20% to 40% of narcoleptics is **automatic behavior**, which is characterized by the subconscious performance of activities. Often these activities appear to be performed deliberately. A common example of automatic behavior is speaking on a subject matter that is completely out of context for the situation.

Excessive daytime sleepiness is the most common symptom of narcolepsy. EDS can manifest itself in many ways, including difficulty concentrating, difficulty remaining awake during normal waking hours, decreased cognition, napping, hallucinations, memory loss, and decreased performance in work-related tasks. Memory loss and difficulty concentrating as a result of

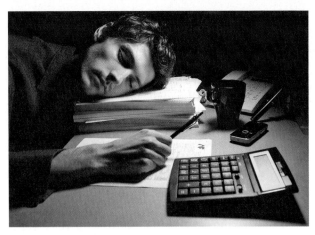

FIGURE 2-13 Individuals with narcolepsy often experience severe Excessive Daytime Sleepiness, which can lead to poor performances in school or at work.
© Cristi Lucaci/Shutterstock.

EDS often lead to poor performance in school or work (see **Figure 2-13**). Excessive daytime sleepiness can also negatively affect one's personal relationships. Individuals experiencing profound EDS are also at an increased risk for automobile accidents and work-related accidents. Nearly half of narcoleptics have reported falling asleep at the wheel.[5] Narcoleptic patients are often able to detect an oncoming sleep attack in time to fight it off. Narcoleptics, however, are known to fall asleep unintentionally and at inappropriate times, such as in the middle of a conversation, while laughing, or during sexual activity. Even those who fight off sleep attacks may experience periods of **microsleep**. Microsleep is a brief lack of consciousness or awareness. Often, the microsleep period is so brief the individual may not be aware that it occurred. Scheduled nap periods may help narcoleptic patients momentarily with feelings of EDS and the occurrence of periods of microsleep.

One of the most well-known and disruptive symptoms of narcolepsy is *cataplexy*. Cataplexy comes from the Greek words *kata*, meaning down, and *plexis*, meaning stroke or seizure. Cataplexy is sometimes mistaken for seizure activity and is characterized by a bilateral loss of muscle tone, usually provoked by strong emotion. It manifests itself as muscle weakness that can range from a mild feeling of weakness to complete limb atonia with a resulting fall. Patients suffering from cataplexy may drop items they are holding, which can cause embarrassment or be hazardous. Periods of cataplexy usually last only a few seconds, but if prolonged they may lead to a period of REM sleep. Cataplexy is seen in approximately 70% of narcoleptics, but often these individuals are able to control the symptoms by controlling emotional stimuli. **Narcolepsy type I** includes the diagnosis of narcolepsy with the complaint of cataplexy. This type was formerly called *narcolepsy with cataplexy*.

Sleep paralysis, another symptom of narcolepsy, is characterized by a partial or total paralysis of skeletal muscles that occurs on awakening or at sleep onset. When occurring at sleep onset, this is called **hypnagogic**; when it occurs on awakening, it is referred to as **hypnopompic**. The average REM latency for a normal, healthy adult sleeper is 90–120 minutes; in contrast, narcoleptics with sleep paralysis may enter REM sleep immediately or almost immediately after sleep onset. Sleep paralysis occurs in approximately 25% of narcoleptic patients and is also often associated with hypnagogic or hypnopompic hallucinations, which are seen in approximately 30% of narcoleptic sufferers. Hallucinations experienced by narcoleptic patients are characterized by vivid, dreamlike experiences occurring at sleep onset or on awakening. They are often accompanied by intense feelings of fear. Sleep paralysis and hypnagogic and hypnopompic hallucinations may also be seen in patients other than narcoleptics who are severely sleep deprived.

Typical onset for narcolepsy is during the late teen years or early twenties. It is now established that narcolepsy type I is caused by a deficiency in hypocretin signaling in the hypothalamus. In some cases, severe head injuries and brain tumors have been known to cause narcolepsy.

Narcoleptic patients often suffer from depression, possibly as a result of the inability to carry out certain normal activities, and they are often underachievers. This can also lead to low self-esteem.

Because of the large number of sleep disorders with resulting symptoms similar to those of narcolepsy, diagnosing the disorder may be difficult. Physicians suspecting narcolepsy may have the patient complete certain sleepiness scales or a sleep diary. Most importantly, the physician should order an MSLT preceded by an overnight diagnostic sleep study. The overnight diagnostic sleep study is to rule out the presence of other sleep disorders such as OSA or periodic limb movement disorder, which are often the underlying causes of certain narcoleptic symptoms. The MSLT is performed the following day and consists of a series of five short nap opportunities. The patient is given 20 minutes to fall asleep. If the patient does not sleep, the nap opportunity is ended and the patient is moved out of the bed. If the patient falls asleep, he or she is monitored for the next 15 minutes. Whereas the average sleep latency for normal sleepers usually ranges from 5 minutes to 20 minutes and REM latency falls between 60 minutes and 120 minutes, more than 80% of narcoleptic patients have an average sleep latency of less than 5 minutes and experience significantly reduced REM latencies. During the MSLT, the 15-minute sleep period is evaluated for two main outcomes: sleep latency and the presence of a **sleep-onset REM period (SOREMP)**. The diagnostic criteria for narcolepsy include the irresistible need to sleep or daytime lapses into sleep for at least 3 months and either (1) a mean sleep latency of 8 minutes or less during an MSLT and at least two sleep-onset REM periods during the five MSLT naps and previous night's diagnostic study or (2) hypocretin-1 concentrations ≤110pg/mL. Narcolepsy type I patients report cataplexy but narcolepsy type II patient do not. Ultimately, the final diagnosis must consider medical history, physical examination, patient questionnaires, and sleep study results.

Narcolepsy currently has no known cure, but certain behavioral and medical treatments have been shown to be effective in treating its symptoms. A behavioral treatment that has been shown to be highly effective in narcoleptics is taking short, regularly scheduled naps during the daytime. Narcoleptics also may find it helpful to discuss their disorder and its associated symptoms with friends, family members, and coworkers. Doing so can help relieve some of the embarrassment and stress that may occur with EDS and some of the other symptoms of narcolepsy.

Perhaps the most significant behavioral treatment for narcoleptics is to practice proper sleep hygiene. Sleep hygiene techniques include practices that are beneficial to the quality of one's sleep, and they have been shown to be effective in improving a patient's ability to initiate and maintain sleep and remain awake and alert during the daytime. Examples of sleep hygiene practices include retiring and awakening at consistent times from day to day; avoiding caffeine, alcohol, and sedatives; getting regular exercise but avoiding heavy exercise within 4 hours of retiring; avoiding reading or watching television while in bed; and avoiding greasy or fatty foods and snacks. Consistently practicing proper sleep hygiene techniques can greatly improve the quality of sleep and the quality of life for both narcoleptics and normal sleepers.

In addition to behavioral modifications, narcoleptics may use certain medications to treat the disorder and its symptoms. The most common medications used to treat narcolepsy are central nervous system (CNS) stimulants such as Provigil, Ritalin, and dexedrine. Amphetamine-like stimulants such as methylphenidate and methamphetamine are also commonly used to treat narcolepsy. CNS stimulants are the most commonly prescribed drugs for treating narcoleptics with excessive daytime sleepiness; REM suppressants and antidepressants are often used to treat narcoleptics with cataplexy, hypnagogic hallucinations, and sleep paralysis. In recent years, fluoxetine and monoamine oxidase inhibitors have also been shown to be useful in treating cataplexy.

Narcolepsy Type II

Narcolepsy type II is characterized by a diagnosis of narcolepsy as defined in the ICSD-3 but without the presence of cataplexy. An additional diagnostic criterion for narcolepsy type II requires that either cerebrospinal fluid hypocretin-1 concentration was not measured or that it is measured at >110 pg/mL.

Idiopathic Hypersomnia

Idiopathic hypersomnia is characterized by daily periods of the irrepressible need to sleep for at least 3 months, nonrefreshing naps, decreased sleep latency (mean sleep latency less than or equal to 8 minutes on an MSLT), an absence of cataplexy, and a 24-hour sleep period of at least 11 hours. Although many of these symptoms may be common symptoms of other sleep disorders, the diagnostic criteria for this disorder require that other relevant sleep disorders be ruled out.

Kleine-Levin Syndrome

Also referred to as **recurrent hypersomnia** or **periodic hypersomnolence**, **Kleine-Levin syndrome** is a rare disorder that occurs when a patient experiences repeating episodes of **hypersomnia** (excessive sleeping). Episodes can range from 2 days to 5 weeks, with an average episode lasting approximately 10 days and recurring at least once a year. During the episodes, patients may sleep 16–18 hours a day and have associated symptoms, including hallucinations, confusion, excessive eating, and disinhibited behaviors. Between episodes the patients exhibit normal levels of alertness, mood, behavior, and cognitive function. Kleine-Levin syndrome typically occurs first during adolescence and lasts 14 years on average. Males are twice as likely to be affected. The underlying cause is not fully understood, but several risk factors have been identified, including birth and developmental issues and having a Jewish heritage. Treatment of this disorder is mainly supportive.

Hypersomnia Due to a Medical Disorder

This disorder exists when a primary medical condition is the underlying cause for hypersomnia. Various medical conditions can cause excessive sleepiness include neurologic, endocrine, and metabolic disorders.

Hypersomnia Due to a Medication or Substance

This disorder is present when the use or abuse of a drug or medication is responsible for extended periods of sleepiness or excessive sleep. This can occur as a result of drug abuse or prescribed use of certain medications.

Hypersomnia Associated with a Psychiatric Disorder

Patients with this disorder meet the diagnostic criteria for hypersomnolence, but the daytime sleepiness is associated with an underlying psychiatric disorder. This is most common among those with mood disorders such as depression, bipolar disorder, and seasonal affective disorder.

Insufficient Sleep Syndrome

An extremely common sleep disorder in today's busy world, **insufficient sleep syndrome** is characterized by not sleeping long enough to satisfy physical and psychological needs. Common alternate terms include *chronic sleep deprivation* and *sleep restriction*. Diagnostic criteria for insufficient sleep syndrome include daytime lapses into sleep, a total sleep time less than expected for the patient's age for a period of at least 3 months, and an absence of another sleep disorder, medication, or mental or physical disorder that may cause the symptoms. Sleep patterns, durations, and times are often recorded in a sleep log or with actigraphy. Although insufficient sleep syndrome has many possible causes, it is common during the teenage years when the need for sleep is high but the subject's lifestyle is not conducive to adequate sleep periods.

Circadian Rhythm Sleep–Wake Disorders

The **circadian rhythm** is an internal biological sleep–wake clock that all living organisms possess. In humans, this cycle is slightly longer than 24 hours but is entrained (maintained on a 24 hour cycle) daily by exposure to sunlight. When an individual's sleep period matches his or her underlying circadian rhythm, optimal sleep is most likely to be achieved. A **circadian rhythm sleep–wake disorder (CRSWD)** is characterized by a disturbance or disruption to the normal sleep–wake rhythm, either because of internal alteration or misalignment with what is required by the individual's environment. A CRSWD can cause the patient to experience excessive daytime sleepiness, insomnia, or both, and its impact can extend to other adverse health consequences, including detriments to physical, social, emotional, or educational well-being. The complaints of CRSWDs must be reported for a period of at least 3 months, and the sleep disturbance cannot be attributed to another sleep or medical disorder. Diagnoses of CRSWDs are often aided by the use of sleep diaries or **actigraphy** monitoring. Actigraphy monitoring has the ability to track trends in the sleep–wake cycle over time, usually 7 days to 3 weeks, through the use of a wearable sensor that tracks motion.

Delayed Sleep–Wake Phase Disorder

Delayed sleep–wake phase disorder is characterized by a significant delay in the primary sleep period compared to what is expected or desired. A patient with this disorder is unable to fall asleep at the desired time or at a time that is considered normal but is successful at a later time in the night. As a result, the patient often sleeps until late in the morning in an effort to achieve the required sleep time. Delayed sleep–wake phase disorder is common in adolescents or young adults who develop habits of staying up late at night.

Advanced Sleep–Wake Phase Disorder

Advanced sleep–wake phase disorder is characterized by a significant advance in the primary sleep period compared to what is expected or desired. A patient with this disorder has difficulty staying awake until the normal or expected bedtime, often falling asleep by 7 in the evening. As a result, the patient awakens extremely early in the morning. This is common in older adults who develop the lifestyle of eating and sleeping at earlier times than they did at younger ages.

Irregular Sleep–Wake Rhythm Disorder

Irregular sleep–wake rhythm disorder is characterized by an abnormal and undefined circadian rhythm of sleep and wake times. Although the total sleep time during the 24-hour cycle is comparable with normal sleepers, the sleep periods come in the form of variable sleep episodes rather than one primary sleep period. Patients with irregular sleep–wake rhythm disorder often experience periods of insomnia and EDS relevant to the sleep–wake pattern they are experiencing. Although considered rare, irregular sleep–wake rhythm disorder is experienced most commonly in patients with neurological or developmental disorders.

Non–24-Hour Sleep–Wake Rhythm Sleep Disorder

Formerly called **free-running disorder**, **non–24-hour sleep–wake rhythm sleep disorder** is characterized by a sleep–wake cycle that is not entrained to the 24-hour light–dark cycle. The patient's circadian rhythm is often longer than 24 hours and marked by a delay in the main sleep episodes each night. Over time, this creates a pattern that seems to "free run" across the 24-hour period. Symptoms of non–24-hour sleep–wake rhythm sleep disorder can vary over time. When the sleep–wake cycle is misaligned with the external environment, symptoms of insomnia and EDS can be severe. Conversely, when the cycle eventually aligns to external cues, the patient will be free from symptoms. Many patients with this disorder are blind.

Shift Work Disorder

Patients with **shift work disorder** have work schedules that overlap with the normal sleep period. Shift workers often work during the late night, overnight, or extremely early morning hours. As a result of the disturbance of the underlying circadian rhythm, patients typically experience EDS during their shifts and insomnia during the daytime hours when they attempt to sleep. Many shift workers experience a variety of other detriments, including poor work performance, impaired judgment, and episodes of drowsy driving, as well as other health consequences.

Jet Lag Disorder

Jet lag disorder occurs when an individual experiences reduced sleep time and symptoms of EDS or insomnia as a result of travel across two or more time zones. This disorder is also associated with impairments in daytime function, fatigue, and gastrointestinal disturbances. Duration and severity of symptoms depends on the direction of travel, number of time zones crossed, and individual tolerance.

Circadian Rhythm Sleep Disorder Not Otherwise Specified

This disorder is characterized by a disturbance to the normal circadian rhythm that does not meet the criteria for other disorders in this class of sleep disorders. Most of these are secondary to medical conditions or medication or substance use. Examples of medical conditions associated with this condition include disturbances from dementia, Alzheimer's disease, and movement disorders such as Parkinson's disease.

Parasomnias

A **parasomnia** is an unwanted physical movement or action during sleep. Commonly occurring parasomnias include walking and talking in sleep. This group of sleep disorders is subdivided into disorders of arousal from NREM sleep, those associated with REM sleep, and other parasomnias. Parasomnias can affect the patient or bedpartner and often result in injuries, disruption in sleep, and other health consequences.

Disorders of Arousal from NREM Sleep

Disorders of arousal from NREM sleep are characterized by incomplete awakenings from sleep that are associated with limited or absent responsiveness to the environment, dream imagery, or recollection of the event. Most episodes occur during stage N3 sleep and in the first third of the sleep period. In general, disorders of arousal from NREM sleep are common in children but tend to decrease in prevalence with age.

Confusional Arousals

A **confusional arousal** occurs when a person awakens from sleep in a confused state. On awakening, individuals exhibit confusion about who they are, where they are, and what is happening around them. During the event, speech and cognition may be delayed, slurred, or slow. Confusional arousals are not associated with fear or movement to leave the bed. Other sleep disorders such as insomnia or hypersomnia can increase the prevalence of confusional arousals, as can shift work or sleep deprivation.

Sleepwalking

Sleepwalking, also called **somnambulism** (*somna*, associated with sleep, and *ambulate*, to move) is a disorder characterized by sitting up in bed, walking, or jumping up and running from the bed. Sleepwalking can range from common behaviors such as walking calmly through the bedroom or house to other complex behaviors occurring out of the bed.

Sleep Terrors

Sleep terrors, also known as **night terrors**, are characterized by awakenings from slow-wave sleep with feelings of intense fear that often begin with a loud scream or cry. Other signs consistent with fear will be evident such as sweating and increased heart and respiratory rates. During a sleep terror episode, individuals will often have their eyes open but are not responsive to the environment. When returning to sleep after a sleep terror, the patient will usually return directly to slow-wave sleep and have no recollection of the event in the morning.

Sleep-Related Eating Disorder

Sleep-related eating disorder is characterized by repeated episodes of eating or drinking during arousals from sleep. In most individuals affected, this disorder occurs on a nightly basis. Often the patient chooses junk foods that are not typically eaten during the day. Most patients with this disorder are exceptionally difficult to awaken during these episodes and have no recollection of the episode in the morning. Patients with this disorder will often gain weight as a result of the high volume of junk foods eaten during the night. They may also injure themselves while cooking during sleep or by eating strange combinations of foods or toxic substances.

REM-Related Parasomnias

Unlike NREM-related parasomnias, **REM-related parasomnias** occur during episodes of stage R. Because episodes of REM sleep tend to be shorter in the beginning of the sleep period and progressively lengthen throughout the course of the night, REM-related parasomnias are often reported to occur in the early morning hours.

REM Sleep Behavior Disorder (RBD)

REM sleep behavior disorder (RBD) consists of physical events or activities occurring during REM sleep. In normal sleepers, muscle atonia occurs during REM. However, in patients with RBD, muscle tone is maintained during REM sleep. As a result, **isomorphism** often occurs, where the muscles move in response to the patient's dream content. On awakening, the patient is likely to remember the dream he or she acted out. Occasionally, the patient may act out violently, performing such acts as flailing arms, hitting, kicking, yelling, and so on. For this reason, sleep-related injuries to both individuals and bed partners are common with this disorder. Periodic limb movements also frequently occur during REM in patients with RBD. Polysomnograms with corresponding video are important to diagnose RBD by documenting the lack of muscle atonia and associated movements. Typically, additional arm and EEG leads are used to detect movements and rule out seizure activity. RBD is most common in men 50 and older. Recent research has come to identify the association of RBD with various neurological disorders such as Parkinson's disease.

Recurrent Isolated Sleep Paralysis

Sleep paralysis, a symptom sometimes associated with narcolepsy, refers to the inability to move at sleep onset (hypnagogic) or on awakening (hypnopompic). The experience is quite frightening, and thus sleep paralysis is often associated with anxiety and stress surrounding the bedtime period. Episodes of sleep paralysis may last a few seconds to several minutes. Because sleep paralysis is a common symptom of narcolepsy, diagnostic criteria for **recurrent isolated sleep paralysis** requires that narcolepsy be ruled out. Sleep paralysis occurring outside the diagnosis of narcolepsy is often caused by periods of sleep deprivation or shifting sleep times or habits.

Nightmare Disorder

A **nightmare** is a common occurrence in which a person has an intense, frightening dream that causes an awakening. Often on awakening, the person is still frightened because of the intensity of the nightmare. Nightmares are common in children and are considered normal for this age group. As a person grows into adolescence, nightmares typically reduce in frequency and intensity. Nightmare disorder is diagnostic when the dreams or sleep disturbance causes significant distress to emotional, social, physical, or occupational well-being. Nightmare disorder is common in patients with **posttraumatic stress disorder (PTSD)**. A patient with PTSD is likely to experience nightmares that relive or cause the patient to reexperience whatever event led to PTSD. Nightmares occur during REM sleep, which is when most dreaming occurs, and often cause the person to delay falling back to sleep.

Other Parasomnias

This subcategory includes those parasomnias that are not reported as being associated with specific sleep stages.

Exploding Head Syndrome

Exploding head syndrome is a sleep disorder characterized by an imagined loud noise or sense of explosion in the head while falling asleep or awakening. Occasionally,

the patient may believe that he or she sees a flash of bright light. The episodes are not associated with complaints of pain, usually last a few seconds, and can vary in frequency from many in one night to infrequent events. The disorder is more commonly reported in women, with an age of onset averaging 58 years. Most patients report that symptoms resolve spontaneously over several years.

Sleep-Related Hallucinations

Like sleep paralysis, **sleep-related hallucinations** are common features of narcolepsy. Hypnagogic and hypnopompic hallucinations often occur in patients with narcolepsy; the patient experiences a visual hallucination either just before sleep onset or at awakening. These hallucinations are often related to sleep-onset REM periods and may be frightening and vivid enough to cause patients to jump out of bed and occasionally injure themselves. Diagnostic criteria for sleep-related hallucinations require the absence of other sleep disorders such as narcolepsy that could be the primary cause. These episodes occur more frequently in adolescents and young adults, with frequency decreasing with age.

Sleep Enuresis

Also called **nocturnal enuresis** or **bedwetting**, **sleep enuresis** is characterized by repeated episodes of involuntary urination during sleep. Because bladder control is a normal developmental milestone, this diagnosis is reserved for patients 5 years of age and older. Diagnostic criteria for sleep enuresis require that the events occur at least twice a week for at least 3 months. In primary sleep enuresis, patients have never demonstrated the ability to stay dry during sleep, while in the secondary disorder patients have demonstrated at least a 6-month period where they have stayed dry over the course of the night. Secondary sleep enuresis can occur in patients with PTSD, those who are victims of abuse, or those who are experiencing the enuresis as a result of a medical condition such as diabetes. Secondary enuresis has been highly correlated to sleep apnea relevant to the respiratory disturbance index. For this reason, sleep-related breathing disorders should be considered as underlying in a patient 5 or older who exhibits bedwetting but who was previously dry.

Parasomnias Due to a Medical Disorder

These disorders are diagnosed when a medical condition can be identified as the cause of a parasomnia. For example, certain neurological disorders such as Parkinson's disease or dementia can lead to sleep-related parasomnias.

Parasomnias Due to a Medication or Substance

These disorders are diagnosed when a parasomnia can be attributed to a drug, medication use, or abuse. Various medications have the potential to prompt parasomnias. For example, some tricyclic antidepressants and treatments for Alzheimer's disease can cause RBD. Sedative hypnotics and beta adrenergic medications have also been associated with various NREM parasomnias.

Isolated Symptoms and Normal Variants

Talking during sleep can occur at any age, during any stage of sleep, and in people who are otherwise normal and healthy. **Sleep talking**, also called **somniloquy**, is often considered benign unless it disturbs the sleep of the talker or the bed partner or is associated with other behaviors in sleep. Many people talk in their sleep without knowing it until they begin to share their room with someone else.

Sleep-Related Movement Disorders

Sleep-related movement disorders are a class of sleep disorders characterized by simple, often repetitive movements during sleep or the onset to sleep. These movements disrupt the sleep of the patient, the bed partner, or both. As a result, patients with sleep-related movement disorders report disturbed nocturnal sleep and excessive sleepiness during the day. Diagnosis of these disorders often necessitates overnight sleep testing with video.

Restless Legs Syndrome (RLS)

Restless legs syndrome (RLS) is a disorder characterized by the irresistible urge to move the body while at rest. Most patients report having uncomfortable sensations in their legs in the evening or at night, although between 21% and 57% of patients report arm sensations as well. The unusual feelings are described as creeping, crawling, itchy, burning, or tingling and tend to increase during periods of relaxation, such as while watching television, reading, or attempting to fall asleep. Individuals suffering from RLS often find themselves rubbing or slapping their legs, twitching their muscles, bouncing their feet, jerking their legs, and getting up to walk around the room to alleviate feelings of restlessness. The amount of time required to alleviate the symptoms of RLS can vary and often causes a delay in sleep onset. As a result, RLS is often associated with complaints of insomnia at night, excessive sleepiness during the day, and other psychosocial or occupational impairments.

The onset of RLS can occur at any age. RLS in children is often misdiagnosed as hyperactivity or growing pains. Most RLS sufferers begin experiencing symptoms by young adulthood and continue to experience these symptoms throughout their lives. RLS affects more than 5% of the total population in the United States. The severity and frequency of RLS symptoms tend to vary with stress, pain, illness, or other factors. Symptoms can appear during pregnancy and disappear immediately after. The most common medical condition associated with RLS is iron deficiency. Obstructive sleep apnea, Parkinson's disease, diabetes, renal failure, and rheumatoid arthritis are other conditions associated with RLS. Certain medications such as antihistamines, antidepressants, and antipsychotics can worsen the symptoms of RLS. Medications used to treat RLS often include dopamine agonists, opioids, benzodiazepines, and anticonvulsants. Massage and musculoskeletal manipulations have also been found to be helpful in some cases.

Sleep technicians should watch their patients carefully for signs of RLS and make note of them for the physician. Because patients are often not aware of this disorder, the technician should ask the patient appropriate questions to help the physician determine if RLS is present. Many patients with RLS also have periodic limb movement disorder.

Periodic Limb Movement Disorder (PLMD)

Periodic limb movement disorder (PLMD), also called **periodic limb movements in sleep**, and formerly known as *nocturnal myoclonus*, is a common sleep disorder affecting approximately one-third of adults 60 and older. This disorder occurs when the patient involuntarily moves the limbs (usually the legs) during sleep. The movements are repetitive, occur in periodic episodes, and are seen mostly in stage N2. Periodic leg movements are not usually seen during REM sleep because of the muscle atonia that occurs during REM.

The most common PLMD symptoms include frequent EEG arousals, fragmented sleep architecture, daytime sleepiness, and other psychosocial or occupational impairments. The symptoms of PLMD tend to increase with stress and certain medications such as tricyclic antidepressants. A periodic limb movement disorder not only affects the sleep of the individual suffering from the disorder but also can affect the sleep of the bed partner who is being kicked during the night. As a result, PLMD patients are often referred to a physician by the spouse or bed partner.

Diagnosis of PLMD requires the use of overnight sleep testing. To be scored, limb movements must last between 0.5 and 5 seconds and have an amplitude of least 8 μV higher than the resting electromyogram (EMG) amplitude. Periodic limb movements occur within 5–90 seconds of each other, and at least four of these movements must occur to create a series. A **PLM index** is calculated by dividing the total number of periodic limb movements by the total sleep time in hours, giving an average number of periodic limb movements per hour of sleep time. PLMD is diagnosed if the patient has a PLM index greater than 15 per hour in adults or greater than 5 per hour in children.

The sample shown in **Figure 2-14** shows a series of six periodic limb movements on a 300-second epoch. They are not associated with respiratory events, and they occur during NREM sleep.

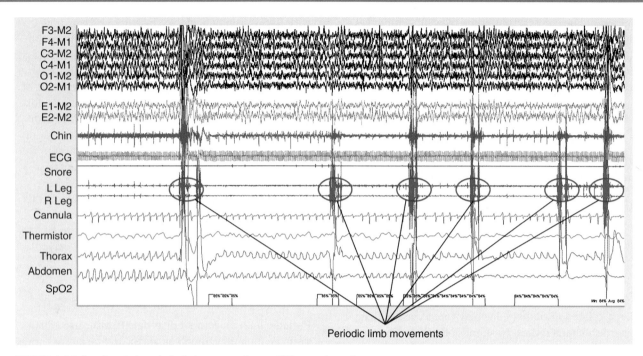

FIGURE 2-14 A series of six periodic limb movements on a 300-second epoch.

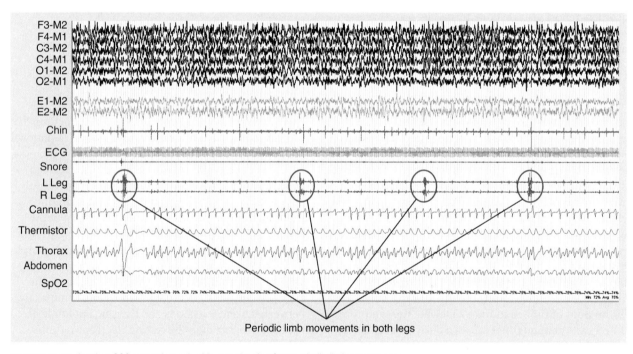

FIGURE 2-15 Another 300-second epoch, this one showing four periodic limb movements.

The sample in **Figure 2-15** shows another 300-second epoch in which four periodic limb movements occur. In this example, both legs are showing movement.

Other sleep disorders that could cause the limb movements (for example, sleep-related breathing disorders) should be ruled out or treated before making a diagnosis of PLMD. **Figure 2-16** shows limb movements (outlined with dark circles) in a 300-second epoch. In this case, the limb movements are preceded by respiratory events (outlined with lighter circles on the line

below). Because the respiratory events appear to be the primary cause of the limb movements, PLMD would not be initially diagnosed. If periodic limb movements persist after the sleep-disordered breathing is corrected, then the patient would likely be diagnosed with PLMD.

The most common treatments for PLMD include the use of certain medications. Benzodiazepines, which suppress the muscle contractions, are perhaps the most commonly prescribed medications for PLMD. Dopaminergic agents have been shown to regulate

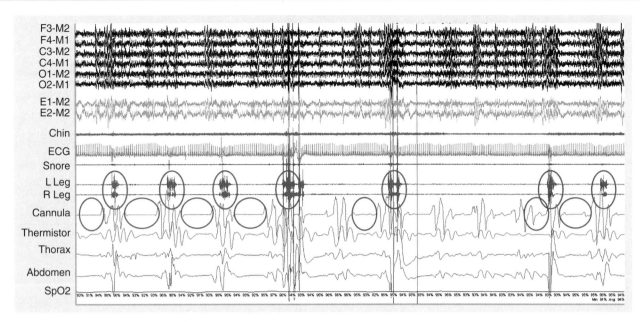

FIGURE 2-16 Limb movements in a 300-second epoch preceded by respiratory events.

muscle movements during sleep. Anticonvulsant agents have also been effective in inhibiting the muscle contractions, and GABA agonists also help relax muscle contractions.

Sleep-Related Leg Cramps

This disorder is characterized by intense and sudden muscle cramps in the legs during sleep. These muscle cramps can last up to several minutes, are often painful, and result in the patient waking up from sleep, thereby disturbing the sleep period. **Sleep-related leg cramps** are common in the elderly and have been reported less frequently in children and adolescents. This disorder has been associated with numerous underlying conditions, including diabetes, peripheral vascular disease, neuromuscular disorders, and dehydration, as well as medications including oral contraceptives, diuretics, and statins.

Sleep-Related Bruxism

Bruxism is grinding the teeth or clenching the jaw. **Sleep-related bruxism** occurs when the sleeping patient has **rhythmic masticatory muscle activity** or repeated or sustained jaw muscle contractions. The unusual and grating sound can cause the patient to awaken or disrupt the bed partner. The symptoms of sleep-related bruxism include muscle soreness in the face, locking of the jaw, and morning headaches. Over time, bruxism can wear away tooth enamel, predisposing the patient to cavities and tooth sensitivity. Bruxism is most commonly seen among children and adolescents, who typically grow out of the disorder; however, some people experience bruxism their entire lives. The disorder is usually discovered or initially suspected by the patient's dentist, who may see evidence of the teeth grinding.

For many, a dental appliance such as a mouth guard is appropriate and can be effective in preventing further damage to the teeth.

The sample epoch in **Figure 2-17** shows a patient with sleep-related bruxism. The events directly under the arrows show disruptions in the EEGs, electrooculograms, chin EMG, and snore channel. When a patient clenches his or her jaw or grinds teeth, many muscles in the face, head, jaw, and neck will tighten, causing disruption in several channels, as shown in the figure. Heavy snoring can cause the same effect, so it is important that the technician make note of snores. In this case, the technician saw these events and noted that no snoring was present.

The arrows in the sample shown in **Figure 2-18** point to episodes of bruxism or grinding of the teeth or clenching of the jaw.

The sample epoch in **Figure 2-19** shows another example of sleep-related bruxism. The episodes of jaw clenching or teeth grinding are shown underneath the arrows. Again, the muscle activity is shown throughout all the leads on the head.

Sleep-Related Rhythmic Movement Disorder

Sleep-related rhythmic movement disorder is characterized by repetitive and rhythmic body movements during drowsiness or sleep, and it often includes **body rocking** or **head banging**. As the names suggest, *body rocking* refers to the entire body moving back and forth, whereas *head banging* refers to movements of the head. The movements usually begin near sleep onset and typically persist for as long as 15 minutes. It is common for infants and young children to have sleep-related rhythmic movements. However, by age five, the prevalence declines significantly. At any age, diagnostic

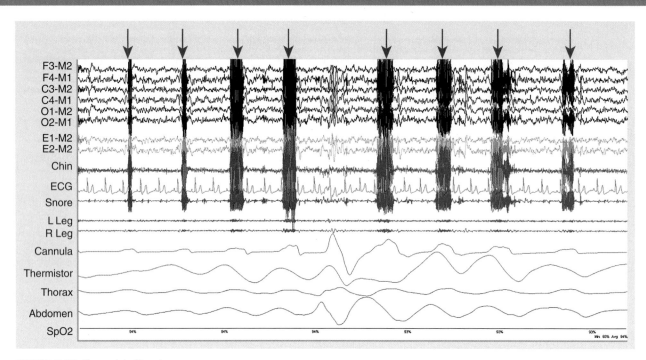

FIGURE 2-17 Sleep-related bruxism.

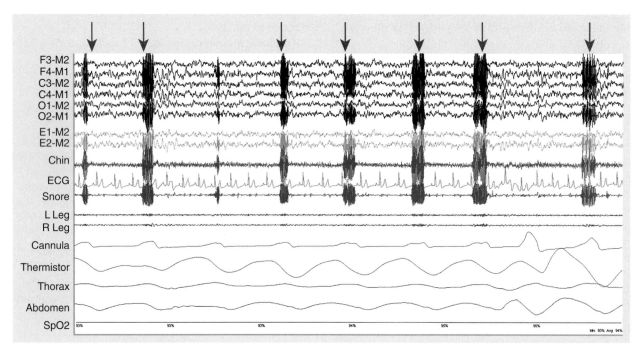

FIGURE 2-18 Another episode of bruxism.

criteria for this disorder require that the behavior causes disturbance to sleep, impaired daytime function, or has caused harm to the individual.

Benign Sleep Myoclonus of Infancy

Myoclonus describes limb jerks or movements. **Benign sleep myoclonus of infancy** is a rare disorder that occurs when repetitive leg jerks or movements in sleep occur during infancy, typically from birth to 6 months of age.

The condition is often confused with seizure activity and may prompt further investigation. However, it does not appear to pose any serious threat to the infant's sleep or health other than occasional arousals from sleep.

Propriospinal Myoclonus at Sleep Onset

Propriospinal myoclonus at sleep onset is an event similar to a sleep start but mainly involves body movements in the abdominal, trunk, and neck areas. They typically

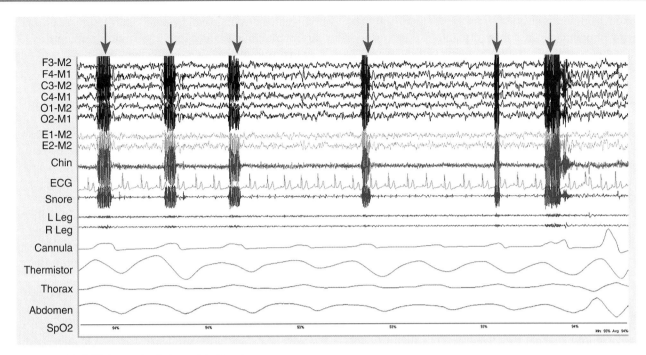

FIGURE 2-19 A third example of sleep-related bruxism.

occur at sleep onset or during brief arousals from sleep and result in sleep-onset insomnia.

Sleep-Related Movement Disorder Due to a Medical Disorder

This disorder is classified as movement disorders that disturb sleep and caused by an underlying medical condition. Various neurological conditions, such as Parkinson's disease, can cause involuntary muscle movements during sleep and disrupt the sleep period.

Sleep-Related Movement Disorder Due to a Medication or Substance

This category is reserved for movement disorders in sleep that are caused by drug use, abuse, or withdrawal.

Isolated Symptoms and Normal Variants

Excessive Fragmentary Myoclonus

Excessive fragmentary myoclonus (EFM) is characterized by frequent small twitches of fingers, toes, or muscles of the mouth during wake or sleep. On a polysomnogram, the movements appear as isolated brief increases in EMG, which usually ranges from 50 to more than 100 microvolts. They are typically insignificant and benign in nature. They occur during NREM sleep and may persist from 10 minutes to several hours. EFM has been associated with various sleep disorders, including sleep-related breathing disorders, narcolepsy, and PLMD.

Hypnagogic Foot Tremor and Alternating Leg Muscle Activation

Hypnagogic foot tremor is characterized by rhythmic leg or foot movements at sleep onset. **Alternating leg muscle activation** is similar but presents itself as a movement by one leg followed by a movement in the other leg. These events can cause brief arousals or awakenings from sleep but are typically benign in most patients who have no complaint of the movements or associated daytime impairments.

Sleep Starts (Hypnic Jerks)

A **sleep start**, also called a **hypnic jerk**, is a sudden muscle jerk or movement at sleep onset often accompanied by feelings of surprise, fear, or falling. Sleep starts are common and affect individuals of all ages but are typically benign. They may disturb the sleep of the bed partner and sometimes cause difficulty returning to sleep.

Other Sleep Disorders

These disorders are not classified in other categories because either they overlap categories or are relatively new or proposed disorders with limited data. Although the ICSD-3 does not specifically list any sleep disorders in this category, the ICSD-2 listed **environmental sleep disorder** here. Environmental sleep disorder can consist of many different factors, including a disorder held by the bed partner that is causing a disruption. For example, if a person has PLMD, the bed partner is likely to experience sleep disruptions, causing EDS, fatigue, or insomnia. This would be considered an environmental sleep disorder. Other factors in the environment can cause these disruptions, such as poor room temperature or lighting, music, or leaving the television on.

Chapter Summary

Seven main classes of sleep disorders have been identified by the American Academy of Sleep Medicine and are outlined and detailed in the ICSD-3. The main classes of sleep disorders are (1) insomnia, (2) sleep-related breathing disorders, (3) central disorders of hypersomnolence, (4) circadian rhythm sleep–wake disorders, (5) parasomnias, (6) sleep-related movement disorders, and (7) other sleep disorders.

Insomnia is the inability to initiate or maintain sleep or restful, restorative sleep. Insomnia can be caused by a wide variety of factors ranging from stress and anxiety to poor sleep hygiene. The complaint of the inability to fall asleep is a symptom and does not always preclude the diagnosis of insomnia. For example, some patients experience sleep state misperception and believe that they do not sleep or sleep little, when in actuality they are sleeping. Frequently, after evaluating these patients further, it is discovered they have other underlying sleep disorders that reduce the quality of sleep. In these cases, the underlying sleep disorder is diagnosed, not the symptom of insomnia. Poor sleep hygiene can be a common contributor to insomnia, but it is easily corrected. Proper sleep hygiene refers to practices such as maintaining a comfortable bedroom temperature, not consuming caffeine shortly before bedtime, and not watching television in bed.

Sleep-related breathing disorders are pervasive and occur most frequently in overweight and obese individuals. Obstructive sleep apnea occurs when an individual is unable to maintain an open airway during the night and suffers periods of no breathing. Chronic sleep apnea can lead to excessive daytime sleepiness, morning headaches, frequent awakenings during the night, hypertension, memory loss, and other symptoms. Central sleep apnea differs from OSA in that the patient is not attempting to breathe during the events. Rather than an obstruction in the upper airway causing the apnea, the central nervous system is the underlying cause.

Central disorders of hypersomnolence cause excessive daytime sleepiness and include disorders such as narcolepsy that can be debilitating and disruptive to normal daytime functions. Narcolepsy is characterized by periods of REM at times when REM should not present itself, including during wakefulness. Symptoms of narcolepsy can include excessive daytime sleepiness, hypnagogic hallucinations, sleep paralysis, and cataplexy.

Circadian rhythm sleep–wake disorders are characterized by disruptions to the normal 24-hour sleep–wake cycle. These disruptions may be self-induced, externally induced, or caused by medical conditions

Case Study Example

A 21-year-old women reports to the sleep disorders center complaining of severe excessive daytime sleepiness that has progressively gotten worse over the last 5 years. She reports difficulty staying awake in her college classes and episodes of "sleep attacks" daily.

Think about what other questions or information you would like to collect from this patient to narrow down which sleep disorders are relevant.

Physical exam reveals a patient with a BMI of 21 and a neck size and oral anatomy within normal limits. No nasal congestion or deviation is observable. The patient's sleep diary demonstrates a regular and sufficient nighttime sleep routine, and a subjective sleep assessment reveals moderate daytime sleepiness. On further questioning, the patient describes vivid lifelike dreams at sleep onset and times when she wakes up but feels like she cannot move.

These features are consistent with which sleep disorder or disorders?

This patient reports chronic EDS, episodes of sleep paralysis, and hypnogogic hallucinations. These clinical features are highly suggestive of narcolepsy. Alternatively, hypersomnia is also possible. The patient's history does not indicate a high risk for sleep-related breathing disorder, but it cannot be ruled out at this time.

What type of testing is indicated?

To confirm a diagnosis of narcolepsy, an overnight sleep study followed by a multiple sleep latency test is indicated. In this case, testing revealed an overnight sleep study within normal limits with the exception of short sleep onset and REM latencies. There were no abnormal respiratory events observed. The MSLT revealed three SOREMPs and a mean sleep latency of 5 minutes.

What Is the Most Likely Final Diagnosis?

The overnight testing ruled out the presence of sleep-related breathing disorders. The presence of SOREMPs on the MSLT also rules out hypersomnia. Instead, the MSLT findings support the diagnosis of narcolepsy type II because the patient does not report cataplectic episodes.

or drugs. One of the most common circadian rhythm sleep disorders is jet lag disorder. This occurs when a person experiences insomnia or excessive daytime sleepiness as a result of traveling across two or more time zones. Shift work is another common cause of circadian rhythm disorder. Individuals who work shifts that overlap into their normal sleep schedule are more likely to experience fatigue, EDS, insomnia, and lack of concentration.

Parasomnias are sleep disorders in which an individual performs some sort of undesirable or unwanted action during sleep. These can cause disturbances to the individual's sleep and can put the patient and those nearby in physical danger. Sleepwalking is a parasomnia in which the individual will arise from bed during NREM sleep to walk, run, or perform other normal activities. In some cases, the individual may jump out of a high window or assault the bed partner. Sleep enuresis is a parasomnia in which the individual has limited or no bladder control during sleep.

Sleep-related movement disorders are a class of sleep disorders that cause smaller, less significant, and often rhythmic or repetitive movements during sleep. Perhaps the most common of these is periodic limb movement disorder. Patients with PLMD exhibit frequent, repetitive movements of the limbs during sleep. These movements can disturb the sleep of the patient or the bed partner. Sleep-related bruxism is another common movement disorder in which the individual grits or grinds his or her teeth or clenches the jaw during sleep. This can disrupt the sleep period and can damage the individual's teeth.

The final class of sleep disorders is called *other sleep disorders* and is reserved for disorders that may overlap other classes or that need to be researched further before being properly classified.

Chapter 2 Questions

Please consider the following questions as they relate to the material in this chapter.

1. What are the classes of sleep disorders? Why are they grouped the way they are?
2. What are some important features of sleep hygiene? Why are these important practices for everyone to follow?
3. Why is OSA important to diagnose and treat quickly and effectively?
4. What is narcolepsy? What social impacts might narcolepsy have on an individual?
5. How do delayed sleep–wake phase disorder and advanced sleep–wake phase disorder differ from each other?
6. What is a night terror? In what ways can a night terror be dangerous?
7. How does RLS differ from PLMD? In what ways are they similar?
8. What are hypnic jerks, and how can they affect a person's sleep?

Footnotes

1. Dickens, C. (1873). *The posthumous papers of the Pickwick Club*. New York: Harper & Brothers.
2. Rechtschaffen, A., & Kales, A. (1968). *A manual of standardized technology techniques and scoring systems for sleep stages of human subprojects*. Los Angeles: UCLA Brain Information Service.
3. American Academy of Sleep Medicine. (2014). *The international classification of sleep disorders* (3rd ed.). Darien, IL: American Academy of Sleep Medicine.
4. Maeder, M. T., Schoch, O. D., & Rickli, H. (2016). A clinical approach to obstructive sleep apnea as a risk factor for cardiovascular disease. *Vascular Health and Risk Management, 12*, 85.
5. Pizza, F., Jaussent, I., Lopez, R., Pesenti, C., Plazzi, G., Drouot, X., . . . & Dauvilliers, Y. (2015). Car crashes and central disorders of hypersomnolence: A French study. *PLoS One, 10*(6), e0129386.

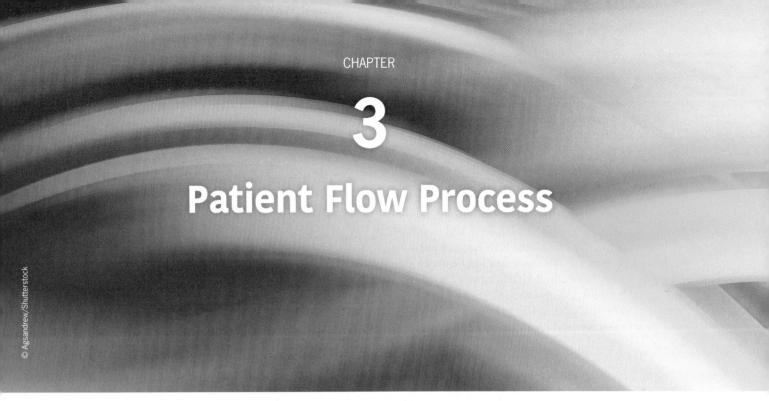

3

Patient Flow Process

CHAPTER OUTLINE

Living with a Sleep Disorder
Physician Screening
The Referral Process
Patient Scheduling and Billing
The Sleep Study Process
Patient Education
The Scoring and Interpretation Process
Second Night Studies
DME Setup
PAP Machines
Patient Follow-Up
Chapter Summary

LEARNING OBJECTIVES

1. Understand the difficulties associated with living with a sleep disorder.
2. Learn how to calculate body mass index.
3. Gain insights into the screening process.
4. Learn about risk factors for common sleep disorders.
5. Learn about commonly used screening tools.
6. Discuss the importance of selecting a sleep lab.
7. Learn about the scheduling and billing processes.
8. Discuss the importance of patient education and some of the resources available.
9. Explain the process of scoring and interpreting sleep studies.
10. Learn about the many different mask styles and machine features.
11. Discuss the importance of following up with patients being treated for sleep disorders.

KEY TERMS

body mass index (BMI)
durable medical equipment (DME)
Epworth Sleepiness Scale (ESS)
Berlin Questionnaire
Stanford Sleepiness Scale (SSS)
Pittsburgh Sleep Quality Index (PSQI)
sleep history questionnaire
vital signs
Mallampati classification
standard polysomnogram (PSG)
positive airway pressure (PAP) titration

split night study
Alert, Well, And Keeping Energetic (AWAKE)
National Sleep Foundation (NSF)
nasal mask
chin strap
full face mask
nasal pillow
oral mask
hybrid mask
Respironics
Resmed
Fisher & Paykel

Living with a Sleep Disorder

Jim is a 28-year-old male with obstructive sleep apnea (OSA) syndrome. His job of cleaning carpets can be physically challenging. The manual labor takes a toll on his body, and the shifting hours (much of his work is done at night) make it impossible to keep a normal, steady sleep schedule. Jim is 5'10" tall and weighs 310 pounds, with a **body mass index (BMI)** of 44.5. BMI is calculated by multiplying a person's weight in pounds by 703 and then dividing by the height in inches squared. If measuring in metric units, the BMI equals a person's weight in kilograms divided by his or her height in meters squared. For example, if a person is 5'6" tall and weighs 200 pounds, the first step in calculating BMI would be to multiply the weight in pounds (200) by 703 to obtain the numerator:

$$200 \times 703 = 140,600$$

Then take the height in inches, which in this case is 66, and square it to get a denominator of 4,356:

$$140,600/4,356 = 32.3$$

Then divide the numerator by the denominator. For this example, the resulting BMI is 32.3. BMI categories for severity are included in **Table 3-1**. A BMI between 18.5 and 24.9 is considered optimal. The preceding example of Jim falls into the obese category.

A high BMI can increase the likelihood of obstructive sleep apnea. In Jim's case, he did not experience the symptoms of OSA until young adulthood when he became overweight. His symptoms included snoring, choking, and gasping for breath during sleep, excessive daytime sleepiness, fatigue, irritability, hypertension, morning headaches, frequent daytime naps, difficulty concentrating, memory loss, loss of libido, and poor job performance.

Jim's loud snoring kept his wife, Nancy, awake. She was concerned about his long breathing pauses during sleep. Often at the end of his apneas, Jim would kick his legs and his body would jerk, disturbing Nancy's sleep. Nancy was worried about Jim's health, and her job performance was also beginning to suffer as a result of his snoring. She eventually talked Jim into discussing his breathing problems during sleep with his physician. Jim's physician referred him to a

sleep center where he was diagnosed with OSA. He returned for a second night study with continuous positive airway pressure (CPAP). From the CPAP titration, Jim's physician determined that the optimal treatment pressure for him was 12 cm H_2O. Jim was referred to a **durable medical equipment (DME)** company, which set him up at home with a CPAP machine set at 12 cm H_2O and a nasal mask.

Both Jim and Nancy immediately saw progress. His snoring, choking, and gasping were almost completely corrected. He had more energy during the daytime. He slept throughout the night almost completely undisturbed, and he had enough energy during the day to perform his job well without having to take naps. The air from the CPAP machine often dried his upper airway, so he got a heated humidifier with his machine to correct the dryness. The mask occasionally caused redness and sore spots on his face, but simple adjustments of the straps allowed him to correct this.

Jim's story is not uncommon for those who suffer from obstructive sleep apnea. Unfortunately, many people with sleep disorders are never diagnosed or treated, either because they do not realize they have a problem with their sleep, or they do not know that their sleep disorder can be treated. In some cases, a patient may present the symptoms to his or her physician, only to be misdiagnosed or given an inappropriate treatment. For example, if Jim had told his physician of his excessive daytime sleepiness without revealing his other symptoms, his physician may have prescribed a sleep aid for him. However, this could have made his apnea worse by further relaxing the muscles and tissues in his upper airway.

Some patients who are referred to a sleep center for evaluation are unable to make the copayments their insurance requires for a sleep study, and others get lost in the scheduling process. The process of identifying patients with sleep disorders and accurately diagnosing and treating those disorders can be complex, time consuming, and expensive. The purpose of this chapter is to discuss these processes and some of the challenges they present.

Physician Screening

Physicians are often faced with the challenge of determining a diagnosis or the appropriate test necessary for diagnosis based on fairly brief visits with their patients. During the typical visit, there is a great deal to accomplish: A physician must establish rapport with the patient, obtain information about the patient's medical history, and understand what prompted the patient's visit. In addition, he or she must obtain additional details about the issue the patient is experiencing and make decisions about how to proceed. Physicians screen their patients for as many health problems, diseases, and disorders as possible to try to help them

Table 3-1
BMI Scale[1]

BMI Category	BMI Range
Underweight	<18.5
Normal	18.5–24.9
Overweight	25–29.9
Obese	>30

obtain better health. However, as a result of the time constraint, sleep health is often not sufficiently discussed. In addition, many patients attribute the signs and symptoms of a sleep disorder to having a busy lifestyle and do not see them as a problem worth raising. This is an important factor as to why so many sleep disorders remain undiagnosed and untreated.

Screening tools are valuable to optimize the physician's time and provide a means for focused identification of risk factors for various sleep disorders. Rather than trying to remember to ask each and every patient relevant questions to help identify sleep disorders, a physician can have her or his patient complete a screening questionnaire while in the waiting room and then follow with a discussion while in the visit if the screening is positive. Some of the most widely used and scientifically validated questionnaires include the Epworth Sleepiness Scale, the Berlin Questionnaire, the Stanford Sleepiness Scale, and the Pittsburgh Sleep Quality Index.

The **Epworth Sleepiness Scale (ESS)**[2] is a short questionnaire designed to determine a patient's subjective level of daytime sleepiness. It has the advantage of being short and simple enough for patients to complete without assistance. It provides the physician with a quick insight into the level of sleepiness experienced by a patient. In this questionnaire, a patient is asked to rate the likelihood that he or she would fall asleep in given situations. The patient rates each situation on a scale of 0 to 3, with 3 being a high chance of dozing or falling asleep and 0 being never dozing or sleeping in the given situation. The following situations are presented to the patient:

- Sitting and reading
- Watching TV
- Sitting inactive in a public place
- Being a passenger in a car for an hour or more
- Lying down in the afternoon
- Sitting and talking to someone
- Sitting quietly after lunch without alcohol
- Stopped for a few minutes in traffic while driving

The scores are then totaled. ESS scores range from 0 to 24 with the following severity ranges:

0–5	Normal daytime sleepiness
6–10	Mild daytime sleepiness
11–17	Moderate daytime sleepiness
18–24	Severe daytime sleepiness

ESS scores outside of the normal range indicate a possible sleep disorder and should prompt further evaluation, preferably by a sleep specialist. This tool is useful not only for screening purposes but also for measuring the effectiveness of treatment. Many sleep specialists will ask their patients to complete the ESS before treatment and at regular intervals after treatment for comparison.

The ESS does have limitations. First, it is a subjective tool; as such, it is dependent on the patients' perception of their level of sleepiness. While assigning scores for each situation, a patient may not perceive him- or herself as sleepy or may not be honest about his or her tendency to fall asleep. Second, in completing the ESS, the patient must consider how they feel during the given situations *in general*, *on a typical day*, rather than how they feel right now. For example, if a patient completes the assessment at 3 P.M. after a long day at work and responds based on how she or he is feeling at that time, a patient will likely assign high values to each situation and overestimate the score. Alternately, if a patient completes the assessment at 9 A.M. and responds based on how they are feeling at that time, they will likely assign low values and underestimate the score. A final limitation of the ESS is that a small percentage of patients with sleep disorders may not be symptomatic or feel extremely sleepy. This is more common with younger individuals, those with mild cases of a sleep disorder, and those with some parasomnias. Despite these limitations, the ESS continues to be a trusted and reliable screening tool.

The **Berlin Questionnaire**[3] consists of three categories related to the risk of having obstructive sleep apnea: snoring, daytime sleepiness, and hypertension. The questions are grouped according to these three categories, and the risk of sleep apnea is determined by the responses in each category. Scoring the Berlin Questionnaire can be complicated, but the final score can be quite useful for the physician.

The patient is first asked for his or her height and weight. From this, BMI is calculated. The questions are as follows:

Category 1

1. Do you snore?
   a. Yes
   b. No
   c. Don't know
   If yes,

2. Your snoring is:
   a. Slightly louder than breathing
   b. As loud as talking
   c. Louder than talking
   d. Very loud—can be heard in adjacent rooms

3. How often do you snore?
   a. Nearly every day
   b. 3–4 times/week
   c. 1–2 times/week
   d. 1–2 times/month
   e. Never or nearly never

4. Has your snoring ever bothered other people?
   a. Yes
   b. No
   c. Don't know

5. Has anyone noticed that you quit breathing during your sleep?
   a. Nearly every day
   b. 3–4 times/week
   c. 1–2 times/week
   d. 1–2 times/month
   e. Never or nearly never

Category 2

6. How often do you feel tired or fatigued after your sleep?
   a. Nearly every day
   b. 3–4 times/week
   c. 1–2 times/week
   d. 1–2 times/month
   e. Never or nearly never

7. During your wake time, do you feel tired, fatigued, or not up to par?
   a. Nearly every day
   b. 3–4 times/week
   c. 1–2 times/week
   d. 1–2 times/month
   e. Never or nearly never

8. Have you ever nodded off or fallen asleep while driving a vehicle?
   a. Yes
   b. No
   If yes,

9. How often does this occur?
   a. Nearly every day
   b. 3–4 times/week
   c. 1–2 times/week
   d. 1–2 times/month
   e. Never or nearly never

Category 3

10. Do you have high blood pressure?
    a. Yes
    b. No
    c. Don't know

The Berlin Questionnaire is scored in the following manner:

Category 1 Scoring

- Item 1 is assigned one point if the answer is Yes.
- Item 2 is assigned one point if the answer is c or d.
- Item 3 is assigned one point if the answer is a or b.
- Item 4 is assigned one point if the answer is a.
- Item 5 is assigned two points if the answer is a or b.

Category 1 is positive if the total score is two or more points.

Category 2 Scoring

- Item 6 is assigned one point if the answer is a or b.
- Item 7 is assigned one point if the answer is a or b.

- Item 8 is assigned one point if the answer is a.
- Item 9 is noted separately.

Category 2 is positive if the total score is two or more points.

Category 3 Scoring

Category 3 is positive if the answer to Item 10 is Yes or if the patient's BMI is 30 or higher. The patient is considered to be at a high risk of OSA if two or more categories have a positive score. The patient is considered to have a low risk of OSA if 0–1 categories have a positive score.

The Berlin Questionnaire is considered to be one of the most valid questionnaires for identifying patients with obstructive sleep apnea. The detailed questions also help patients discover their own symptoms, understand that these symptoms are not normal, and greatly increase the likelihood of seeking treatment.

Perhaps the main criticism of the Berlin Questionnaire is that it is specific only to identify patients with obstructive sleep apnea while making little attempt to discover other sleep problems.

The **Stanford Sleepiness Scale (SSS)**[4] is similar to the ESS in that it seeks to identify patients who have excessive daytime sleepiness. The main difference, however, is that the SSS asks the patient to assign a level of sleepiness for how they are feeling *at the time of the assessment*. The SSS has the advantage of being a quick and easy way for a patient to identify his or her own sleepiness at several given points in time. This can help physicians who would like to get insights into a circadian rhythm disorder or the effects of poor sleep hygiene. It is also frequently used during a sleep study to assess how the patient is feeling before bedtime or nap opportunities. The Stanford Sleepiness Scale is shown in **Table 3-2**.

Table 3-2
Stanford Sleepiness Scale

Degree of Sleepiness	Scale Rating
Feeling active, vital, alert, or wide awake	1
Functioning at high levels, but not at peak; able to concentrate	2
Awake but not relaxed; responsive but not fully aware	3
Somewhat foggy, let down	4
Foggy; losing interest in remaining awake; slowed down	5
Sleepy, woozy, fighting sleep; prefer to lie down	6
No longer fighting sleep, sleep onset soon; having dreamlike thoughts	7
Asleep	X

Like the Epworth Sleepiness Scale, the Stanford Sleepiness Scale has its limitations. Specifically, although the SSS can identify when a patient is sleepy and the perceived severity of the sleepiness, it is a subjective assessment and does not identify the specific cause of the patient's sleepiness.

Finally, the **Pittsburgh Sleep Quality Index (PSQI)**,[5] developed in 1989 by doctors at the University of Pittsburgh Medical School, was designed to be a more comprehensive screening tool for a broader range of sleep disorders. Using this tool, the patient rates his or her own sleep over a one-month period. It asks patients questions about their quality of sleep and the type of sleep disturbances they are experiencing. The results give numbers in seven categories: sleep duration, sleep latency, quality of sleep, sleep efficiency, sleep disturbances, sleep medications, and daytime dysfunction. The PSQI asks the patient the following questions:

1. During the past month, when have you usually gone to bed?
2. During the past month, how long (in minutes) has it usually taken you to fall asleep each night?
3. During the past month, what time have you usually gotten up in the morning?
4. During the past month, how many hours of actual sleep did you get at night? (This may be different than the number of hours you spent in bed.)
5. During the past month, how often have you had trouble sleeping because you . . .
   a. Cannot get to sleep within 30 minutes
   b. Wake up in the middle of the night or early in the morning
   c. Have gotten up to use the bathroom
   d. Cannot breathe comfortably
   e. Cough or snore loudly
   f. Had cold feet
   g. Were too hot
   h. Had bad dreams
   i. Had pain
   j. Other reasons (please describe)
6. During the past month, how often would you rate your overall sleep quality?
7. During the past month, how often have you taken medicine (prescribed or over the counter) to help you sleep?
8. During the past month, how often have you had trouble staying awake while driving, eating meals, or engaging in social activity?
9. During the past month, how much of a problem has it been for you to keep up enough enthusiasm to get things done?
10. Do you have a bed partner or share a room?
11. If you have a bed partner or share a room, ask him or her how often in the past month you have had . . .

   a. Loud snoring
   b. Long pauses between breaths while asleep
   c. Legs twitching or jerking while you sleep
   d. Episodes of disorientation or confusion during sleep
   e. Other restlessness during sleep (please describe)

The PSQI has the ability to empower patients to take control of reporting their own sleep problems. Numerous studies have shown the PSQI to have high validity and reliability. It offers physicians a broad viewpoint of potential sleep problems in patients. However, like other subjective screening tools, the PSQI is reliant on a patient's honest and accurate reporting.

Besides the utilization of questionnaires, screening for sleep disorders relies heavily on the recognition of various risk factors. Risk factors for sleep-related breathing disorders include being male; being overweight; having a thick neck; advancing age; loud snoring, gasping or choking during sleep; and having high blood pressure, diabetes, or a family history of sleep apnea. Risk factors for insomnia include being female, pregnant or menopausal, advancing age, being under significant stress, having depression, doing shift work, and having a family history of insomnia.

As mentioned previously, sleep disorders tend to be underdiagnosed. Therefore, it is important for physicians to use the various screening tools available like the ESS, learn to recognize signs and symptoms of sleep disorders, and ask appropriate questions regarding a patient's sleep habits, wakefulness, and alertness. If a sleep disorder is suspected, then referral to a sleep specialist is recommended.

The Referral Process

Once a physician recognizes that a patient may have a sleep disorder, most often he or she will refer that patient to a sleep specialty center for further evaluation. In some cases, the physician may feel comfortable managing the patient's sleep issue and refer to a sleep center for the testing only. In both cases, the physician will often indicate several options of local sleep centers for the patient to consider. Less frequently, a patient may self-refer to a sleep center (if allowed by the patient's insurance coverage) after recognizing that he or she is having sleep difficulties. Ultimately, the choice of facility depends on the answers to several questions:

- Is the center able to accept the patient's insurance? Sleep studies are expensive procedures. If the lab is not contracted with the patient's insurance, then it is unlikely the patient will be able to afford the study.
- Is the lab accredited? Although accreditation does not mean perfection, it can give a strong indication that the lab is organized, well-kept, and run according to proper protocol.

- Is the lab reputable? Physicians can often learn a lot about a sleep center by asking other physicians about their experiences. Similarly, patients can consult with people in their community to help inform their choice.
- Is the lab located conveniently for the patient? Although a sleep center may be close to the physician's office, it is not necessarily close to the patient's home or work. Location can be key for patients with a busy lifestyle.
- Does the lab have facilities to accommodate the patient's needs? Facilities such as showers, private restrooms, and a clean, comfortable bed can make an otherwise unpleasant sleep study much more tolerable.
- Can the lab schedule the patient quickly? Patients with sleep disorders need to be diagnosed and treated in a timely manner. Failing to do so can be extremely dangerous to the patient and may expose the physician and lab to potential lawsuits.
- Does the lab have a quick turnaround time? Just as important as scheduling the patient in a timely manner is getting results back to the physician quickly. Although some labs may be backlogged for several months, others have a 24-hour turnaround time for scoring and interpretation.
- Is the staff at the sleep lab qualified, reputable, and professional? Physicians should take the time to meet the recording technicians and scoring technologists. The clinical staff should be credentialed and licensed (if applicable) and have an excellent bedside manner. Sleep technologist credentials include the Registered Polysomnographic Technologist (RPSGT)[6] and Registered Sleep Technologist (RST)[7] credential.
- What is the patient-to-technician ratio? This is an important factor to preserve patient safety. The American Academy of Sleep Medicine (AASM) recommends a patient to technician ratio of 2:1, although in some cases a 3:1 ratio is acceptable. Because of the complicated and detailed processes involved in performing a sleep study, one technician should never be expected to perform more than three sleep studies at once.
- Is the lab secure? Sleep labs should be in a secure location. Patients should be able to feel comfortable knowing they and their valuables will be safe.

Although ease of referral should not be the determining factor, it benefits a sleep-disorder center to make the referral process as quick and easy as possible for the physician's office. Referrals should always include the patient's name, contact information, date of birth, Social Security number, and the physician's signature. Any medical records, information, or sleep questionnaires completed by the patient should be included with the referral.

The Consultation

The first visit to the sleep-disorder center begins with a consultation appointment with the sleep specialist, unless the primary care physician is only using the facility for the testing. In the latter case, the patient's first visit will be for overnight sleep testing. When booking the consultation appointment, the facility will often send the patient information and paperwork to be completed and brought with the first visit. These documents usually include a **sleep history questionnaire**, paperwork for basic demographics and insurance information, various screening instruments (described previously in the chapter), and a sleep diary to record the sleep routine over a period of at least one week.

The sleep history questionnaire typically includes a brief medical history; patient demographics such as age, height, and weight; and various questions related to the patient's sleep habits. The purpose of the sleep questionnaire is to get an understanding of the patient's sleep routine, habits, and symptoms related to any sleep disorders he or she may have. The sleep questionnaire often contains questions relating to the patient's sleep hygiene, such as watching television in bed or drinking excessive amounts of caffeine. The following example questions are typically found in a sleep history questionnaire:

- What prescribed medications are you currently taking?
- Do you smoke?
- Do you drink alcohol to help you fall asleep?
- What time do you normally go to bed? Wake up?
- How long does it normally take you to fall asleep at night?
- About how many times do you normally wake up at night?
- Do you usually wake up feeling refreshed?
- Do you snore?
- Do you kick your legs in your sleep?
- Do you have feelings of restlessness in your legs while trying to fall asleep?
- Do you awaken with headaches?
- Do you grit or grind your teeth at night?
- Do you awaken choking or gasping for breath?
- Do you sweat at night?
- Do you have difficulty initiating or maintaining sleep?
- Do you walk in your sleep?
- Do you talk in your sleep?
- Are you tired during the daytime?
- Do you fall asleep unintentionally?
- Do you have difficulty concentrating?
- Do you take naps during the day?
- Do you follow the same sleep schedule on weekends that you do during the week?

During the consultation, the screening tool, the sleep history questionnaire, and the sleep diary are used to prompt discussion on the various sleep issues the patient may be experiencing and highlight signs of a possible sleep disorder. The sleep specialist will likely perform a brief physical exam that can include measuring height, weight, neck size, and **vital signs** (heart rate, respiratory rate, blood pressure, pulse, and oxygen saturation), as well as an assessment of external and internal oral anatomy. External facial features are observed for features such as small or recessed jaw, nasal septum deviation, and other craniofacial abnormalities that are risk factors for sleep-disordered breathing. The inside of the mouth, tongue, palate, and back of the throat are also assessed for features that can indicate airway crowding. These include an enlarged tongue, a narrow and high arched palate, and enlarged tonsils or adenoids. Some physicians will use standardized assessment tools—for example, the **Mallampati classification**[8] to classify crowding of the oral airway. The Mallampati score is based on the ability to visualize the soft palate, uvula, and tonsillar pillars. This tool was developed originally for use in anesthesia to assess how difficult an intubation will be. However, a Mallampati class III and IV airway have also been associated with a higher incidence of sleep apnea. The Mallampati classification is shown in **Figure 3-1**.

At the conclusion of the consultation, and based on clinical and medical history, screening tools, and physical exam, the physician will determine if the patient is a candidate for sleep testing and, if so, what type of test is indicated. Several different types of sleep tests are available. The diagnostic overnight study, also called a **standard polysomnogram (PSG)**,

is ordered most frequently and is used to diagnose numerous sleep disorders including sleep-related breathing (SRB) and movement disorders. The **positive airway pressure (PAP) titration** study, also an overnight test, provides treatment to those patients diagnosed with a SRB disorder. A **split night study** combines the diagnostic study and the PAP study in an effort to accomplish both assessments in one night. In rare cases, the PSG, PAP, or split night study may be done during the daytime period for those patients who are shift workers and normally sleep during the day.

Other sleep-testing procedures include the multiple sleep latency test (MSLT), maintenance of wakefulness test (MWT), actigraphy, limited channel studies, and home sleep testing. These will be discussed in subsequent chapters of the text. Finally, for some patients, sleep testing may not be indicated and the physician may be able to make a diagnosis based on history and symptoms alone. In these cases, treatment options and a follow-up plan will be discussed.

Patient Scheduling and Billing

When scheduling the patient for overnight sleep testing, it is helpful to discuss the purpose of a sleep study, the testing process, and the facility itself. This will help the patient feel a little more at ease and know what to expect. It is important to determine if the patient has specific scheduling requirements or needs for the overnight procedure. For example, patients who work long hours may require that the study take place on a weekend night. Some patients may require a private bathroom with a shower, whereas others may require handicap-accessible facilities.

The scheduler will also inquire about the patient's insurance information and verify that the facility participates with the insurance and that the sleep testing is an allowed coverage. The billing department and insurance company will need to know the type of sleep study performed and will require documentation afterward that the study was completed. When verifying insurance benefits for a PAP titration, it may be necessary to provide documentation from the diagnostic study to show that the PAP titration is medically indicated.

Once the insurance is verified and the study is scheduled, the patient should be given information about what to bring and what to expect at the lab. Many facilities mail or email patients written instructions. Alternately, some labs may have a website in place for the patients to verify how to prepare for the study, what to expect, and where the lab is located.

The Sleep Study Process

Michael, a 55-year-old businessman with obesity, hypertension, and heavy snoring, was referred by his primary care physician to a sleep lab for a diagnostic

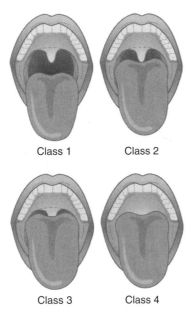

Class 1   Class 2

Class 3   Class 4

FIGURE 3-1 The Mallampati Classification. In classes III and IV, there is limited visibility of the palate and uvula, which indicates a crowded airway and a higher risk for obstructive sleep apnea.

polysomnogram to rule out obstructive sleep apnea. After Michael scheduled his sleep study, the scheduler emailed him directions to the lab and a sheet of instructions. He was instructed to bring his pajamas, clothes and toiletries for the next day, and any medications he normally takes at night.

As he drove to the sleep lab, Michael was nervous about his study. When he got closer, he noticed a well-lit sign clearly marking the sleep center. The parking lot was well-lit, and he was able to park close to the front entrance of the lab. He approached the entrance and noticed a security camera and a small sign that instructed him to ring the buzzer below. He did as instructed, and the technician's voice came over the intercom asking for his name and date of birth. After he provided the necessary information, the technician buzzed him in. Upon entry, Michael noticed that the facility appeared homey rather than like a business office or a medical clinic. The technician introduced herself confidently with a friendly smile and firm handshake. She was well-groomed and professional in her appearance and mannerisms (see **Figure 3-2**). The technician then asked Michael to provide two forms of identification. She walked Michael to his room where he saw a large comfortable bed, a nightstand similar to his at home, and a private restroom with a shower. The technician handed Michael several health and sleep-related questionnaires and instructed him to change into his pajamas. She left the room and closed the door behind her, giving him the privacy he needed. After filling out the necessary forms and changing into his pajamas, Michael was again greeted by the technician,

who introduced him to several wires and electrodes. The technician explained that these wires were used to gather the information necessary for his doctor to determine if he has sleep apnea or any other sleep disorder. She explained that the wires were connected to an amplifier that communicated with a computer in the technician room where she would stay throughout the night. She showed him an intercom in his room and explained that she would be accessible if he needed anything during the night.

The technician began measuring Michael's head for the proper electrode placement, cleaning the electrode sites, and applying electrodes to his scalp and skin. As she placed the wires, she explained the purpose of each wire, and what she would be monitoring with it. She also used this time to teach Michael about sleep apnea, its signs and symptoms, and the most common treatments. By the time the hookup was completed, Michael had well over 20 wires and electrodes on him; however, they were gathered in such a way that he did not feel like he would get tangled up in them. He was also comforted in knowing why each wire was necessary and that the technician was nearby if he needed anything.

The lights were turned off and the technician left the room. After a series of brief tests that involved Michael looking in different directions, moving each foot separately, and so on, Michael was instructed to try his best to fall asleep. It took him a little longer to fall asleep than normal, but eventually he was able to relax and drift off. Because the bed and the atmosphere of the lab were so comfortable (see **Figure 3-3**), Michael was able to sleep throughout most of the night.

Shortly after Michael awoke in the morning, the technician entered the room and congratulated him on completing a successful sleep study. After removing the wires and electrodes, she gave him several

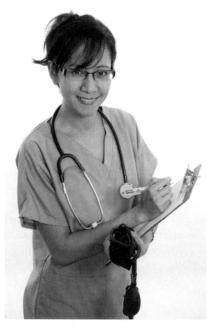

FIGURE 3-2 A warm, friendly greeting from the sleep technician can improve a patient's experience at the lab.
© Geo Martinez/Shutterstock.

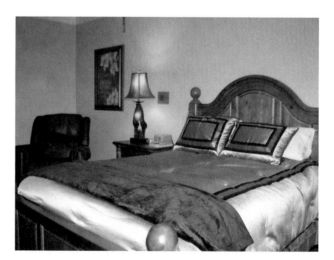

FIGURE 3-3 This suite at Sleep Healers in Dallas, Texas, is designed to help patients feel comfortable and at home. By reducing the clinical feel of the lab, patients are better able to relax and have a more positive experience in the sleep lab.

questionnaires to complete and said that his study was completed. She left the room, and Michael showered and got ready for work. He left feeling like his study was successful. He was confident that the technician was capable, knowledgeable, and qualified. He was comfortable enough to sleep throughout the night and felt that the study reflected his typical night's sleep at home. When he got to work, he emailed his physician to let him know about the positive experience he had at the lab.

Michael's experience is quite common for sleep patients. Although his apprehension about the sleep study could have prevented him from getting quality sleep at the lab, the friendly technician and the warm atmosphere helped him relax enough to sleep well. Using data from the sleep study, Michael's physician diagnosed him with obstructive sleep apnea and asked him to return for a PAP titration study. Michael was disappointed to learn that he had sleep apnea but was willing to go back to the lab because of the positive experience he had during the first study.

During the PAP titration study, Michael learned more about sleep apnea and the effect it could have on his health if left untreated. His technologist explained all aspects of PAP therapy and how it would help treat his disorder and benefit his health. The mask and air pressure were somewhat difficult to get used to, but because he understood its importance to his health, he was willing to make it work. Michael had a successful PAP titration study and was eventually set up with CPAP at home. He uses it every night, and now sleeps soundly.

Patient Education

A vital aspect of the sleep study process is educating patients. Patients who know more about their sleep disorder, the potential consequences, and the various treatment options are more likely to schedule a sleep study, complete the sleep study, and comply with therapy. There are numerous opportunities to provide patient education, including at the physician's office during the consult or follow-up appointments, during the sleep study, through the sleep lab's website, and when the durable medical equipment (DME) company sets the patient up with the PAP therapy.

Although improved public awareness has helped to increase the number of patients treated for sleep apnea and other disorders, many remain untreated. Some refuse treatment despite being diagnosed with a sleep disorder. Sleep technicians and technologists have the opportunity to help prevent this by educating those they see in the sleep lab. It is important to discuss topics such as healthy sleep habits, relevant sleep disorders, and the importance of complying with therapy. In providing education to patients, it should be done in a manner approved by the medical director and should not include providing a diagnosis before the patient has received this from his or her physician.

Patient education and support groups such as **AWAKE**[9]—Alert, Well, and Keeping Energetic—help patients on PAP learn more about sleep apnea, the use of PAP therapy, and its effectiveness in treating sleep apnea. It also offers a form of support in navigating the equipment, supplies, and any issues new patients face. The AWAKE network of sleep apnea support groups was founded in 1988 by the American Sleep Apnea Association. Hundreds of AWAKE groups have been formed all over the United States to help people with sleep apnea. Guest speakers are often invited to come and teach participants about the latest innovations in sleep apnea treatment, weight loss, or similar topics.

The **National Sleep Foundation (NSF)**[10] is a worldwide leader in sleep-disorder education for patients and members of the public. Operating primarily from grants, sponsorships, memberships, and other contributions, the NSF provides extensive information to the public regarding sleep and its importance to all aspects of health and wellness. The NSF produces patient-focused informative brochures about sleep apnea, PAP therapy, narcolepsy, and many other sleep-related topics. Many physicians and sleep labs use these resources to educate patients. Other sleep organizations and sleep labs produce informative brochures, flyers, and pamphlets to increase public awareness of sleep and sleep disorders.

The Scoring and Interpretation Process

When a sleep study has been concluded, the data collected are archived in a manner directed by the lab and prepared for the scoring process. The scoring technologist—who is often an RPSGT or an RST—carefully reviews the sleep study epoch by epoch. With a typical sleep study lasting a minimum of 720 epochs (6 hours), the scoring process can be time consuming. Each 30-second epoch is assigned a stage of sleep and significant events are marked. Events commonly seen in sleep studies include snores, leg movements, electroencephalogram arousals, apneas, hypopneas, and others. The scorer reads through the patient questionnaires, histories, and notes from the consult and the sleep study to get to know the patient better. A detailed report is generated that compiles all of the staging and significant events. The technologist also includes a brief subjective assessment of the study and patient to help the interpreting physician.

The interpreting physician reviews the raw data and the reports generated by the scorer. The physician thoroughly reviews all patient charts, histories, questionnaires, and notes made by the recording technician and scoring technologist. The physician will then write a detailed interpretation of the sleep study based on all of this information. Although both the structure and content of the interpretation can vary greatly from one physician to the next, the core of a sleep study interpretation includes specific findings and recommendations dictated by the AASM.

At the follow-up appointment, the physician reviews the findings of the sleep study and discusses recommendations with the patient. Following a diagnostic polysomnography that is positive for sleep-disordered breathing, the physician will often recommend a second study with a PAP titration. For those patients diagnosed with other sleep disorders, PAP therapy will not be indicated. Instead, patients may be referred for additional sleep testing such as an MSLT, an MWT, or actigraphy testing or be initiated on a treatment plan.

Second Night Studies

In the case of a patient with a sleep-related breathing disorder, a new referral is sent to the sleep lab, and the process for scheduling and completing a sleep study is repeated. In some cases, the referring physician may initially send a diagnose-and-treat referral, which is sufficient for both the diagnostic and therapeutic sleep studies given certain parameters.

During the PAP titration, the patient arrives at the lab and is hooked up with the same wires and electrodes as during the first study, with the addition of a PAP mask. The technologist often has the responsibility of being the first to introduce PAP to the patient. This often begins with educating the patient on the benefits, potential side effects, and methods to counteract the side effects of PAP therapy. The lab should have a variety of mask types and sizes available for the patient to try, and the technologist should be knowledgeable enough to choose an appropriate mask for the patient. Having a positive first-time experience can greatly improve the patient's response to PAP therapy and will result in better treatment compliance and improved outcomes.

Before the study begins, the technologist should instruct the patient how to breathe with the positive pressure. Patients often have difficulty falling asleep the first time they use PAP therapy. The technologist should be sensitive to the needs of the patient during this time while helping the patient relax and breathe calmly and comfortably. Often a patient will need to sit up on the side of the bed with the lights on for several minutes before feeling comfortable lying down with the lights off. This desensitization process can help patients cope with the unfamiliarity of PAP. Patients with claustrophobia, sinus problems, or posttraumatic stress may have great difficulty with PAP.

Technologists should start the patient on a low, comfortable pressure, according to the lab's protocol, and encourage the patient as they acclimate to the therapy. They should also explain to the patient that they will periodically change the pressure during the night according to the patient's needs. As breathing

disturbances persist, the pressure will be increased to correct these disturbances. If the patient is unaware of these changes, he or she will likely awaken during the night confused and alarmed at the increased pressure. The patient should also be informed that the maximum pressure reached during the night of the study will not necessarily be the pressure recommended by the interpreting physician. A variety of pressures are needed during the titration to determine the most appropriate for each patient, which may include pressures above and below the optimal level for treatment. When the PAP titration is completed, the patient is discharged and the scoring and interpreting processes are repeated.

DME Setup

If the interpreting physician recommends home PAP therapy after reviewing a titration study, the order for PAP equipment is sent to a DME company. An order for PAP includes the recommended pressure and humidification, and it may or may not include the specific brand of mask or machine. The DME company that carries the PAP equipment contacts the patient, verifies the insurance for payment, and schedules a time to meet with the patient for setup. DME companies often meet with patients in their home, at the DME office, or in the sleep lab where the patient had his or her sleep studies. The DME representative brings a variety of masks and machines to find the most appropriate fit for the patient. Because of the many different mask types and styles, finding the best fit for each patient can be tricky. The following are among the most common mask styles. Because of the wide variety of masks and frequent innovations, specific brands and models of masks will not be discussed here.

Nasal Masks

As the name suggests, a **nasal mask** covers only the nose. These masks fit from the bridge of the nose down to just above the upper lip and just beyond the outside of each nare (see **Figure 3-4**). Traditionally, nasal

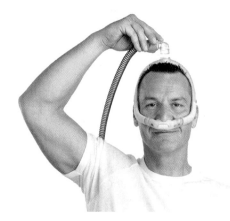

FIGURE 3-4 Nasal PAP masks cover only the nose.
Courtesy of ResMed.

masks have been the most commonly used type of PAP mask. Most patients find this style of mask to be comfortable and to provide an appropriate seal, as long as it properly fits.

Many patients with OSA breathe through their mouth while untreated but are able to keep their mouth closed during sleep while on PAP. When they are unable to keep their mouth closed, a nasal mask with a **chin strap** may be appropriate. Chin straps are placed under the chin and reach above the head to help keep the mouth closed.

Full Face Masks

Many patients who are unable to keep their mouth closed while on PAP therapy may require the use of a **full face mask**. A full face mask covers both the nose and mouth (see **Figure 3-5**). These are typically large, bulky masks that are used as a second or third option. Although uncomfortable for many patients, these masks are critical for some. Patients who have difficulty breathing through their nose because of congestion, a deviated septum, or other problems often prefer full face masks. Patients who require high PAP settings often have difficulty keeping their mouth closed during treatment and may perform better with a full face mask.

Nasal Pillows

A modification of the nasal mask is the **nasal pillow**. Nasal pillows rest on the end of the nose and have two soft conelike pieces that rest just inside or on the end of each nare (see **Figure 3-6**).

Nasal pillows have become popular in the past several years because they are small, lightweight, and comfortable. Occasionally, nasal pillows may cause mild discomfort inside or on the ends of the nares. Technologists and clinicians have expressed concern over a nasal pillow mask's ability to provide a proper seal, particularly at higher pressures. However, studies have

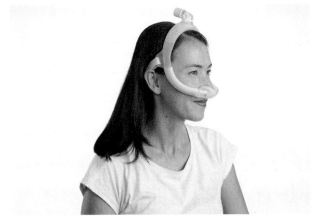

FIGURE 3-6 Nasal pillows rest on the end of the nose.
Courtesy of ResMed.

shown that nasal pillows produce similar air leakage to nasal masks.

Oral Masks

Oral masks cater to patients who are purely mouth breathers and who may not have been successful with the full face mask. An oral mask fits on the mouth and is usually held in place by a small device that reaches under the tongue (see **Figure 3-7**).

Other Mask Types

New technologies in PAP masks are consistently being released in an effort to improve compliance and make PAP treatment more comfortable and tolerable. Some examples of some less commonly used interfaces include the **hybrid mask**, which is an oral mask with a nasal pillow (see **Figure 3-8**). This interface aims to provide a more comfortable and less bulky solution to the full face mask. Other masks cover the entire face, providing a solution for many claustrophobic patients who prefer not to have a mask directly over their nose.

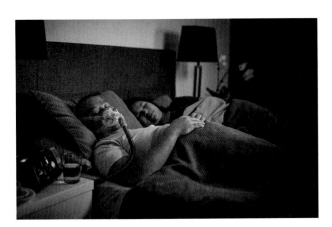

FIGURE 3-5 Full face masks cover the nose and mouth.
Courtesy of ResMed.

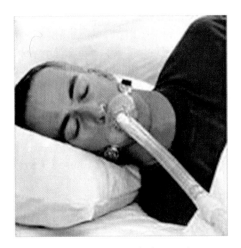

FIGURE 3-7 Oral PAP masks cover only the mouth.

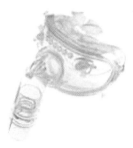

FIGURE 3-8 The hybrid mask.

PAP Machines

In addition to masks, patients also have many different PAP units from which to choose. PAP machine manufacturers such as **Respironics**,[11] **Resmed**,[12] **Fisher & Paykel**,[13] and others, are constantly working to improve capabilities to help patients tolerate and respond better to treatment. PAP units have progressively gotten smaller, sleeker, and quieter in an effort to integrate well into the bedroom environment. Advances in technology such as expiratory pressure relief, heated humidification, and mask fit feedback capabilities have also helped alleviate some of the common patient complaints of therapy. Whatever the specific needs of the patient, it is important that the physician, along with the DME representative, understand how to meet these needs with the technology available. Doing so can greatly increase the likelihood the patient will comply with treatment.

Patient Follow-Up

An important aspect of the patient flow process that should never be overlooked is patient follow-up. After patients are diagnosed and initial treatment begins, they should be followed periodically to address issues that develop and encourage good compliance. Unfortunately, compliance to therapy is generally low, especially in the case of PAP therapy. Many patients who start treatment do not stick to it. To address this issue, patients using PAP therapy should receive phone calls at regular intervals to check in, confirm that they are still complying with therapy, and to help them through any problems that they have encountered. A follow-up sleepiness assessment is a great tool to use to confirm symptomatic improvements with the use of therapy.

Improved technologies in PAP machines now allow access to usage information to add to the discussion at the patient follow-up. Units are able to connect to the patient's wireless internet and transmit compliance data to the DME company or physician. These data may include time spent on the device per night, weekly patterns of usage, and residual respiratory and arousal events. This information is often discussed at the follow-up appointment to address residual issues, set future usage goals, and achieve full compliance with therapy.

Over time, a patient's PAP pressure requirements may change. Some factors that may be responsible include weight gain, weight loss, and aging. For this reason, once patients are consistent in their usage of therapy, they should be instructed to schedule a follow-up at least once a year and contact their physicians sooner should any symptoms return.

Finally, wear and tear of the masks or interfaces, headgear, tubing, and so on occur and may create problems with usage. Therefore, patients should be informed of their eligibility for replacement equipment as needed.

Chapter Summary

Sleep disorders can greatly impair an individual's livelihood and ability to function during normal daytime activities, and they can be detrimental to overall health. Many people living with a sleep disorder do not even know they have one. It is important for physicians to take the time to screen their patients for sleep disorders to assist in identifying those who are effected. Using screening tools such as the Epworth Sleepiness Scale, the Berlin Questionnaire, or the Pittsburgh Sleep Quality Index, can provide greater insight into a patient's sleep habits and whether or not a sleep consultation or study is appropriate.

The process of diagnosing and treating patients with sleep disorders begins with physician screening and referral. When deciding on a sleep lab, the patient and physician should consider lab accreditation, the physical appearance of the lab, the location, the qualifications and friendliness of the staff, the turnaround time, the security of the lab, and the patient-to-technician ratio. After the referral is received by the lab, the lab contacts the patient to get him or her scheduled and to verify the patient's insurance. The scheduler should ensure the patient is aware of how to get to the lab, what to bring, and what to expect during the consultation or study. A confirmation call can help ensure that the patient arrives on time.

The consultation appointment is an opportunity for the sleep specialist to learn about the patient's sleep habits and the sleep issues he or she is experiencing. The physician will evaluate the patient's signs and symptoms, do a brief physical exam, any consider all of the patient's risk factors. If necessary, further testing may be indicated and ordered. Alternatively, diagnosis and treatment options will be discussed.

In the case that overnight sleep testing is indicated, the technician should always greet the patient with a smile, introduce him- or herself, and ask the patient for two identifiers. After completing medical history questionnaires and changing into pajamas, the patient will be hooked up to the equipment. During the setup, the technician should inform the patient of the purpose of each wire and what to expect during the study. In addition, this time is a good opportunity to provide patient education on proper sleep habits and relevant sleep disorders. The patient should be made to feel comfortable during the overnight testing with the goal of recording a quality study that is close to the patient's typical night sleep.

After the study is completed, it is reviewed in detail by a scoring technologist and an interpreting physician. Reports are generated, including the final interpretation, which includes findings from the study and recommendations for treatment. If OSA is diagnosed, the interpreting physician often recommends a second overnight study with a PAP titration. The process is repeated and an optimal PAP level is determined.

If home PAP is indicated by the physician, an order is sent to the DME company and the patient is set up at home with the appropriate PAP equipment. Because of the wide variety of facial features and the specific needs of patients, equipment manufacturers have developed a multitude of PAP masks, machines, and devices. DME companies must have knowledgeable staff and a surplus of this equipment available to ensure the treatment is as effective as possible. Choosing the wrong mask for a patient can greatly decrease the likelihood that he or she will comply with treatment.

After the patient is set up at home with the proper equipment, a detailed follow-up process should be practiced to ensure the patient continues with treatment, is aware of new technologies and treatment options, and is notified when a re-titration may be needed.

Chapter 3 Questions

Please consider the following questions as they relate to the material in this chapter.

1. How is BMI calculated? If a patient is 5′11″ tall and weighs 180 pounds, what is his BMI?
2. What are some advantages and disadvantages to using the Epworth Sleepiness Scale? The Berlin Questionnaire?
3. What are some points to consider when choosing a sleep lab to refer patients to?
4. What should a scheduler discuss with the patient when scheduling a sleep study? What should not be discussed?
5. When building a lab, why might it be important to choose a nice carpet and large beds over laminate flooring and hospital beds? How can a lab with a homelike feel help when performing a sleep study?
6. Why is it important to educate patients throughout the sleep study process?
7. What are some of the latest technologies in PAP masks?
8. When might it be appropriate to use a full face mask on a patient?
9. Why is it important to follow up with patients after they have been set up on PAP therapy?

Footnotes

1. Centers for Disease Control and Prevention. (2017). Healthy weight: About adult BMI. Accessed from https://www.cdc.gov/healthyweight/assessing/bmi/adult_bmi/index.html
2. Johns, M. (1991). The Epworth Sleepiness Scale. Accessed from http://epworthsleepinessscale.com/
3. Netzer, N. C., Stoohs, R. A., Netzer, C. M., Clark, K., & Strohl, K. P. (1999). Using the Berlin Questionnaire to identify patients at risk for the sleep apnea syndrome. *Annals of Internal Medicine, 131*(7), 485–491.
4. Hoddes, E., Zarcone, V., Smythe, H., Phillips, R., & Dement, W. C. (1973). Quantification of sleepiness: A new approach. *Psychophysiology, 10*(4), 431–436.
5. Buysse, D. J., Reynolds III, C. F., Monk, T. H., Berman, S. R., & Kupfer, D. J. (1989). The Pittsburgh Sleep Quality Index: A new instrument for psychiatric practice and research. *Psychiatry Research, 28*(2), 193–213.
6. Board of Registered Polysomnographic Technologists. (2018). The RPSGT credential. Accessed from https://www.brpt.org/rpsgt/
7. American Board of Sleep Medicine. (2018). RST certification. Accessed from https://absm.org/rst-certification/
8. Nuckton, T. J., Glidden, D. V., Browner, W. S., & Claman, D. M. (2006). Physical examination: Mallampati score as an independent predictor of obstructive sleep apnea. *Sleep, 29*(7), 903–908.
9. American Sleep Apnea Association. (2017). A.W.A.K.E. Accessed at https://www.sleepapnea.org/community/all-about-awake/
10. National Sleep Foundation. (2018). Accessed from https://www.sleepfoundation.org/
11. Philips Respironics. (2018). Sleep therapy solutions. Accessed from https://www.usa.philips.com/healthcare/solutions/sleep
12. Resmed. (2018). Sleep apnea treatment options. Accessed from https://www.resmed.com/us/en/consumer/diagnosis-and-treatment/what-is-sleep-apnea/sleep-apnea-treatment.html
13. Fisher & Paykel Healthcare. (2018). Sleep apnea. Accessed from https://www.fphcare.com/us/homecare/sleep-apnea/

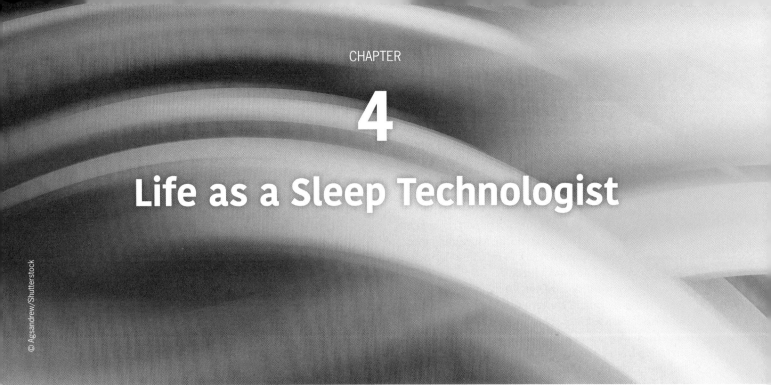

4

Life as a Sleep Technologist

© Agsandrew/Shutterstock

CHAPTER OUTLINE

Shift Work
Responsibilities as a Healthcare Worker
Professional Training and Credentialing
Chapter Summary

LEARNING OBJECTIVES

1. Learn the impact of shift work and methods to effectively work night shifts.
2. Understand the responsibilities of a healthcare professional.
3. Learn strategies to prevent the spread of infection in the sleep lab environment.
4. Understand the importance of protocols for responding to patient adverse medical events and other emergencies.
5. Discuss professionalism and its ethical principles.
6. Increase quality in the lab.
7. Learn techniques to help pass the sleep technologist board examination.

KEY TERMS

shift work
night shift
graveyard shift
International Agency for
    Research on Cancer
material safety data
    sheet (MSDS)
disaster plan
infection control
universal precautions
Control III
Occupational Safety and
    Health Administration
    (OSHA)
cleaning log
patient confidentiality
Health Insurance Portability
    and Accountability
    Act of 1996 (HIPAA)
quality assurance

interscorer reliability
School of Sleep Medicine
Accredited Sleep
    Technologist
    Education Program
Board of Registered
    Polysomnographic
    Technologists (BRPT)
Registered
    Polysomnographic
    Technologist (RPSGT)
Registered Sleep
    Technologist (RST)
Sleep Disorders Testing
    and Therapeutic
    Intervention credential
American Association of
    Sleep Technologists
continuing education
    unit (CEU)

Shift Work

The term **shift work** is used to describe work hours that occur on a schedule outside of the traditional 9 A.M. to 5 P.M. day. It can include early morning, evening, or overnight hours or a combination of these in rotating shifts. According to the National Health Interview Survey, 28% of all U.S. workers in 2010 worked a shift other than a regular day shift.[1] More recent data from 2015 show similar statistics.[2]

The 24-hour lifestyle has grown in popularity and has become somewhat of a societal norm. More and more businesses are beginning to cater to this lifestyle, including the fast-food industry and retail.

Healthcare workers have long been assigned to shift work. This is a primary concern for many sleep technologists, because a large majority of sleep studies are performed at night. Sleep technologists typically work anywhere from 10- to 12-hour shifts during the night. Unfortunately, in an effort to stay awake during the shift, many develop poor sleep and nutrition habits. For example, the tendency is to eat fatty or sugary foods and to drink caffeinated beverages and energy drinks throughout the night in attempts to stay alert. These habits, and shift work in general, can have profoundly negative consequences to one's health. Working a **night shift**, also known as a **graveyard shift**, is suspected of increasing the likelihood of cancer and ischemic heart disease. In 2007, the **International Agency for Research on Cancer** listed night work as a "probable cause" of cancer.[3] Because healthy sleep habits are difficult to maintain while working outside of the traditional 9 A.M.–5 P.M. hours, many shift workers suffer from insomnia, excessive daytime sleepiness (EDS), impaired alertness and cognition, and difficulty maintaining wakefulness during work. Drowsiness in a healthcare worker is a risk to both the individual and his or her patients. It can pose dangers that include patient care errors, poor judgment, delayed reaction, and even drowsy driving on the ride home from a work shift. Therefore, it is important to pay careful attention to signs of sleepiness, such as blinking, yawning, dry or tired eyes, nodding off, and so on. These signs should alert you to get up, walk around, drink some water, and take a break. To improve sleep and wakefulness in shift workers, the National Sleep Foundation recommends the following[4]:

1. Bedtime rituals:
   a. Take a warm bath.
   b. Lower the room temperature. Cool environments are associated with better sleep quality.
   c. Avoid prebedtime tasks such as balancing the checkbook or reading an exciting novel that would make it more difficult to fall asleep.
2. Light:
   a. Darken the bedroom and bathroom.
   b. Install light-blocking and sound-absorbing curtains or shades.
   c. Wear eyeshades.
3. Sound:
   a. Wear earplugs.
   b. Use a white noise maker or fan.
   c. Install carpeting and drapes to block out noise.
   d. Unplug the telephone.
4. Food:
   a. Avoid caffeine for at least 5 hours before bedtime.
   b. Do not drink alcohol before bedtime.
5. Exercise:
   a. Do not exercise heavily within 3 hours of bedtime.
6. Sleep schedule:
   a. Avoid long naps, even on weekends.
   b. Taking short naps (20 minutes) can be especially helpful.
   c. Try to maintain a consistent sleep schedule, even on days or nights when not working.
7. Driving home:
   a. Loud music and windows down do not help a person stay awake while driving. Doing these things are signals that you are sleepy, and you should pull over and rest for a few minutes.
   b. Taking a short nap at work at the end of your shift may help you stay awake while driving home.
   c. If driving home in the morning, wear dark sunglasses. Overexposure to light after working a night shift can damage your eyes and make it more difficult to fall asleep.
   d. Carpool or use public transportation when possible.
8. Staying alert at work:
   a. Take short breaks throughout the shift.
   b. Talk with coworkers when possible. Conversations with coworkers can help you stay awake and alert.
   c. Use breaks to get away from the desk or computer; go outside, exercise, walk, climb the stairs, or the like.
   d. Eat three normal, healthy meals. Avoid fatty foods that may make you tired or upset your stomach.
   e. Caffeine consumption should be kept to a minimum; consume only during the first part of the shift.
   f. Do not leave the most tedious or boring tasks for the end of the shift when you are most likely to be tired.
   g. Night shift workers hit their lowest point of alertness at 4 A.M., so plan breaks at that time.
   h. Turn on all the lights in your work area. Encourage your employer to install bright lights.

These strategies can help improve performance in the workplace, ensure a better quality of life, and reduce the risk of health complications associated with shift work.

Responsibilities as a Healthcare Worker

Healthcare workers are responsible for the well-being of their patients. Sleep technologists are often exclusively responsible for their patients during the overnight sleep study. As such, it is important for sleep technologists to reduce risks to their patients and be prepared to act should dangerous situations occur. In addition, as healthcare professionals, sleep technologists are expected to abide by certain standards of professionalism. The next sections of this chapter will provide details on these important responsibilities.

Patient Safety

Maintaining patient safety in the sleep lab environment is best achieved through the use of facility protocols. Facility protocols help to maintain safe practices to reduce the risk of preventable harm. They also help to prepare a healthcare professional for action when there is a risk by offering guidance on what actions to take. Some of the most commonly addressed safety measures in the sleep lab environment are presented in the following sections.

Electrical Safety

There are several concerns with electrical safety in the sleep lab. Sleep technologists use a variety of electrical devices and equipment to diagnose and treat sleep disorders in the lab. All of these present potential dangers to the patient if not used appropriately. Equipment such as continuous positive airway pressure machines, differential amplifiers, and other ancillary equipment should be properly grounded to the building's main electrical ground and should always be used according to the manufacturer's specifications. Technologists should check all electrical cables to ensure there are no exposed, bare, or frayed wires. If damaged wires are noted, they should be taken out of use and replaced. All electrical outlets and switches should be installed and inspected according to building code and have proper covers on them. Medical equipment should be inspected for safety by a professional electrician at least once a year. All electrodes and wires should be checked frequently to ensure they are in good condition.

Chemical Safety

All chemicals in the sleep lab must have a **material safety data sheet (MSDS)** available. This important resource contains detailed information on the chemical properties, warnings, safety precautions, and exposure information of a substance and are typically kept in a binder or a digital location that is accessible to the staff. Products frequently used in the sleep lab environment that require an MSDS include collodion, electroencephalogram (EEG) paste, prepping solutions and gels, alcohol, and cleaners.

Falls

Precautions should be taken in the sleep lab to identify situations that can increase the risk of falls. Specifically, technologists should assist older patients and those who have difficulty walking. In addition, the lab environment should be designed so that few obstructions stand in common walkway areas. Plants or decorative items on the floors in hallways and bedrooms are cautioned against. Because patients may need to use the bathroom during the night, lighting should be in place to illuminate the way. Finally, when appropriate, bed rails should be used to help prevent at-risk patients from falling out of bed. This is of particular importance when testing pediatric patients. Some sleep centers will perform a *falls assessment* before performing a sleep study to determine risk and make appropriate accommodations for the patient.

Disaster Planning

Every sleep lab should have written emergency protocols and a **disaster plan** in place for loss of power, fires, tornadoes, hurricanes, floods, bomb threats, explosions, gas leaks, and other potential emergent situations. The plans should make clear how to announce the emergency, who is responsible for responding, and procedures for technologists to follow to ensure the safety of patients. All employees should be knowledgeable about the facility's emergency protocols, including where emergency equipment is stored and how to use it (for example, fire extinguishers). In addition, technologists should actively participate in practice drills and trainings on a periodic basis. A list of emergency numbers such as poison control, police, and fire should be posted and clearly visible. When they arrive at the sleep lab, patients should be shown all emergency exits and pathways for evacuation in case of a crisis.

Patient Medical Events

Sleep technologists must be properly trained and prepared to respond to various patient medical events, including cardiac arrest. Other examples of patient medical emergencies include severe breathing difficulties, prolonged seizure activity, and symptomatic cardiac arrhythmias. Training and certification in basic life support and cardiopulmonary resuscitation is a critical part of this preparation. Additional training in cardiac rhythm recognition is also extremely important to help recognize a patient whose status is deteriorating. Sleep-testing facilities should have clear and specific protocols in place for each of these medical emergencies. Like disaster preparedness, these written protocols should outline the role of the sleep technologist, including how to announce the emergency, who will be responding to assist, and the procedures for the technologist to follow to ensure the safety of the patient. Technologists and all clinical staff who would be involved should be well versed in the policies, know where the emergency equipment is stored, and understand how to use it (e.g., defibrillator, code cart). Further, management should ensure that all clinical staff participate in emergency drills and successfully complete competency assessments or certifications on a periodic basis where applicable.

Note that medical emergency protocols will differ greatly between hospital-based sleep centers and private sleep-testing facilities. Sleep centers housed within a hospital or medical center have access to vital resources in responding to a patient medical event. These include having immediate access to hospital physicians, nurses, other clinical staff, and medical equipment for diagnosing and addressing the condition. In contrast, private sleep centers have to rely on local first responders through 911 emergency calls. This can add a great deal of responsibility on the sleep technologist who may be the only clinician on site during the testing. In this case, the sleep technologist may be faced with delivering lifesaving care over an extended period of time until first responders arrive. This emphasizes the importance of certification and competence in basic life support, use of a defibrillator, and cardiopulmonary resuscitation.

Infection Control

Infection control refers to a set of guidelines and principles used to help prevent the spread of disease. Infection control is of particular importance in the healthcare industry, where direct contact between employee and patient are frequent, and exposure to blood, saliva, or other bodily fluids may occur. Sleep technologists are not typically at risk of infection as much as other clinicians who take blood samples, give injections, and the like. However, it is important for sleep technologists to be aware of the dangers of exposure and to practice **universal precautions**. Universal precautions refers to the practice of avoiding contact with patients' bodily fluids by wearing gloves, and goggles or face shields when appropriate.

Hand Washing

A sleep study set-up includes the application of electrodes to the scalp, face, and body of the patient. As a result, sleep technologists have a great deal of contact with their patients through their hands. To avoid the spread of infection, sleep technologists should wash their hands with an antibiotic soap before and after contact with each patient.

Gloves

Technologists should wear nonlatex gloves when working with patients. This protects both the patient and the technologist from exposure to pathogens. Gloves should fit comfortably and be changed for each patient.

Disposable Equipment

Disposable equipment should be used when possible to prevent the spread of disease from patient to patient. Airflow sensors placed directly under a patient's nose are subject to droplet exposure, which can spread to the next patient if not properly cleaned. Disposable airflow sensors can decrease the risk of this occurring.

Equipment Cleaning

All nondisposable equipment should be thoroughly and properly cleaned after each use. Hospital based sleep labs have the ability to use the central sterilization department for assistance with equipment cleaning. Most private sleep-testing facilities will use disinfectants such as **Control III** to clean wires, electrodes, equipment, and surfaces. Nondisposable sensors, such as respiratory effort belts or pulse oximeter sensors that cannot be submersed in liquid, should be cleaned with a disinfectant wipe or according to the manufacturer's recommendations.

Linen Cleaning and Storage

According to accreditation standards, all sleep labs should have separate storage for clean and soiled linens. The soiled linen area should be closed off and separate from the areas containing clean equipment and linens. When laundering linens, facilities should be sure to follow **Occupational Safety and Health Administration (OSHA)** standards.

Lab Cleaning

The sleep lab environment and the patient testing rooms should be kept clean at all times. The responsibility of cleaning the patient rooms will vary depending on whether the facility is hospital based or privately owned. Often, hospital-based centers rely on their internal housekeeping department to complete this task, whereas private facilities frequently place the responsibility on the sleep technologist. Whichever the case, lab surfaces and floors should be cleaned with a disinfectant cleaner, furniture and fixtures should be dusted regularly, and items left behind by patients such as pillows should be removed. A **cleaning log** should be used to document each time the lab and equipment are cleaned and what cleaning agents were used.

Case Study

A 40-year-old female patient arrives at a dimly lit sleep lab for her study. She was unsure if this was the location where she was supposed to report. She was the only person in the small room past the entrance. Eventually, a young man appearing untidy and poorly groomed introduced himself as the sleep technologist. He shows the patient her room and, as he leaves the room, instructs her to change into her pajamas. The patient notices a camera in the room and begins to worry that the technologist might be watching her change from the monitoring station.

How could this initial patient interaction be improved? How could this patient be made to feel more comfortable?

This initial patient interaction could have been improved in the following ways:

1. The sleep lab environment could be made to appear more inviting (better lighting, better signage, more welcoming atmosphere, etc.).

2. To make the female patient feel more comfortable, the supervisor could have ensured that she was not left alone in the lab with a male technologist.

3. The technologist could have presented himself in a more professional manner in several ways. First, he should have introduced himself with his name and with a friendlier, more welcoming demeanor. Next, the technologist's untidy appearance is not particularly comforting to a patient who is trusting him to care for her. Professional attire and grooming is an important part of acting professionally, and he should have spent more time on his appearance before reporting to work.

4. The technologist could have pointed out the camera to the patient on her arrival to the bedroom and suggested she change in the restroom.

Professionalism

Healthcare professionals are expected to conduct themselves in a professional manner and abide by a high standard of ethical principle.[5] As such, sleep technologists should treat all patients with kindness, respect, and empathy. They are expected to advocate for quality care and support positive health outcomes for their patients. As part of the healthcare team, sleep professionals should work collaboratively with other clinicians and perform their duties with honesty, integrity, and accountability. In addition, acting in a professional manner includes dressing in appropriate attire and according to their facility's protocol. This typically includes donning scrubs and a white lab coat if in a clinical or entry-level role, or business attire if in a managerial role. Acting in a professional manner can greatly increase a patient's comfort level and confidence that his or her care and the testing is being performed by a knowledgeable and trusted professional.

Patient Confidentiality

When patients seek medical care, they share private health information so that physicians can appropriately diagnose and treat them. In doing so, the expectation is that the information will remain confidential and only be shared with the necessary people or entities involved in their care. **Patient confidentiality** refers to the right of an individual to have this personal medical information kept private. In 1996, the U.S. Department of Health and Human Services issued a privacy rule to protect the health information of consumers. This rule, called the **Health Insurance Portability and Accountability Act of 1996 (HIPAA)**, sets the standards for privacy and protection of patient records, and all healthcare workers in the United States are expected to comply fully. HIPAA laws instruct healthcare workers on appropriate use and protection of medical information. For example, a patient coming to the sleep lab for an overnight polysomnography may have human immunodeficiency virus. Although it may be helpful for the physician to know this information in order to provide adequate health care for the patient, this information is private and should not be shared. Another example is a delivery driver who does not want his boss to know about his obstructive sleep apnea because it might put his job in danger. Patient privacy guidelines also include not leaving a patient chart or form open and available in waiting areas, having conversations with patients using a quiet voice, and avoiding talking about the results of one patient's sleep study with another patient. These guidelines also include more complex practices such as the proper methods of storing and transferring electronic records.

HIPAA laws should be carefully researched by sleep technologists, lab managers, and all healthcare professionals. Failing to properly abide by patient privacy practices can result in lawsuits, fines, and arrests.

Quality Assurance

Sleep-testing facilities should have a system in place to ensure quality and improvements in quality for all processes. Scoring technologists are prime candidates to give feedback to sleep technicians regarding study quality, because they carefully review every epoch of data recorded. Scoring technologists can give subjective ratings of the quality of each signal, the titration, the notes, procedures, and patient questionnaires. In large facilities, this information can be entered into a database so trends can be followed, and appropriate training and quality-control techniques can be put into place.

Quality assurance can also be used to ensure consistency and accuracy of scoring by technologists. The digital polysomnogram now makes it easy to compare multiple score masks of the same study. Scorer A and Scorer B can score the same study, and their score sets can be compared in several ways. A commonly used standard is that if two scorers score 85% of the epochs of a sleep study the same, it is considered acceptable. This can vary according to lab protocol. The American Academy of Sleep Medicine (AASM) offers an online **interscorer reliability** program in which a scoring technologist can enter scoring information for a sample study. The answers are then graded against an established gold standard and a grade is given. A sleep facility can create an account and customize a minimum acceptable grade on the exam. The lab can then use these data as evidence of quality-improvement measures for scoring sleep studies when it applies or reapplies for accreditation. The scoring technologist can also use this information as evidence of scoring competency.

The AASM dictates that accredited centers collect four quality-control measures and report on them quarterly, every 6 months, and annually. Interscorer reliability, as previously discussed, must be one such measure. Other measures are left up to the manager of the facility and can include measures such as patient satisfaction, technical quality, or test result turnaround time. Administrative measures should also be put in place for processes such as scheduling, billing, and managing.

Professional Training and Credentialing

Historically, many sleep technicians were hired with no healthcare experience and were expected to perform sleep studies with little training. In these instances, there is the tendency for poor-quality sleep studies and lack of confidence in the results. More recently, steps have been taken to help ensure that sleep professionals are properly trained and that lab managers have plenty of available resources for training and continuing education.

In 1982, Mary Carskadon, William Dement, and Sharon Keenan developed the first formal training program for sleep technologists and physicians—the **School of Sleep Medicine**—at Stanford University. Since then, many other sleep-training programs have developed across the United States and around the world. Some of these are independent, some are affiliated with hospitals or sleep labs, and some exist as part of respiratory therapy or other programs at colleges and universities.

The American Academy of Sleep Medicine has become a great resource for various sleep training programs, including the **Accredited Sleep Technologist Education Program** and online training modules. These programs are useful for basic training and in helping technologists prepare for the national sleep credentialing examinations. The most common credentialing path is offered by the **Board of Registered Polysomnographic Technologists (BRPT)**. After meeting the requirements to sit for the BRPT examination and successfully passing it, the sleep technologist may use the **Registered Polysomnographic Technologist (RPSGT)** credential. The AASM has also developed the **Registered Sleep Technologist (RST)** credential for sleep technologists. The examination for the RST credential has eligibility requirements that include previous experience in the field. Finally, there is the **Sleep Disorders Testing and Therapeutic Intervention credential** offered by the National Board for Respiratory Care. This credential was designed specifically for respiratory therapists who chose to specialize in sleep diagnostics and therapeutics and is designated by the acronyms CRT-SDS or RRT-SDS.

Credentialing Exam Preparation

Credentialing exams are often a source of great stress and fear for many sleep technologists. The following list outlines helpful tips for preparing for the sleep technologist credentialing examinations:

- *Study frequently and consistently*. Good time management is critical for preparing for a board examination. It is important for candidates to develop a timeline for studying several months before the exam date and make every attempt to stick to it. Eligible candidates should map out frequent blocks of time to review content, take practice examinations, and review the results.
- *Study from a variety of sources*. Sleep technologists should use the many resources available to them through the national organizations and library resources. These can include online training modules, exam-prep resources, polysomnography textbooks, and books specific to EEG, electrocardiogram, or respiratory care. Sleep technologists who are well versed in these fields will be well prepared for the board exam. Technologists should also become familiar with medical

terminology and abbreviations as this information will be especially helpful in taking the exam.

- *Consider a visit to a sleep school.* Sleep schools and formal sleep-education programs are now available in most states and nearly every region of the country. Online sleep-training programs are becoming more prevalent now as well. These can be valuable resources in board exam preparation.
- *Practice working with the variety of technical equipment used for sleep testing.* Exposure and hands-on experience working with various technologies can greatly expand a technologist's skill set and improve his or her ability to identify and troubleshoot technical issues.
- *Take practice exams.* Practice examinations are available from various sources, including the national credentialing bodies, the **American Association of Sleep Technologists**, as well as other private companies that specialize in exam preparation. These can be valuable in preparing for the board exam. These are usually written in the same format as the board exam and can help technologists become accustomed to the style of questions asked in the exam. Taking these exams can also help technologists discover the areas in which they need further study. Practice examinations can be one of the most powerful tools for preparing a technologist for the board exam.
- *Do not cram.* Given the amount of knowledge and experience required to pass the sleep board exam, trying to cram for the test during the last few days or weeks before the exam is not likely to help.
- *Find a partner to study with.* Reviewing the material with a partner can be especially useful. Choose a partner who has a good study ethic and will challenge you. Have your partner pose short verbal quizzes to test your recollection. If possible, find a fellow sleep professional to help you review and understand challenging topics.
- *Use flash cards.* Flash cards and similar quick reference tools can be great visual study guides. Flash cards are available for purchase or can be made.

Test-Taking Tips

The following tips can help when taking the sleep board exam or any multiple-choice test:

- Read the question thoroughly before looking at the possible answers.
- Come up with the answer in your head before looking at the possible answers.
- Eliminate answers you know are incorrect.
- Read all choices before choosing your answer.
- If you do not know the answer, make the most educated guess possible and mark the answer.

Make a note for yourself to come back to this question if you have time at the end of the test.

- Do not keep changing your answer. Usually your first answer is correct unless you misread the question.
- Bring a watch to the test and pace yourself. Make sure you know ahead of time how many questions are on the exam and how long you have to take it. Allow yourself extra time at the end of the exam to review the questions you were unsure of.
- Keep a positive attitude and try to relax. If you feel stressed during the test, stop and take a few deep breaths or get up and take a break, get a drink of water, or the like.
- Eat before taking the test but avoid foods that will make you sleepy.
- Get a full night of sleep before the test. Try to keep the same sleep schedule for several nights before the exam to improve your chances of feeling rested and alert during the test.
- Go to the bathroom right before taking the exam so you do not waste time doing this during the test.

Continuing Education

All healthcare professionals are expected to engage in lifelong learning and seek out opportunities to continue to learn in their field. This expectation extends to sleep technologists. There are numerous ways to obtain a **continuing education unit (CEU)**. Sleep technologists can attend local, state, or national sleep conferences; participate in CEU approved in-services; or complete webinars offered by approved providers. Depending on the credential, the number of CEUs required per year will vary. However, in all cases, proof of continuing education (e.g., certificate of completion) will be requested to renew the credential.

Chapter Summary

Sleep technologists face a variety of challenges and opportunities. One main challenge is that of working nights. Shift work may increase the likelihood of several health problems and can cause EDS, insomnia, and poor work performance and concentration. Alertness while working nights can be improved by several techniques, including using bright lights, exercising, and avoiding caffeine.

As healthcare professionals, sleep technologists have a wide array of responsibilities. One of the most important is infection control. The spread of infection can be reduced by practicing universal precautions such as handwashing, wearing gloves, and properly cleaning equipment after each use.

Patient safety is another responsibility of sleep technologists. Part of this is reducing the risk of electrical shock by routinely inspecting equipment and electrical cables and cords. Furniture and decor should be placed in appropriate locations to reduce the patients' risk of falling. Each lab should also have its own written emergency management plans in place, including those for responding to various patient adverse medical events, electrical outages, and fire. Practice drills and annual competencies should be completed on a regular basis.

Sleep technologists are responsible for creating and maintaining a professional appearance and attitude. They are expected to dress and act in a professional manner and uphold the ethical principles of professional conduct.

Quality assurance involves selecting a set of measures that provide feedback on the quality of care. For sleep-testing facilities, this can include measures of interscorer reliability or technical quality of the sleep study. Quality-assurance processes are useful at reducing errors and increasing efficiency.

The field of polysomnography has grown rapidly over the past few decades. Sleep schools and training programs are available in nearly every region, and online training programs are available as well. In addition, there has been a trend toward standardizing educational programs to ensure a minimum competency.

After certain requirements have been met, sleep technologists have the opportunity to take a credentialing exam. Technologists can use several techniques to help them study, including using study groups, taking practice exams, and using a variety of study materials. Other techniques can improve performance, including getting a full night's sleep before the test, pacing oneself, and keeping a positive attitude.

Chapter 4 Questions

Please consider the following questions as they relate to the material in this chapter.

1. What negative impacts can shift work have on an employee? What are some ways to combat these effects?
2. How should linens be stored in the lab to reduce the spread of infection?
3. How often should electrical equipment in the lab be inspected? Why is this important?
4. How can a technologist's professional appearance and attitude impact a patient's treatment?
5. What quality-assurance measures should a sleep lab have in place?
6. What opportunities for training do sleep technologists have available to them?
7. What studying techniques are effective at improving success on the credentialing exams?

Footnotes

1. Centers for Disease Control and Prevention (CDC). (2011). National Health and Nutrition Examination Survey: 2009–2010 Documentation, Codebook, and Frequencies Occupation Questionnaire (OCQ_F). Accessed from http://www.cdc.gov/nchs/nhanes/nhanes
2. CDC. (2015). NHIS-Occupational Health Supplement (NHIS-OHS). Accessed from https://wwwn.cdc.gov/Niosh-whc/chart/ohs-workorg/work?OU=WORKSCHD_RCD&T=GE&V=R
3. International Agency for Research on Cancer. (2007). IARC monographs programme finds cancer hazards associated with shiftwork, painting, and firefighting. Lyon, France: World Health Organization.
4. National Sleep Foundation. (2019). Shift work and sleep. Accessed from https://www.sleepfoundation.org/articles/shift-work-and-sleep
5. National Association for Healthcare Quality. (n.d.). NAHQ Code of Ethics for Healthcare Quality Professionals and Code of Conduct. Accessed from https://nahq.org/about/code-of-ethics.

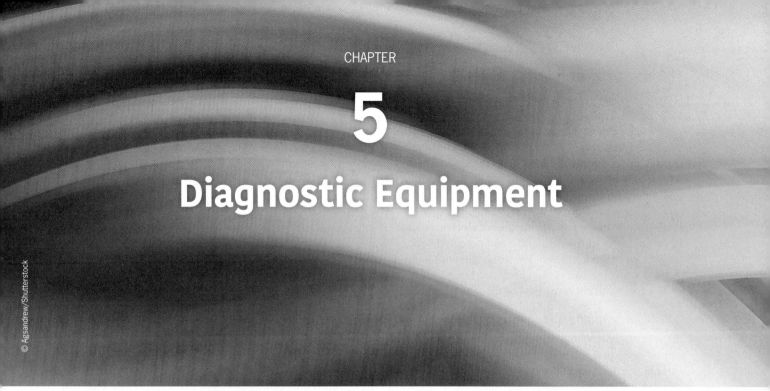

CHAPTER

5

Diagnostic Equipment

© Agsandrew/Shutterstock

CHAPTER OUTLINE

Basics of Electricity
Signal Pathways
Monitoring Devices
Differential Amplifiers
Electrical Grounding
Digital Polysomnography
Chapter Summary

LEARNING OBJECTIVES

1. Learn the basic concepts of electricity.
2. Understand the differences among voltage, current, and resistance.
3. Be able to identify unsafe electrical conditions.
4. Understand the pathway of signals from the patient to diagnostic equipment.
5. Learn about monitoring devices used in polysomnography.
6. Understand how differential amplifiers work.
7. Understand how electrical grounding occurs.
8. Discuss the impacts of digital polysomnography.

KEY TERMS

current
voltage
resistance
impedance
transmembrane potential
polarity
common mode rejection
common mode rejection
  ratio (CMRR)
snap electrode
cup electrode
snore microphone
snore sensor
oximeter
oxyhemoglobin
deoxyhemoglobin
arterial blood gas
body position sensor
thermal airflow sensors
apneic events
thermocouple
thermistor
polyvinylidene fluoride
  (PVDF) airflow sensors
pressure transducer
pneumotachography
hypopneic events

respiratory effort–
  related arousals
capnography
capnograph
capnogram
transcutaneous CO_2 monitor
esophageal balloon catheter
esophageal manometry
pleural pressure
respiratory inductive
  plethysmography (RIP)
pH probe
actigraphy
motion detector
differential amplifier
frequency response curve
ground
ground loop
international 10/20 electrode
  placement system
monopolar or referential
  recording montage
bipolar recording montage
automatic scoring
digital polysomnography
analogue polysomnography
sampling rate

Basics of Electricity

Sleep technologists work with various types of electronic equipment for diagnostic and therapeutic purposes. They can experience problems in the lab such as power failures, frayed cabling, and equipment malfunctions. Understanding the basic principles of electricity not only helps the sleep technologist troubleshoot equipment problems but also helps keep the patient and technologist safe from electrical harm. This chapter will discuss some of the basic principles of electricity and how they apply to the diagnostic equipment, devices, and sensors used in the lab. We will begin with a few basic electrical terms.

Electrical **current** is the flow or movement of an electrical charge. Just as the current of a river refers to movement of its water, electrical current refers to movement of electricity. In electric shock, it is the current that causes harm to the subject. Results from electric shock can range from a small tingling feeling to cardiac arrest and death. Current is measured in amperes, or amps. The flow of biologic potentials is usually measured in microamps (μA), or millionths of an amp. Ohm's law states that the current (I) equals the voltage (V) divided by the resistance (R). Therefore, the mathematical formula for current is:

$$I = V/R$$

Ohm's law can be used to predict the effect that changes in voltage or resistance can have on current. For example, as voltage increases and resistance decreases, current increases. An increased current results in greater effects from electrical shock. The flow of electricity will always follow the path of least resistance. This grounding effect will be discussed later in this section.

Voltage, or electrical tension, refers to the difference in electrical potential between two points. Voltage is measured in volts, although biologic potentials are usually measured in microvolts (μV), or millionths of a volt. The word *potential* is key when discussing voltage. A point has a certain electrical potential based on the potential of its reference point. However, it may not reach that potential because of electrical resistance to the current or flow. Using Ohm's law, voltage can be determined using the following equation:

$$V = IR$$

As mentioned previously, a higher voltage presents an increased risk for the user of the equipment. Diagnostic equipment should be checked regularly by an electrician for safety of use. It should also be marked as either extra low voltage, low voltage, high voltage, or extra high voltage. Equipment with high or extra high voltages present the danger of electric shock, and are labeled with the international safety symbol shown in Figure 5-1.

FIGURE 5-1 The international safety symbol.
© Aleksandrs Bondars/Shutterstock.

Electrical **resistance** refers to the degree to which an object opposes or resists electrical current. Resistance is measured in ohms and is calculated using Ohm's law:

$$R = V/I$$

According to Ohm's law, increased resistance under conditions of constant voltage will result in a decreased current. Conversely, decreased resistance under conditions of constant voltage will result in an increased current. Sometimes electrical resistance is desired, while other times it is intentionally minimized. For example, when cutting or splicing an electrical cord, an electrician will take precautions such as wearing rubber gloves to increase resistance to the flow of electricity (decrease the current) through his or her body. In polysomnography, we try to minimize electrical resistance in order to increase the current of certain biologic potentials from the brain, eyes, muscles, and other parts of the body. The term **impedance** is used to refer to electrical resistance in bioelectric signals. As the resistance, or impedance, increases in the pathway from the patient to the diagnostic equipment, the signal quality decreases, and it becomes more difficult to determine various waveforms derived from the patient.

Electrical resistance has a variety of sources. In polysomnography, electrical resistance is often caused by debris or hair on the skin, insufficient conductive solution between the skin and electrode, a fray in the housing of a lead wire or cable, or a poor connection between the lead wires, the head box, or the cabling to the polysomnograph.

Physiological electrical activity is based on the concentration and flow of ions across the cell membrane. The **transmembrane potential** is based on the concentration of ionic charges inside the cell compared with charges outside the cell. The transmembrane potential of a resting neuron is 60–80 mV (millivolts), and the interior of the cell is negative with respect to the exterior.

In polysomnography, the term **polarity** refers to the positive or negative nature of an electrical signal. In this case, the terms *positive* and *negative* are relative. An electrical potential by itself cannot be negative until it is compared to another potential that is greater. One electrical input from the differential amplifier is characterized as either positive or negative with respect to the other input and is based on the concentration and flow of ionic charges. In other words, if the potential at point A is greater than the potential at point B, then point A is positive with respect to B. If the potential at point A is less than the potential at point B, then A is negative with respect to B.

Electricians have many standards and codes when designing circuits in a building. When a main power line enters a building, it passes through an electrical substation where it is transformed into a low voltage for safe use. The electricity is then distributed throughout the building using a distribution panel. Three wires are used for each branch, which translate into the three-hole electrical sockets most small electrical equipment plugs into. The first of the three branches is the earth ground, which is represented by a green wire. The ground provides a stable, consistent reference point for all electrical potentials to use, and provides a path of least resistance to a safe location. The second wire is neutral, and is represented by a white wire. The third and final wire is the hot wire, or the positive wire, and is represented by a black wire. Using this standard coding allows for maximum electric safety and minimizes the risk of incorrect outlet wiring.

Healthcare workers are responsible for the safety of their patients and themselves. This includes protecting against electrical shock from the diagnostic equipment. To accomplish this, the sleep technologist should always be certain that all diagnostic and other electrical equipment is properly grounded and in good condition. In addition, all equipment should be periodically tested according to the facility's requirements.

Signal Pathways

Understanding the function of the diagnostic equipment and how the electrical signals flow from the patient to the end recording device, technologists are better able to troubleshoot issues and therefore provide quality recordings. Diagnostic sleep equipment may be set up a in variety of ways. For example, one equipment manufacturer may use an external direct current (DC) device whereas another builds the DC amplifier into the same box as the alternating current (AC) amplifier. Also, some may use a separate head box that is connected to the main amplifier through a cable, whereas another company may combine the head box and amplifier into one unit. Regardless of the setup however, a few general principles are common with regard to the general flow of electrical potentials originating from the patient and ending at the recording device:

1. An electrical signal is produced by activity in or from the patient's body.
2. A bioelectrical signal transmits through the skin to the electrode. The bridge between the skin and the electrode is the most common cause of impedance.
3. The signal transmits from the electrode through the lead wire to a head box placed close to the patient's bed.
4. The signal passes straight through the head box to the differential amplifier, usually via a shielded cable.
5. The differential amplifier measures and amplifies the *difference* between two signal inputs (G1–G2), subtracting the main reference and ground signal. The term **common mode rejection** is frequently used to refer to the ability of the differential amplifier to eliminate signals that appear simultaneously and in-phase in both G1 and G2 inputs. Common mode rejection reduces background artifact and electrical interference and helps produce a cleaner, more accurate waveform. The **common mode rejection ratio (CMRR)** measures the ability of the amplifier to reject input signals that are common to both inputs. The higher the CMRR, the better the amplifier is able to reject unwanted signals. High-quality amplifiers have a high CMRR. Most electroencephalogram (EEG) amplifiers have a CMRR of 5,000 to 10,000.
6. Ancillary equipment, like respiratory effort sensors, thermocouples, and pressure transducers, convert movement, pressure, or change in temperature to an electrical signal that is interfaced through the headbox and sent as an output to the software.
7. Filter, polarity, and sensitivity settings are applied to the channel properties according to AASM recommendations and for optimal sleep data output.
8. DC devices such as positive airway pressure (PAP) devices or capnography units send other data about the patient's activities during the night. These signals are sent through a DC amplifier rather than through the differential amplifier, but they are then sent to the polysomnograph to be viewed on the same page as the AC channels.
9. Output signals are then transmitted via a CAT-5 or similar data cable. Some newer sleep systems use the lab's Internet to transmit the data wirelessly.

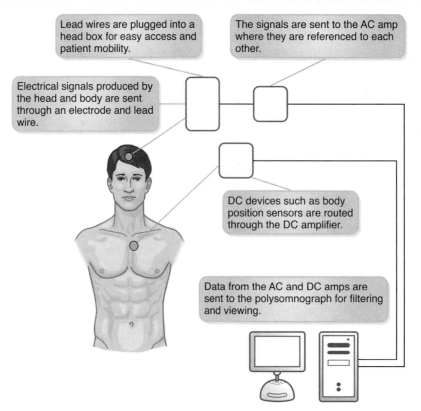

Lead wires are plugged into a head box for easy access and patient mobility.

The signals are sent to the AC amp where they are referenced to each other.

Electrical signals produced by the head and body are sent through an electrode and lead wire.

DC devices such as body position sensors are routed through the DC amplifier.

Data from the AC and DC amps are sent to the polysomnograph for filtering and viewing.

FIGURE 5-2 Signal pathways.

The diagram in **Figure 5-2** illustrates these general principles of signal pathways.

Monitoring Devices

To diagnose and treat many sleep disorders, sleep testing is necessary. A standard diagnostic sleep study includes the collection of biological data, including brain waves (electroencephalogram), muscle activity (electromyogram), heart rate and rhythm (electrocardiogram), eye movement (electrooculogram), and various respiratory parameters. To accomplish this, a variety of sensors and electrodes are used. These sensors are each designed with a specific purpose, although some can be used in place of others. This section will discuss some of the most commonly used electrodes, sensors, and other monitoring and recording devices used in polysomnography.

Snap Electrodes

Snap electrodes (see **Figure 5-3**) are most frequently used on the face and body to record electromyograms (EMGs) and electrocardiograms (ECGs). They can also be used to record electrooculograms (EOGs). These sensors snap onto a disposable sticky electrode patch that is placed firmly against the patient's skin. The center of the patch is electrically conductive and transmits the signal through the buttonlike attachment at the end of the lead wire. Snap leads are easier to attach to the skin than **cup electrodes** but are not ideal for EEG

signals because they cannot attach to the scalp through the hair. They are typically easier to use and less expensive than cup electrodes. However, the ongoing cost of these electrodes is increased by the need to purchase the disposable electrode patches.

Cup Electrodes

The cup electrode (see **Figure 5-4**) is also used frequently in polysomnography and EEG. Cup electrodes are ideal for recording brain waves because they are small and can be placed firmly against the scalp through the hair. Their unique cuplike shape allows them to hold electrically conductive gels or pastes, decreasing the amount of electrical resistance and thereby increasing signal quality. Cup electrodes are plated with a highly conductive metal, usually

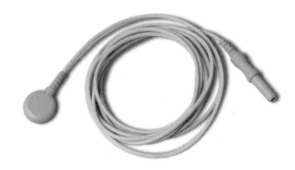

FIGURE 5-3 A snap electrode.

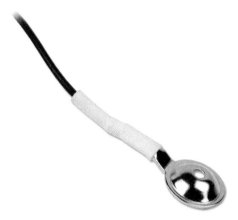

FIGURE 5-4 A cup electrode.

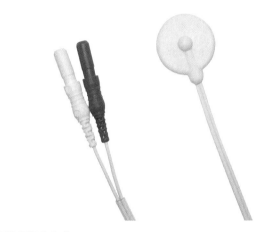

FIGURE 5-5 Snore sensor.

gold, and therefore tend to be rather expensive. They are placed against the scalp using gauze and an electrically conductive EEG paste to hold the electrode in place throughout the recording. Cup electrodes may also be used for recording EOGs and EMGs; when used for these parameters, they can be taped onto the surface of the skin.

Snore Sensors and Microphones

Snore microphones and **snore sensors** are used to monitor a patient's snoring. Snore sensors (see **Figure 5-5**) do this by using the vibrations from the upper airway to produce an electrical signal. Snore microphones detect the noise from the snores and convert this noise into a waveform, which is then sent to the amplifier. With either type, bursts of increased amplitude in the waveform indicate snoring.

Oximeters

The **oximeter** (see **Figure 5-6**) is an external diagnostic device that estimates the amount of hemoglobin in a patient's blood that is saturated by oxygen. This is displayed as a percentage, with a higher percentage

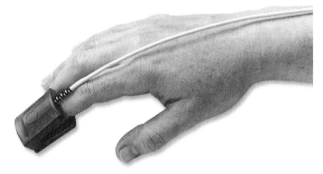

FIGURE 5-6 An oximeter.

indicating an increased level of oxygen in the blood. The device is placed on the patient's finger so that a red light shining on one side can be detected through the patient's finger by the sensor on the opposite end. Hemoglobin saturated with oxygen (**oxyhemoglobin**) absorbs more infrared light, whereas deoxygenated blood (**deoxyhemoglobin**) absorbs more red light. The oximeter measures and compares how much red and infrared light is absorbed by the blood versus the amount that reaches the light detector. The reading produced by the oximeter is called the SpO_2, which is an abbreviation for the oxygen saturation as measured by a pulse oximeter. The SpO_2 in a normal healthy adult should be 95% or greater. For the most accurate readings, the sensor, the finger, and the nail must be clean. Nail polish can cause the light to dim as it passes through the finger, giving a false low reading. If the sensor cannot be placed on a finger, then a toe or earlobe can be used. The SaO_2 is a measurement of oxygen saturation in the arterial blood and is measured by performing an invasive **arterial blood gas** test, which is not routinely done during sleep testing. Technologists should be careful to refer to the patient's blood oxygen level as read by the pulse oximeter as SpO_2 rather than SaO_2.

Body Position Sensors

Body position sensors are DC devices that detect the position in which the patient is lying. These sensors are usually attached to the thoracic belt via a Velcro strip and are displayed on the recording as either supine, left, right, prone, or upright. The body position sensor shown in **Figure 5-7** has a Velcro strip on the back that sticks to the respiratory effort belt (described later in this chapter). Other body position sensors wrap around the belt or are placed directly on the patient.

Thermal Airflow Sensors

Thermal airflow sensors are recommended by the AASM[1] for identification of respiratory events characterized by cessation (lack) of airflow, also known as

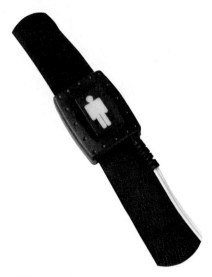

FIGURE 5-7 A body position sensor.

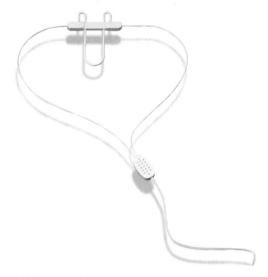

FIGURE 5-9 A thermistor.

apneic events. Thermal devices should be placed on the upper lip with the nasal sensors at the openings of the nares and the oral sensor hovering over the opening of the mouth. The sensor can be taped on to keep it in place. Thermal sensors include thermistors, thermocouples, or polyvinylidene fluoride (PVDF) airflow sensors. These are described in the following section.

Thermocouples

Nasal–oral **thermocouples** (see **Figure 5-8**) are used in polysomnography to detect airflow. Thermocouples work by detecting the rate of temperature change. Thermocouples are made from two dissimilar metals with different levels of expansion. This temperature-sensitive change in the metals is then converted into an electrical signal and sent to the polysomnograph. The signal from

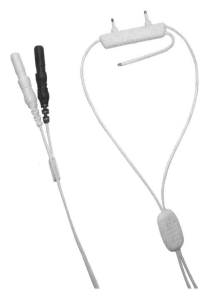

FIGURE 5-8 A thermocouple.

the thermocouple appears as a sinusoidal waveform that indicates inspiratory and expiratory flow. Total cessation of airflow, or apnea, is well detected with this sensor because there will be no temperature change. Nasal–oral thermocouples are sometimes assembled from four sensing elements so airflow can be recorded on separate channels from both nares and both sides of the mouth, or they can be combined into one channel displaying oral and nasal airflow.

Thermistors

Thermistors (see **Figure 5-9**) are also used in polysomnography to detect airflow. Nasal–oral thermistors are typically made of three thermistor ends so the airflow can be recorded at both nares and in front of the mouth. They do this by detecting changes in temperature between room air and expired air. As these temperature changes occur, an electrical signal is produced. This signal is amplified with a Wheatstone bridge circuit. The signal is then calculated with respect to ground or another specified reference. The output signal is also sinusoidal and corresponds to respiratory inspiration and expiration. Similar to a thermocouple, apneic respiratory events are well detected with this sensor.

PVDF Airflow Sensors

Polyvinylidene fluoride is a specialized plastic used for many applications, including piping, insulation, and electronic components. The intrinsic properties of the compound make it useful for use in biomedical sensors. **Polyvinylidene fluoride airflow sensors** (see **Figure 5-10**) work by generating an electrical signal in response to changes in temperature and pressure. This sensor type has gained popularity for use in sleep diagnostics, and recent research has shown high comparisons between PVDF, thermal airflow monitoring, and nasal pressure sensors.

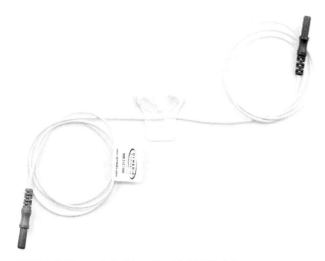

FIGURE 5-10 A polyvinylidene fluoride (PVDF) airflow sensor.

TriplePlay PVDF Reusable Airflow Sensor, Ped., White, Dymedix Diagnostics Inc., Retrieved from https://www.electramed.com/neurology/sleep-sensors/dymedix-pediatric-disposable /nr36400301-tripleplay-pvdf-reusable-airflow-sensor-ped-white

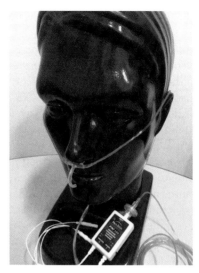

FIGURE 5-11 A pressure transducer with nasal–oral pressure cannula.

Pressure Transducers

Pressure transducers measure airflow from the nose and mouth via an oral–nasal cannula. Pressure transducers were developed to help detect partial airway obstruction and flow limitation because traditional thermal sensing devices were unable to do so accurately.

As the patient breathes, the pressures that are created with inspiration and expiration are detected in the cannula and used by the device to produce an electrical signal that depicts airflow. Pressure transducers provide highly accurate measurements of flow and correlate highly with the traditional reference standard for flow, **pneumotachography**. This correlation makes them ideal for measuring reductions in flow, flow limitation, and snoring. Nasal pressure transducers are recommended by the AASM[1] for identification of **hypopneic events** and **respiratory effort–related arousals**.

Data recorded from the pressure transducer device can be collected by AC or DC inputs. In a DC input set up, the unit sends a signal to the DC amplifier with a voltage that corresponds to the amount of airflow measured, and it is translated as a flow volume tracing. In an AC input setup, the device plugs directly into the headbox. In this case, the signal must be filtered appropriately so that low-frequency waveforms can appear.

When placing the nasal pressure cannula, the nasal prongs are placed at the openings of the nares while the oral prong should hover over the opening of the mouth. If needed, the prongs may be trimmed for patient comfort. The cannula is then draped over the patient's ears to keep it in place and is secured under the chin (see **Figure 5-11**).

Capnography

Capnography is the measure of concentration or partial pressure of carbon dioxide (CO_2) in the respiratory gases. Capnography relies on the principle of absorption. Because CO_2 has the ability to absorb infrared light, a **capnograph** passes infrared light through a gas sample and measures the light passing through to the sensor. As CO_2 levels change with inspiration and expiration, the device measures the changes in light absorption. This, in turn, produces varying voltages that are depicted as a waveform of CO_2 over time. This waveform is referred to as a **capnogram** (see **Figure 5-12**). The normal capnography waveform[2] begins with a baseline phase where the partial pressure of carbon dioxide (PCO_2) is zero. This is followed by the initial portion of exhalation where there is a sharp rise in CO_2 as alveolar

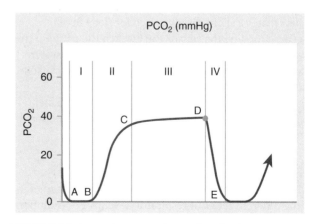

FIGURE 5-12 A normal capnography waveform tracing.

gas is mixed with dead space gas. The waveform then levels off and forms a plateau for the remaining portion of exhalation. This portion of the signal represents flow from the alveoli and is called the *alveolar plateau*. At this point in the waveform the end-tidal CO_2 ($ETCO_2$) value is measured. Normal values for $ETCO_2$ are between 35 and 45 mm Hg. Finally, the waveform drops off drastically with the inspiratory phase because CO_2 is usually absent in inspired air.

CO_2 values provide important information about a patient's ventilatory status. Changes in respiratory rate and tidal volume are displayed quickly as changes in the waveform and $ETCO_2$ value. Higher than normal $ETCO_2$ values indicate that ventilation is not effective at eliminating CO_2 (hypoventilation) and can be associated with obesity, pulmonary disease, or respiratory distress. Lower than normal $ETCO_2$ values indicate hyperventilation and can be seen with anxiety or diabetic complications.

In sleep diagnostics, capnography can be measured externally or transcutaneously. External measures are accomplished by using a nasal–oral cannula connected to an external capnography unit. This method tends to be favored because of ease of use. To eliminate placing yet another cannula on the upper lip, many vendors produce split cannulas for collection of both nasal pressure airflow and capnography. The external capnography device is interfaced with the sleep software as a DC device, and the waveform is incorporated into the digital polysomnogram.

Transcutaneous CO_2 monitors measure the gases in the blood using a heated sensor that is placed on the skin. The heat from the sensor causes the blood to concentrate at the sensor, allowing gas from arterialized capillary blood to reach the sensor. Proper application and cleaning of the test site are important, and the electrode attachment to the skin must be airtight. The sensor is heated to approximately 42 degrees Celsius (107.6 degrees Fahrenheit) and must be repositioned occasionally throughout the night to prevent burning. This creates a slight disadvantage for sleep testing because moving the sensor can awaken the patient. The capnography unit is interfaced with the sleep system as a DC device. Like many DC devices, most transcutaneous CO_2 monitors require calibration.

Capnography is currently recommended as a standard for pediatric diagnostic sleep testing but is considered optional for adults.

Respiratory Effort Technology

Measuring respiratory effort is important for characterizing different types of respiratory events. For example, if a patient is attempting to breathe but his or her upper airway is collapsed (an obstructive apnea), there will be a period of no airflow accompanied by continued respiratory effort. Conversely, if a patient makes no attempt

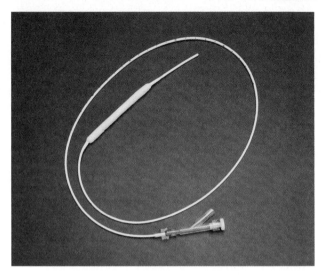

FIGURE 5-13 An esophageal balloon catheter.
Courtesy of CooperSurgical, Inc.

to breathe (a central apnea), there will be a period of no airflow and no effort to breathe. Differentiating these types of breathing events is critical to diagnosis and treatment.

Historically, there have been numerous different technologies used to measure the effort to breathe—for example, mercury strain gauges, piezoelectric crystals, and intercostal electromyography. However, currently the AASM[1] recommends the use of either esophageal manometry or dual thoracoabdominal respiratory inductance plethysmography technology for collection of this parameter. Thoracoabdominal PVDF belts are offered as an acceptable alternative. We will discuss these recommended technologies in detail in the following paragraphs.

Esophageal balloon catheters are most commonly used to record respiratory effort in clinical research of upper-airway resistance. These sensors consist of a narrow tube with a thin flaccid balloon at the open end (see **Figure 5-13**). The catheter is inserted through the nose into the lower third of the esophagus and connected to a pressure transducer outside of the body. As the patient breathes, **esophageal manometry** measures changes in the esophageal balloon pressure in cm H_2O pressure. The measures from this technology closely reflect **pleural pressure** (pressure surrounding the lung) and the effort to breathe. The resulting waveform is sinusoidal (qualitative) and provides numeric pressure measures (quantitative). Although this method is considered highly accurate of effort detection, it is not often chosen for use in diagnostic sleep testing because it is invasive and must be properly placed into the esophagus by an experienced clinician before testing.

Respiratory inductive plethysmography (RIP) is the most common recent technology chosen for the measurement of respiratory effort. It includes the use of two

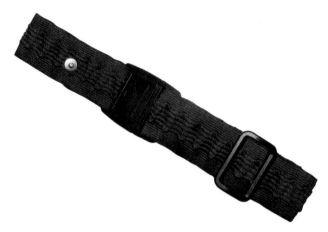

FIGURE 5-14 Reusable respiratory inductive plethysmography (RIP) effort belts.

SleepSense RIP Reusable Inductive Kit, © Sleep Sense, Retrieved from https://www.mvapmed.com/sleepsense-rip-reusable-inductive-kit.htm

elastic belts that are placed snuggly around the patient's chest and abdomen. The belts contain a coiled wire and are attached to a device that produces an AC current (see **Figure 5-14**). The current that is applied to the loop of wire creates a magnetic field. As the patient breathes, changes in the cross-sectional area of the thorax and abdomen occur. This changes the shape of the magnetic field and *induces* an opposing current that can be measured and is directly proportional to the change in area that occurred. The resulting RIP waveform is sinusoidal and semiquantitative. Further, the waveform can mimic the pressure transducer waveform in that the shape, phase, and amplitude of the signal provides information about the patient's breathing. For example, the upstroke of the signal is associated with inspiration while the down stroke is associated with exhalation. Also, a low-amplitude effort signal indicates more shallow breathing, and the appearance of flattening in shape of the waveform can indicate flow restriction.

With RIP technology, the correct placement of the belts is important. The thoracic belt should be placed at or below the fourth intercostal space while the abdominal belt should be placed just above the umbilical. This ensures the greatest accuracy and depiction of respiratory effort.

Other Monitoring Devices

The following devices are not included in a standard diagnostic polysomnogram but may be used either alone or in conjunction with the overnight sleep test to monitor additional parameters. To detect acidity levels in the esophagus, **pH probes** can be inserted into the esophagus through the nose. Normal pH levels in the esophagus should be around 7, indicating a neutral environment. Sudden reductions in pH to values of 4 or below indicate the occurrence of gastroesophageal reflux disease. Integrating the measurement of pH into

a sleep study can be useful to determine the association of reflux events with sleep-disordered breathing as well as to guide treatment regimens.

Actigraphy is a noninvasive method used to track sleep–wake patterns over time. Actigraphy devices contain accelerometers to record motion and are usually worn on the wrist. The output simply depicts periods of motion, assumed to be when the patient is awake, from periods of no or little motion, periods assumed to be sleep. Actigraphy is most useful in sleep diagnostics to assess for various circadian rhythm disorders in which patients have disturbances to the normal biological sleep clock. Various types of actigraphy devices have recently become popular in the sporting and fitness industry because they can be useful in monitoring levels of physical activity during the day.

Motion detectors work similar to body position sensors but are most often used in polysomnography to record periodic limb movements during sleep. Motion detectors detect movements through a piezoelectric crystal contained within straps that can be attached to the arms or legs. When motion is detected, stress is applied to the crystal and a signal is produced.

Differential Amplifiers

A **differential amplifier** is a specific type of electronic amplifier that multiplies the difference between two inputs by a common factor called the *differential gain*. In polysomnography, the differential amplifier converts two input signals recorded from the patient's head, face, or body; amplifies the difference between the two signal inputs, subtracting the main reference and ground signal; and sends a resulting output signal to the polysomnograph. This process is illustrated in **Figure 5-15**. V+ refers to the first input or voltage signal, which is also called *G1* (gate 1) or the exploring electrode. This is the electrode site that contains the biologic potentials of interest (active). V−, the second input, is called *G2* (gate 2) or the reference electrode. This is the electrode site that provides a relatively stable or consistent signal voltage so it can be used as an appropriate reference for the exploring electrode.

To record EEGs, sensors are used to detect extremely small electrical impulses from the brain. While these potentials are being recorded, many other electrical potentials from external sources may enter the signal pathway. These sources may include signals from the patient such as muscle activity, body

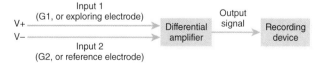

FIGURE 5-15 How a differential amplifier works. Output voltage = G1 – G2.

movements, pulses from the heart, or electrical leakage from nearby devices such as computers, lamps, cell phones, or other diagnostic equipment. The differential amplifier uses two inputs for each channel to help eliminate unwanted signals. For example, a channel with inputs from the C3 and M2 electrode sites records all signals from the C3 electrode site and subtracts the signals from the M2 site. In theory, M2 will detect the same undesired electrical signals from other sources that C3 is detecting with the exception of the desired EEGs in the C3 area. After these two inputs are differentiated through the amplifier, the resulting signal will be the true EEG waves in the left central hemisphere of the brain.

To further explain this process, assume that the electrode at G1 receives a signal input of 10µV. At the same time, the reference electrode at G2 receives a signal input of 5µV. G2 is subtracted from G1, and the output voltage is 5µV. If the signal at G2 is greater than the signal at G1, then the output signal is negative. This is why a differential amplifier is an alternating current amplifier because the signals alternate quickly from positive to negative voltages.

To focus on specific waveforms of interest to polysomnography, frequency filters are used. Standard sleep diagnostics include the recording of channels for brain waves, eye movement, muscle activity, cardiac rhythm, and airflow channels. The recording of activity of interest in each of these parameters differs. For example, in muscle channels, it is important to detect high-frequency muscle activity, while in the airflow channels, the focus is on slow-frequency breathing activity. The use of low- and high-frequency filters provides a window of focus for the specific and relevant waveforms for each channel. Frequency filters allow the system to focus on a defined range of frequencies by greatly reducing or attenuating the amplitude of unwanted signals with frequencies above the high-frequency filter (HFF) and below the low-frequency filter (LFF). Compare this to the tuner of a radio that focuses on a specific frequency range to detect signals from a desired radio station. Similarly, the sensitivity or gain setting of an amplifier can be compared to the volume knob of a radio, which amplifies the signals to a desired level for easier detection.

To illustrate the function of the LFF and HFF in attenuating and eliminating unwanted waveforms, it is useful to consider the following example.

A channel is set with the LFF at 0.5 Hz. As a result, the amplifier will attenuate the amplitude of signals at 0.5 Hz to approximately 70% and attenuate signals below 0.5 Hz to a greater degree. As incoming signals move further below the LFF setting (e.g., 0.4 Hz, 0.3 Hz) they will be attenuated further until signals greatly below 0.5 Hz (e.g., 0.05 Hz) are completely eliminated. Conversely, all frequencies above 0.5 Hz and up to the setting of the HFF will be allowed into the recording. This same concept is true for the HFF.

A channel is set with the HFF at 35 Hz. As a result, the amplifier will attenuate the amplitude of signals at 35 Hz to approximately 70% and attenuate signals above 35 Hz to a greater degree. As incoming signals move further above the HFF setting (e.g., 45 Hz, 60 Hz) they will be attenuated further until signals greatly above 35 Hz (e.g., 100 Hz) are completely eliminated. Conversely, all frequencies below 35 Hz and down to the setting of the LFF will be allowed into the recording.

A **frequency-response curve** is a graphical display of an amplifier's ability to eliminate unwanted signals through the use of the filters. **Figure 5-16** is an example of a differential amplifier's frequency response curve for typical EMG settings (LFF 10 Hz, HFF 100 Hz). On the left side is the percentage that the signal is amplified, and at the bottom are the frequencies. Note that the waveforms of greatest amplitude lie between the settings of the LF and HF filters—in this case, 10 Hz and 100 Hz, respectively. All others are greatly

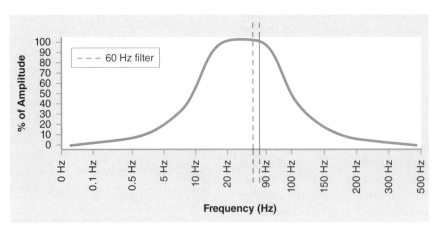

FIGURE 5-16 A frequency response curve.

reduced in amplitude. Also of note is the 60-Hz filter shown in the middle of the chart. Background electrical noise in the United States emits frequencies of 60 cycles per second. When artifacts from background electrical activity become a problem, a 60-Hz filter, also known as the *notch filter*, may be applied. This effectively eliminates all frequencies in the 60-Hz range from the recording.

Electrical Grounding

In electrical engineering, the term **ground** can have multiple meanings. The ground is a reference point in an electrical circuit by which other electrical signals or voltages are measured. The electrical ground can also refer to the common return path for an electrical current or a physical connection to the earth. As previously discussed in this chapter, electrical current follows the path of least resistance. When a circuit is connected to the ground, this becomes the path of least resistance and provides a safe place for electricity to flow without being hazardous to the user. In the sleep lab, the amplifiers, computers, PAP machines, and other electrical equipment should always be plugged into a grounded outlet. If there is no ground connected, the risk of electrical shock is extremely high.

In polysomnography, we often refer to the *patient ground*. This refers to an electrode that stands as a common reference for all other electrodes, similar to an electrical ground in a circuit. The ground lead provides a common point for all EEG and EOG electrodes to compare signals to, providing a consistent and realistic depiction of the patient's true EEG and EOG activity.

In **Figure 5-17**, a boy is flying a kite 200 feet above his head. One could not determine the elevation of the kite without knowing the elevation of the spot of land on which the boy is standing. In this case, let us assume

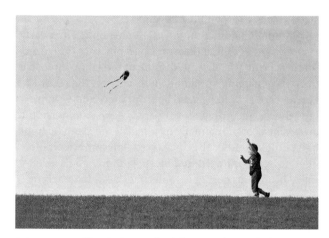

FIGURE 5-17 Electrical grounding is better understood when comparing it to a boy flying a kite.

that the boy is standing in a field that has an elevation of 500 feet above sea level, which makes the elevation of the kite 700 feet. Here, the sea level would be comparable to our patient ground because it is the reference point we use to measure everything else.

Using the principle of grounding as shown in the kite example, we will now discuss how electrical grounding and referencing are used in polysomnography. Suppose that the O1 electrode records an electrical signal of 25 µV, and M2 simultaneously records an electrical signal of 40 µV. Using the equation OV (output voltage) = G1 – G2, we determine that the output voltage is –15 µV. Without a patient ground lead to use as a reference, these signals could not exist in the first place. A 25 µV signal in the O1 electrode is not 25 µV by itself but is 25 µV more than the voltage recorded in the patient ground site at that exact same moment. Similarly, the 40 µV signal in M2 is actually 40 µV more than the signal received in the ground lead at that exact moment. Therefore, the output voltage is not –15 µV by itself but 15 µV less than the signal at the ground lead.

Because all EEG and EOG leads are referenced to the ground electrode, this becomes perhaps the most important electrode in the patient hookup. When the ground lead is loosely attached and records 60-Hz signals from outside sources, these signals will be recorded in all the EEG and EOG channels. Therefore, it is vital that the ground electrode site is properly cleaned and that the electrode is firmly attached to the skin, thereby minimizing electrical impedances.

Depending on the brand of amplifier used, the patient ground lead may require its own reference lead. Using a main reference to the ground helps ensure reliability of the signals received by the ground lead. This practice should not be confused with using two grounds. If a technologist were to use two ground leads on a patient, it could create a **ground loop**. Ground loops occur when the electrical signals loop from one ground lead to the other through the patient's body or head. An electrical ground loop can be caused when multiple pieces of diagnostic equipment are connected to a patient and each uses its own ground reference that is dissimilar from the ground of the opposing diagnostic equipment. This type of ground loop can cause severe electrical shock to the patient and can be extremely hazardous.

In polysomnography, and in any type of bioelectric recording, electrode placement is crucial to visualize relevant waveforms and to ensure accurate recordings. To record EEG activity, or brain waves, electrodes must be placed on the scalp using the **international 10/20 electrode placement system**.[3] This system is an internationally recognized and standardized measurement system used to determine the correct location for scalp electrode placement. The system relies on skull landmarks, uses measures along different planes of the head, and employs various percentage measures (10%, 20%, 50%) along those planes. Locations are described by letters associated with the underlying area of the brain and numbers based on location and hemisphere. This system will be described in detail in Chapter 6.

The standard EEG convention (also called the *polarity convention*) states that positive voltages result in a downward pen deflection, whereas negative voltages result in an upward pen deflection. This standard is maintained throughout EEG and polysomnography recordings for consistency and validity in tracings.

When recording EEGs, it is important to select an appropriate montage, or signal distribution and channel setup. In electroencephalography, there are two main types of recording montages: **monopolar or referential recording montages** and **bipolar recording montages**. Monopolar or referential montages are characterized by an active or exploring electrode referenced to a common reference electrode. For example, in a standard polysomnogram, active electrodes are placed at the O1, C3, and F3 site locations over the brain. Each electrode is referenced to the M2 electrode placed at the mastoid. Referential EEG montages are commonly used in polysomnography.

Bipolar montages are characterized by having two active or exploring electrodes existing at each input. For example, a bipolar montage might include a channel that references O1 to O2 and another channel that references O2 to C4. Bipolar recordings are more commonly used in neurodiagnostics and standard full EEG recordings and are useful for locating seizure activity in the brain.

As previously discussed in this chapter, impedance is a resistance to the flow of electricity or current. Having high impedance values during the recording of the sleep study will result in artifact and poor signal quality. Thus, every effort should be made to minimize electrode impedances in each polysomnography channel by properly cleaning the electrode site and applying the electrode firmly against the skin. Impedance values must be measured as part of the standard procedures at the beginning and end of the sleep study and as needed over the course of the night. The AASM[1] recommended standard for impedance values is less than 5,000 ohms.

Digital Polysomnography

For the first few decades of sleep testing, polysomnographic recordings were performed with analogue machines (see **Figure 5-18**). These large, complex machines included stacks of individual amplifiers for each channel collected with manual dials for LFF, HFF, and sensitivity control. There were pens with an inkwell for each channel, continuously scrolling paper, and seemingly countless other gauges and dials. Today,

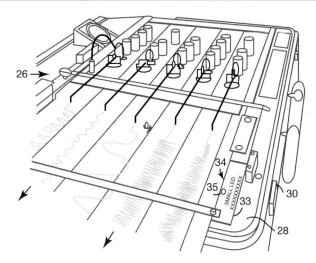

FIGURE 5-18 For decades, sleep data were recorded on analogue polysomnographs like the one shown here. Today, most sleep data are recorded using digital systems.

most sleep studies are recorded digitally, and the filter, sensitivity, and polarity settings as well as customizable properties can be adjusted by using the computer's keyboard and mouse. Videos of the patients can now be recorded digitally and integrated into the sleep study itself, allowing the scoring technologist and interpreting physician to see exactly what the patient is doing while simultaneously viewing the EEGs and other signals from the patient. PAP pressures are often adjusted by controls on the computer, and two-way intercoms between the technologist and the patient are often built into the computer as well.

The ability to record signals from the patient digitally has revolutionized the polysomnography industry. Sleep studies are now transferable to anywhere in the world for scoring and interpreting procedures. The scoring process has become much faster and easier, with the computer generating reports and making the necessary calculations after the scorer has marked the appropriate sleep stages and significant events.

Automatic scoring modules are now built into nearly every brand of digital polysomnography software. Automatic scoring has alleviated some of the labor-intensive process of tagging all significant events on the record. However, it should be used appropriately and within guidelines. According to standards, sleep studies should always be scored manually by a registered sleep technologist holding either the Registered Polysomnographic Technologist or Registered Sleep Technologist credential. Automatic scoring is sometimes used to generate a preliminary report for the physician to have a quick glance at a patient's sleep study before a qualified individual is able to review the scoring and make changes as necessary. Also, automatic scoring can be used to mark certain events rather than to score the entire study. For example, if a patient is snoring the entire night, marking each individual snore can become quite cumbersome. It may be appropriate in this case to allow the software to detect the snores and then manually make corrections to the scored snoring events as necessary. Always follow the sleep lab's protocols and AASM recommendations regarding automatic scoring.

Digital polysomnography, like any digital system, has certain drawbacks when compared to analogue systems. Analogue systems make an actual recording of the event. In the case of **analogue polysomnography**, the pen constantly touches the paper, and is adjusted up and down based on the signals it receives. Digital polysomnography, however, records only one tiny bit of information at a time and displays that bit as a dot on the screen. A good digital system will have a high **sampling rate**, meaning it has the ability to record and display many bits of information per second. Compare this to an audio recording device. An audio record contains recordings of the actual soundwaves and plays those sounds as a continuous stream. A compact disc digitally records bits of music at a time, converts them to a digital format, and puts the bits of information together. If the digital recording has a poor sampling rate, the sound quality decreases. Higher sampling rates increase the file size but also increase the quality of the recording. The same is true of digital polysomnography. Higher sampling rates in digital polysomnography allow the viewer to more accurately detect high-frequency activity such as EEGs or muscle movements. If the sampling rate is decreased, certain fast activity is lost in the recording. The AASM recommends a minimum sampling rate of 200 Hz for EEGs, EOGs, EMGs, and ECGs, with a sampling rate of 500 Hz listed as desirable.

Chapter Summary

An understanding of some basic principles of electricity is essential for sleep technologists. *Voltage* refers to the difference in concentration of ionic charges at two different points. *Current* refers to the flow of electricity. *Resistance* refers to anything that restricts or defers the flow of a current and is measured in ohms. In polysomnography, we often refer to resistance in terms of impedance.

Electrical safety is key in polysomnography for both the technologist and the patient. It is essential that all equipment is properly grounded and that all wiring is appropriately housed.

Electrical signals generated by the patient are transmitted through the electrodes to a differential amplifier, where they are referenced to each other and to a common ground. An amplifier's *common mode rejection ratio* refers to its ability to reject unwanted signals.

Amplifiers with a higher CMRR are better at referencing signals and rejecting unwanted signals.

Many different types of monitoring devices help us detect electrical signals produced by the different parts of the body. Cup electrodes are highly conductive and are good for placement on the scalp for recording EEGs. Snap electrodes snap onto disposable electrodes that stick to the patient's skin. These are good for recording EKGs or EMG activity. Snore microphones and sensors help us detect vibrations in the upper airway, and oximeters detect the amount of oxygen in the blood. Respiratory effort belts stretch around a patient's abdomen and thorax and let us know when and if the patient is trying to breathe. Thermistors and thermocouples detect airflow by reading changes in temperature at the nose and mouth, and pressure transducers measure the volume of air inhaled and exhaled by the patient to display a flow tracing.

Differential amplifiers determine an output signal by subtracting the voltage received by the reference electrode from the voltage received by the exploring electrode. Technologists should be able to calculate output voltages based on exploring and reference voltages.

Filters enable the user to view a desired range of signals while attenuating signals outside the desired range. A frequency-response curve shows the amplifier's ability to attenuate unwanted signals outside filter ranges.

AC signals are referenced to a common ground placed on the patient. Voltages are based on the differences between exploring signals and the common ground. It is essential that the ground electrode have minimal impedance so all other signals have the ability to record accurately. Ground loops can occur when two ground leads are used, which can cause poor tracings and pose a danger to the patient.

Two EEG montages commonly used in polysomnography are referential and bipolar montages. Bipolar montages use two exploring electrodes as inputs, whereas referential montages use common references in each channel.

The international 10/20 electrode placement system is the standard for measuring and placing EEG electrodes. Sleep technologists use this system to locate the appropriate locations on the patient's head for applying the EEG electrodes.

The field of polysomnography has taken a dramatic leap forward with the development of digital sleep-recording devices. Digital polysomnography allows for faster diagnosis and treatment, and it allows the physician to view data trends during the entire night. Digital polysomnography also allow physicians to import mass quantities of data from thousands of patients to help in their research.

Chapter 5 Questions

Please consider the following questions as they relate to the material in this chapter.

1. What is voltage? Current? Resistance?
2. Why is a signal's polarity important in polysomnography?
3. What pathway does a signal take to get from the patient to the polysomnograph?
4. What monitoring devices are optimal for recording EEGs? EMGs?
5. What advantages does a pressure transducer have over a thermistor or thermocouple?
6. If the exploring electrode receives a signal of $-20\ \mu V$ at the same time the reference electrode receives a signal of $30\ \mu V$, what is the output signal?
7. What is a ground loop, and what causes it?
8. What might be some advantages and disadvantages to a bipolar montage? A referential montage?
9. How has the conversion of analogue to digital recordings impacted the field of polysomnography?

Footnotes

1. American Academy of Sleep Medicine. (2017). *The AASM manual for the scoring of sleep and associated events: Rules, terminology, and technical specifications*, version 2.4. Darien, IL: Author.
2. American Thoracic Society. (2018). Waveform capnography. Accessed from https://www.thoracic.org/professionals/clinical-resources/video-lecture-series/critical-care/waveform-capnography.php
3. Transcranial Technologies. (2012). *10/20 system positioning manual*. Accessed from http://chgd.umich.edu/wp-content/uploads/2014/06/10-20_system_positioning.pdf

6

Patient Hookup Procedures

CHAPTER OUTLINE

International 10/20 System
Electrode Placement for Sleep Studies
Electrode Application
Impedance Checks
Helpful Strategies for Sleep Technologists
Chapter Summary

LEARNING OBJECTIVES

1. Understand the importance of the international 10/20 system.
2. Learn the EEG measurements for sleep studies and full EEG montages.
3. Learn the electrode sites for the face and body.
4. Learn how to properly apply electrodes for optimal recording.

KEY TERMS

International 10/20 electrode placement system
nasion
inion
pre-auricular points
canthus
anterior tibialis
impedance

International 10/20 System

Dr. Herbert H. Jasper developed the **international 10/20 electrode placement system** in 1949 as a standard measurement tool for placing electrodes on the head for recording electroencephalograms (EEGs). This system of measurement uses anatomical features such as the ears and the bridge of the nose as landmarks to begin measurement. Electrode sites are then found by measuring distances between these landmarks and using percentages of those distances rather than specific lengths. This allows for accurate and consistent electrode placement across varying head shapes and sizes from pediatrics to adults. The name of the measurement system was derived from the percentages used in the measurements. Most of the sites are found by marking 10% or 20% of the measurements between anatomical features of the head and skull. When measuring for a full EEG hookup, as many as 256 electrode sites may be used. However, for a standard sleep study, only six electrode sites are used for exploring electrodes, and another three or four sites are used as references or ground, depending on the type of equipment used.

This section will explore two options for electrode placement. The first option will show the standard electrode placements for an overnight sleep study. The second will show a more detailed option for electrode placements, including a 24-lead hookup for a sleep study with a full EEG montage.

Electrode Placement for Sleep Studies[1,2]

When measuring for electrode placement for a standard sleep study, the American Academy of Sleep Medicine (AASM)[2] recommends the following electrode sites:

- F3
- F4
- C3
- C4
- O1
- O2
- M1
- M2
- Cz, Fz, or Fpz (often used as ground and main reference)

In addition to these standards, alternative acceptable variations are presented in the *AASM Manual for the Scoring of Sleep and Associated Events*.[2] Please note the diagrams in **Figures 6-1** and **6-2** and the following instructions for measurement.

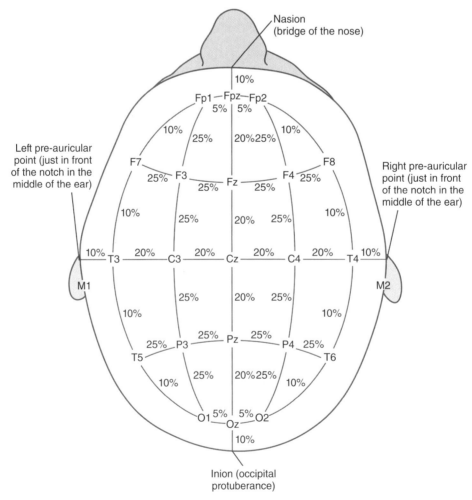

FIGURE 6-1 International 10/20 electrode placement system.

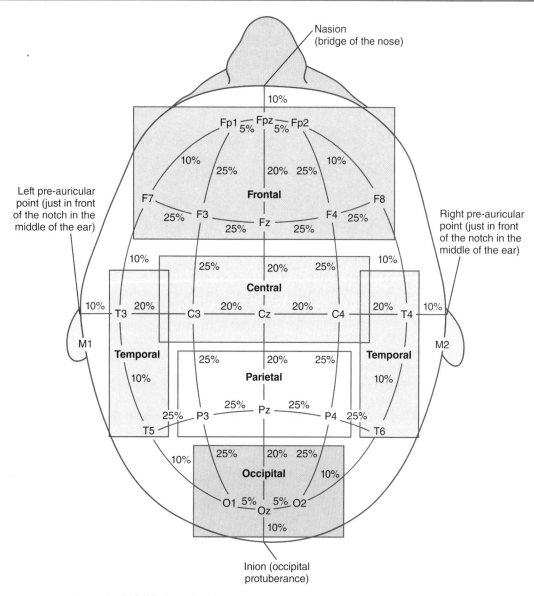

FIGURE 6-2 International 10/20 electrode placement system by section.

Option 1: Placement for EEG Electrodes in a Standard Sleep Study

Step 1: Locate the Four Landmarks

The EEG measurement process begins by locating four landmarks on the head:

1. Nasion
2. Inion
3. Left pre-auricular point
4. Right pre-auricular point

The **nasion** is a landmark found midline at the intersection of the frontal and nasal bones. It is found just superior to the bridge of the nose and is marked by a bony depression between the eyes. The **inion** is the most prominent point of the occipital bone at the back of the skull. The **pre-auricular points** are found by locating the notch in the middle of the front part of each ear. Directly in front of this notch is the pre-auricular point. All three points are shown in **Figures 6-3** and **6-4**.

Step 2: Measure and Mark Between the Nasion and Inion

Measure the distance from the nasion to the inion across the top of the head. Mark 10% of the total distance up in the front and back. Assume this distance is 30 cm. In this case, marks would be placed 3 cm up from the nasion and inion. Mark the halfway or 50% point (15 cm in this example). Mark 20% down in the front (6 cm in this example). This is the first mark for locating Fz. Visual representations of these measurements are shown in **Figures 6-5** through **6-8**.

Step 3: Measure and Mark Between the Pre-auricular Points

Measure the distance from the left pre-auricular point to the right pre-auricular point, with the tape measure passing through the 50% mark made previously at the top of the head. Mark 10% of this distance up on each

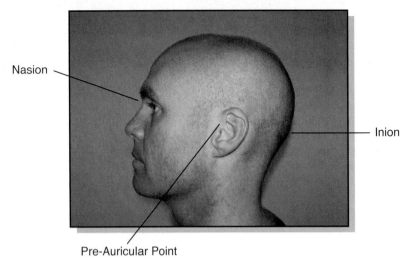

Nasion

Inion

Pre-Auricular Point

FIGURE 6-3 Head left view starting points.

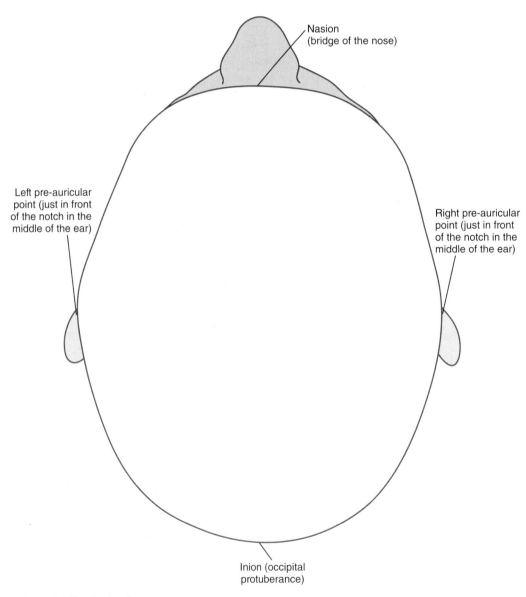

Nasion
(bridge of the nose)

Left pre-auricular
point (just in front
of the notch in the
middle of the ear)

Right pre-auricular
point (just in front
of the notch in the
middle of the ear)

Inion (occipital
protuberance)

FIGURE 6-4 Four landmarks.

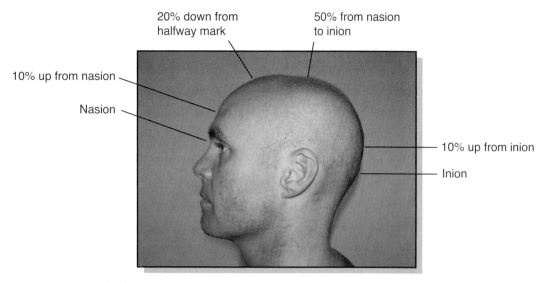

FIGURE 6-5 Head left view, step 2.

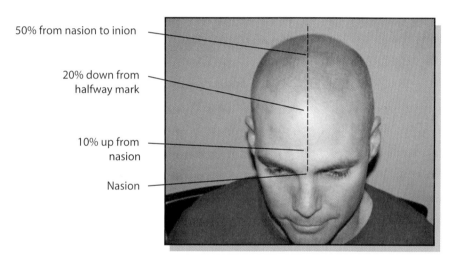

FIGURE 6-6 Head front view, step 2.

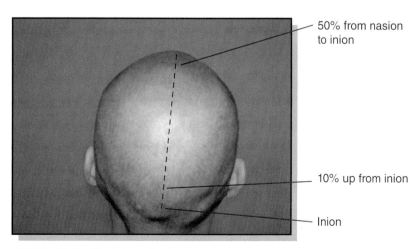

FIGURE 6-7 Head back view, step 2.

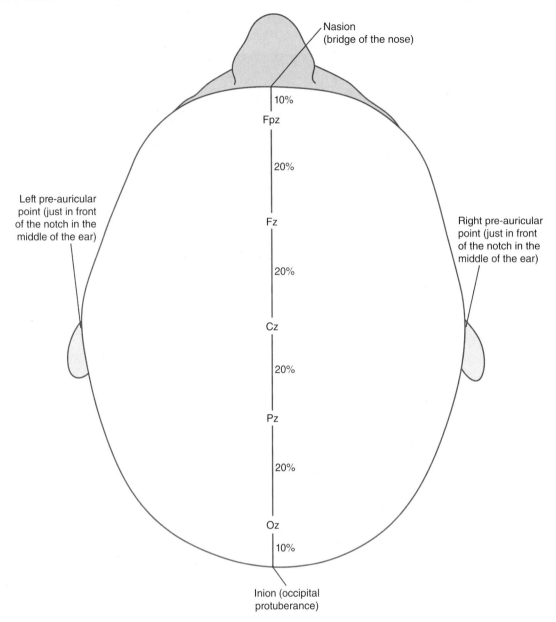

Nasion
(bridge of the nose)

10%
Fpz

20%

Left pre-auricular
point (just in front
of the notch in the
middle of the ear)

Fz

Right pre-auricular
point (just in front
of the notch in the
middle of the ear)

20%

Cz

20%

Pz

20%

Oz

10%

Inion (occipital
protuberance)

FIGURE 6-8 Step 2 drawing.

side. In this example, we will use 34 cm as our measurement. Therefore, the marks will be made 3.4 cm up from the left and right pre-auricular points. Mark 50% of the total distance—in this example, at 17 cm (this 50% mark will intersect the other 50% mark, indicating the exact point for Cz). Mark 20% of the total distance down on each side (6.8 cm in this example). These 20% marks are the first marks for locating C3 and C4. These points are shown in **Figures 6-9** and **6-10**.

Step 4: Measure and Mark the Circumference of the Head

Make a vertical mark aligned with the middle of the nose through the mark that is 10% up from the nasion. Then, starting at the intersection of these two marks (which

gives us the exact location for Fpz), measure the circumference of the head while passing the tape measure over each of the 10% marks. In this example, we will assume the circumference of the head is 60 cm. Mark 50% at the back of the head—in this example, 30 cm. This gives us the location for Oz. Mark 5% of the circumference (3 cm in this example) on the left and right side of Fpz and Oz. Extrapolate the line that is 10% up from the nasion to intersect with these points. The intersection of this line and the mark 5% to the left gives the location for Fp1. The intersection of this line and the mark 5% to the right gives the location for Fp2. Do the same on the back of the head, revealing the locations for O1 and O2. In the front of the head, measure 10% to the left of the newly discovered Fp1 point (or 15% of the circumference to the left of Fpz) and place a mark. In this example, the

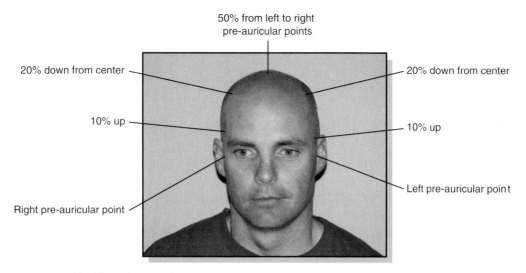

50% from left to right
pre-auricular points

20% down from center

20% down from center

10% up

10% up

Left pre-auricular point

Right pre-auricular point

FIGURE 6-9 Head front view, step 3.

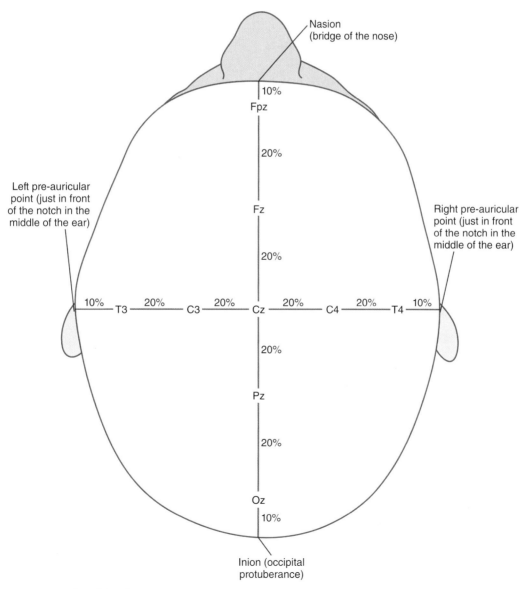

Nasion
(bridge of the nose)

10%

Fpz

20%

Left pre-auricular
point (just in front
of the notch in the
middle of the ear)

Fz

Right pre-auricular
point (just in front
of the notch in the
middle of the ear)

20%

10% — T3 — 20% — C3 — 20% — Cz — 20% — C4 — 20% — T4 — 10%

20%

Pz

20%

Oz

10%

Inion (occipital
protuberance)

FIGURE 6-10 Step 3 drawing.

mark would be 6 cm to the left of Fp1 or 9 cm to the left of Fpz. Do the same on the right side of the head. These two marks, with the horizontal line from Fp1 and Fp2 extended, will show the locations for F7 and F8. These points are all shown in **Figures 6-11** through **6-13**.

Step 5: Measure and Mark from Fp1 to O1 and from Fp2 to O2

Measure from Fp1 to O1, passing the tape measure over the mark that is 20% down on the left side from Cz (the first mark made for C3). Assume this measurement is 24 cm. Mark 50% of this measurement—in this example, 12 cm. This mark should intersect the mark that is 20% down to the left of Cz. The intersection of these two marks is the exact location for C3. Mark 25% of this measurement, or halfway between Fp1 and C3. This is the first mark for F3. Do the same on the right side to find C4 and the first mark for F4. See **Figures 6-14** through **6-16** for these marks.

Step 6: Measure and Mark from F7 to F8

Measure from F7 to F8, passing the tape measure directly over the first mark made for Fz in step 2 and for F3 and F4 in step 5. Assume this measurement is 16 cm. Mark 50% of this measurement—8 cm in this example. This line will intersect the first mark made for Fz, and the intersection will mark the exact location for Fz. Mark 25% on each side—in this example, 4 cm. These marks will intersect the first marks made for F3 and F4, and the intersection of these marks will give the exact locations of F3 and F4. (See **Figures 6-17** and **6-18**.)

After completing these steps, the following electrode sites have been marked: Fpz, Fp1, Fp2, Fz, F3, F4, F7, F8, Cz, C3, C4, Oz, O1, and O2. For the staging of sleep, electrodes are placed at the following six EEG locations: F3, F4, C3, C4, O1, and O2. M1 and M2 are reference electrodes that are placed behind the ears high on the

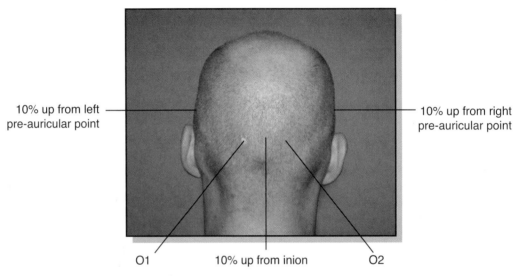

FIGURE 6-11 Head back view, step 4.

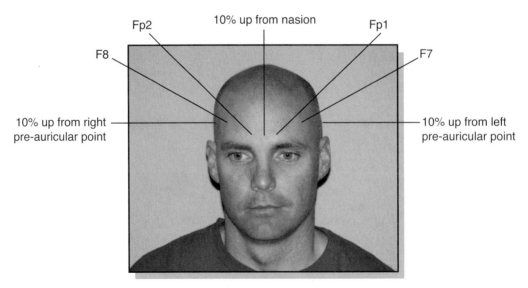

FIGURE 6-12 Head front view, step 4.

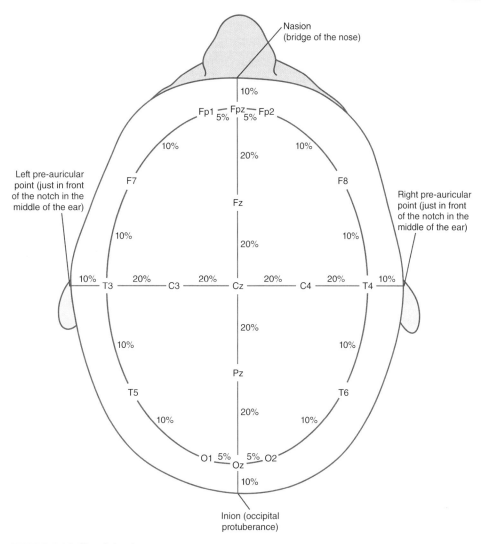

FIGURE 6-13 Step 4 drawing.

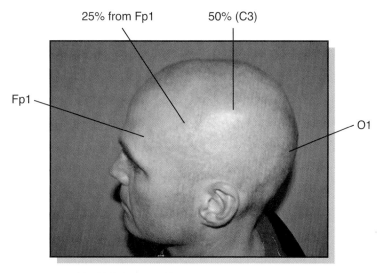

FIGURE 6-14 Head left view, step 5.

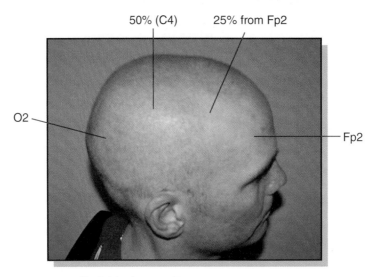

FIGURE 6-15 Head right view, step 5.

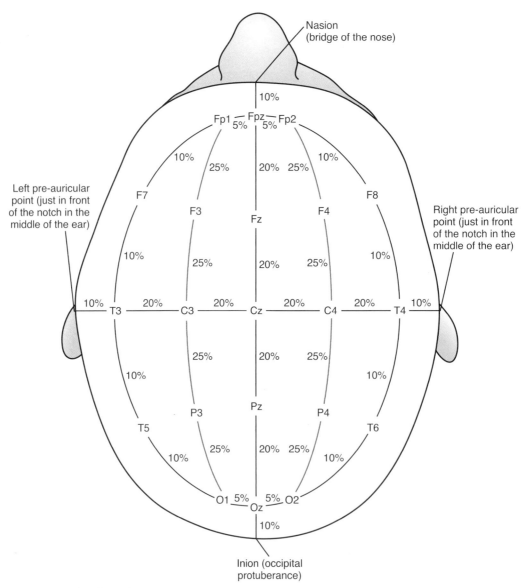

FIGURE 6-16 Step 5 drawing.

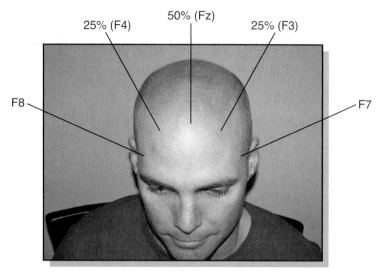

25% (F4)   50% (Fz)   25% (F3)

F8   F7

FIGURE 6-17 Head front view, step 6.

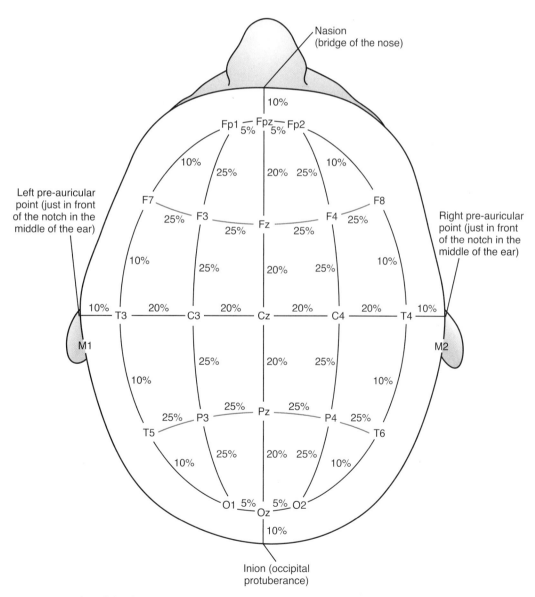

Nasion
(bridge of the nose)

10%

Fp1 Fpz Fp2
     5%   5%

10%   10%
      25%   20% 25%

Left pre-auricular
point (just in front
of the notch in the
middle of the ear)

F7   F8

25%   F3   Fz   F4   25%
      25%   25%

Right pre-auricular
point (just in front
of the notch in the
middle of the ear)

10%   25%   20%   25%   10%

10%   T3 20% C3 20% Cz 20% C4 20% T4 10%

M1   M2

25%   20%   25%

10%   10%

25%   25%
T5 25% P3   Pz   P4 25% T6

10%   25%   20% 25%   10%

O1 5% Oz 5% O2

10%

Inion (occipital
protuberance)

FIGURE 6-18 Step 6 drawing.

mastoid process. Alternatively, M1 and M2 can be placed on the earlobes. Ground electrodes (and main reference if needed) are often placed at Cz, Fz, or Fp1 locations.

Option 2: Placement for EEG Electrodes for Full EEG Hookup

For a full EEG hookup in a sleep study, the steps are the same but with additional marks. The following additions are made to the standard sleep hookup when performing a full EEG hookup with a sleep study. EEG hookups may vary according to protocol and individual requests by physicians.

Step 1: Step 1 remains the same in the full EEG hookup as it is for locating the six EEG electrode sites when performing a standard sleep study.

Step 2: In step 2, an additional mark is placed 20% of the measurement down in the back from Cz. This is the first mark for locating Pz.

Step 3: Step 3 remains the same. The marks placed 10% up from the pre-auricular points are the first marks for locating T3 and T4.

Step 4: In step 4, additional marks are placed at the 25% points, which will be almost directly over the pre-auricular points. These will intersect with the marks that are 10% up from the pre-auricular points, giving the exact locations for T3 and T4. Additional marks made in the back of the head are similar to the marks made for F7 and F8. In the back of the head, these are the locations for T5 and T6.

Step 5: In step 5, an additional mark is placed on the back of the head, 25% of this measurement up from O1. This gives the first mark for P3. This is repeated on the right side for P4.

Step 6: In step 6, a measurement is made on the back of the head from T5 to T6, similar to the measurement made in the front of the head from F7 to F8. The 50% mark intersects with the mark placed 20% down in the back from Cz, and gives the exact location for Pz. The 25% marks intersect with the first marks made for P3 and P4 and give the exact location for these two electrodes.

With these additions, the following electrode sites have been marked: Fpz, Fp1, Fp2, Fz, F3, F4, F7, F8, Cz, C3, C4, T3, T4, Pz, P3, P4, T5, T6, Oz, O1, and O2. These electrode sites may be used in various combinations and montages for more advanced electroneurodiagnostics.

Other Electrode Sites

The international 10/20 system provides measurements to find sites for EEG electrodes in adults and children. Following are instructions for locating each required

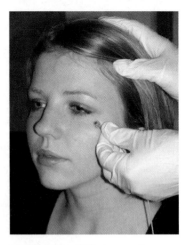

FIGURE 6-19 EOG placement.

electrode site on the face and body. Nuances between the adult and pediatric patient are discussed where applicable, otherwise the placement is the same regardless of patient age or size.

Electrooculogram (EOG) Electrodes

The electrooculogram (EOG) leads are placed 1 cm laterally and 1 cm up or down from the outer **canthus** (see **Figure 6-19**). The canthus is the corner of the eye, or the point at which the eyelids meet. The recommended placement for adult patients is to place the right EOG (termed E2) 1 cm laterally and 1 cm up from the right outer canthus, and the left EOG lead (E1) 1 cm laterally and 1 cm down from the left outer canthus. These are both referenced to the same lead, usually M2. An alternate EOG hookup is to place both EOG leads 1 cm laterally and 1 cm down from the outer canthus of each eye. In children, the EOG electrode placement may be reduced to 0.5 cm laterally on each side because of the smaller size of the face.

Chin Electromyogram (EMG)

The EMG channels used in polysomnography have bipolar derivations in that the signal is derived from two active (exploring) electrodes. This differs from an EEG channel that derives its signal from one active and one reference electrode (a referential channel). To record muscle activity at the chin, three chin electromyogram (EMG) leads are placed. Two of these provide the primary signal for the chin EMG while the third serves as a backup in case either of the other leads detaches during the night. The first lead is placed in the middle of the chin, 1 cm above the inferior edge of the mandible (the electrode marked "A" in **Figure 6-20**). The other two are placed below the inferior edge of the chin ("B" and "C"). One should be placed 2 cm down and 2 cm to the left of the midline,

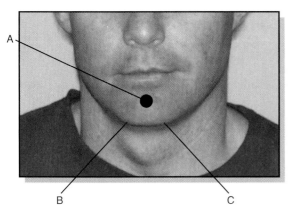

FIGURE 6-20 Chin lead placement.

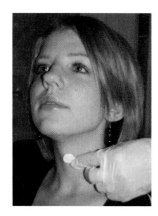

FIGURE 6-21 Snore sensor placement.

and the other 2 cm down and 2 cm to the right of the midline. For optimal chin EMG recordings, one of the two active inputs should be above the chin and the other one below. In the example in Figure 6-20, the chin EMG channel would be derived of electrode A and B or C. If B or C were to come unattached during the recording, the other could be used. This would ensure that the recording can continue without disturbing the patient. For pediatric patients, the measurements are often reduced to 1 cm above and below the mandibular edge and 1 cm to the right and left of the midline.

Airflow Sensors

Two airflow sensors—a thermal device and a pressure transducer cannula—are placed directly in front of the nose and mouth. These devices detect airflow from both the nose and the mouth.

Snore Sensor/Microphone

The snore sensor or microphone is usually placed directly on the center of the patient's throat (see **Figure 6-21**). The patient is asked to cough lightly while the technologist feels for these vibrations on the throat. The technologist then places the snore sensor on the location where the vibrations are the strongest. Snore microphones detect the sound of the snore and should be placed at a location where the snoring can be heard. Often technologists choose to place a snore microphone near the nose or mouth as opposed to on the throat.

Electrocardiogram (ECG) Leads

Sleep study montages must use at least a single-channel, two-lead electrocardiogram (ECG). The ECG provides a display of the electrical activity of the heart. In a two-lead ECG hookup, one lead is placed directly under the middle of the right collarbone (see **Figure 6-22**), and

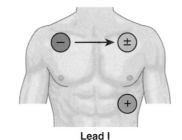

Lead I

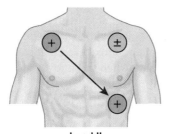

Lead II

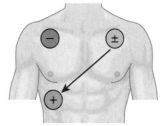

Lead III

FIGURE 6-22 ECG lead placement.

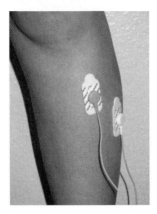

FIGURE 6-23 Leg lead placement.

the other is placed on the lower left side of the ribcage. The exploring electrode is the lead on the lower left, and the reference is the lead on the upper right collarbone. This provides an upright lead II monitoring ECG signal. An additional ECG lead may be placed under the middle of the left collarbone. This can serve as a backup electrode should one of the other two become dislodged during the study. Using three electrodes provides the opportunity to display two additional waveforms of the heart rhythm (leads I and III). All three waveforms will portray upright p waves, QRS complexes, and T waves in patients with normal heart rhythms.

Leg EMG Leads

Two electrodes are placed on the outside of the lower half of each leg. Specifically, they should be applied to the middle of the **anterior tibialis** muscle so they are 2–3 cm apart (see **Figure 6-23**). Foot and leg movements are best detected from this muscle. It is strongly recommended to have separate channels for each leg. However, if not enough channels are available for separate leg channels, one electrode can be placed on each leg, and these two electrodes can be referenced to each other. This is not ideal because it does not allow right and left movements to be differentiated.

Respiratory Effort

Detection of respiratory effort is most commonly accomplished with the use of effort belts that are stretched around the chest and abdomen. The AASM currently recommends the use of belts that use either respiratory inductive plethysmography (see **Figure 6-24**) or polyvinylidene fluoride technology.[2] The technologist should take care to avoid pulling the belts so tight that they restrict the patient's breathing or are uncomfortable.

Oximeter Finger Sensor

The finger sensor for the oximeter is placed on the tip of any of the three middle fingers. On one side of the device is a red light; on the other side is a sensor that reads the red light. These two must be aligned with

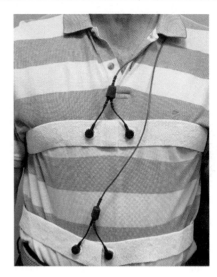

FIGURE 6-24 Respiratory belt placement.

each other, on opposite sides of the fingertip. Any fingernail polish should be removed because it can inhibit the oximeter's ability to accurately detect the oxygen level in the blood.

Electrode Application[2]

This section will discuss the proper methods of applying an electrode. Although the examples and pictures used in this section refer to EEG electrode placement, the same principles apply to other electrode sites.

Locate the Electrode Site

Locating the proper electrode site is perhaps the most important step in electrode application. Although obtaining clean artifact tracings is important, acquiring the desired signals is perhaps more important. Placing an electrode—whether it be an EEG, EOG, EMG, or other channel type—in the wrong location can lead to misdiagnosis and treatment of the patient. To locate EEG electrode sites, the technologist should always measure the head using the international 10/20 system of electrode placement discussed previously in this chapter (see **Figure 6-25**). Many experienced technologists believe they can acquire the desired EEGs by approximating electrode site locations; however, this is not the case. Careful EEG measurement is always required when performing a patient hookup. After each EEG electrode site has been located, the technologist marks these sites with a grease pencil. The pencil is made from a nontoxic wax that can easily be removed from the skin when the study is completed.

Prepare the Electrode Site

Once the electrode sites have been located and marked through proper measuring techniques, the technologist cleans and prepares the site. Electrode impedances must be minimized to achieve optimal recordings. Among

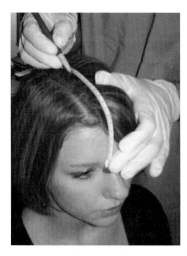

FIGURE 6-25 Locating the electrode site.

the most common causes of high electrode impedances are dirt, debris, and dead skin at the bridge between the electrode and the skin. Therefore, proper cleaning of the site can greatly reduce impedances and increase the quality of the recording.

The technologist prepares the site by removing the marker, dead skin, dirt, and other debris from the scalp at the site with a cotton swab and a skin prep solution (see **Figures 6-26** and **6-27**). Many of the skin preparation solutions used for this purpose contain a mild abrasive to help remove oils and dead skin from the site. The size of the scrubbed area should be no larger than the size of the cup of the electrode. When preparing an electrode site on the face or body, the same method applies; an alternate method is simply cleaning the site with an alcohol pad. Other electrode sites, such as the legs and the chest, may require shaving to allow the electrodes to stick to the skin.

Prepare the Electrode

After prepping the electrode site, the cup of the electrode is filled with an electrically conductive paste or gel (see **Figure 6-28**). The paste should completely fill the cup electrode to allow the bioelectric signals to enter the signal pathway with little resistance. When using snap leads, the wire lead is snapped to a sticky button-like electrode that contains its own conductive medium.

Place the Electrode

The electrode is now placed in the location that was located and cleaned (see **Figure 6-29**). The hair should be moved to allow for a space on the scalp big enough for the cup electrode to be placed against the scalp. When placing the EEG electrode, it is important to

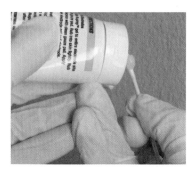

FIGURE 6-26 Prep gel.

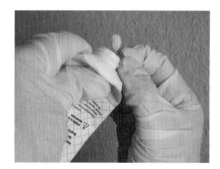

FIGURE 6-28 Electrode paste.

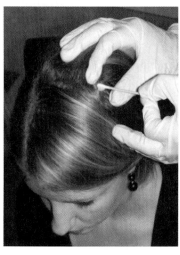

FIGURE 6-27 Prepping the electrode site.

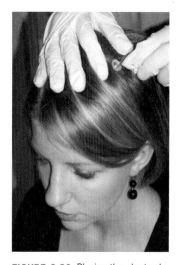

FIGURE 6-29 Placing the electrode.

press firmly against the scalp so that all sides of the metal cup are in direct contact with the skin. This minimizes electrode impedances and the likelihood of a 60-Hz artifact contaminating the signal. If the paste completely fills the electrode like it should, it is not uncommon for some of it to squeeze out the sides and the top hole of the electrode. When placing a snap electrode on the face or body, the center of the sticky electrode must be in direct contact with the skin and pressed firmly to record the desired signals. All electrode wires should be directed toward the back of the head so they can be gathered out of the way of the patient's face.

Adhering the Electrode

Cup electrodes are adhered to the scalp using a square piece of gauze and additional EEG paste. The gauze is placed diagonally over the cup, with the center of the gauze directly over the center of the cup and the lower edge of the gauze extending down onto the wire (see **Figure 6-30**). A relatively small amount of EEG paste is applied to the bottom of the gauze and resides between the gauze and the cup or scalp. While holding the gauze and cup in place, the technologist presses the paste against the cup and scalp using a fingernail or tongue depressor. This pressing motion begins at the center of the cup and moves outward. The paste will hold the gauze tight against the cup and the skin when performed properly. When adhering a cup electrode to the face or body, tape or sticky gauze is used. Snap electrode stickers adhere easily to any skin surface free of hair. Many technologists find it helpful to add small pieces of tape to the electrodes on the face and body to help secure the edges (see **Figure 6-31**).

Although it is not used as widely as it once was, some labs still use collodion and similar glues rather than EEG paste to secure cup electrodes to the patient's

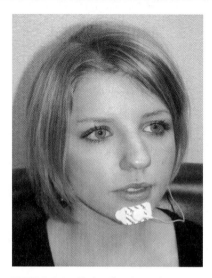

FIGURE 6-31 Taping the electrode.

scalp. EEG glue is sometimes used in place of paste because it holds the cup electrodes against the scalp very securely throughout the night, regardless of how much the patient moves. EEG glue is being used less frequently for sleep testing because of its noxious smell, which can cause the patient and technologist to feel lightheaded and dizzy. When using an EEG glue, it is important to complete the setup in a room that is well ventilated and separate from the patient bedroom. Even with these precautions, most technologists highly prefer EEG paste, even though the likelihood of electrode movement increases with paste.

Impedance Checks

Impedances are measures of electrical resistance. Electrode impedances are checked after the patient hookup is completed. The AASM recommends that electrical impedances for EEGs and EOGs be below 5,000 ohms.[2] High impedances increase the chance of poor quality signals. This can make the scoring of the study difficult and could possibly affect the diagnosis or treatment of the patient. Electrodes with impedances higher than 5,000 ohms should be removed, the site cleaned, and the electrode reapplied or replaced. Impedance checks should be performed at the beginning and end of the study. Additional impedance checks may be performed as needed or according to lab protocol. For example, some labs require one impedance check every hour during the recording to ensure the quality of the study.

Helpful Strategies for Sleep Technologists

Following are helpful strategies that many technologists have found helpful in the patient hookup process.

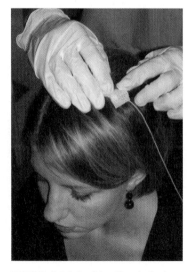

FIGURE 6-30 Applying the electrode.

Antiperspirant

To decrease the prevalence of sweat artifact, some technologists apply small amounts of antiperspirant to certain electrode sites before applying the electrode. Impedances should be carefully monitored when using this method, because the use of antiperspirant may decrease signal quality.

Ponytailing

Because of the large number of wires used in a hookup, many patients tend to get tangled during the night as movement occurs. When this happens, it creates tension on the wire and often causes the electrode to disconnect from the skin. To prevent this, most sleep technologists use a method of "ponytailing," or grouping the wires in a common location on or near the patient. When applying the electrodes, the wires should be faced toward the location where the grouping will take place to decrease the likelihood of the electrodes detaching when pulled. Many technologists group the wires together at the patient's chest, shoulder, or top of the head or on the bed close to the patient.

Patient Questionnaires

Many labs require technologists to perform two or three patient hookups in a shift, which challenges the technologist's time and abilities. Many technologists find it helpful for the patient to complete the questionnaires during the hookup to maximize efficiency. Further, if the patient has questions about the forms as they are completing them, the technologist is readily available to address the questions.

Positive Airway Pressure Desensitization

Many patients have difficulty tolerating continuous positive airway pressure (CPAP) the first time they use it. Some technologists find it helpful to have the patient breathe with the CPAP mask on and the pressure set at a low level before the patient hookup begins. This better uses the technician's time and allows him or her to work with other patients while the first patient is becoming desensitized to CPAP. It also decreases the amount of time spent at the beginning of the study working out tolerance issues with the patient.

Chapter Summary

The patient hookup is one of the most important steps in performing a sleep study. A properly performed patient hookup provides accurate recordings of the patient's EEGs, EOGs, EMGs, and other parameters, with minimal artifact. Putting forth the extra time and effort to perform a quality hookup at the beginning of the night can save the technologist a lot of unnecessary work later during the night.

The international 10/20 electrode placement system was designed in 1949 to locate the proper electrode sites for recording EEGs. This system of measurements of the head uses specific landmarks as the beginning points for all measurements. Distances between the measurements are divided by certain percentages to find electrode sites. In polysomnography, six electrode sites are used to identify sleep stages. In EEG studies and sleep studies with full EEG montages, many electrode sites are identified using the international 10/20 system.

In addition to the EEG electrode sites, the technologist must be able to identify and locate electrode sites on the face and body. These include the sites for EOG electrodes, chin EMG electrodes, airflow sensors, snore microphones and sensors, ECG leads, respiratory effort belts, leg EMG electrodes, oximeter finger probes, and others.

Electrodes are placed on the skin differently, depending on the type of electrode used. All electrodes should be thoroughly cleaned before application. The electrode sites also need to be cleaned, removing dirt and dead skin. The electrode is filled with an electrically conductive paste and pressed firmly against the skin. It is then held in place by tape or gauze.

After the patient hookup, impedance checks are performed on all channels. Optimal impedances for EEG and EOG channels are less than 5,000 ohms.

Chapter 6 Questions

Please consider the following questions as they relate to the material in this chapter.

1. Why are percentages used in the international 10/20 system rather than uniform distances?
2. What electrode site is 20% of the distance from the nasion to the inion in front of Cz?
3. Why are three electrodes placed on the chin?
4. What muscle are the leg EMG electrodes placed on?
5. Why is it important to clean and prepare a site before placing an electrode?
6. What is an impedance? Why is it important to keep impedances low?

Footnotes

1. Trans Cranial Technologies. (2012). 10/20 system positioning manual. Accessed from http://chgd.umich.edu/wp-content/uploads/2014/06/10-20_system_positioning.pdf
2. American Academy of Sleep Medicine. (2017). *AASM manual for the scoring of sleep and associated events: Rules terminology and technical specifications*, Version 2.4. Darien, IL: Author.

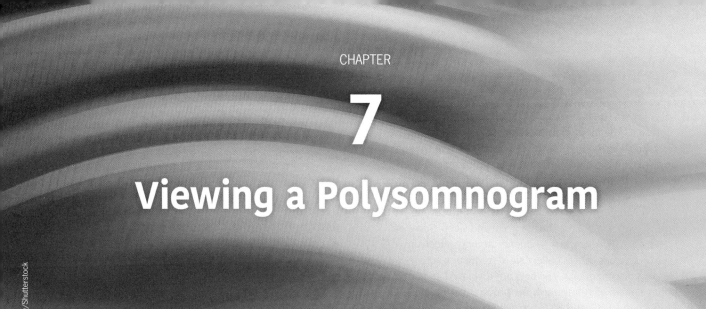

Viewing a Polysomnogram

CHAPTER OUTLINE

Display of Data
EEG Channels
EOG Channels
EMG Channels
ECG Channel
Respiratory Channels
Oxygen Saturation (SpO₂)
Body Position
Chapter Summary

LEARNING OBJECTIVES

1. Identify the various parameters recorded in polysomnography.
2. Understand how these parameters are collected and displayed on the record.
3. Learn the value that each parameter adds to the interpretation of the study.
4. Understand the significance of certain recorded events.

KEY TERMS

polysomnogram
paper speed
epoch
electroencephalogram
  (EEG)
brain waves
montage
amplitude
frequency
morphology
EEG arousal
seizure activity
beta spindles
referential montage
electroocculogram (EOG)

outer canthus
E1
E2
conjugate eye movements
electromyogram
  (EMG)
bipolar channel
electrocardiogram (ECG)
electrokardiogram (EKG)
ECG arrhythmia
atria
ventricles
SpO₂
oxygen saturation
oxygen desaturation

Display of Data

The term **polysomnogram** is derived from Greek and Latin roots. The first part, *poly*, indicates *many* and represents the many channels of data collected. *Somno* refers to sleep, and *gram* or *graphy* refers to the writing or display of the data. Various parameters are collected as part of a diagnostic sleep study, and the data are displayed as lines, or channels, on the record. The channels are viewed simultaneously to show activity from several parts of the body at one time during wake and sleep. Some of the channels portray fast frequency activity (electromyogram), whereas others collect slow-frequency activity (respiratory channels). The data are displayed at a rate, or **paper speed**, of 10 mm/sec. For polysomnography, EEG, EOG, chin EMG, and EKG activity is optimally viewed as a 30-second "page," most often referred to as an **epoch**. For slower-frequency channels like airflow, several epochs can be combined to display windows of larger time segments. Common window widths range from 120 seconds (4 epochs) to 300 seconds (10 epochs).

EEG Channels

The first type of channel on a polysomnograph is the **electroencephalogram (EEG)**. EEG leads are placed on the head to detect impulses, or **brain waves**, from specific areas of the cortex. Because these signals alternate quickly from positive to negative deflections, they are directed through an alternating current (AC) differential amplifier. The standard EEG electrodes used during a sleep study, as recommended by the American Academy of Sleep Medicine (AASM)[1] are as follows:

- F3
- F4
- C3
- C4
- O1
- O2
- M1 (reference)
- M2 (reference)

Although a standard sleep study requires only three EEG channels (one frontal, one central, and one occipital), six exploring electrodes are most often placed to serve as backups if necessary. In this text, all six EEG channels are shown. **Figure 7-1** reviews the scalp location sites for these electrodes.

The sample epoch in **Figure 7-2** shows a typical layout or **montage** for a standard diagnostic sleep study. This layout may change according to individual preferences. In this example, the top six channels are EEG channels. EEG data are used in sleep primarily for

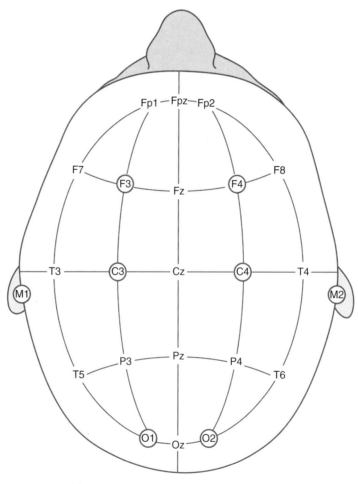

FIGURE 7-1 EEG sites.

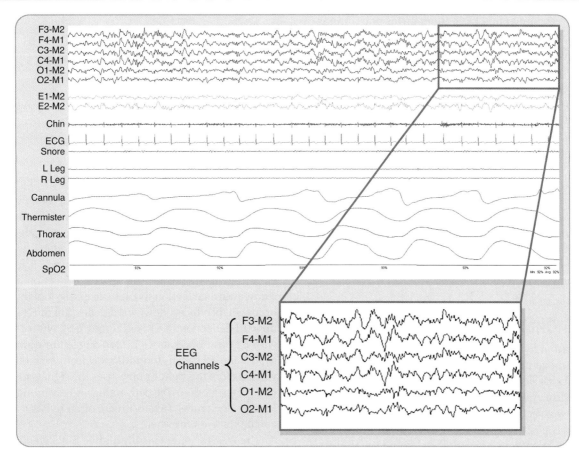

FIGURE 7-2 Sleep study montage.

determining wakefulness versus sleep and to distinguish the various stages of sleep. The **amplitude**, **frequency**, and **morphology** (shape) of the waves help the reader determine the stage of sleep (see **Figure 7-3**).

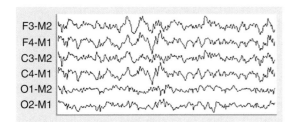

FIGURE 7-3 EEG sample waves.

EEGs are also recorded to detect **EEG arousals**. An EEG arousal is an abrupt shift in brain wave frequency lasting at least 3 seconds, and preceded by at least 10 seconds of sleep.[1] EEGs are also beneficial in detecting other events such as **seizure activity** and **beta spindles**.

Figure 7-4 is a sample from a sleep study that shows an EEG arousal. Here the patient was asleep and then had an abrupt shift in EEG frequency for at least 3 seconds. An EEG arousal may occur spontaneously, in response to external stimuli such as a loud noise, or because of abnormal events such as periodic limb movements or respiratory events.

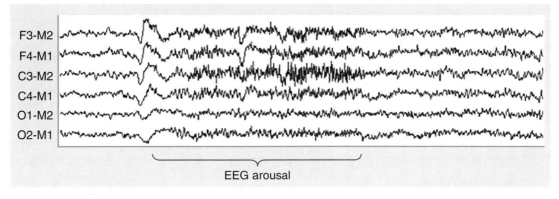

FIGURE 7-4 EEG arousal.

The recommended EEG montage for polysomnography is a **referential montage**. Referential montages use one active electrode and one reference electrode for each channel. For EEG channels collected in a standard diagnostic sleep study, the electrodes on the left side of the head—namely, F3, C3, and O1—are all referenced to the opposite mastoid, M2. Therefore, any signal produced at the M2 site or detected by the M2 electrode will manifest itself in all three of these channels. Conversely, the electrodes on the ride side of the head—namely, F4, C4, and O2—are all referenced to M1. The signals derived at F3 and F4 should be similar because they lay over the same area of the frontal cortex on each side. However, they will not be identical because they have different reference electrodes. This is also true of the C3 and C4 electrodes as well as the O1 and O2 electrodes.

EOG Channels

In addition to brain wave activity, the presence and type of eye movements during sleep are also used to identify the various sleep stages. The **electrooculogram (EOG)** is the display of eye movements. The signal is derived from two electrodes placed near the eyes. Because the cornea is positively charged with respect to the retina, when a patient looks toward the electrode, a positive charge is sent to the polysomnograph, resulting in a downward pen deflection. When a patient looks away from the EOG electrode, a negative charge results, creating an upward pen deflection.

Proper placement of the EOG electrodes requires identifying the **outer canthus**, the junction of the upper and lower eyelids on the outside perimeter of the eye. Electrode placement recommended by the AASM[1] for the left EOG is 1 cm lateral to the outer canthus and 1 cm below the eye, and the right-eye electrode is placed 1 cm laterally to the outer canthus and 1 cm above the eye. The left EOG electrode is referred to as **E1**, and the right EOG electrode is **E2** (see **Figure 7-5**). This placement allows the reader to see both horizontal and vertical eye movements.

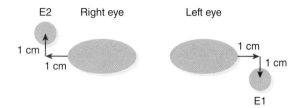

FIGURE 7-5 EOG placement.

EOG Example 1: E2 Up, E1 Down

As previously mentioned, when a patient looks away from the EOG electrode, an upward pen deflection is produced, whereas looking toward the electrode will produce a downward signal. Therefore, when the EOG electrodes are placed as depicted in Figure 7-5, looking left or down will produce an upward deflection in E2 and a downward deflection in E1. Conversely, looking right or up will produce a downward deflection in E2 and an upward deflection in E1 (see **Figure 7-6**). Notice that with E2 positioned above E1, looking left or down causes the E1 and E2 signals to move away from each other, whereas looking right or up causes the signals to move toward each other. The converging and diverging of the E1 and E2 channel waveforms are often referred to as **conjugate eye movements**.

The AASM[1] offers an alternative EOG electrode placement that is also acceptable for use in collecting eye movements. Specifically, the E1 electrode can be placed 1 cm below and 1 cm laterally to the outer canthus of the left eye and the E2 electrode 1 cm below and 1 cm laterally to the outer canthus of the right eye (see **Figure 7-7**).

EOG Example 2: E1 Down, E2 Down

In this example, E1 and E2 are both placed 1 cm out from and below the eyes as shown in Figure 7-7. When looking directly left or right, the channels will respond similarly to the preceding example (see **Figure 7-8**). However, when the eyes look up, both channels will receive negative signals resulting in upward pen deflections. When both eyes look down, both channels

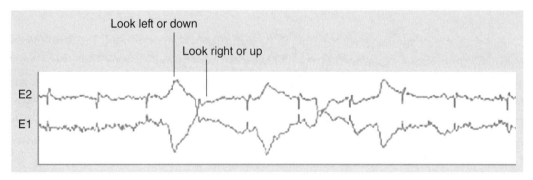

FIGURE 7-6 EOG Example 1.

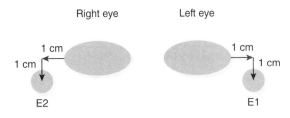

FIGURE 7-7 EOG alternative placement.

will receive positive signals resulting in downward pen deflections (see **Figure 7-9**).

EMG Channels

The **electromyogram (EMG)** portrays the recording of muscle activity and tone. Muscle tone, particularly of the chin and jaw area, is an important criterium used in determining sleep stages. Muscle tone decreases in amplitude from wake to sleep, and it decreases further during rapid eye movement (REM) sleep. Further, many sleep disorders are characterized by movements of specific muscle groups during sleep.

For the purpose of polysomnography, it is not necessary to identify specific wave forms or shapes in EMGs, but rather amplitude changes. Sharp, abrupt changes

in amplitude may indicate muscle movement such as a leg jerk or twitch. Gradual, subtle changes in EMG amplitude may indicate a change in muscle tone, such as when the muscles in the chin relax at sleep onset.

EMGs recorded in sleep testing include the chin, legs, and, in some cases, the arms. Other muscle groups may be recorded depending on lab protocol or special patient needs. The EMG channels are set up as **bipolar channels** that use two exploring electrodes rather than an exploring and a reference electrode.

Three electrodes are used in recording the chin EMG activity. The channel is derived using two of the three electrodes. The third serves as a backup electrode because a quality chin EMG is important in determining sleep stages. The amplitude of the chin EMG is set relatively high at the beginning of the night, so subtle decreases in tone at sleep onset and REM onset can more easily be detected.

EMG Examples 1 and 2

In **Figures 7-10** and **7-11**, the chin EMG is relatively high during non-rapid eye movement (NREM) and will decrease during REM. The leg EMG channels show no movement or activity during these epochs.

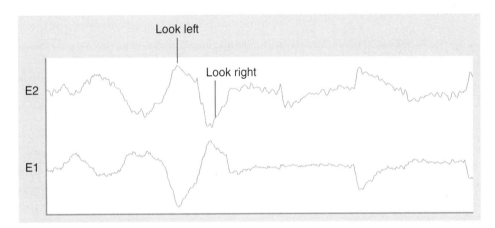

FIGURE 7-8 EOG Example 2.

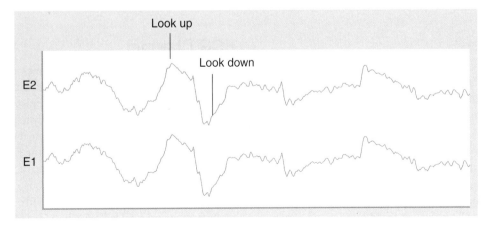

FIGURE 7-9 EOG Example 2.

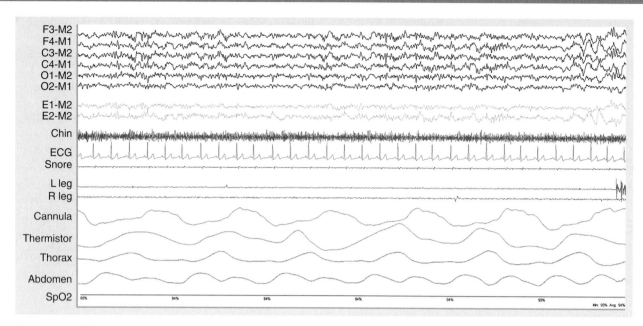

FIGURE 7-10 EMG Example 1.

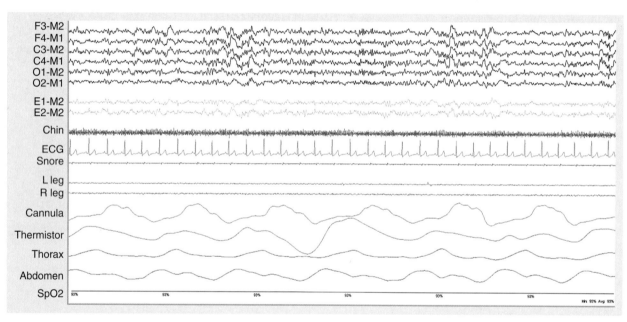

FIGURE 7-11 EMG Example 2.

EMG Example 3

At the beginning of the epoch shown in **Figure 7-12**, the chin EMG amplitude is low. A few seconds into the epoch, the chin EMG amplitude increases dramatically. In this case, this change results from the end of a REM period.

EMG Example 4

In **Figure 7-13**, increased amplitude is noted at the end of hypopnea in the chin EMG channel, the snore microphone, and the leg EMG channels. This represents an arousal from sleep accompanied by a leg movement and an audible snore.

ECG Channel

The **electrocardiogram (ECG)**, sometimes spelled **electrokardiogram (EKG)** because of its German roots, is a recording of the heart's electrical impulse activity. The ECG is recorded as part of a sleep study to provide information about the heart rate and rhythm and to ensure a patient's safety throughout the night. The ECG provides the ability to identify abnormal electrical activity that may occur. Some sleep disorders, like obstructive sleep apnea (OSA), where patients have periods of reduced or no breathing and reduced oxygenation, add stress to the cardiovascular system. This additional strain on the heart

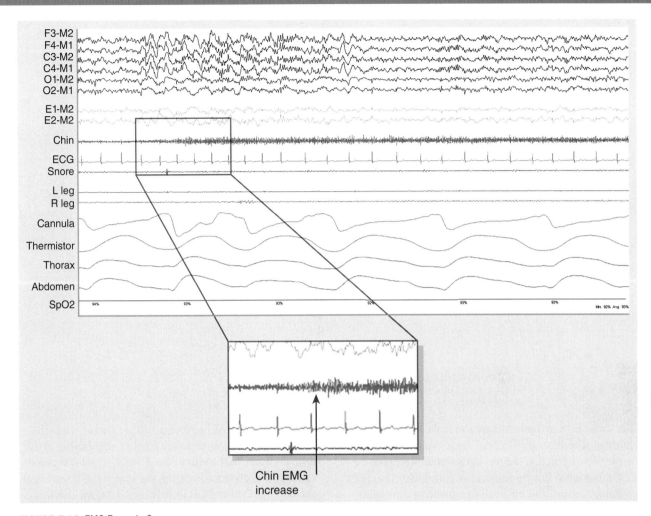

FIGURE 7-12 EMG Example 3.

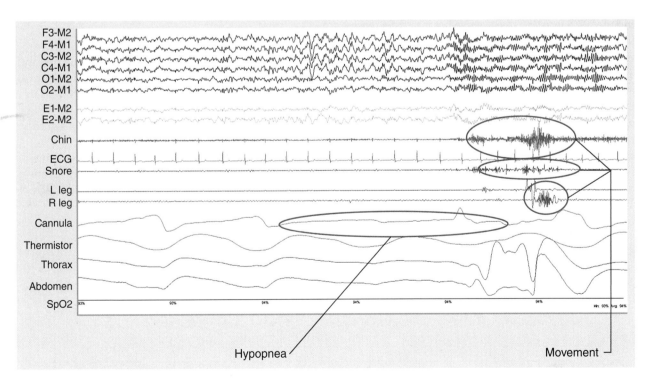

FIGURE 7-13 EMG Example 4.

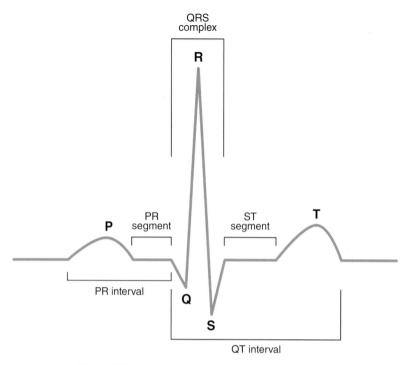

FIGURE 7-14 Normal ECG.

Created by Agateller (Anthony Atkielski), converted to svg by atom. - SinusRhythmLabels.png, Public Domain, https://commons.wikimedia.org/w/index.php?curid=1560893

may cause **ECG arrhythmias**, or abnormal heart rates or rhythms. Therefore, it is critical that sleep technologists be properly trained in the mechanics and interpretation of ECGs and know how to respond in emergency situations.

Rate, rhythm, and intervals between the different waves are all important factors to consider when interpreting an ECG and can help identify abnormalities. The normal adult heart rate while awake is 60–100 beats per minute.[2] While asleep, the average heart rate decreases by 10–20 beats per minute. The normal ECG rhythm is made up of a P wave, a QRS complex, and a T wave (see **Figure 7-14**). Each waveform corresponds to a portion of the heart's electrical and mechanical activity. The P wave indicates the contraction of the **atria**, or upper chambers of the heart. The QRS complex corresponds to the contraction of the **ventricles**, or lower chambers of the heart. Lastly, the T wave indicates the repolarization of the ventricles. Segments and intervals of the waveform can also provide important information. The PR interval refers to the distance from the beginning

of the P wave to the beginning of the Q wave while the QT interval refers to distance from the beginning of the QRS complex to the end of the T wave. The PR segment refers to the distance between the end of the P wave and the beginning of the QRS while the ST segment refers to the distance from the end of the QRS complex to the beginning of the T wave.[3] Normal values and interpretation of ECG rhythms will be discussed later in the text.

ECG Example 1

The ECG in **Figure 7-15** shows a normal sinus rhythm. Each beat has a P wave, a QRS complex, and a T wave. This 30-second sample shows 33 beats, which tells us the rate is 66 beats per minute (bpm). This falls within normal range for adult patients. There are no significant artifacts in the tracing.

The ECG sample in **Figure 7-16** does not have any significant artifact, but the tracings of the P waves are not as visible as in Figure 7-15. This 30-second epoch shows 27 beats, which is a rate of 54 bpm.

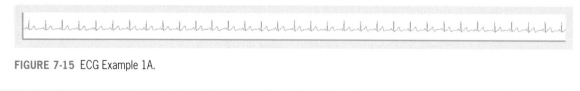

FIGURE 7-15 ECG Example 1A.

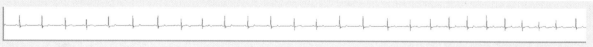

FIGURE 7-16 ECG Example 1B.

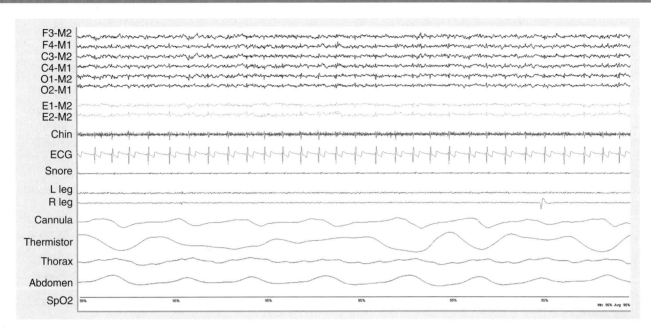

FIGURE 7-17 ECG Example 2A.

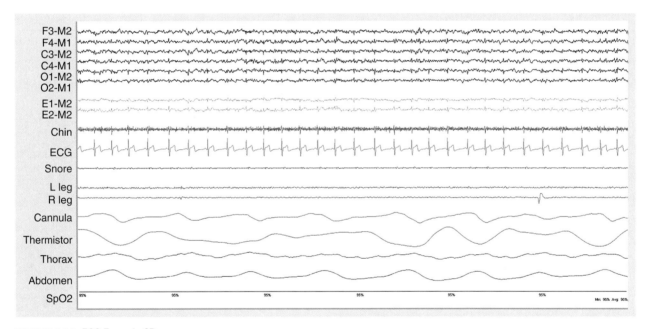

FIGURE 7-18 ECG Example 2B.

ECG Example 2

The ECG tracing in the sample in **Figure 7-17** is upside down. This occurs when the positive and negative leads are plugged into the wrong inputs. This is easily corrected by switching the plugs in the head box or changing the polarity settings. In **Figure 7-18**, the problem has been corrected.

Respiratory Channels

Respiratory parameters recorded in polysomnography include airflow and respiratory effort. Most often this is accomplished via a thermal sensor, a pressure transducer, and respiratory effort belts. Respiratory channels are the slowest of the AC channels on the polysomnograph. The waveform is sinusoidal in nature, and the frequency is determined by the speed of the breath. The faster the patient breathes, the faster the wave oscillates. The amplitude of the wave is determined by the volume of air inhaled and exhaled. A deeper breath results in a higher amplitude wave. During a continuous positive airway pressure (CPAP) titration, the airflow is often recorded by the CPAP machine as a direct current (DC) channel. The resulting waveform looks similar to the airflow waveform as read by a thermal sensor or pressure transducer. Airflow is recorded primarily to detect apneas, hypopneas, and other respiratory disturbances.

Respiratory events can occur as a result of airway obstruction (obstructive apnea or hypopnea) or the central nervous system telling the body not to breathe (central apnea). To distinguish between obstructive and central events, data on respiratory effort must be collected. Respiratory effort data are collected most often from belts placed around the abdomen and thorax to determine whether the patient is attempting to breathe. A lack of respiratory effort is characterized by a flattening in amplitude in the respiratory effort channels, whereas continued effort is marked by continuous excursions on the waveform.

Respiratory Channels Examples 1 and 2

The examples provided in **Figures 7-19** and **7-20** portray respiratory channels that are included as part of a diagnostic sleep study. Note there are two airflow channels—one from a nasal pressure transducer and one from a thermistor, and two effort channels—one from the thoracic belt and one from the abdominal belt. Note the sinusoidal signal pattern and synchrony between the channels.

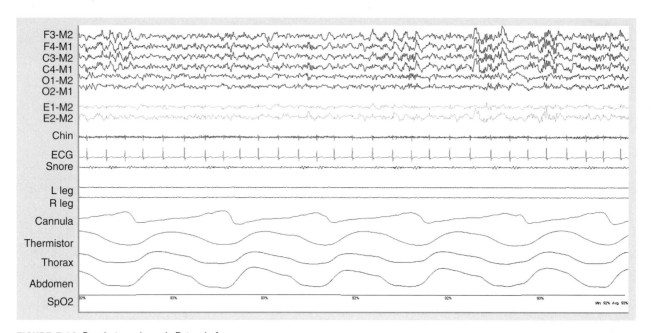

FIGURE 7-19 Respiratory channels Example 1.

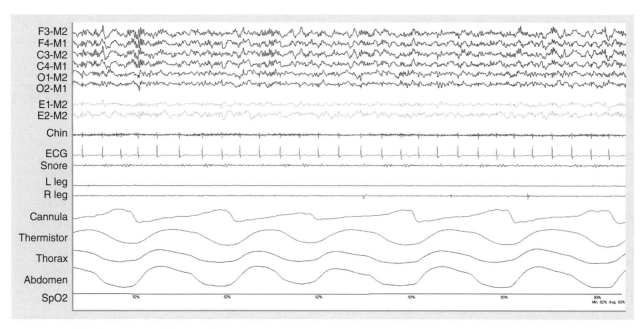

FIGURE 7-20 Respiratory channels Example 2.

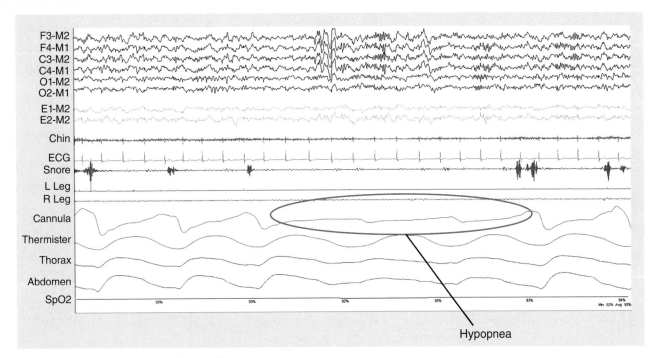

FIGURE 7-21 Respiratory channels Example 3.

Respiratory Channels Example 3

The sample in **Figure 7-21** shows a hypopnea. Hypopneas are characterized by a decrease in airflow by at least 30% for 10 seconds or more, followed by an arousal or desaturation. In this image, note the decreased amplitude in the pressure transducer airflow channel during a period of approximately 20 seconds.

Oxygen Saturation (SpO$_2$)

SpO$_2$ is a measurement of the saturation of oxygen in the blood as read by a pulse oximeter. In polysomnography, pulse oximetry allows a continuous measure of **oxygen saturation** throughout the night without disturbing the patient's sleep. Collecting information about oxygen saturation helps identify respiratory events and serves to monitor patient safety. It is typically displayed with a channel on the montage with periodic labels to show the saturation at certain intervals.

In sleepers without respiratory disturbances, the saturation remains fairly constant throughout the night. The SpO$_2$ in a normal healthy adult should be 95% or greater. Oxygen saturation decreases with respiratory disturbances such as apneas and hypopneas.

There is typically a delay of a few seconds from the beginning of an apnea or hypopnea to the beginning of an **oxygen desaturation**. An oxygen desaturation in response to a respiratory disturbance may vary anywhere from 1% to 40% or more. In other words, one patient whose baseline oxygen saturation is 95% may desaturate to 90% in response to an apnea, whereas another patient may desaturate to 60% in response to an apnea of the same length. These variances, along with the frequency of respiratory disturbances, often define the severity of the case. Certain hypopnea definitions include oxygen desaturations of specified levels. Because of the role of oxygen desaturations in OSA and other sleep-related breathing disorders, obtaining an accurate SpO$_2$ reading throughout the night is extremely important. It becomes the recording technologist's responsibility to ensure the validity of the SpO$_2$ tracings throughout the night. The following sections provide some SpO$_2$ samples.

SpO$_2$ Example 1

The oxygen saturation in the sample shown in **Figure 7-22** remains steady throughout the epoch. The patient is breathing normally, so the oxygen saturation remains the same.

As shown in the enlarged section, many digital systems show SpO$_2$ statistics while the study is running. This system displays the minimum and average SpO$_2$ during the epoch.

SpO$_2$ Example 2

The sample in **Figure 7-23** shows changes in oxygen saturation in response to a hypopneic respiratory event. Note that during the duration of the event the oxygen saturation decreases from 95% to 89%.

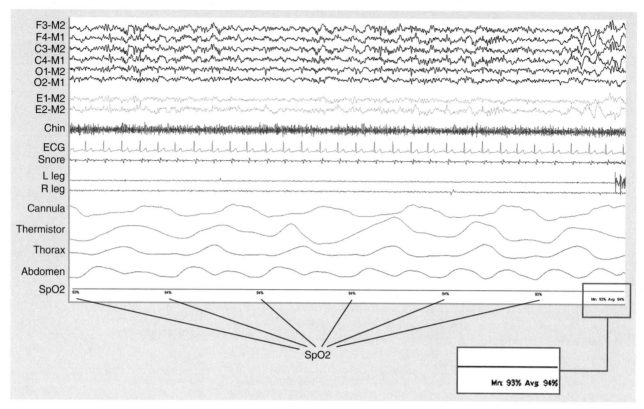

FIGURE 7-22 SpO$_2$ Example 1.

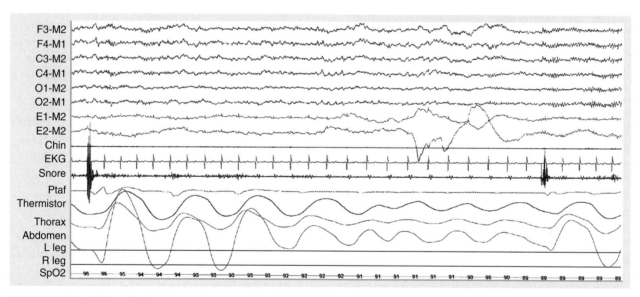

FIGURE 7-23 SpO$_2$ Example 2.

Figure by Lisa M. Endee; produced from a sleep study provided to Stony Brook University School of Health Technology and Management Polysomnographic Technology Program by Dr. Kala Sury.

SpO$_2$ Example 3

The sample in **Figure 7-24** shows a full night of SpO$_2$ readings in a patient without significant sleep-disordered breathing. The oxygen saturation remains fairly constant throughout the night. Note the section in which the SpO$_2$ dropped to 0% after approximately 2 hours of recording. This is when the oximeter was removed so the patient could use the restroom.

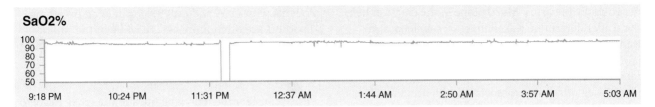

FIGURE 7-24 SpO$_2$ Example 3.

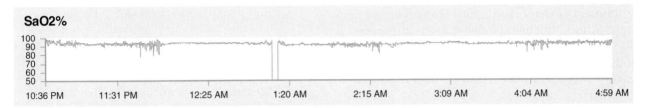

FIGURE 7-25 SpO$_2$ Example 4.

SpO$_2$ Example 4

The sample in **Figure 7-25** shows a full night of SpO$_2$ readings in a patient with mild to moderate OSA. The oxygen desaturations are reflective of periods of respiratory disturbances.

Body Position

The body position channel is a DC channel that displays the position in which the patient is laying determined by readings from the body position sensor. The body position sensor is placed in the middle of the chest and typically displays the body position as supine, left, right, prone, or upright. The sleep technologist and scoring technologist usually have the option of overriding the reading from the body position sensor.

The body position is particularly important in patients with sleep-disordered breathing. Many patients with obstructive sleep apnea have more severe symptoms while in the supine position. Therefore, it is important to document information on body position during the diagnostic sleep study to identify positional trends. In addition, when titrating PAP, it is important to correct the sleep-disordered breathing while the patient is in the supine position.

The body position is usually displayed on the polysomnograph in text format and sometimes includes a line that adjusts as the patient moves. The sample in

Figure 7-26 shows a full night's reading of a patient's body position. The patient begins the night in the supine position, moves to the right, to the left, and to the right again, and finally settles down in the left position for the final few hours of the test.

Chapter Summary

A polysomnogram is a combination of readings of several different biological parameters throughout the night. These parameters help us determine such things as wakefulness, sleep stages, EEG arousals, eye movements, muscle tone, muscle movements, ECG rate and rhythm, respiratory rate and disturbances, decreases in oxygen saturation, and body position. Each parameter has its own role in helping to identify sleep problems and disorders.

EEG leads are placed on the head to record brainwaves. These help us determine wakefulness versus sleep, sleep stages, EEG arousals, seizure activity, and other EEG events. EOG leads are placed near the eyes to record eye movements. Eye blinks can be seen during wakefulness, slow eye movements are often seen at sleep onset, and rapid eye movements can be seen during REM sleep.

EMG channels record tone and activity in specific muscle groups. The muscle groups typically recorded in polysomnography include the chin and legs, and

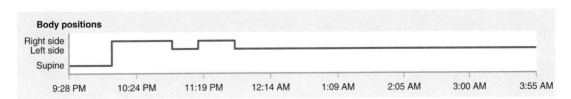

FIGURE 7-26 Body position example.

occasionally the arms. Muscle tone in the chin can help the reader determine wakefulness versus sleep, and REM versus NREM. Muscle activity in the chin and jaw area can help identify teeth grinding or head movements. Recording muscle activity in the legs can help identify leg movements associated with events such as apneas, or disorders associated with limb movements.

ECG channels are recorded to help the reader identify rate or rhythm problems associated with the heart during sleep.

Respiratory channels recorded in a polysomnogram typically include a thermal device, a pressure transducer, and respiratory effort belts or bands recorded at the thorax and abdomen. Respiratory effort information can help identify apneas as either obstructive or central.

SpO_2, or the recording of oxygen saturation in the blood by a pulse oximeter, is recorded in polysomnography to help identify the effects of respiratory disturbances. The oxygen level in the blood often decreases as a result of obstructive apneas and hypopneas.

Body position is recorded in polysomnography by a body position sensor and is verified visually by the sleep technologist. This is important primarily in patients with suspected sleep-disordered breathing.

Patients with OSA and other sleep-related breathing disorders are often more severe while in the supine position.

Chapter 7 Questions

Please consider the following questions as they relate to the material in this chapter.

1. What does EEG stand for? Why are EEGs recorded in polysomnography?
2. How does the placement of EOG leads affect how the tracings are displayed?
3. What can a gradual decrease in the amplitude of the chin EMG channel indicate?
4. Why is respiratory effort recorded?
5. What does a decrease in SpO_2 often indicate?
6. Why is the patient's body position significant?

Footnotes

1. American Academy of Sleep Medicine. (2017). *AASM manual for the scoring of sleep and associated events: Rules terminology and technical specifications*, version 2.4. Darien, IL: Author.
2. American Heart Association. (2019). All about heart rate. Accessed from https://www.heart.org/
3. ACLS Medical Training. (2019). The basics of ECG. Accessed from https://www.aclsmedicaltraining.com/basics-of-ecg/

8

Artifacts and Troubleshooting

CHAPTER OUTLINE

Artifacts
ECG Artifact
Movement Artifact
Slow-Wave Artifact
Snore Artifact
Sixty-Hz Interference
Muscle Artifact
Electrode Popping
Pen Blocking
Improper Gain or Sensitivity Settings
Improper Filter Settings
Correcting Artifacts
Chapter Summary

LEARNING OBJECTIVES

1. Define artifacts and discuss their significance.
2. Identify several of the most common types of artifacts.
3. Learn multiple methods of correcting the artifacts discussed.
4. Learn general troubleshooting techniques.

KEY TERMS

artifact
impedance check
high impedance
ECG artifact
hypertension
re-referencing
double referencing
jumper cables
movement artifact
slow-wave artifact
sweat artifact
respiratory artifact
sway artifact

low-frequency filter (LFF)
snore artifact
electrical noise
60-Hz interference
60-Hz filter
notch filter
line filter
high-frequency filter (HFF)
muscle artifact
electrode popping
pen blocking
gain setting
sensitivity setting

Artifacts

The term **artifact** refers to an extraneous signal appearing in a recording channel on the polysomnograph. Artifacts are electrical signals recorded in a channel that cause the desired signal to become harder to read—for example, vibrations from a patient's snoring that are seen in channels other than the snore channel, such as the chin electromyogram (EMG) or electroencephalograms (EEGs). Another type of recording artifact could occur if the electrical activity of the heart (ECG) invades the leg EMG or snore channel.

The most likely cause of signal artifact is poor electrode application. Thus, care should be taken to thoroughly prepare the skin surface before applying electrodes. After electrodes are placed on the patient, an **impedance check** should be performed to assess the quality of the signals. Electrical impedance refers to resistance to a current. When electrical flow is impeded or resisted, a signal is more likely to be contaminated with artifact or extraneous electrical activity. Impedance values should be low and fairly equal in measurement. The AASM recommends that impedance values below 5 kiloohm be achieved.[1] Low and equal impedance values are associated with higher-quality recordings that are less likely to contain artifacts. Conversely, **high impedance** values are associated with an increased chance of contamination with artifacts and occur when an electrode is not securely placed against the skin or scalp, when the electrode site has not been properly cleaned, or when the sensor is faulty, broken, or dirty.

Ultimately, the recording technologist is responsible for properly identifying recording artifacts and taking action to correct them when appropriate. Artifacts can originate from the patient, the equipment, or external sources, and corrective methods vary. Some artifacts must be addressed immediately to maintain the collection of pertinent information. For others, it may be suitable to simply monitor and note the artifact. In general, artifacts that are identified at the initial patient setup should be corrected by replacing the electrode, re-prepping the skin, or adjusting the placement of the electrode. If artifacts are identified after the patient falls asleep, every effort should be made to use troubleshooting techniques that are the least intrusive to the patient's sleep.

ECG Artifact

ECG artifact is a fast-wave activity that depicts the electrical activity of the patient's heart and appears in a channel other than the ECG channel. This is a common artifact in patients with **hypertension**. The increased blood pressure in hypertensive patients causes the pulse to be felt easily in areas of the body away from the heart. Hence, electrodes placed for a standard sleep study may be more susceptible to recording the ECG in hypertensive patients than in patients with normal or low blood pressure.

ECG artifact is most commonly seen in the EEG, electrooculogram (EOG), chin EMG, and leg EMG channels and presents itself as a single fast wave appearing approximately every second, depending on the underlying heart rate. The artifact can be easily identified by lining up the extraneous signal with the patient's QRS complex in the ECG channel. **Figure 8-1** shows an example of ECG artifact appearing in the chin EMG channel (top). Notice how there are periodic fast waves superimposed on the EMG activity that occur at the same time as the QRS complex of the ECG channel (bottom).

The primary cause of ECG artifact is poor electrode placement. An electrode that is placed directly over a large vein or an artery is likely to detect the pulse and transmit this signal to the polysomnograph.

ECG artifact rarely presents itself for the first time in the middle of the recording. Rather, it is likely to appear at the initial hookup. The sleep technologist should always assess for ECG artifact at the beginning of the study and correct the issue before the patient falls asleep.

Correction of ECG artifact relies on identification of the source electrode. Because the artifact is usually associated with poor electrode placement, the best method of correction is to move any affected electrode to an appropriate alternate location. For example, the reference electrodes M1 and M2 are usually placed on the mastoid process behind the ear. If they are recording the ECG, these electrodes can be moved higher up behind the ear or to the earlobes.

If ECG artifact is identified after the patient falls asleep, it can be corrected by either **re-referencing** or **double referencing**. Re-referencing is accomplished by changing one of the channel's inputs (G2) to an alternate electrode. For example, the chin EMG channel is derived from two out of three electrodes placed on the chin. If an

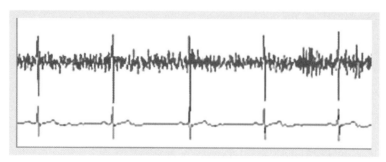

FIGURE 8-1 ECG artifact appearing in the chin EMG channel.

ECG artifact appears in the chin EMG channel, the G2 electrode can be changed to the third (alternate) electrode. This can be accomplished within the software channel properties and without entering the patient's room. In this example, the EMG channel has been re-referenced.

When ECG artifact appears in more than one channel, the technologist should identify which reference electrodes the channels have in common. This is an important troubleshooting strategy. Identifying the common variable between the channels points to the origin of the artifact. For example, ECG artifact seen in every other EEG and EOG channel can be attributed back to the common reference electrode to those channels, either M1 or M2. If the M1 electrode is thought to be the source, the affected channels can be re-referenced by changing all of the G2 inputs to M2. ECG artifact seen in all EEG and EOG channels points to problematic M1 and M2 electrodes. If placement of these electrodes is deemed ideal or the patient is already asleep, then the artifact can be appropriately corrected by double referencing. *Double referencing* refers to a method of troubleshooting that links the M1 and M2 reference electrodes together before their use as references for other electrodes to eliminate common artifacts between them. Traditionally, technologists used wires called **jumper cables** on the head box to physically link the inputs. Currently, most software applications provide the ability to double reference within the channel properties. In this later case, the EEG and EOG channels would be referenced to both M1 and M2. In doing so, the differential amplifier uses the property of common mode rejection and "rejects" or eliminates signals that appear in both M1 and M2, in this case the ECG artifact.

Note that for ECG artifact, reducing the gain setting in the affected channel would not be an appropriate correction technique because this will obscure the relevant waveforms of interest. For example, if this was done in the chin EMG channel, subtle amplitude changes in muscle tone as the patient enters rapid eye movement sleep would be obscured.

Examples of ECG artifact can be seen in the next few sections.

ECG Artifact Example 1

The sample in **Figure 8-2** shows ECG artifact in the chin EMG channel. The fast single waves in the chin EMG channel occur regularly and simultaneously with the QRS complex in the ECG channel. Because the patient is asleep, this artifact in the EMG channel is best addressed by re-referencing the EMG channel to the alternate chin electrode. If the patient wakes to use the bathroom, the affected chin electrodes can then be more optimally corrected. This would include removing the electrode, re-prepping the surface of the skin, and replacing the electrode. In this example, note that the ECG artifact is also seen subtly in the O1, O2, E1, E2, and snore channels.

ECG Artifact Example 2

The sample in **Figure 8-3** shows ECG artifact in the EEG channels, the EOG channels, and the chin EMG. Note the fast single waves appearing in the top seven channels,

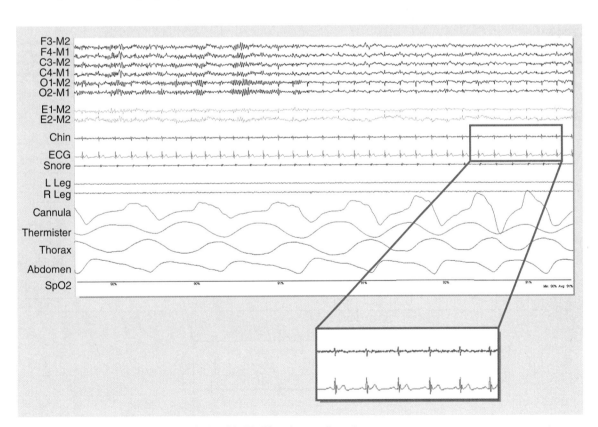

FIGURE 8-2 ECG artifact in the chin EMG, O1, O2, E1, E2 and snore channels.

which line up directly with the ECG waves. Because the ECG artifact appears in all of the EEGs and EOGs, the source of the artifact lies in the electrodes these channels have in common—namely, M1 and M2. Appropriate correction would include either replacement and repositioning of the M1 and M2 electrodes or double referencing as described in the previous section. The ECG artifact in the chin EMG channel would be addressed similarly to the description in ECG Artifact Example 1.

ECG Artifact Example 3

The sample in **Figure 8-4** shows an ECG artifact in the snore channel. The QRS complex can be seen between the snore bursts. This is usually correctable by moving the snore microphone toward the center of the throat. However, because the patient is asleep, the technologist must consider the consequence of waking the patient and the effect it will have on the sleep study. In this case, the snore activity remains easily visible on

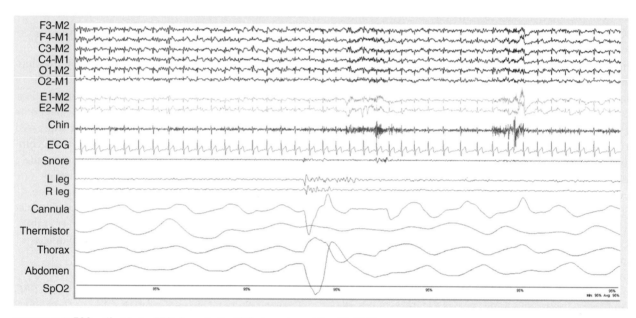

FIGURE 8-3 ECG artifact in the EEG channels, the EOG channels, and the chin EMG.

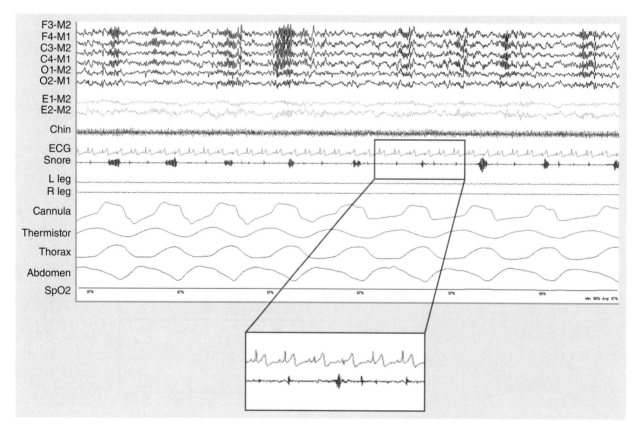

FIGURE 8-4 ECG artifact in the snore channel.

the channel making it appropriate to simply document the artifact and continue to monitor the signal.

ECG Artifact Example 4

The sample in **Figure 8-5** shows ECG artifact in the EEG channels, the EOG channels, and the chin EMG. Again, because the ECG artifact appears in all of the EEGs and EOGs, the source of the artifact lies in the reference electrodes M1 and M2. In this case, the patient is awake.

Therefore, the most appropriate corrective technique is to replace and reposition the M1 and M2 electrodes.

The ECG artifact in the chin EMG channel would be addressed by re-referencing the EMG channel to the alternate chin electrode.

ECG Artifact Example 5

The sample in **Figure 8-6** shows another example of ECG artifact in the chin EMG. Because the patient is

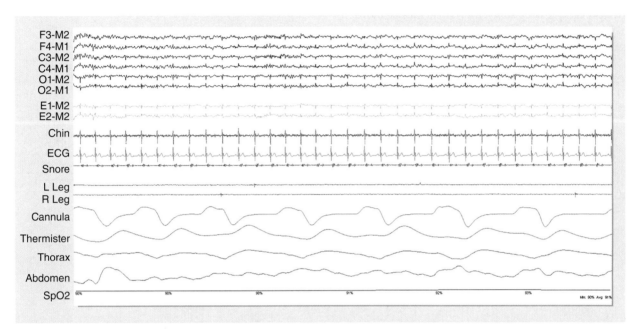

FIGURE 8-5 ECG artifact in the EEG channels, the EOG channels, and the chin EMG.

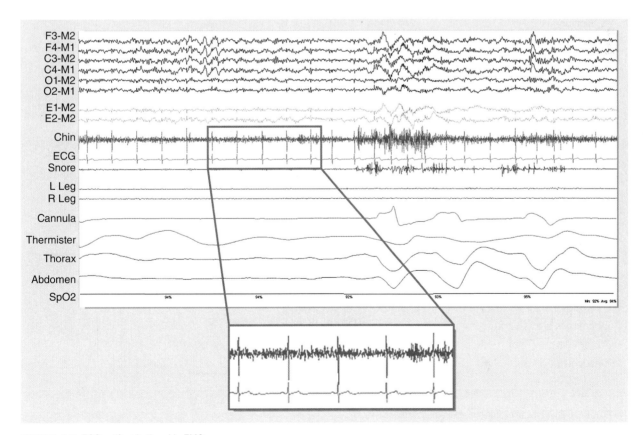

FIGURE 8-6 ECG artifact in the chin EMG.

asleep, the most appropriate method of correction would be re-referencing the EMG channel until the patient awakens and the electrode can be replaced.

Movement Artifact

Movement artifact is characterized by high-amplitude, high-frequency signals that obscure many or all of the channels and occur as a result of a body movement. Movement is probably the most frequently occurring artifact during a sleep study. Even small muscle movements can cause high-amplitude, high-frequency changes as the skin moves across the tissues underneath it.

Movement artifact is most often seen during the beginning of the night as the patient adjusts body positions frequently (see **Figure 8-7**). During impedance checks and calibration procedures, the technologist should instruct the patient to lie still, preferably in the supine position, reducing or eliminating movement artifact. Patients with obstructive sleep apnea and sleep-related movement disorders tend to move frequently during the night, causing artifact.

Technologists should always evaluate signal quality after movements take place to ensure artifact-free tracings. Examples of movement artifact can be seen in the next several sections.

Movement Artifact Example 1

The sample shown in **Figure 8-8** illustrates a typical example of movement artifact. Here, the patient's major body movements from a positional change are causing

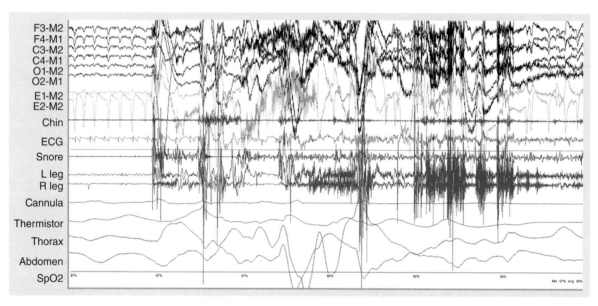

FIGURE 8-7 Movement artifact is common in polysomnography, particularly at the beginning of the study while the patient finds a comfortable position.

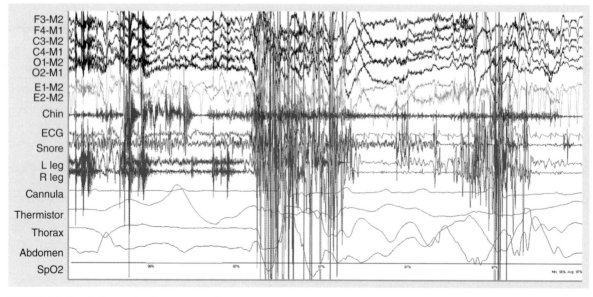

FIGURE 8-8 A typical example of movement artifact.

high-amplitude, high-frequency activity in all channels. This activity makes it nearly impossible to determine specific waveforms or details in any of the channels. However, because the patient is changing positions and was awake before the large movements, it is assumed the patient is also awake during the activity.

Movement Artifact Examples 2 and 3

The samples in **Figures 8-9** and **8-10** show another example of movement artifact. Note the high-amplitude activity in many of the channels that obscures the

relevant waveforms of interest. By the end of these epochs, the patient settles down, movements cease, and the signals become readable again.

Movement Artifact Example 4

The sample in **Figure 8-11** shows another example of movement artifact. Note that the patient is not moving in the initial portion of this epoch but begins movements after approximately 5 seconds. As with the other samples, the period of movement is easy to identify because of the heavily obscured signals.

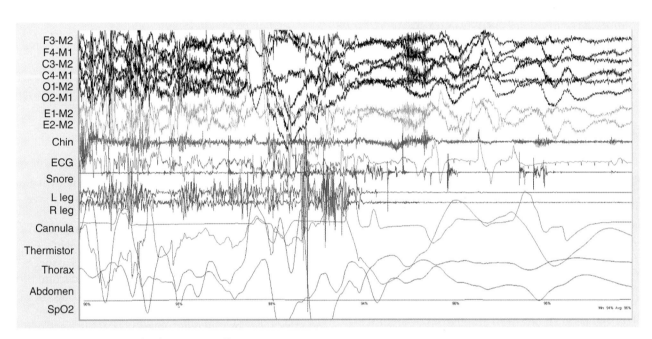

FIGURE 8-9 Another example of movement artifact.

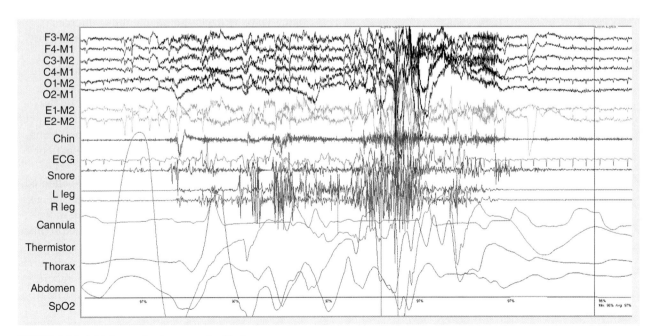

FIGURE 8-10 A third example of movement artifact.

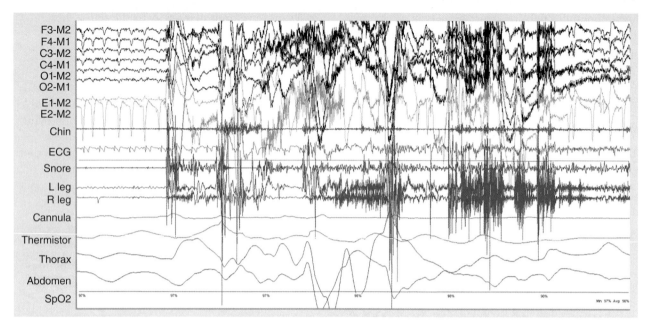

FIGURE 8-11 Movement artifact can obscure most or all of the signals.

Slow-Wave Artifact

Slow-wave artifact can be subdivided into several types that include sweat, respiratory, and sway artifact. Slow-frequency artifacts are characterized by a slow-frequency, usually high-amplitude waveforms intruding into one or several channels (see **Figure 8-12**). **Sweat artifact** is a type of slow-frequency artifact caused by sweat on the patient's skin. Salt from sweat causes a chemical reaction that, in turn, causes slow changes in the frequency of electrical signals. The EOG and EEG channels are most frequently affected by sweat artifact. As the patient sweats from the forehead, often the ground lead is affected, which serves as a reference for all the EOG and EEG channels. When sweat artifact appears as a slow wave in the EEG channels, it can be mistaken

for slow-wave sleep. However, these frequencies are much slower than EEG slow waves and tend to move synchronously with each other.

Not all slow-wave artifacts are caused by perspiration. **Respiratory artifact** is a slow-frequency artifact that it caused by slow, subtle head movements associated with breathing. This can be differentiated from sweat artifact by comparing the slow-wave artifact to the patient's breathing pattern. **Sway artifact** is commonly caused by swinging movements of the electrode wires or the headbox. This artifact is usually recognized by ruling out the other two causes or visualizing motion of the head box.

Slow-wave artifacts can be masked by increasing the **low-frequency filter (LFF)**. However, the most appropriate method of correcting the artifact is to correct the source of the problem. For example, if a patient is sweating and slow artifact is noted, it is appropriate to remove electrodes affected by the sweat, dry the area, replace them, and use a fan to keep the patient cool. If the artifact is caused by breathing, as in a respiratory artifact, repositioning the patient's head on the pillow can be helpful. In some cases of respiratory artifact, only certain channels are affected. For example, if a patient is lying on his or her side and leaning on the M1 electrode, then slight head movements during breathing can cause a slow-wave artifact in all the channels referenced to M1. In this example, the technologist can re-reference the affected channels to M2 to avoid waking the patient. Lastly, re-securing the head box can effectively eliminate sway if that is the source of the artifact.

The following sections show samples of slow-frequency artifacts.

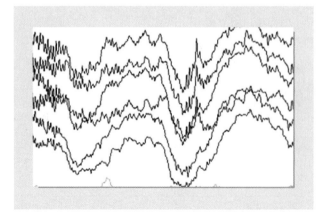

FIGURE 8-12 Slow-wave artifact appears as a low-frequency, often high-amplitude signal that can obscure relevant waveforms.

Slow-Wave Artifact Example 1

The sample in **Figure 8-13** shows a slow-wave artifact in the EEG and ECG channels. This is most likely due to sweat. The EEG waveforms in this sample should not be confused with slow-wave EEG waveforms seen in stage N3.

Slow-Wave Artifact Example 2

The sample in **Figure 8-14** is the same epoch as the previous example but with the low-frequency filter on the EEGs increased from 0.3 to 1 Hz. By increasing the LFF, much of the slow-frequency artifact has been eliminated. The EEGs are much easier to read; at 1 Hz,

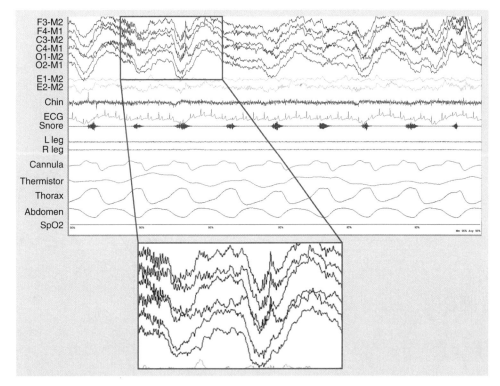

FIGURE 8-13 A slow-wave artifact in the EEG channels and ECG channel.

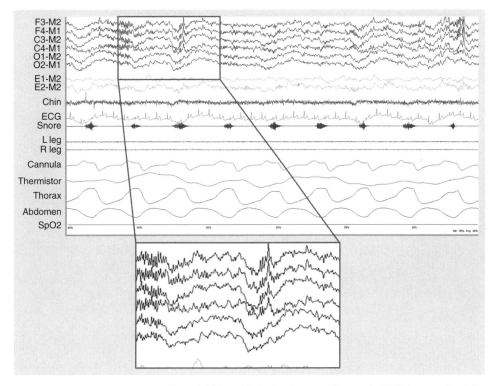

FIGURE 8-14 The same epoch as Figure 8-13 but with the low-frequency filter on the EEGs increased to 1 Hz.

it is unlikely that any relevant EEG waveforms have been eliminated or significantly attenuated.

Slow-Wave Artifact Example 3

Figure 8-15 is another example of a slow-wave artifact in the EEGs and ECG. Note that the EEG waveforms are greatly obscured by the artifact, making identification of sleep stage difficult, if not impossible.

Slow-Wave Artifact Example 4

The sample in **Figure 8-16** is the same epoch as shown in **Figure 8-15** but with the low-frequency filter increased to 1 Hz. As with the first example, the EEG waveforms are much easier to identify now, making sleep staging possible. The LFF in the ECG channel was also increased to 1 Hz in this sample.

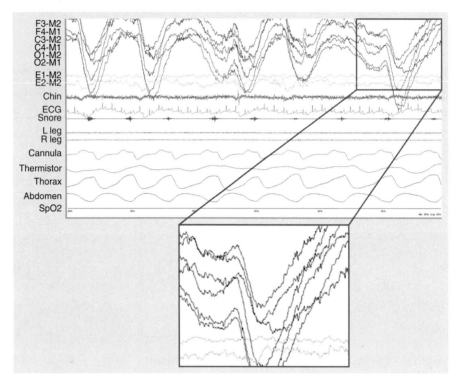

FIGURE 8-15 Another example of a slow-wave artifact in the EEGs and ECG.

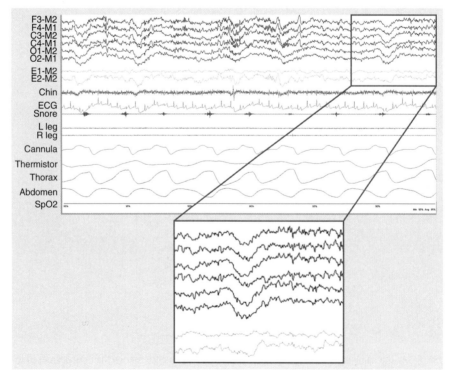

FIGURE 8-16 The same epoch as Figure 8-15 but with the low-frequency filter increased to 1 Hz.

Slow-Wave Artifact Example 5

The slow-wave artifact seen in **Figure 8-17** occurs in the F3 channel. Note that the waveform activity corresponds with the respiratory rate as seen in the airflow and respiratory effort channels. As a result, this slow-wave artifact is classified as a respiratory artifact. Because the artifact occurs in only one channel, the source is the exploring electrode, F3, most likely a result of the patient's head moving marginally during breathing. This artifact can be corrected by asking the patient to reposition his or her head on the pillow. However, because in this example the patient is asleep and the artifact only occurs in the one channel, it can simply be documented. Frontal brain waveform activity can instead be viewed in the alternate F4 channel so that the patient does not have to be awakened.

Snore Artifact

Snore artifact is an artifact caused by snoring. This usually appears in the EEG channels or in the chin EMG. Snore artifacts appear as high-amplitude, high-frequency bursts of activity for a short period of time, corresponding with and ending when the snore ends.

Snore artifact is not correctable by changing filter or gain settings, but it will correct itself when the patient stops snoring. This is commonly seen in obstructive sleep apnea (OSA) patients who snore heavily during the night.

The next two sections show examples of snore artifact.

Snore Artifact Example 1

The sample in **Figure 8-18** shows an example of snore artifact appearing in the EEG, EOG, and chin EMG channels. The patient has two large snores in this epoch, both of which appear as high-frequency, high-amplitude bursts in the EEG, EOG, and chin EMG channels.

Snore Artifact Example 2

The sample in **Figure 8-19** shows another example of snore artifact. Here, the patient has one long snore that results in high-frequency, high-amplitude waveforms in the EEG, EOG, and chin EMG channels. This immediately corrects itself after the snore ends.

Sixty-Hz Interference

When an electrode is broken or disconnected from the patient or head box, it works as an antenna and detects electrical activity from external sources. This electrical activity is often referred to as **electrical noise** and is usually in the frequency range of 60 Hz, because this is the frequency used by most electrical devices and outlets in the United States. This high-frequency, usually high-amplitude signal appears to dominate any affected channel (see **Figure 8-20**), obscuring relevant waveforms. Occasionally **60-Hz interference** may be present when all connections are stable, but an electrical device resides close to the diagnostic equipment.

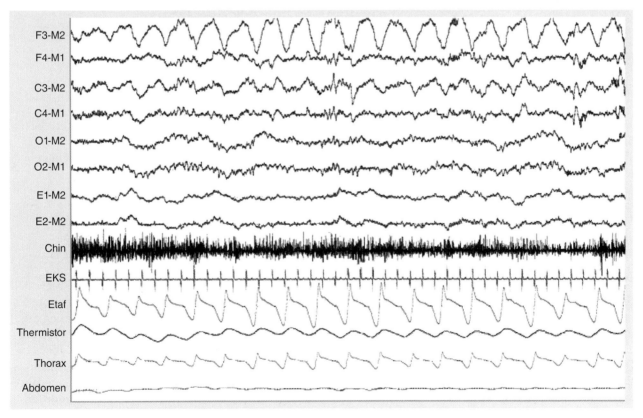

FIGURE 8-17 A respiratory artifact in the F3 channel.
Figure by Lisa M. Endee; produced from a sleep study provided to Stony Brook University School of Health Technology and Management's Polysomnographic Technology Program by Dr. Kala Sury.

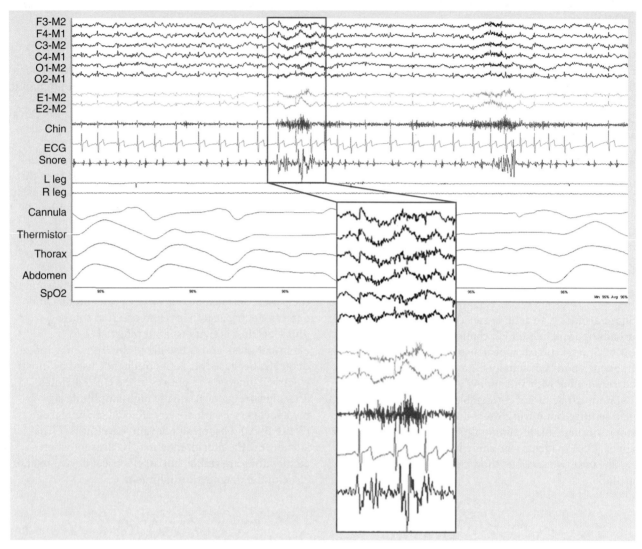

FIGURE 8-18 A snore artifact appearing in the EEG, EOG, and chin EMG channels.

Today's sleep diagnostic systems include a built-in **60-Hz filter**, also called a **notch filter** or a **line filter**. This sets a special frequency filter from 59 Hz to 61 Hz to help reduce 60-Hz artifact. However, frequency filters merely attenuate signals outside the filter ranges rather than completely eliminate them. Therefore, if a 60-Hz signal is present, it will likely affect the quality of the tracing even if the notch filter is applied. As with other artifacts, the optimal method of correction is at the source.

Determining the source of 60-Hz artifact can sometimes be difficult, because there are many potential reasons this type of artifact could appear in the recording. The most common cause of 60-Hz artifact is poor electrode application or improper cleaning of the site. Faulty, broken, or disconnected electrodes can permit the entrance of 60-Hz signals into the pathway, as can loose cable connections or electrical devices sitting close to the diagnostic equipment. Metal jewelry and other metal items touching the electrode also can be potential sources of 60-Hz interference.

The next several sections show examples of high impedances and 60-Hz activity.

Sixty-Hz Interference Example 1

The sample in **Figure 8-21** shows 60-Hz interference occurring in both leg EMG channels. The channels show a high-frequency "buzzing" waveform that obscures all muscle activity. Because leg EMG channels are bipolar channels, there are no alternate electrodes to re-reference to. Although decreasing the **high-frequency filter (HFF)** can make the signal appear clean, it will not correct the problem. Because the patient is awake, the most appropriate method of correction is to reapply the leg electrodes. High impedance values can help identify the problematic electrode for each leg.

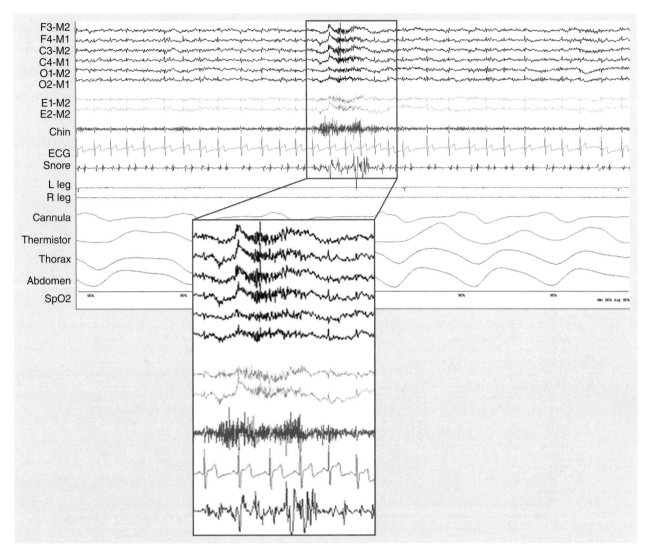

FIGURE 8-19 Another example of snore artifact.

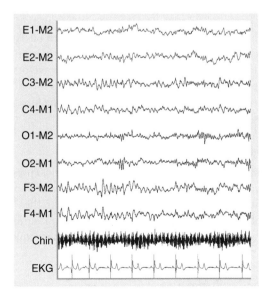

FIGURE 8-20 Sixty-Hz artifact seen in the chin EMG channel.

Figure by Lisa M. Endee; produced from a sleep study provided to Stony Brook University School of Health Technology and Management's Polysomnographic Technology Program by Dr. Kala Sury.

Sixty-Hz Interference Example 2

The sample in **Figure 8-22** shows the same epoch above with the 60-Hz notch filter applied for demonstration purposes. Note that the high-frequency buzzing activity has been eliminated and the true muscle activity of the channel is now visible. The notch filter could be used to correct 60-Hz artifact temporarily until an opportunity for electrode reapplication presents itself (e.g., if the patient wakes to use the bathroom). Coincidentally, ECG artifact is also now visible in the leg channels shown.

Sixty-Hz Interference Example 3

The sample in **Figure 8-23** illustrates 60-Hz interference artifact in each channel that is referenced to M2. Although it is possible that all of the exploring electrodes referenced to M2 are the culprits, it is much more likely that the reference electrode M2 is the source of the artifact and needs to be reapplied. Notice that the

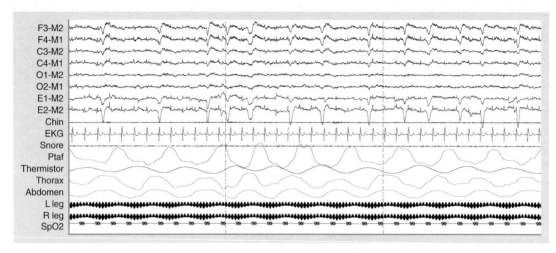

FIGURE 8-21 This sample shows 60-Hz interference occurring in both leg EMG channels.

Figure by Lisa M. Endee; produced from a sleep study provided to Stony Brook University School of Health Technology and Management's Polysomnographic Technology Program by Dr. Kala Sury.

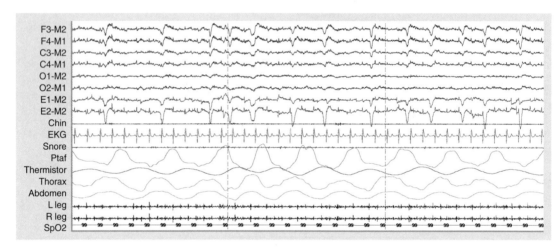

FIGURE 8-22 The same epoch as Figure 8-21 with the 60-Hz notch filter applied to leg EMG channels.

Figure by Lisa M. Endee; produced from a sleep study provided to Stony Brook University School of Health Technology and Management's Polysomnographic Technology Program by Dr. Kala Sury.

same channels afflicted with 60-Hz artifact also contain ECG artifact. When electrodes are poorly applied, as in the case of the M2 electrode in this example, it increases the likelihood of all types of artifacts contaminating the channel signal.

Sixty-Hz Interference Example 4

In the epoch shown in **Figure 8-24**, the EMG channel exhibits a 60-Hz artifact. If the technologist has performed the proper hookup with a backup chin lead, this problem is easily corrected by re-referencing to an alternate chin electrode with a lower impedance value. The backup chin lead allows the technologist to correct problems such as this without waking the patient.

Sixty-Hz Interference Example 5

In the epoch shown in **Figure 8-25**, the patient is awake and has pulled several leads off, including a chin lead and the snore microphone. The patient is also moving

his or her head, causing movement artifact in the EEGs. The chin EMG channel is contaminated with 60-Hz artifact that has obscured all the other channels, making it nearly impossible to determine any true waveforms in this epoch. In this case, the technologist has no choice but to enter the patient room and reapply the leads that the patient has removed.

Sixty-Hz Interference Example 6

The sample in **Figure 8-26** shows only electrical noise. The technologist has unplugged the head box to allow the patient to use the restroom, so no signals from the patient are displayed here. Some channels look similar to true signals from the patient because of the frequency filters that are applied.

Muscle Artifact

Muscle artifact occurs when high-frequency muscle activity contaminates a channel that is not designed to collect muscle activity. The artifact appears to mimic

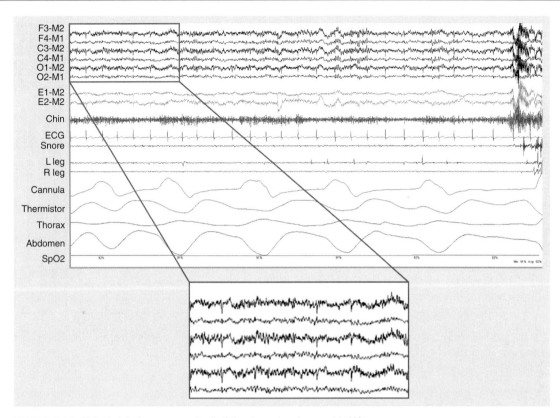

FIGURE 8-23 Sixty-Hz interference seen in all of the channels referenced to M2.

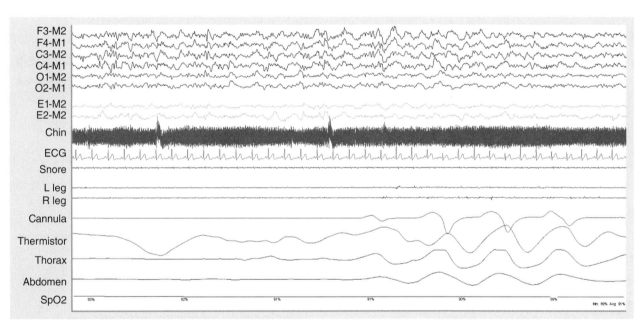

FIGURE 8-24 A poorly applied chin EMG leads exhibiting 60-Hz artifact.

the activity that is collected in the EMG channels. On a sleep study, muscle artifact is commonly seen in the EEG and EOG channels when a patient is anxious or clenches the jaw or grinds his or her teeth. Muscle artifact is most often observed when the patient is awake and tends to gradually disappear as the patient relaxes and enters sleep.

Muscle Artifact Example 1

In the sample in **Figure 8-27**, muscle artifact is observed in the C4 channel. Note the discrepancy of the activity in this channel from the other EEG channels and the similarity to the EMG channel, which records muscle activity. The patient is awake during this epoch, which is when muscle artifact most often occurs. This artifact will likely disappear

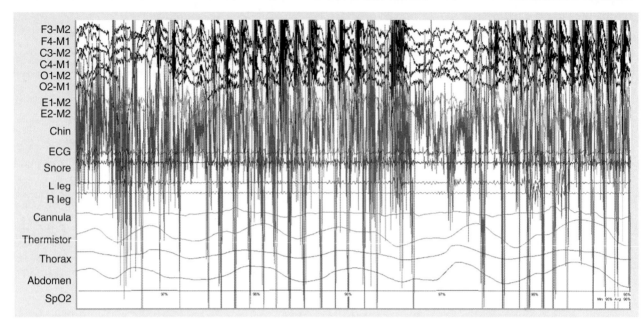

FIGURE 8-25 The patient is awake and has pulled several leads off, including a chin lead and the snore microphone. The patient is also moving his head, causing movement artifact in the EEGs.

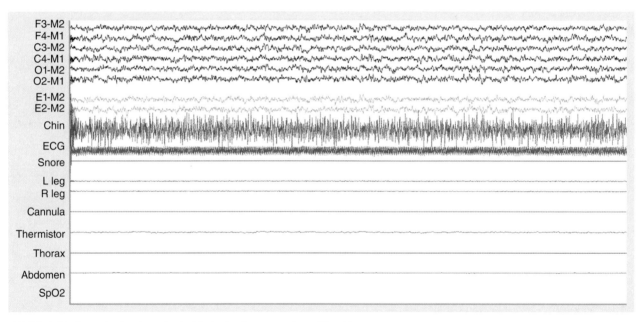

FIGURE 8-26 A sample showing only electrical noise from an unplugged head box.

as the patient relaxes and falls asleep. In the meantime, central EEG activity can be viewed from the C3 channel.

Muscle Artifact Example 2

In the sample in **Figure 8-28**, muscle artifact is observed in the EEG and EOG channels at the end of the epoch. Notice the tag at the bottom of the screen that indicates the technologist asked the patient to grind his or her teeth as part of the calibration procedures. Because teeth grinding or jaw clenching increases muscle activity in the face and cranial muscles, increased muscle activity is often recorded in the electrodes overlying those

areas—in this case, the EEG and EOG electrodes. When the patient stops grinding, the activity disappears.

Muscle Artifact Example 3

In **Figure 8-29** muscle artifact is observed in all of the EEG and EOG channels. The chin EMG channel is also contaminated with 60-Hz artifact, which makes reading muscle activity extremely difficult. Lastly, movement artifact is seen in all channels at the end of the epoch. Because the patient is awake during this epoch, the artifacts should be addressed appropriately before the patient goes back to sleep.

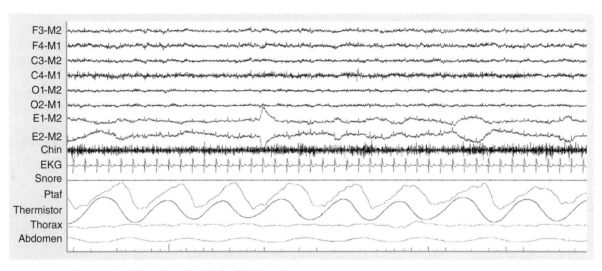

FIGURE 8-27 An example of muscle artifact in the C4 channel.

Figure by Lisa M. Endee; produced from a sleep study provided to Stony Brook University School of Health Technology and Management's Polysomnographic Technology Program by Dr. Kala Sury.

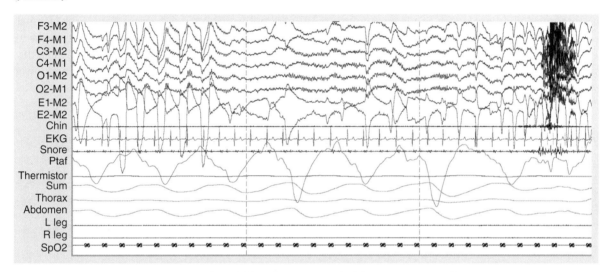

FIGURE 8-28 Muscle activity seen in the EEG and EOG channels at the end of the epoch corresponding with teeth grinding.

Figure by Lisa M. Endee; produced from a sleep study provided to Stony Brook University School of Health Technology and Management's Polysomnographic Technology Program by Dr. Kala Sury.

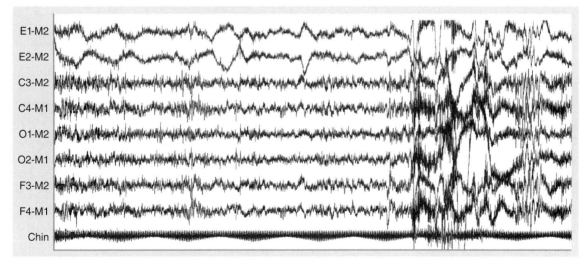

FIGURE 8-29 An example of muscle artifact in the EEG and EOG channels, 60-Hz artifact in the chin EMG channel, and movement artifact in all channels at the end of the epoch.

Figure by Lisa M. Endee; produced from a sleep study provided to Stony Brook University School of Health Technology and Management's Polysomnographic Technology Program by Dr. Kala Sury.

Electrode Popping

Electrode popping is characterized by occasional pops or bursts of 60-Hz activity in a channel (see **Figure 8-30**). This is usually caused by a loose connection in the signal pathway or a faulty or broken wire. Electrode popping often displays itself as just one fast high-amplitude wave, or it may pop for a few seconds at a time before returning to normal. Occasionally, electrode popping may present itself as a slow-wave artifact.

Electrode popping has been known to occur when the electrode is not securely attached to the scalp or when the lead wire is not plugged firmly into the head box. A lead wire that fits loosely over a pin on the head box will not make a solid connection, which can allow signals from external sources to enter the signal pathway. Another potential source of electrode popping could be an external electrical device that sends a periodic signal, such as a baby monitor. Like other artifacts, the optimal method of correcting electrode popping is at the source of the problem. This usually requires replacing or reapplying the electrode.

Electrode Popping Example 1

The epoch in **Figure 8-31** shows electrode popping in the snore channel. These fast, high-amplitude waves (marked by the arrows) are too short in duration to be snores, and they do not occur in association with the patient's respiratory rate. Because this artifact is unlikely to affect the ability to score the study, it is appropriate to wait until the patient wakes to enter the room and reapply the snore microphone.

Electrode Popping Example 2

In **Figure 8-32**, an electrode on the leg displays a single pop halfway through the epoch. This is unlikely to cause any problems in the study unless it persists.

Pen Blocking

Pen blocking is characterized by a blocking of the pens at the highest and lowest points of the channel parameters (see **Figure 8-33**). This artifact occurs when the gain setting in a channel is too high, causing the pen to attempt to reach beyond the upper and lower parameters of the channel. Certain models of digital

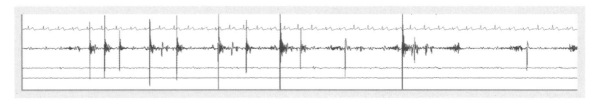

FIGURE 8-30 Electrode popping occurs when 60-Hz signals periodically, and usually briefly, enter the signal pathway.

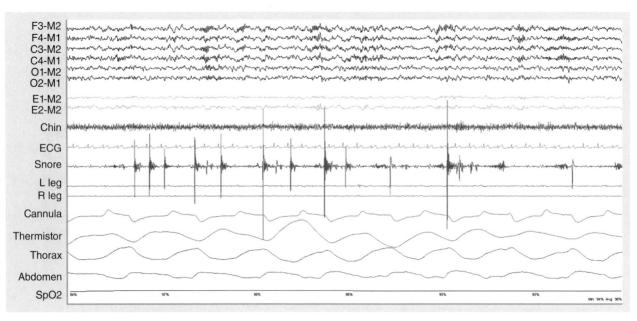

FIGURE 8-31 Electrode popping in the snore channel.

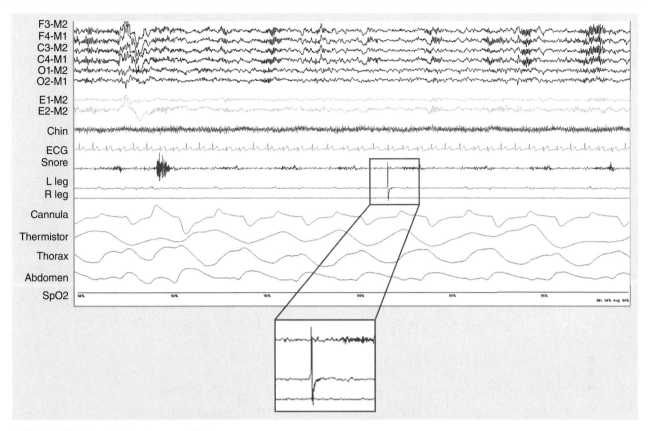

FIGURE 8-32 A single electrode pop on the leg.

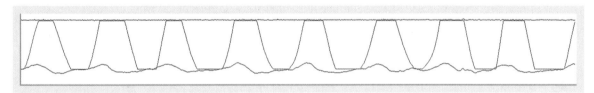

FIGURE 8-33 Pen blocking occurs when the gain is set too high to allow the pen to remain within the channel's upper and lower parameters.

polysomnographs allow the pens to deflect as far as necessary to display the entire waveform, even if it intrudes into other channels. In this case, pen blocking will not occur, but the gain should still be decreased to keep the signals from overlapping each other.

Frequently, a fast, deep breath taken by a patient can cause the pens to block in the airflow and respiratory effort channels. The respiratory channels should be set to a sensitivity level that is high enough for subtle changes to be detected but low enough that pen blocking rarely occurs. Pen blocking is a common artifact that is easily identified and corrected. Pen blocking for more than a single 30-second epoch may indicate that an adjustment to the sensitivity level may be necessary.

Pen Blocking Example 1

In the example in **Figure 8-34**, the patient's sweat artifact has become so severe that the signals are reaching well beyond what the channel is set to display. The sweat artifact is causing the pen blocking. The technologist should not change the sensitivity or gain settings but should try to cool the patient to stop the sweating.

Pen Blocking Example 2

In the example shown in **Figure 8-35**, the gain setting for the airflow is set too low and the thorax is set too high, causing the pen to block at the top and the bottom of the channel. This problem is easily resolved by adjusting the gain or sensitivity settings in these two channels.

Improper Gain or Sensitivity Settings

Gain and *sensitivity* are two terms used interchangeably to describe the amplitude settings on the polysomnograph. Although the actual amplitude of the signal remains unchanged and is defined at the source of the signal (the patient), the display of the height of

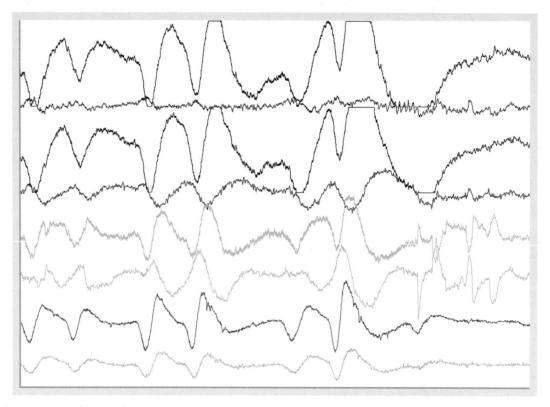

FIGURE 8-34 Sweat artifact causing the signals to reach well beyond what the channel is set to display.

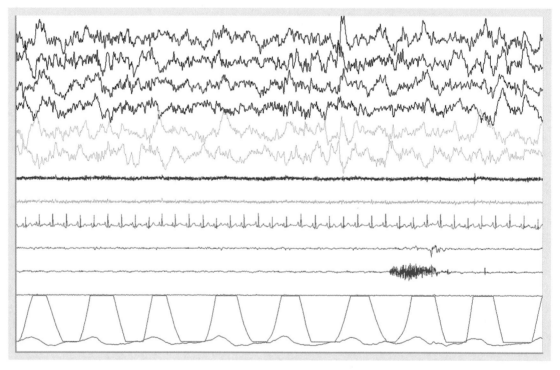

FIGURE 8-35 The gain setting for the airflow is set too low and the thorax is set too high.

the signal can be adjusted. When the **gain setting** is increased, the height of the waveform display increases. The **sensitivity setting** is measured in terms of microvolts per vertical millimeter (µV/mm). When the sensitivity setting is increased, the waveform appears shorter in height. Some polysomnographs use a gain setting, some use a sensitivity setting, and some have options to use either one or both. For example, the sensitivity can be set at 20 µV/mm and the gain set at 1. Changing the gain setting from 1 to 2 would double the height of the waveform, while changing the sensitivity from 20 to 40 µV/mm would half the display of the waveform.

An improper gain or sensitivity setting can diminish the quality of the signal collected at the channel and impede the technologist's ability to interpret the study. Most digital systems have the ability to adjust these settings after the recording has taken place, but the technologist should optimize these settings at the beginning of the study to ensure that accurate data are being obtained. The next sections show examples of improper gain or sensitivity settings.

Improper Gain or Sensitivity Settings Example 1

In the epoch shown in **Figure 8-36**, the gain setting for the thermistor is set too high. Because this digital polysomnograph does not allow pen blocking, the tracing overlaps into the channels above and below it. This can cause some confusion and make it more difficult to identify respiratory disturbances. The technologist should decrease the gain setting to correct this problem.

Improper Gain or Sensitivity Settings Example 2

The gain setting on the chin EMG channel in the sample shown in **Figure 8-37** is set too high, causing the tracings to overlap into the channels above and below it. Changes in muscle tone are difficult to detect, and the ECG and EOG channels are difficult to visualize.

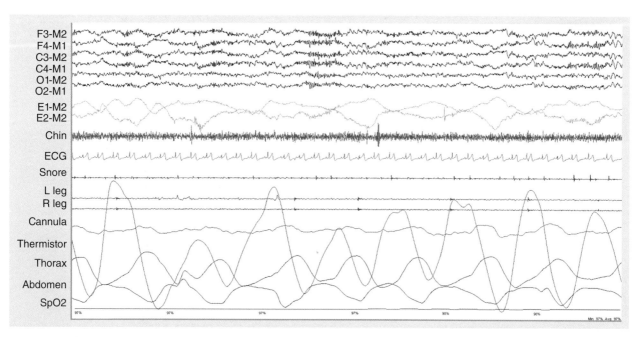

FIGURE 8-36 The gain setting for the thermistor is too high.

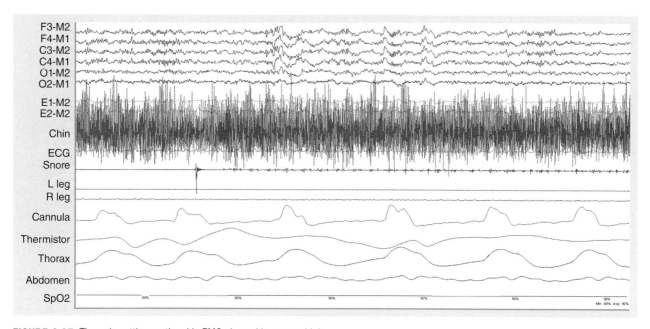

FIGURE 8-37 The gain setting on the chin EMG channel is set too high.

Improper Gain or Sensitivity Settings Example 3

In the sample in **Figure 8-38**, the sensitivity setting is incorrect in the F3 channel. The AASM recommends a sensitivity setting of 7 μV/mm.[1] In this example, all are correctly set, with the exception of F3, which is set to 20 μV/mm. Note that the waveforms are much smaller in appearance. Staging at this level would be extremely difficult and would result in errors. This is corrected by adjusting the F3 channel sensitivity setting back to 7 μV/mm.

Improper Gain or Sensitivity Settings Example 4

In the example shown in **Figure 8-39**, the gain in the ECG channel is set too high, making the ECG waveforms

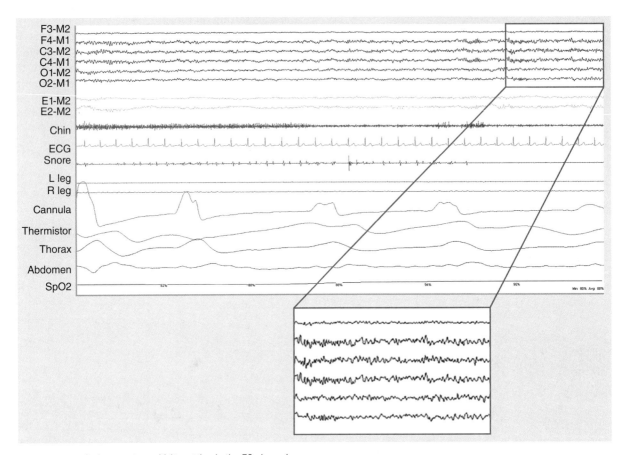

FIGURE 8-38 An incorrect sensitivity setting in the F3 channel.

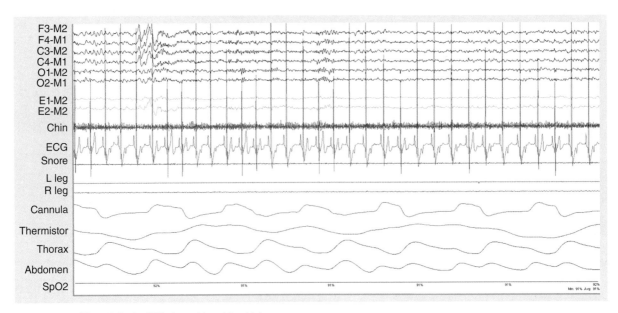

FIGURE 8-39 The gain in the ECG channel is set too high.

difficult to read and causing them to intrude into the other channels. The technologist should decrease the gain setting or increase the sensitivity setting, whichever is applicable in this case.

Improper Filter Settings

Improper filter settings can also negatively affect the signals on a polysomnograph. As a general rule, filters should not be used to correct artifacts because it is likely to eliminate relevant waveforms intended to be recorded from the patient. For example, typical EEG activity ranges from approximately 1 Hz to approximately 14 Hz. If the LFF on an EEG channel is increased from the recommended setting of 0.3 to 3 Hz, it will attenuate the slow EEG waves and delta waves will be missed. If the HFF is decreased from the recommended setting of 35 to 10 Hz, it will attenuate alpha waves, spindles, and other fast EEG waveforms.

Because of the potential effects of over filtering, frequency filters should be used conservatively. The next section shows an example of improper filtering.

Improper Filter Settings Example

In the sample in **Figure 8-40**, the HFF for the first channel, F3, has been decreased from the recommended setting of 35 Hz to 10 Hz, greatly attenuating most of the

EEG activity and making it tough to identify the sleep stage. The technologist can easily correct this by increasing the HFF to allow the fast EEG waves to pass through.

Correcting Artifacts

Correcting artifacts is a skill acquired by sleep technologists through experience. Every experienced technologist should be proficient in identifying and correcting artifacts. When determining the type of artifact that is present, the technologist should analyze the intruding signal to determine its approximate amplitude and frequency and whether the artifact affects one or more channels. If the artifact affects only one channel, then the source is likely the exploring electrode. If the artifact affects more than one channel, then the source is likely a common reference. If the artifact is present in all channels, then the patient may be moving, the source could be an external electrical device, or the ground or main reference electrode may be problematic.

The most effective method of correcting artifacts is to follow the signal pathway starting at the patient and moving toward the recording equipment, checking connections, cables, equipment, and settings along the way. The most common source of artifacts is improper electrode application or preparation. If the technologist is

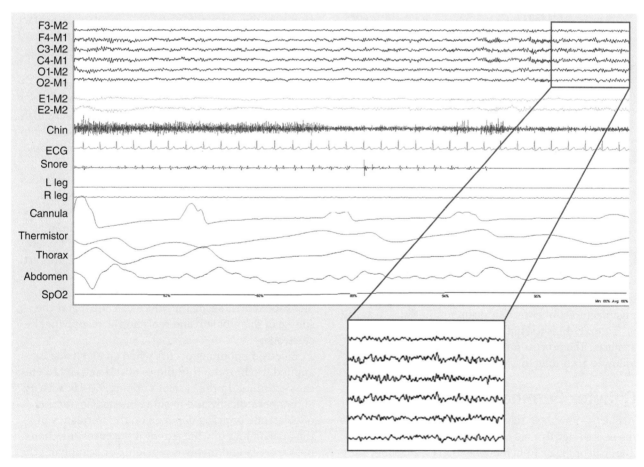

FIGURE 8-40 The HFF for the F3 channel has been decreased from 35 to 10 Hz, greatly attenuating most of the EEG waveforms and making it extremely difficult to identify the sleep stage.

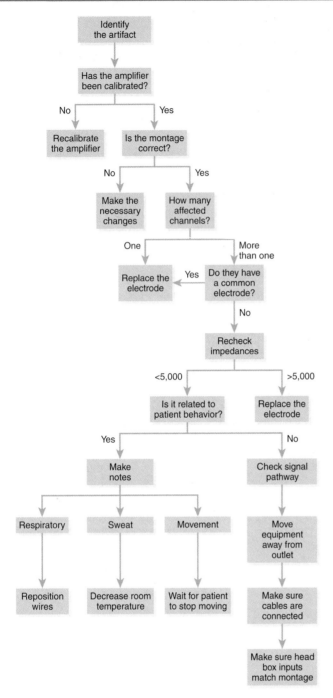

FIGURE 8-41 Eliminating artifact.

unable to troubleshoot the issue, most sleep equipment manufacturers offer technical support hotlines to assist.

Figure 8-41 is a sample flowchart for eliminating artifacts. The process for eliminating artifacts should be followed according to the lab's protocol.

Chapter Summary

Artifacts—unwanted signals altering the ability to identify the desired signals—are common in polysomnography. They can originate from multiple sources, including the patient, the equipment, or outside sources. There are different types of artifacts, but the most common are discussed in this chapter.

ECG artifact is a common artifact that occurs when the ECG waveforms intrude into other channels. This is often seen if an electrode is placed too close to a large vein or artery. ECG artifact is characterized by a single fast wave appearing in a channel other than the ECG channel at the same time as the QRS complex. This is often seen in patients with high blood pressure. The best method of correcting ECG artifact is moving the affected electrode farther away from the source of the ECG signal.

Movement artifact is probably the most common artifact in polysomnography and occurs when a patient moves. When the skin moves over the tissues, high-amplitude, high-frequency signals are displayed. When the patient moves his or her entire body, all signals on the polysomnograph are usually obscured. Movement artifact is corrected by waiting for the patient to stop moving. Large body movements can often result in electrodes coming loose or detaching from the skin.

Slow-wave artifacts, often called *sway artifacts*, are characterized by a low-frequency, usually high-amplitude waveform intruding into other signals. This is often seen in the EEGs and EOGs when the patient sweats. Sweating can cause a slow-wave artifact to occur in multiple channels. Slow-wave artifacts are usually correctable by increasing the low-frequency filter. However, the optimal method for correcting an artifact is always at the source. In the case of sweat artifact, the patient should be cooled to decrease the sweating, which is the source of the artifact.

Snore artifact occurs when a patient's heavy snoring can be detected in channels other than the snore channel. This appears as periodic high-frequency, high-amplitude bursts of activity. This artifact is common in OSA patients and is corrected when the patient stops snoring.

Sixty-hertz interference occurs when the electrodes pick up electrical signals from outside sources. This often occurs when high impedances are present, allowing electrical noise to intrude into the desired signal. Faulty or broken electrodes, or those attached loosely to the skin, can also cause 60-Hz interference. This artifact often obscures all relevant waveforms and should always be corrected. Proper correction of 60-Hz artifact should include locating the electrode that is the source of the problem and replacing or reapplying the electrode.

Electrode popping occurs when an electrode is applied too loosely. This allows 60-Hz activity to enter the recording. In the case of popping, 60-Hz activity enters periodically and in short bursts. Correction of electrode popping depends on the frequency of the artifact and to what extent it obscures the channel's activity and involves replacing or reapplying the electrode.

Pen blocking occurs when a signal reaches the maximum or minimum points of the channel. On an analogue polysomnograph, the pens can reach only a certain limit before stopping. When the signal goes beyond the point the pen can reach, a square wave appears, which is called *pen blocking*. Some digital systems mimic the analogue systems by causing the signals to block; others allow the signals to intrude into other channels. Pen blocking can be corrected by decreasing the gain setting. However, if the signal is capping because of sweat artifact, the source of the artifact should be addressed rather than simply altering the filters and gain settings to cover up the artifact.

Troubleshooting artifacts on the sleep study begins with identification of the artifact as the first and most important step. Once an artifact is identified, the technologist should determine which input or inputs are affected. When an artifact affects one channel, it is likely that the exploring electrode is the origin of the issue. When multiple channels are affected, the source is likely a common reference shared. Correcting the most common causes of artifacts, such as poor electrode application, should be attempted first. The technologist should then follow the signal pathway from the patient to the polysomnograph to discover and troubleshoot additional sources of the artifact.

Case Study

The technologist has just completed the setup of a patient for a diagnostic sleep study. An impedance check is performed and reveals the following impedance values:

- F3   2.8 kohms
- F4   3.1 kohms
- C3   2.4 kohms
- C4   2.2 kohms
- O1   2.4 kohms
- O2   2.6 kohms
- E1   3.0 kohms
- E2   2.9 kohms
- M1   8.1 kohms

- M2   7.8 kohms
- Chin EMG electrode 1   4.4 kohms
- Chin EMG electrode 2   18.4 kohms
- Chin EMG electrode 3   4.2 kohms

1. **Which of the channels are likely to be problematic? Why?**
   The technologist reviews the signal waveforms and notes the epoch seen in Figure 8-42.
2. **Which artifacts are seen? In which channels?**
3. **What is the likely reason for the presence of these artifacts?**
4. **What is the most appropriate method to correct these artifacts?**

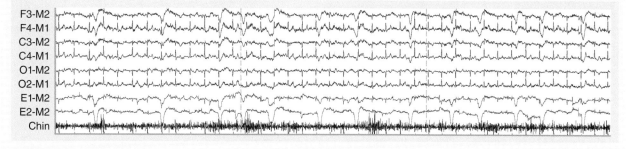

FIGURE 8-42 Case study example.

Figure by Lisa M. Endee; produced from a sleep study provided to Stony Brook University School of Health Technology and Management's Polysomnographic Technology Program by Dr. Kala Sury.

Chapter 8 Questions

Please consider the following questions as they relate to the material in this chapter.

1. What is an artifact?
2. What is the best way to correct ECG artifact?
3. How will increasing the LFF affect sweat artifact? What is the best method to correct sweat artifact?
4. How is 60-Hz artifact identified? What are some likely sources of 60-Hz activity?
5. What is pen blocking? Why can it occur on some polysomnographs but not on others?
6. How can an HFF setting of 10 Hz affect an EEG signal?

Footnote

1. American Academy of Sleep Medicine (2017). *AASM Manual for the Scoring of Sleep and Associated Events. Rules Terminology and Technical Specifications.* Version 2.4.

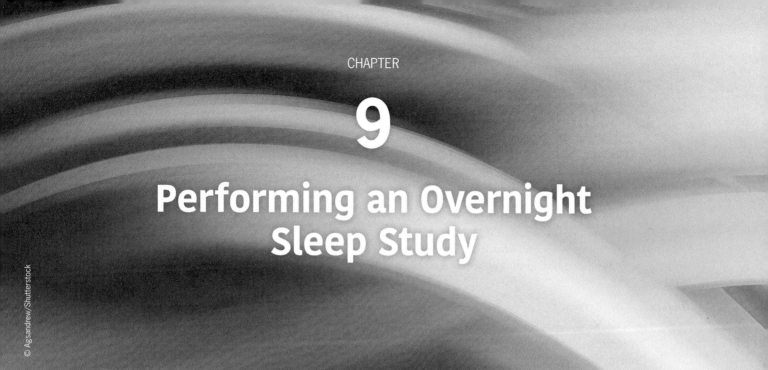

CHAPTER

9

Performing an Overnight Sleep Study

CHAPTER OUTLINE

Order of Operations
Reviewing the Patient Chart
Preparing the Patient Tray
Preparing the Patient Room
Connecting the Diagnostic Equipment
Selecting a Montage
Amplifier Calibrations
Patient Paperwork
Patient Hookup and Education
Impedance Check
Physiologic Calibrations
Maintaining Patient Safety and the Integrity of the Recording
Technologist Notes and Documentation
Ending the Study
Patient Discharge
Chapter Summary

LEARNING OBJECTIVES

1. Learn how to prepare for a sleep study before the patient arrives.
2. Discuss multiple options for sleep study montages.
3. Understand amplifier calibration waveforms.
4. Learn how to properly educate a patient.
5. Discuss physiologic calibrations.
6. Learn how to take detailed technologist notes.

KEY TERMS

patient chart
physician order
patient tray
ambulatory sleep study
montage
sampling rate
baseline study montage
CPAP montage
multiple sleep latency
   test (MSLT) montage
rapid eye movement
   (REM) behavior disorder
   study montage
nocturnal seizure disorder
   study montage
tidal volume
amplifier calibrations
machine calibrations
rise time
fall time

time constant
frequency
hertz (Hz)
cycles per second
amplitude
morphology
shape
high-frequency filter (HFF)
low-frequency filter (LFF)
sensitivity
gain
mechanical baseline
electrical baseline
time axis
consent form
pretest questionnaire
posttest questionnaire
impedance check
physiologic calibrations
biocalibrations

Order of Operations

In many sleep-testing facilities, the sleep technologist is the sole clinician responsible for patient care during the overnight period. The typical overnight shift begins between 6 P.M. and 7 P.M. and the first third of the night is often the busiest. Therefore, the technologist should make as many pretest preparations as possible to ensure a smooth flow of operations when the patient arrives. The following is a proposed order of operations for the sleep technologist. This will, of course, vary according to lab procedure and protocol. Each step will be discussed in more detail in the subsequent sections of this chapter.

Before Patient Arrival

1. Review the patient chart.
2. Prepare the patient tray.
3. Prepare the patient room.
4. Connect the diagnostic equipment.
5. Select an appropriate montage.
6. Perform pretest amplifier calibrations.

After Patient Arrival

1. Provide and explain patient questionnaires.
2. Perform patient hookup and provide patient education.
3. Perform pretest physiologic calibrations.

During the Study

1. Maintain patient safety and the integrity of the recording.
2. Keep thorough and accurate technologist notes and documentation.
3. Finish the study.

After the Study

1. Discharge the patient.

Reviewing the Patient Chart

On arrival at the sleep lab, one of the first things the technologist should do is become familiar with any patient he or she will be working with that night. The **patient chart** should include the patient demographics, a brief medical history, a description of the patient's primary sleep complaints and sleep habits, the details of a physical examination, a list of the patient's current medications, and a notation of any special needs the patient may have. The technologist should carefully review this paperwork to be prepared to care for the patient appropriately. A patient who has difficulty initiating sleep and is nervous about the study should be placed in a room that is least prone to outside noises or disruptions. Patients who are overweight should be placed in rooms and beds that can accommodate them safely and comfortably. The technologist should also review the medical history to be prepared for any potential emergent situations. For example, a patient with a history of heart disease and bypass surgery should be monitored closely during the night.

Perhaps the most important piece of the patient chart to review is the **physician order**. The technologist should always review the physician order before performing a sleep study. He or she should ensure that the order makes sense for this patient and that it matches up with instructions from any other source such as the lab manager. If the lab manager's notes instruct the technologist to perform a diagnostic polysomnography and the physician's order calls for a continuous positive airway pressure (CPAP) titration, the technologist should clarify this with both the lab manager and the physician to ensure that the appropriate study is performed.

In addition, the technologist should look for special instructions on the order such as requests for supplemental oxygen or split night studies if certain criteria are met. Often, the scheduler will have notes about the patient for the technologist. When the scheduler calls the patient, he or she obtains information that is pertinent to the technologist. For example, a diabetic patient may request to be awakened during the night to have a snack, or a patient with back or neck problems may request a particular type of mattress or recliner to sleep in. Being prepared for these types of requests can enable the technologist to efficiently handle the flow of work when the patients arrive.

Preparing the Patient Tray

The patient hookup process can be time consuming, so it becomes important for the technologist to use the time spent with the patient as efficiently as possible. Preparing a **patient tray** before the patient arrives can greatly reduce the time spent on the hookup process. The patient tray includes all the items needed for the patient hookup. **Figure 9-1** shows a utility cart that has

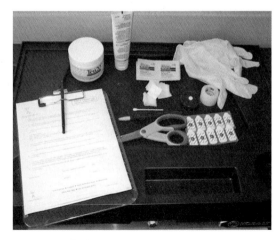

FIGURE 9-1 Patient tray.

been converted for use in the sleep lab. The supplies are stored inside the drawers when not in use and organized on top when performing a hookup. The cart rolls from the patient room to the storage closet. The supplies typically used on a patient cart or tray include:

- Clipboard with patient questionnaires and handouts
- Gloves
- Electroencephalogram (EEG) marker or pen
- Measuring tape
- Alcohol prep pads
- Cotton swabs
- Prepping gels and pastes
- EEG conductive paste
- Electrodes, sensors, and lead wires
- Tape
- Precut gauze pads
- Hair clips
- CPAP masks

Preparing the Patient Room

Before the patient arrives, the testing room should appear clean, orderly, and welcoming. The bed should be made up, the floors clean, the television turned off, and the equipment hidden so that the patient enters the room feeling as comfortable as possible. Patients are usually uneasy about having a sleep study and often do not know what to expect. A patient who enters the testing room to see a nicely decorated room with a comfortable feel and a large bed will likely be pleasantly surprised. This could help alleviate some of the patient's fears or concerns about having a sleep study.

Connecting the Diagnostic Equipment

Before patient arrival, it is also important to check the diagnostic equipment to ensure connectivity. Any equipment problems that can be discovered and addressed before patient arrival will help ensure a problem-free night and will help the patient feel more confident in the validity of the study. The technologist should ensure that the amplifiers, CPAP machines, and other devices are plugged in and powered on. The computer should be booted up, and amplifier calibrations should be performed. This process is discussed in detail later in this chapter.

When using a digital polysomnograph, the recording should be started before the patient arrives to allow the technologist to check that all channels are working appropriately and that all direct current (DC) devices are connected. Some facilities instruct the technologist to pause the study while the patient hookup

is completed to keep the file size of the study to a minimum. Others require that the recording continue through the setup process.

As a general rule, it is usually best to keep the hardware equipment connected at all times to avoid technical difficulties. When performing **ambulatory sleep studies**, the technologist must become especially familiar with the equipment, because it is disconnected at the end of each study and reconnected at the beginning of the next.

Selecting a Montage

A **montage** is the configuration of all the channels included in the sleep study. It consists of channel names, the signals to be included in the channel (the exploring electrode and the reference electrode, or positive and negative sites), the filter settings, the sensitivity or gain setting, **sampling rates**, and the color and position of each tracing. Different montages are used with different types of studies, and it is important that the technologist choose an appropriate montage for the type of study being performed.

Most labs have a diagnostic or **baseline study montage**, a **CPAP montage** for CPAP titrations, a **multiple sleep latency test (MSLT) montage**, a **rapid eye movement (REM) behavior disorder study montage**, and a **nocturnal seizure disorder study montage**. These montages are similar in that they all record and display the basic parameters of interest for sleep—that is, EEG, electrooculogram (EOG), chin electromyogram (EMG), and electrokardiogram (EKG). However, they vary in the types of derivations and the reference electrodes used, and they may include additional channels not seen in the other montages. For example, a baseline diagnostic polysomnography (PSG) montage includes those parameters previously listed as well as parameters for airflow, respiratory effort, leg movement, and oxygen saturation. A CPAP montage includes all the same channels as a baseline montage but records airflow from the CPAP machine instead of through thermal and pressure devices. It may also include other parameters from the CPAP machine such as level of positive airway pressure (PAP) treatment, leak, breaths per minute, and **tidal volume**.

Tables 9-1 through 9-5 contain sample montages used in polysomnography. These will vary from lab to lab according to preferences and lab protocol; however, certain parameters are recommended by the American Academy of Sleep Medicine (AASM) as standard for optimal recording. These parameters can be reviewed in the *AASM Manual for the Scoring of Sleep and Associated Events.*[1]

Amplifier Calibrations

Amplifier calibrations, sometimes referred to as **machine calibrations**, are performed to ensure the validity of the signals transmitted from the amplifier to

Table 9-1
Baseline or Diagnostic Montage

Channel	Low-Frequency Filter (Hz)	High-Frequency Filter (Hz)	Sensitivity (μV/mm)	Desirable Sampling Rate (Hz)
F4–M1	0.3	35	7	500
C4–M1	0.3	35	7	500
O2–M1	0.3	35	7	500
E1–M2	0.3	35	7	500
E2–M2	0.3	35	7	500
Chin EMG	10	100	2	500
ECG	0.3	70	20	500
Left leg	10	100	7	500
Right leg	10	100	7	500
Snore	10	100	7	500
Nasal pressure	DC or ≤0.03	100	7	100
Thermal airflow	0.1	15	7	100
Thorax	0.1	15	7	100
Abdomen	0.1	15	7	100
SpO$_2$	N/A	N/A	N/A	25
Heart rate	N/A	N/A	N/A	25
Body position	N/A	N/A	N/A	1

Note: The AASM recommends the hookup include electrode sites F3, C3, O1, M2, and a third site at the chin as a backup. For more information on these alternative acceptable montages, please see the *AASM Manual for the Scoring of Sleep and Associated Events*.[1]

Table 9-2
PAP Montage

Channel	Low-Frequency Filter (Hz)	High-Frequency Filter (Hz)	Sensitivity (μV/mm)	Desirable Sampling Rate (Hz)
F4–M1	0.3	35	7	500
C4–M1	0.3	35	7	500
O2–M1	0.3	35	7	500
E1–M2	0.3	35	7	500
E2–M2	0.3	35	7	500
Chin	10	100	2	500
ECG	0.3	70	20	500
Left leg	10	100	7	500
Right leg	10	100	7	500
Snore	10	100	7	500
Nasal pressure	DC or ≤0.03	100	7	100

Channel	Low-Frequency Filter (Hz)	High-Frequency Filter (Hz)	Sensitivity (µV/mm)	Desirable Sampling Rate (Hz)
Thermal airflow	0.1	15	7	100
Thorax	0.1	15	7	100
Abdomen	0.1	15	7	100
SpO$_2$	N/A	N/A	N/A	25
Heart rate	N/A	N/A	N/A	25
Body position	N/A	N/A	N/A	1
CPAP flow	0.1	15	7	100
CPAP pressure	N/A	N/A	N/A	25
CPAP leak	N/A	N/A	N/A	25

Table 9-3
MSLT Montage

Channel	Low-Frequency Filter (Hz)	High-Frequency Filter (Hz)	Sensitivity (µV/mm)	Desirable Sampling Rate (Hz)
F4–M1	0.3	35	7	500
C4–M1	0.3	35	7	500
O2–M1	0.3	35	7	500
E1–M2	0.3	35	7	500
E2–M2	0.3	35	7	500
Chin	10	100	2	500
ECG	0.3	70	20	500

Note: A diagnostic PSG is performed the night before an MSLT to rule out sleep disorders such as obstructive sleep apnea and periodic limb movements of sleep. The MSLT montage includes only those channels necessary for sleep staging and the ECG for patient safety. Therefore, after completing the PSG, airflow sensors and leg electrodes may be removed before continuing on with the MSLT study.

Table 9-4
REM Behavior Disorder Montage

Channel	Low-Frequency Filter (Hz)	High-Frequency Filter (Hz)	Sensitivity (µV/mm)	Desirable Sampling Rate (Hz)
F4–M1	0.3	35	7	500
C4–M1	0.3	35	7	500
O2–M1	0.3	35	7	500
E1–M2	0.3	35	7	500
E2–M2	0.3	35	7	500
Chin	10	100	2	500
ECG	0.3	70	20	500
Left leg	10	100	7	500

(Continues)

Table 9-4
REM Behavior Disorder Montage (*Continued*)

Channel	Low-Frequency Filter (Hz)	High-Frequency Filter (Hz)	Sensitivity (μV/mm)	Desirable Sampling Rate (Hz)
Right leg	10	100	7	500
Snore	10	100	7	500
Nasal pressure	DC or ≤0.03	100	7	100
Thermal airflow	0.1	15	7	100
Thorax	0.1	15	7	100
Abdomen	0.1	15	7	100
SpO$_2$	N/A	N/A	N/A	25
Heart rate	N/A	N/A	N/A	25
Body position	N/A	N/A	N/A	1

Table 9-5
Seizure Disorder Montage (Sample)

Channel	Low-Frequency Filter (Hz)	High-Frequency Filter (Hz)	Sensitivity (μV/mm)	Desirable Sampling Rate (Hz)
Fp1–F7	0.3	35	7	500
F7–T3	0.3	35	7	500
T3–T5	0.3	35	7	500
T5–O1	0.3	35	7	500
Fp1–F3	0.3	35	7	500
F3–C3	0.3	35	7	500
C3–P3	0.3	35	7	500
P3–O1	0.3	35	7	500
Fz–Cz	0.3	35	7	500
Cz–Pz	0.3	35	7	500
Fp2–F4	0.3	35	7	500
F4–C4	0.3	35	7	500
C4–P4	0.3	35	7	500
P4–O2	0.3	35	7	500
Fp2–F8	0.3	35	7	500
F8–T4	0.3	35	7	500
T4–T6	0.3	35	7	500
T6–O2	0.3	35	7	500
E2	0.3	35	7	500

Channel	Low-Frequency Filter (Hz)	High-Frequency Filter (Hz)	Sensitivity (µV/mm)	Desirable Sampling Rate (Hz)
E1	0.3	35	7	500
Chin	10	70	2	500
ECG	0.3	70	20	500
Leg EMG	10	70	7	500
Arm EMG	10	70	7	500
Snore	10	70	7	500
Nasal pressure	DC or ≤0.03	100	7	100
Thermal airflow	0.1	15	7	100
Thorax	0.1	15	7	100
Abdomen	0.1	15	7	100
SpO$_2$	N/A	N/A	N/A	25
Heart rate	N/A	N/A	N/A	25
Body position	N/A	N/A	N/A	1

Note: Seizure disorder montages require that additional EEG leads be placed. These can be arranged in the montage in multiple ways. The interpreting physician often defines whether a bipolar or referential EEG montage will be used. This sample montage demonstrates a bipolar EEG montage. Notice that each EEG channel is derived from two active EEG electrode sites.

the polysomnograph. The AASM[1] practice guideline requires that an amplifier calibration be documented at the beginning and end of every sleep study.

To perform an amplifier calibration, alternating signals of 50 µV and −50 µV are sent by the amplifier over a 30-second period and received by the polysomnograph. When a −50µV signal passes through the channel, it will rise to an amplitude of 50 µV and then fall back to baseline. The time it takes to reach its peak is termed the **rise time**, and the time it takes to fall back to baseline is the **fall time** or **time constant**. These parameters are directly affected by the filter and sensitivity or gain settings. Therefore, if the machine calibration is completed when each channel is set to identical filter and sensitivity settings, then the resulting signal will be identical in all channels. If the machine calibration is completed when each channel is set to the appropriate filter and sensitivity settings for the sleep study montage, as shown in the sample montages provided previously in this chapter, then the resulting signal will vary between channels with different settings. When the calibration procedure is performed in this way, it allows the technologist to verify that the calibration waveforms are identical in like channels and different in those with dissimilar settings. An experienced technologist is able to estimate the filter and sensitivity settings of each channel and therefore determine the channel type. Moreover, the amplifier calibrations can provide a way to identify channels that

are set improperly. For example, because all EEG channels should have identical filter and sensitivity settings, the resulting 50 µV signal should appear identical in shape, amplitude, and polarity in all EEG channels. An EEG channel that displays a calibration signal that looks dissimilar to all of the others can indicate a setting error and prompt the technologist to investigate further.

Waveform Characteristics

The **frequency** of a wave is characterized by the number of times it repeats or oscillates in a second. Frequency is measured in **hertz (Hz)** or **cycles per second**. A wave that oscillates three times in 1 second (or makes three complete upward and downward motions) has a frequency of 3 Hz. Waves that look wide are slow and have a low frequency. The narrower the wave, the faster it is, and therefore the higher its frequency. In the examples shown in **Figure 9-2**, wave C and wave A have the same frequency, but wave B is twice as fast as both of them. Its frequency is double the frequency of waves A and C.

The **amplitude** of a wave is directly affected by the voltage of the associated signal. When sensitivity and gain settings are identical, a taller wave is derived from a higher voltage signal than a shorter wave. In the examples in **Figure 9-2**, wave B is the same height as wave A, and wave C is half the height of waves A and B. Assuming the sensitivity and gain settings are identical in these

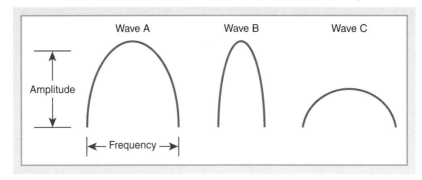

FIGURE 9-2 Sample waveforms.

channels, the amplitudes of these signals are directly correlated with the height of the waves.

Although the frequency and amplitude are typically the most important defining characteristics of a wave, the **morphology** or **shape** of EEG waves can help determine sleep stages and seizure activity. The shape of electrocardiogram (ECG) waves can be critically important in determining dysrhythmias.

Time Constant

In **Figure 9-3**, a calibration wave starts at a baseline level at the vertical center of the channel, which is 0 μV. It quickly rises to the peak as an input signal of −50 μV is received and then slowly falls back to the baseline level. The rise time is defined as the amount of time it takes for the calibration signal to rise from baseline to 63% of its highest point (peak). The rise time of a calibration wave increases and decreases with the **high-frequency filter (HFF)** setting but is most often an incredibly short length of time (usually in the hundredths of a second).

During its fall, a calibration wave falls just below the baseline level before returning to 0 μV. The time constant, also called *fall time* or *fall time constant*, is defined as the amount of time for the calibration wave to fall from its highest point to 37% of its amplitude. The time constant performs the same function as the **low-frequency filter (LFF)** in that both place limits on the amount of slow-wave activity displayed by attenuating the amplitude of the signals with frequencies below the filter setting. A decreased LFF setting allows slower waves to enter the signal. This causes the calibration wave to fall more slowly, therefore increasing the time constant. Conversely, an increased LFF setting attenuates slower waves, causing the calibration wave to fall more quickly back to baseline and decreasing the time constant.

Following the −50 μV calibration signal, an alternating +50 μV calibration signal causes a downward pen deflection. The calibration wave appears exactly the same but is flipped upside down from the sample shown in **Figure 9-3**.

Frequency Filters, Gain, and Sensitivity Settings

Electrical filtering can be compared to a funnel in which materials of various sizes are poured (see the drawing in **Figure 9-4**). The HFF is comparable to the larger top of the funnel because it filters out items that are larger than what we want to enter the funnel. The LFF is comparable to the smaller bottom of the funnel in that it releases only the objects that are smaller than what we want inside the funnel. With the filters in place, the funnel will contain a mixture of the frequencies we would like to view.

The HFF determines the upper limit of frequencies that a channel will display at full amplitude. The amplitude of electrical signals with frequencies higher than the HFF setting will be greatly attenuated, making it difficult to visually detect these waves. Decreasing the high-frequency filter in a channel can make the signal appear cleaner, but decreasing it too much can attenuate or even eliminate many of the desired signals in a channel. For example, many technologists decrease the HFF from the recommended 35 Hz to 15 Hz to "clean up" the appearance of the EEG channels; however, this would make it difficult to detect many EEG arousals.

The LFF determines the lower limit of frequencies that a channel will display at full amplitude. The amplitude of electrical signals with frequencies lower than the LFF setting will be greatly attenuated, making it

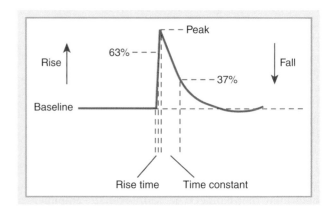

FIGURE 9-3 Calibration wave diagram.

The next few sections contain examples that show how frequency filters and sensitivity settings can affect the waveforms.

Filters Example 1

The first example shows an EEG strip with the typical EEG low- and high-frequency filter settings. This illustration is used as a comparison for the samples that follow, which use the same EEG with different filter settings.

Standard EEG Frequency Filter Settings: 0.3–35 Hz

In this sample (see **Figure 9-5**), the filters are set at 0.3 Hz (LFF) and 35 Hz (HFF), which are standard for EEG channels. Compare all of the following samples to this one and note the changes in the waveforms as the filters are adjusted.

Decreased LFF: 0.05–35 Hz

In this sample (see **Figure 9-6**), the LFF is decreased from 0.3 to 0.05 Hz, allowing more slow waves to enter the signal. Note how these added slow waves cause a wavering appearance in the channel. The true EEG waves are still visible, but they may be more difficult to identify because they are affected by the slow waves.

Increased LFF: 10–35 Hz

In this sample (see **Figure 9-7**), the LFF is increased dramatically from the first sample, eliminating many of the slow waves. At 10 Hz, note that most of the desired EEG waves are filtered out. This is not an acceptable filter setting.

Decreased HFF: 0.3–12 Hz

In this sample (see **Figure 9-8**), the HFF is decreased from 35 to 12 Hz, eliminating many of the faster waves. This cleans up the appearance of the signal but may filter some of the fastest EEG waves that are relevant to sleep staging, such as spindles.

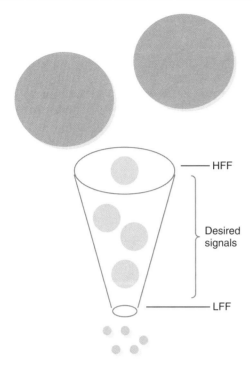

FIGURE 9-4 Filter illustration.

difficult to visually detect these waves. Increasing the LFF in a channel can improve the overall appearance of the signals, but increasing it too much can attenuate or even eliminate many of the desired signals in a channel. For example, if a technologist increases the LFF from the recommended 0.3 Hz to 1 Hz to eliminate slow-frequency artifact it can make it difficult to detect delta waves and slow-wave sleep.

The **sensitivity** setting determines the amplitude of the waveform and is displayed as microvolts per vertical millimeter (µV/mm). A low-value sensitivity setting is associated with a small number of microvolts per millimeter and results in a taller wave. Equally, a high sensitivity setting is associated with a smaller waveform. The **gain** is similar to the sensitivity, but it represents the number of times that the height of the wave is multiplied. A gain setting of 2 will display a wave twice as tall as a gain setting of 1.

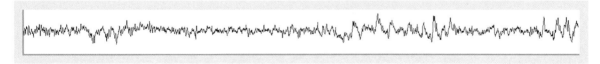

FIGURE 9-5 Filter settings 1.

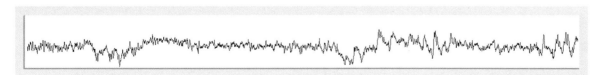

FIGURE 9-6 Filter settings 2.

Increased HFF: 0.3–100 Hz

In this sample (see **Figure 9-9**), the HFF was increased from 35 to 100 Hz, allowing faster waves to enter the channel. These faster signals cause the signal to look darker and can make the shape and details of specific waveforms more difficult to see.

Filters Example 2

Compare the EEGs in the first sample to the other samples in this section. These are all filter variations of the same EEG strip.

Standard EEG Filter Settings: 0.3–35 Hz

This sample (see **Figure 9-10**) shows an epoch of stage N3 with standard EEG filter settings. Compare the rest of the samples on this page to **Figure 9-10** and notice the changes as the filters are adjusted.

Decreased LFF: 0.05–35 Hz

In this sample (see **Figure 9-11**), the LFF is decreased to 0.05 Hz, allowing extremely slow waves to enter the signal. Note the sway in the baseline of the channel.

Increased LFF: 5–35 Hz

In this sample (see **Figure 9-12**), the LFF is increased to 5 Hz, eliminating many slow to midrange EEG signals. Note that none of the delta activity seen in the first strip is visible.

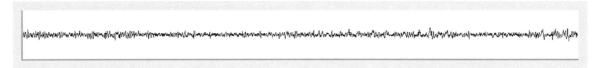

FIGURE 9-7 Filter settings 3.

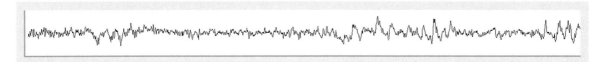

FIGURE 9-8 Filter settings 4.

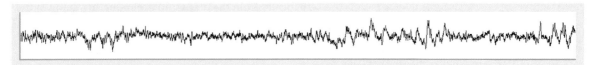

FIGURE 9-9 Filter settings 5.

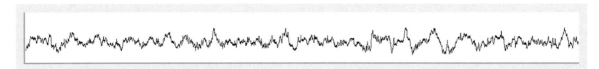

FIGURE 9-10 Filter settings 6.

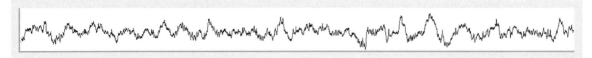

FIGURE 9-11 Filter settings 7.

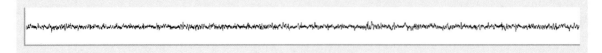

FIGURE 9-12 Filter settings 8.

Decreased HFF: 0.3–15 Hz

In this sample (see **Figure 9-13**), the HFF is decreased to 15 Hz, eliminating or attenuating waves that were previously seen in the 15–35 Hz range.

Increased HFF: 0.3–100 Hz

In this sample (see **Figure 9-14**), the HFF is increased to 100 Hz, allowing fast waves into the channel.

Sensitivity Setting

Compare the sample in **Figure 9-15** with the samples in **Figures 9-16** and **9-17** as the sensitivity to an EEG strip is adjusted. In **Figure 9-16**, the sensitivity setting is increased from 7 to 14 µV/mm. Note that the amplitude of the waveforms decreases. Conversely, when the sensitivity setting is decreased in **Figure 9-17** from 7 to 2 µV/mm, the amplitude of the waveforms increases.

Figure 9-18 is an example of an amplifier calibration. Note that the calibration waves are all identical in polarity, amplitude, rise time, and fall time.

Standard Settings

The sample in **Figure 9-19** shows amplifier calibrations with all channels set to identical filter and sensitivity settings. As a result, all channels look identical to each other in polarity, amplitude, rise time, and fall time. The channels in this sample are set with the following parameters:

Sensitivity: 7 µV/mm
LFF: 0.3 Hz
HFF: 35 Hz
Paper speed: 30 sec/page (10 mm/sec)

Increased Low-Frequency Filter

The sample in **Figure 9-20** shows calibration waves with an increased low-frequency filter. Increasing the

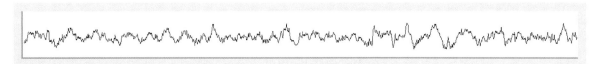

FIGURE 9-13 Filter settings 9.

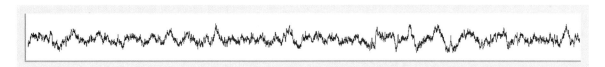

FIGURE 9-14 Filter settings 10.

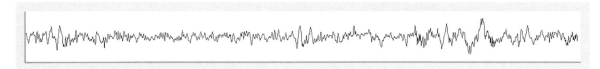

FIGURE 9-15 Filter settings 11. Sensitivity = 7 µV/mm.

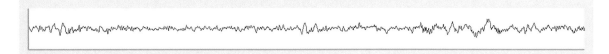

FIGURE 9-16 Filter settings 12. Sensitivity = 14 µV/mm.

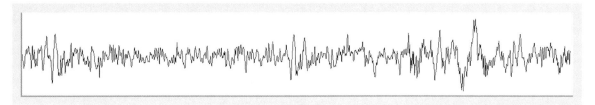

FIGURE 9-17 Filter settings 13. Sensitivity = 2 µV/mm.

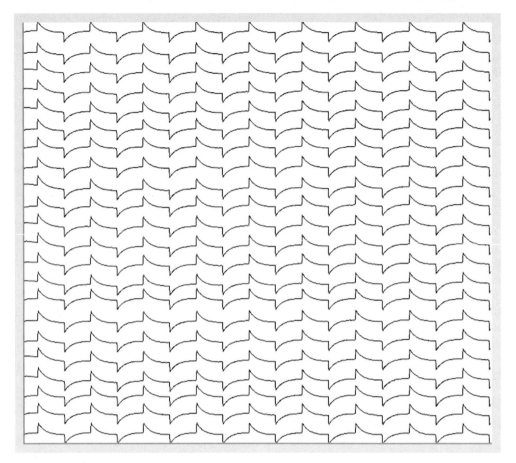

FIGURE 9-18 Amplifier calibrations.

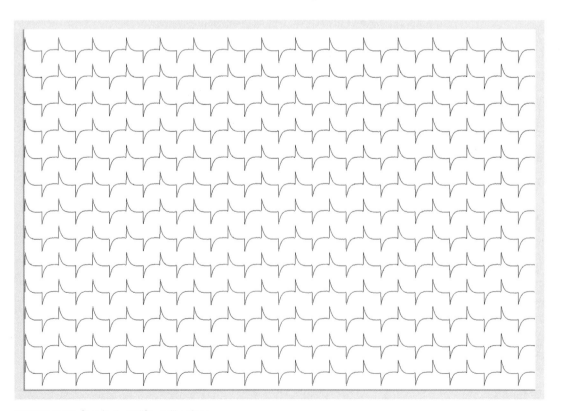

FIGURE 9-19 Standard amplifier calibrations.

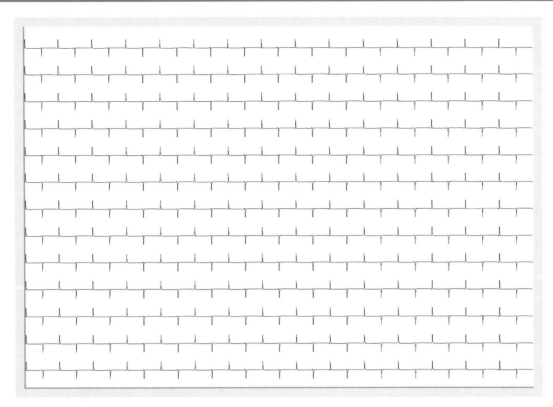

FIGURE 9-20 Increased low-frequency filter.

LFF decreases the time constant, forcing the calibration wave to return to its baseline more quickly. EMG channels have a LFF setting similar to this.

> Sensitivity: 7 µV/mm
> LFF: 10 Hz
> HFF: 35 Hz
> Paper speed: 30 sec/page (10 mm/sec)

Decreased Low-Frequency Filter

In **Figure 9-21** the low-frequency filter has been decreased to 0.1 Hz. This increases the time constant setting, which means the wave has more time to return to baseline.

> Sensitivity: 7 µV/mm
> LFF: 0.1 Hz
> HFF: 35 Hz
> Paper speed: 30 sec/page (10 mm/sec)

Decreased High-Frequency Filter

In **Figure 9-22** the high-frequency filter has been decreased to 15 Hz. This causes the calibration waves to reach their peaks more slowly, which causes a slightly rounded peak. An example showing an increased HFF will not be shown in this text, because the changes in rise time would be too subtle to visually detect.

> Sensitivity: 7 µV/mm
> LFF: 0.3 Hz
> HFF: 15 Hz
> Paper speed: 30 sec/page (10 mm/sec)

Increased Sensitivity Setting (or Decreased Gain)

In **Figure 9-23** the sensitivity has been changed from 7 µV/mm to 10 µV/mm. A higher sensitivity setting or a lower gain makes the waves appear shorter in height.

> Sensitivity: 7 µV/mm
> LFF: 0.3 Hz
> HFF: 35 Hz
> Paper speed: 30 sec/page (10 mm/sec)

Decreased Sensitivity Setting (or Increased Gain)

The sample in **Figure 9-24** shows an amplifier calibration with similar settings to those in **Figure 9-18**, but with a decreased sensitivity value level (or an increased gain setting). Note the increased height of the waveforms.

> Sensitivity: 3 µV/mm
> LFF: 0.3 Hz
> HFF: 35 Hz
> Paper speed: 30 sec/page (10 mm/sec)

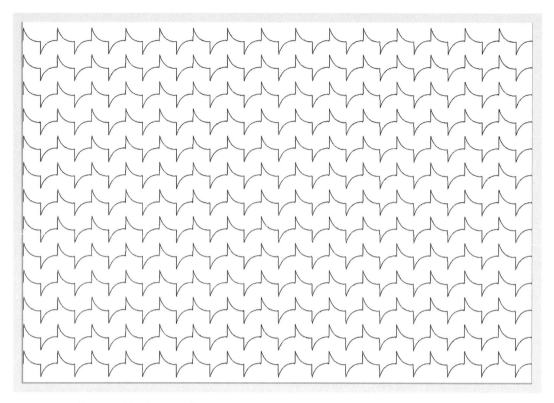

FIGURE 9-21 Decreased low-frequency filter.

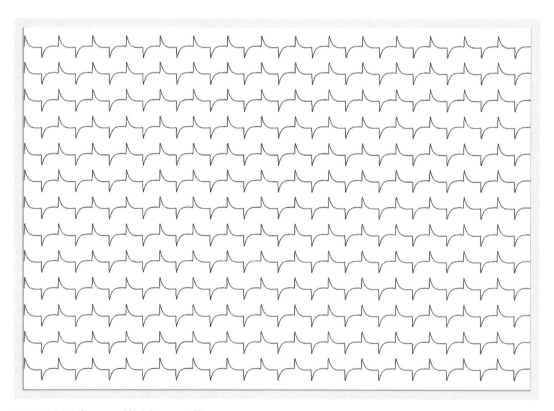

FIGURE 9-22 Decreased high-frequency filter.

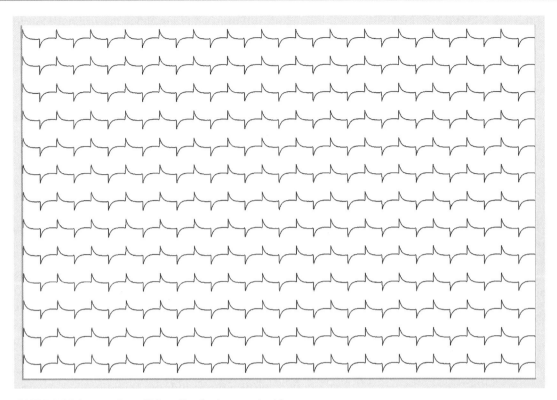

FIGURE 9-23 Increased sensitivity setting (or decreased gain).

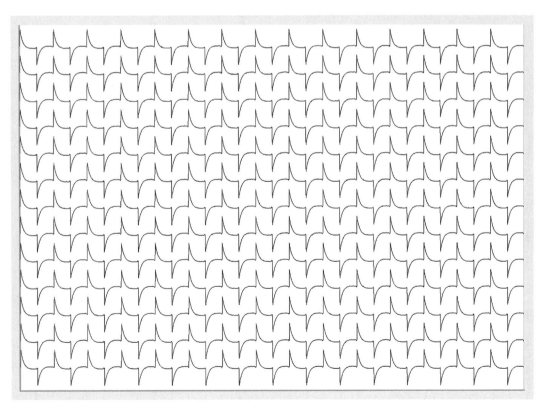

FIGURE 9-24 Decreased sensitivity setting (or increased gain).

Decreased Paper Speed

The sample in **Figure 9-25** shows an amplifier calibration with the same settings as the previous two examples but with a slower paper speed. The paper speed is set at 60 sec/page or 5 mm/sec. The decreased paper speed makes the waves closer together.

> Sensitivity: 7 μV/mm
> LFF: 0.3 Hz
> HFF: 35 Hz
> Paper speed: 60 sec/page (5 mm/sec)

Increased Paper Speed

The sample in **Figure 9-26** shows an amplifier calibration with the same settings as those in **Figure 9-25** but with a faster paper speed. The paper speed is set at 10 sec/page or 30 mm/sec.

> Sensitivity: 7 μV/mm
> LFF: 0.3 Hz
> HFF: 35 Hz
> Paper speed: 10 sec/page (30 mm/sec)

Multiple Channel Settings

The calibration waves in **Figure 9-27** have various HFF, LFF, and sensitivity settings. Note that each channel appears different in the rise time, fall time, and amplitude of the waveforms.

If the channels included in a diagnostic sleep study montage are set with the appropriate filter and sensitivity settings, and an amplifier calibration is performed, then the channels with identical settings will appear identical, while those with different settings will appear dissimilar (see **Figure 9-28**). In **Figure 9-28**, note that the top eight channels appear identical in rise time, fall time, amplitude, and polarity of the waveforms. These channels are the EEG and EOG channels that have identical filter and sensitivity settings. Now compare the calibration signal in the EEG channels to those in the EMG channels (CHIN, LLEG, RLEG). Note that the chin EMG channel appears different than those above and similar to the right and left leg EMG channels. This is because muscle channels have different filter settings from the EEG and EOG channels. Specifically, the EMG channels have higher LFF and HFF settings compared to the EEG and EOG channels, and thus they will have faster rise times and shorter time constants. This means that the signal will rise and fall more quickly back to baseline, giving a spikelike appearance to the waveform. Also note that the pressure transducer airflow and thermocouple airflow channels which measure airflow appear different from the other channels. In this case, the airflow channels have lower LFF and HFF settings compared to the other channels, and thus will have slower rise times and longer time constants. This means that the signal will rise and fall more gradually back to baseline.

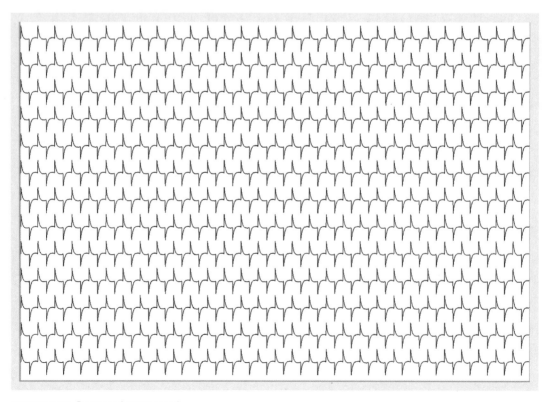

FIGURE 9-25 Decreased paper speed.

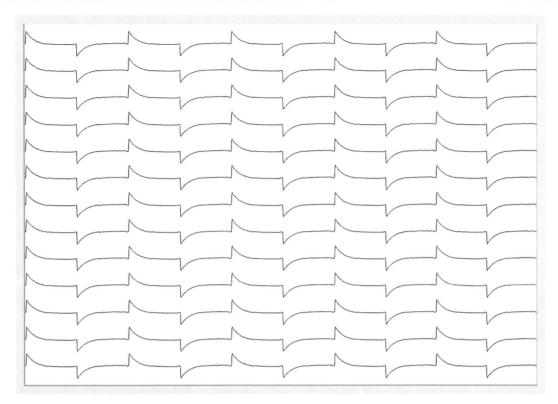

FIGURE 9-26 Increased paper speed.

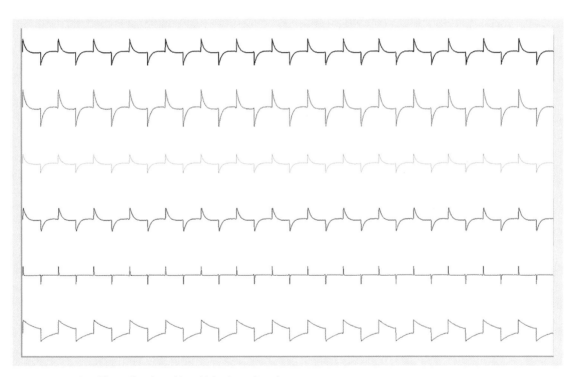

FIGURE 9-27 Amplifier calibration with multiple channel settings.

To be comprehensive, several other calibration procedures associated with traditional methods of data collection for sleep studies are worth noting. Historically, collection of sleep study data was accomplished with analog-based amplifiers that produced paper recordings. For the most part, this method has been replaced by digital technology, although it may still be used in some research-based facilities. When collecting sleep data in this traditional way, it was appropriate to perform calibration procedures that assessed

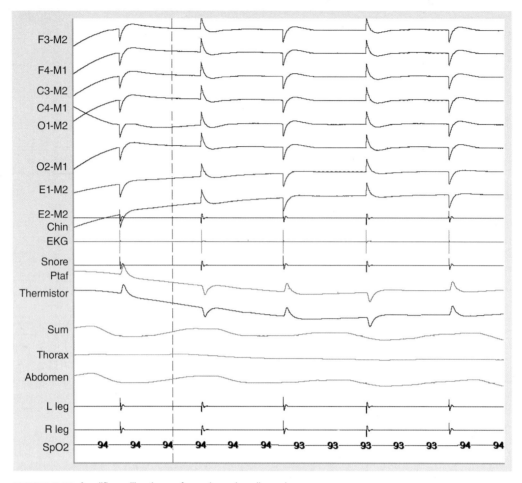

FIGURE 9-28 Amplifier calibration performed on a baseline polysomnogram.

Figure by Lisa M. Endee; produced from a sleep study provided to Stony Brook University School of Health Technology and Management's Polysomnographic Technology Program by Dr. Kala Sury.

the **mechanical baseline**, **electrical baseline**, and **time axis** alignment of the pen tracings on the paper. The mechanical baseline describes the vertical positioning of the pen with the power to the polysomnograph turned off, and the electrical baseline refers to the vertical positioning of the pen with the power to the polysomnograph turned on. The time axis is the horizontal positioning of the pen on the paper recording.

Patient Paperwork

After the patient has arrived, the technologist introduces him- or herself, often provides a brief tour of the lab, and directs the patient to the testing room. The patient is then typically asked to complete a series of questionnaires and consent forms. The content of the patient questionnaires depends on the needs of the lab and physician. In general, the following documents are often completed on the night of the sleep study:

- Consent for sleep testing
- Consent for audio and video recording
- Pretest (bedtime) questionnaire
- Posttest (morning after) questionnaire
- Patient feedback survey

Consent for Testing

A **consent form** is a legal document created by a healthcare facility. Its purpose is to have patients acknowledge that they understand the procedure that will or may occur, understand both the benefits and potential negative consequences of that procedure, have had the opportunity to ask questions, and are consenting to the procedure after having their questions answered. The document is signed by the patient and by a witness. In the sleep center environment, the sleep study consent form accomplishes this, and the sleep technologist is often the witness signatory. Some sleep labs will also include a separate video consent form because standard sleep testing includes a recorded video portion.

Depending on lab protocol, the technologist may be responsible for obtaining a copy of the patient's health insurance card and other related information for billing purposes at this time. However, in most cases this information has already been obtained during the consultation.

Pretest Questionnaire

The **pretest questionnaire**, sometimes referred to as the *bedtime questionnaire*, asks questions about the patient's activities during the day and evening of the test. Questions often included in this document are:

- How many hours did you sleep last night?
- Have you consumed any caffeine today?
- Have you consumed any alcohol today?
- What medications have you taken today?
- Did you take a nap today?

The purpose of this questionnaire is to assess any factors that may affect the patient's ability to sleep during the study.

Posttest Questionnaire

The **posttest questionnaire**, sometimes referred to as the *morning after questionnaire*, is given to the patient in the morning after the study is completed. This questionnaire asks how the patient slept during the overnight study. Questions often included in this document are:

- How long did it take you to fall asleep last night?
- How many times do you remember waking up last night?
- How did your sleep last night compare with your normal night's sleep?
- How many hours do you feel you slept last night?
- Do you feel rested?

The purpose of this questionnaire is to allow the patient to explain anything that may have been unusual during the night of the study. For example, if the patient slept poorly during the night of the study because he or she was nervous but normally sleeps well at home, it would be important to explain this to the physician and the scoring technologist.

Patient Hookup and Education

The patient hookup process can take even an experienced technologist up to an hour to complete. This is valuable time spent with the patient, and the sleep technologist should take advantage of this time to:

- Build a relationship of trust with the patient
- Help the patient feel comfortable with the lab, the technologist, and the sleep study process
- Educate the patient to help ensure compliance with testing and treatment if applicable

The exact method and content used to educate the patient is determined by the sleep lab and the medical director. While educating the patient, the technologist should be careful not to make the patient feel like a diagnosis is being given. For example, the technologist should be able to discuss sleep apnea with the patient without the patient feeling like the technologist is diagnosing him or her with sleep apnea. Only the physician can diagnose the patient, and the technologist should make that clear with the patient. However, the technologist can discuss sleep hygiene techniques,

the importance of adequate sleep, and the dangers of sleep apnea and other disorders. Doing so can help motivate the patient to practice better sleep habits and comply with treatments recommended by the physician.

Impedance Check

After all appropriate electrodes and sensors are placed on the patient, the technologist should plug the electrodes into the headbox and then connect the headbox and ancillary equipment to the amplifier. After visually inspecting the waveform signals, the technologist should perform an **impedance check** to ensure standard values are met and a quality test is obtained. It is recommended by the AASM that impedance values remain below 5 kiloohm (KΩ), although in some cases, leg EMG electrode values may be acceptable below 10 KΩ. Any impedance values that fall above standard recommendations should be corrected before continuing with the study. Impedance checks should be performed before lights out at the beginning of the study, and just after lights on at the end of the study.

Physiologic Calibrations

After impedance values are optimized, the patient should be instructed to lie in bed while the technologist runs **physiologic calibrations**, also known as **biocalibrations**. During this process, the patient is asked to perform certain physical tasks such as moving a foot, clenching the jaw, or blinking to view the associated signals on the polysomnograph. Biocalibration procedures ensure accurate placement of electrodes and sensors; more importantly, they serve as a baseline for scoring the sleep study. For example, asking the patient to close his or her eyes will reveal what the patient's alpha activity looks like in the EEG. Also, a light cough by the patient gives the scorer a general idea of the volume of snores at varying levels. Physiologic calibrations are performed prior to lights out at the beginning of the study, and just after lights on at the end of the study.

The following physiologic calibrations are recommended by the AASM as standard:

- *Close eyes:* The technologist instructs the patient to lie down and relax with eyes closed for 30 seconds. This reveals alpha activity in the occipital EEG channels.
- *Open eyes:* The technologist instructs the patient to lie still with his or her eyes open for 30 seconds (blinking is allowed), moving as little as possible. Alpha activity should be eliminated with the eyes open.
- *Look left and right:* The technologist instructs the patient to look to the left and right at least five times while keeping the head still. Moving the

eyes back and forth mimics the eye movement activity seen during REM sleep.

- *Look up and down:* The technologist instructs the patient to move his or her eyes up and down at least five times while keeping the head still. This mimics eye movements seen during stage N1 and helps differentiate between vertical and horizontal eye movements.
- *Blink:* The technologist instructs the patient to blink five times while keeping the head still. This provides a reference for revealing blinks later in the study.
- *Grind teeth:* The technologist instructs the patient to grind his or her teeth or mimic chewing for at least 5 seconds. This provides a reference for increased chin EMG activity.
- *Snore:* The technologist instructs the patient to simulate a snore or hum for at least 5 seconds. This helps set a standard for snore levels during the night.
- *Breathe normally:* The technologist instructs the patient to breathe normally to ensure that airflow and effort signals are optimal and synchronized.
- *Hold breath:* The technologist instructs the patient to take a deep breath and hold it for approximately 10 seconds. This mimics a central apnea because the patient is not attempting to breathe.
- *Breathe through nose:* The technologist instructs the patient to breathe only through his or her nose for approximately 10 seconds. This ensures that nasal breathing is captured.
- *Breathe through mouth:* The technologist instructs the patient to breathe only through the mouth for

approximately 10 seconds. This ensures that oral breathing is captured.

- *Flex the feet:* The technologist instructs the patient to flex the left foot or raise the toes on the left foot at least five times. This command is then repeated for the right foot. These movements mimic the leg movements seen during wake and sleep and should produce bursts of increased amplitude in each leg EMG.

Figures 9-29 to **9-34** demonstrate physiologic calibration procedures being performed at the beginning of a CPAP study. The epochs shown are sequential epochs covering the entire calibration procedure. Note the epoch numbers on the display.

Figure 9-29 depicts the initiation of physiologic calibrations. Note the technologist tag at the bottom of the screen; it indicates the beginning of the calibrations followed by the request for the patient to close his or her eyes. Eye closure is characterized by a fast frequency activity in the EEG channels (alpha), which is most notable in the occipital channel (O2).

In the first half of **Figure 9-30**, the technologist has directed the patient to open his or her eyes. This is evidenced by the attenuation of the alpha activity seen when the eyes were closed. After the midpoint of the epoch, the technologist directs the patient to move his or her eyes left and right. Note the fast, biphasic, and symmetrical waveforms noted in the EOG channels (E1 and E2).

Figure 9-31 begins with the patient moving his or her eyes up and down as noted by the signal excursions

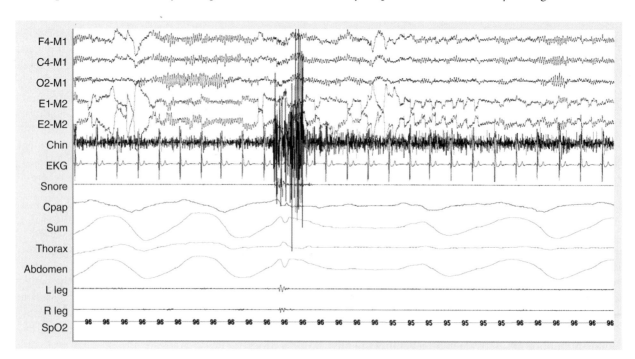

FIGURE 9-29 Physiologic calibrations sample 1. (Patient asked to close their eyes.)

Figure by Lisa M. Endee; produced from a sleep study provided to Stony Brook University School of Health Technology and Management's Polysomnographic Technology Program by Dr. Kala Sury.

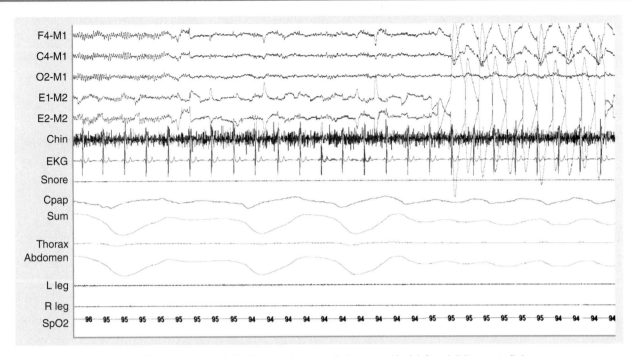

FIGURE 9-30 Physiologic calibrations sample 2. (Patient asked to open their eyes and look left and right repeatedly.)

Figure by Lisa M. Endee; produced from a sleep study provided to Stony Brook University School of Health Technology and Management's Polysomnographic Technology Program by Dr. Kala Sury.

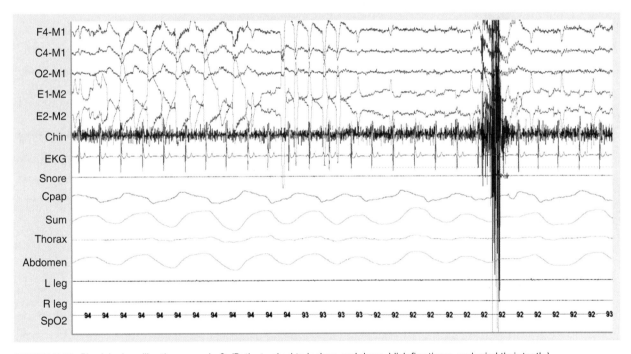

FIGURE 9-31 Physiologic calibrations sample 3. (Patient asked to look up and down, blink five times, and grind their teeth.)

Figure by Lisa M. Endee; produced from a sleep study provided to Stony Brook University School of Health Technology and Management's Polysomnographic Technology Program by Dr. Kala Sury.

in the eye channels. Note that these excursions are not as high in amplitude as the left–right movements. A little before the midpoint of the epoch, the patient is instructed to blink five times. Finally, in the later part of the epoch, the technologist has asked the patient to grind his or her teeth; a corresponding increase in chin EMG activity is seen.

At the end of the epoch in the previous example, the patient is directed to make a snoring noise. An increase in activity in the snore channel can be seen at the beginning of the epoch shown in **Figure 9-32**. Shortly after, the patient is asked to breathe through his or her nose and signal excursion is confirmed in the CPAP flow channel.

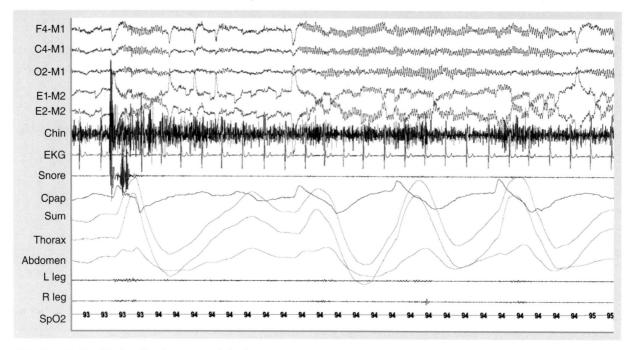

FIGURE 9-32 Physiologic calibrations sample 4. (Patient asked to breath normally.)

Figure by Lisa M. Endee; produced from a sleep study provided to Stony Brook University School of Health Technology and Management's Polysomnographic Technology Program by Dr. Kala Sury.

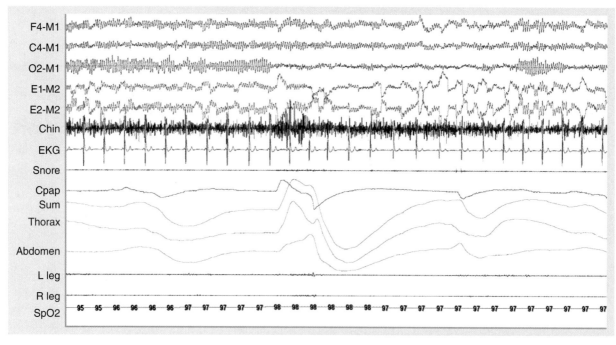

FIGURE 9-33 Physiologic calibrations sample 5. (Patient asked to hold their breath.)

Figure by Lisa M. Endee; produced from a sleep study provided to Stony Brook University School of Health Technology and Management's Polysomnographic Technology Program by Dr. Kala Sury.

Figure 9-33 portrays a directed breath hold in which a flattening of the CPAP flow and respiratory effort channels is noted.

In **Figure 9-34**, the patient is asked to point and flex his or her right foot. Note the burst of increased amplitude activity in the right leg EMG channel (RLEG). This is repeated with the left leg, and a similar burst of activity is seen.

Maintaining Patient Safety and the Integrity of the Recording

After all calibration procedures are performed and the patient is given the final instructions about the sleep study, the technologist documents lights out on the record and the sleep study is begun. The technologist's responsibility for the duration of the study is to maintain the safety of

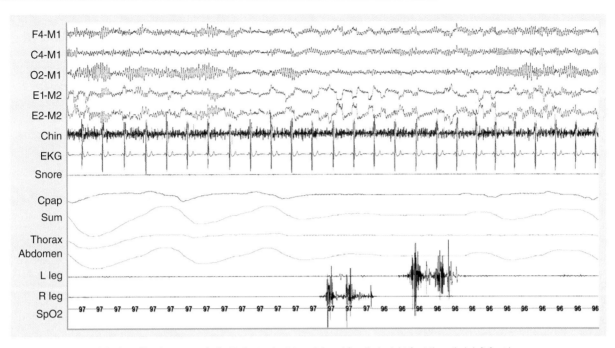

FIGURE 9-34 Physiologic calibrations sample 6. (Patient asked to point and flex their right foot then their left foot.)

Figure by Lisa M. Endee; produced from a sleep study provided to Stony Brook University School of Health Technology and Management's Polysomnographic Technology Program by Dr. Kala Sury.

the patient and the integrity of the recording. Monitoring the patient's EKG, oxygen saturation, and other vital parameters are important to ensuring patient safety, as is certification in basic life support and cardiopulmonary resuscitation. To ensure that quality signals are obtained and maintained throughout the sleep study, the technologist must quickly identify artifacts when they occur and troubleshoot them appropriately and in a timely manner.

Technologist Notes and Documentation

To initiate a sleep study, the technologist must correctly enter the patient's information into the computer so that the record can be properly identified. This information entered by the sleep technologist is translated directly to the scored report. The following patient information should be included:

- Patient's full name
- Patient's height and weight
- Patient's date of birth
- Patient's medical history
- Patient's insurance information
- Patient's current medications
- Referring and interpreting physicians
- Technologist's full name and credentials
- Date of the sleep study
- Type of study being performed
- Montage being used

One primary task of the sleep technologist is to document the activities of the patient throughout the night. The required documentation may vary from lab to lab but is often referred to as the "technologist's notes."

The technologist's notes should include items that are visible on the polysomnograph as well as those that are not. For example, the quality of snoring (soft, medium, or loud) is a helpful detail because the scoring technologist is unable to hear the patient's snore. Also, if the technologist hears bruxism, it is important to make a notation of it on the epochs in which it occurs, because an audible accounting of teeth grinding is a criteria for scoring this event. Every lab's data-acquisition protocol should include the required documentation by the technologist. The following are several items that are often included in the sleep technologist's notes.

- Name of technologist
- Date of the study
- Type of study performed
- Amplifier calibrations
- Physiologic calibrations
- Start and end times of the sleep study
- Technical difficulties and methods of correction
- Times and purposes for entering the patient room
- Level of snoring (mild, moderate, severe)
- Leg movements, respiratory events, EEG arousals, and other significant events noted
- Any EEG or EKG abnormalities noted
- Any abnormal behavioral observations
- Periods of nocturia (patient using the restroom)
- Patient concerns or complaints
- Anything noteworthy on discussion with the patient
- Type and size of PAP interface
- CPAP or bi-level PAP starting, ending, and pressure changes
- Supplemental oxygen flow level
- Any other unusual event or observation that may not be seen by the scoring technologist

Table 9-6 shows an example of technologist's notes during a sleep study.

Posttest Summary

Patient is a 57-year-old male who is 68 inches tall and weighs 245 lbs. He complains of snoring, witnessed apneas, gasping for breath during sleep, and daytime fatigue. His medical history includes hypertension, diabetes, asthma, and congestive heart failure. He has smoked one pack of cigarettes a day for the past 32 years. The diagnostic sleep study started at 2220, and the sleep latency was slightly prolonged at 25 minutes. The patient had frequent obstructive apneas and hypopneas throughout the night and snored

Table 9-6
Sample Technologist's Notes

Patient Name: Jane Doe	**Referring Physician:** Dr. Smith
Technologist Name: John Jackson	**Interpreting Physician:** Dr. Jones
Sleep Study Date: 8/1/18	**Sleep Study Type:** Diagnostic

Time	Epoch No.	Stage	Position	SpO$_2$ (%)	Notes
2210	20	W	Supine	95	Amplifier calibrations
2215	30	W	Supine	95	Physiologic calibrations
2220	40	W	Supine	95	Lights out, patient breathing room air
2245	90	N1	Supine	94	Sleep onset
2358	116	W	Right	95	Patient moving to the right lateral position
0020	160	N3	Right	89	Occasional hypopneas w/ O$_2$ desaturations
0040	200	N2	Left	92	Patient moving to the left lateral position
0115	270	R	Left	84	REM onset, frequent obstructive apneas
0145	330	W	Supine	93	Patient awake, moving to supine position
0210	380	N2	Supine	87	ECG presents occasional unifocal PVCs
0230	420	N3	Supine	88	Persistent hypopneas and oxygen desaturations
0245	450	N2	Supine	90	Leg movements associated with respiratory events
0300	480	R	Supine	81	Frequent severe obstructive apneas
0325	530	W	Upright	0	Nocturia. Patient complained of pain in left leg
0330	540	W	Left	93	Patient back to bed
0345	570	N1	Left	92	Patient asleep, beginning to desaturate
0400	600	N2	Left	89	Occasional hypopneas
0420	640	W	Right	94	Patient awake, moving to right lateral position
0440	680	N2	Right	94	Patient snoring lightly
0500	720	R	Right	83	Pt in REM, frequent obstructive apneas w/ desaturations
0515	750	R	Right	85	Pt still in REM with severe obstructive apneas
0535	790	W	Upright	0	Nocturia
0540	800	W	Supine	95	Patient back to bed
0550	820	W	Supine	94	Patient having difficulty getting back to sleep
0600	840	W	Supine	95	Patient still awake, complaining of pain in left leg
0620	880	W	Supine	95	Lights on
0625	890	W	Supine	95	Posttest physiologic calibrations
0630	900	W	Supine	94	Posttest amplifier calibrations

lightly. The ECG presented occasional unifocal PVCs. REM latency was prolonged at 175 minutes. The patient got out of bed twice during the night to use the restroom and complained of pain in his left leg. Leg movements were few and usually occurred in association with respiratory events. The study ended at 0620.

Ending the Study

At the end of the sleep study, lights on is tagged on the record and the patient is woken up. The technologist must then complete a final impedance check to document that the signal quality was maintained throughout the recording. Posttest amplifier and physiologic calibrations are then performed similarly to those done at the beginning of the study. The technologist then must "unhook" the patient, carefully removing each electrode and wire from the patient's skin. Adhesive remover is often used so the technologist can remove the sticky electrodes without causing harm to the patient. The technologist should assist the patient by cleaning the paste off the electrode sites after the wires have been removed and cleaning the markings caused by the EEG measurements the previous night. The patient completes the required posttest forms and questionnaires and then is allowed to change clothes and prepare for the day.

Patient Discharge

Each lab should have a written procedure in place for patient discharge. Typically, after the patient has completed all morning questionnaires and forms, he or she will shower and get ready to leave. Before the patient leaves, the technologist has a last opportunity to further educate the patient or answer questions. The technologist can also provide the patient with educational pamphlets or brochures about sleep and sleep disorders. Finally, it is important that the patient understand approximately when to expect the results of the study.

Chapter Summary

The sleep technologist has a great deal of responsibility in performing a quality sleep study and caring for patients. Typically, a sleep technologist is responsible for two patients per night, although this can vary slightly per testing facility and depending on the special needs of the patients. The technologist should always be well prepared before patients arrive to ensure a smooth flow process.

The first thing a sleep technologist should do when preparing for the patient to arrive is to review the patient chart. The technologist should become acquainted with the patient's medical history, screening questionnaires, and any notes left by the physician or clerical staff. The technologist should pay extra attention to the physician's orders to ensure that the appropriate study is being performed and that any special requests by the physician are attended to.

Next, the technologist should prepare the patient tray and testing environment. This involves gathering all items needed for the patient hookup, including all wires, electrodes, pastes, tapes, and other supplies. The patient hookup is time intensive and proper preparation can be helpful in spending the time more efficiently. In preparing the testing room, the technologist should ensure the environment is clean and appears inviting. Most diagnostic equipment should be out of sight.

Before the patient arrives, the technologist should also ensure that the diagnostic equipment is in working order. Connection problems should be addressed before the patient arrives.

The technologist then should select an appropriate montage for the type of study ordered. A montage is the setup of signals to be displayed on the polysomnograph, including reference electrodes, filter and sensitivity settings, sampling rates, display settings, and other parameters. Amplifier calibrations can be performed at this time as well. This process gives the technologist a final check to ensure equipment connectivity and confirms the filter and sensitivity settings for each channel; any necessary modifications to these parameters can be made before patient arrival.

When the patient arrives, he or she completes a series of forms and questionnaires according to lab protocol. The technologist should ensure that these are filled out properly and completely, making note of any unusual or significant responses.

The technologist then performs the patient hookup. During this time, the technologist should build a relationship of trust with the patient, help the patient feel comfortable, and provide as much sleep education as possible. Doing so not only helps the patient relax and feel more confident in the validity of the study but also helps ensure the patient will comply with the recommended testing or treatment.

After the patient hookup is completed, an impedance check should be performed to ensure acceptable values and quality signals. Any impedance values that fall above standard recommendations should be corrected before continuing with the study.

Next, the technologist should complete the physiologic calibrations. This is a series of tests in which the patient is instructed to move his or her legs, hold his or her breath, and perform other simple physical tasks. This allows the technologist to verify appropriate placement of electrodes and sensors and serves as a baseline for scoring the sleep study.

During the study, the technologist keeps detailed and accurate notes of anything significant about the patient activities during the night. The requirements of the technologist notes are outlined according to lab protocol but usually include details on the quality of the patient's snoring, any significant events and behavioral observations that occurred, and the study start and end times.

In the morning, at the end of the study, the technologist awakens the patient, performs a final impedance check and both amplifier and physiologic calibrations. The patient is unhooked from the diagnostic equipment and given a series of posttest questionnaires as needed by the lab and physician. The technologist provides further patient education during this time without divulging information from the study.

Case Study

A sleep technologist has just finished loading the diagnostic polysomnogram montage in preparation for a sleep study. She performs an amplifier calibration and notes the tracings shown in **Figure 9-35**.

■ Which channel or channels appear to have incorrect settings? Why?

■ For each incorrectly set channel, which setting do you think is incorrect? Is it set too low or too high? Hint: Use the correctly set channels for comparison.

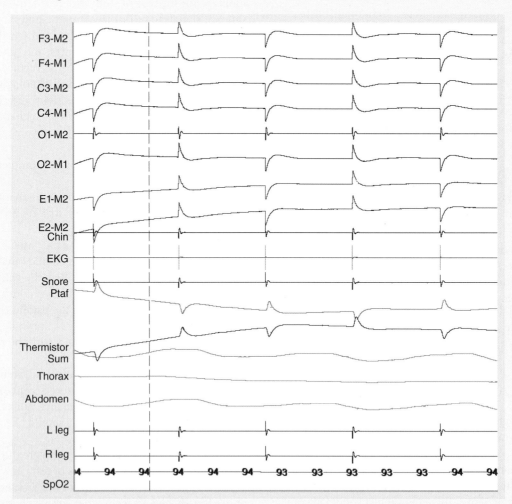

FIGURE 9-35 Case study amplifier calibration.

Figure by Lisa M. Endee; produced from a sleep study provided to Stony Brook University School of Health Technology and Management's Polysomnographic Technology Program by Dr. Kala Sury.

Chapter 9 Questions

Please consider the following questions as they relate to the material in this chapter.

1. What items should be included on the patient tray?
2. What is the recommended sampling rate for EEG channels?
3. What additional channels are usually recorded during an REM behavior-disorder study?
4. What is the time constant, and how is it affected by filter settings?
5. Why do we record eye movements during physiologic calibrations?
6. What are some items recorded in the technologist's notes? Why are these important items to note?

Footnote

1. American Academy of Sleep Medicine (2017). *AASM Manual for the Scoring of Sleep and Associated Events. Rules Terminology and Technical Specifications*. Version 2.4.

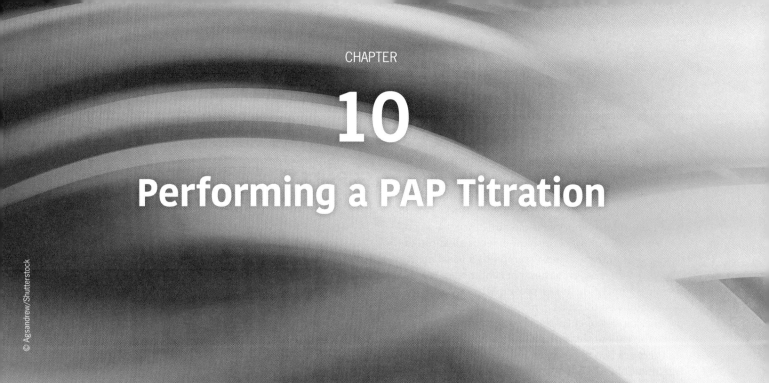

10
Performing a PAP Titration

© Agsandrew/Shutterstock

CHAPTER OUTLINE

LEARNING OBJECTIVES

1. Understand how PAP therapy is used in the treatment of sleep-related breathing disorders.
2. Learn how to choose an appropriate interface.
3. Discover the different types of PAP equipment.
4. Understand the goals of a titration.
5. Know when to use bi-level PAP.
6. Learn how to titrate O$_2$.

KEY TERMS

positive airway pressure (PAP) therapy
sleep-related breathing disorders (SRBDs)
continuous positive airway pressure (CPAP)
bi-level positive airway pressure (bi-level PAP)
respiratory cycle
inspiratory positive airway pressure (IPAP)
expiratory positive airway pressure (EPAP)
hypocapnea
hypoxic respiratory drive
hyperoxemia
hypercapneic respiratory drive
hypercapnea

adaptive support ventilation (ASV)
average volume assured pressure support (AVAPS)
nasal mask
full face mask
nasal pillow interface
auto positive airway pressure (auto PAP)
acclimatization
desensitization
respiratory disturbance index (RDI)
split-night sleep study
first night effect
apnea–hypopnea index (AHI)
supplemental oxygen
hypoxemia

PAP Therapy

Despite many recent technological advancements in both surgical and nonsurgical treatment options, **positive airway pressure (PAP) therapy** remains the preferred and most widely used therapy for the treatment of **sleep-related breathing disorders (SRBDs)**. PAP therapy is noninvasive and includes three main equipment components: a blower unit, corrugated tubing, and an interface (see **Figure 10-1**). The therapy works by pulling in and filtering normal room air (21% oxygen) and applying it to a blower. The blower sends air through the tubing to an interface, most commonly a nasal mask, at a set pressure that is measured in centimeters of water pressure (cm H_2O). The air pressure that is delivered can be adjusted to act as a mechanical splint to hold the patient's airway open, assist with ventilating the patient while the patient sleeps, or both.

There are two main types of PAP therapy for the treatment of SRBDs: **continuous positive airway pressure (CPAP)** and **bi-level positive airway pressure (bi-level PAP)**. The main difference between the two is that pressure applied during CPAP therapy remains consistent, or "continuous," throughout the **respiratory cycle** (inspiration and expiration), whereas bi-level therapy uses pressure applied at two separate levels, hence the term *bi-level*. Specifically, during bi-level therapy, the pressure is higher during the inspiratory phase and lower during the expiratory phase. CPAP therapy and the various forms of bi-level therapies will be discussed in the upcoming sections.

CPAP

CPAP remains the preferred and most widely used therapy for obstructive sleep apnea (OSA). Obstructive sleep apnea is characterized by a complete or partial obstruction in the upper airway during sleep that results in frequent arousals, among other deleterious consequences. The air pressure that is delivered during CPAP therapy serves as a mechanical splint to hold the patient's airway open during the respiratory cycle. With the airway patency maintained, the patient is able to inhale and exhale normally and achieve better quality sleep. See **Figure 10-2** for a depiction of how CPAP works.

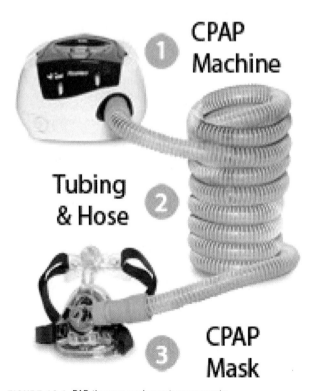

FIGURE 10-1 PAP therapy equipment components.

Retrieved from https://www.cpap.com/cpap-faq/cpap-equipment

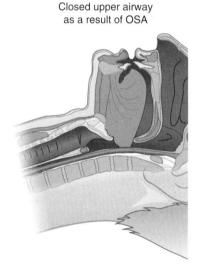

Closed upper airway as a result of OSA

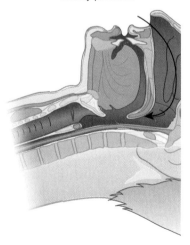

Airway opened by positive airway pressure

FIGURE 10-2 Closed and open airways.

Bi-Level

As previously mentioned, bi-level therapy is characterized by two separate pressures corresponding with inhalation and exhalation. These separate treatment levels are referred to respectively as **inspiratory positive airway pressure (IPAP)** during inhalation and **expiratory positive airway pressure (EPAP)** during exhalation. The EPAP and IPAP settings serve different purposes. Like CPAP, EPAP acts to maintain the patency of the airway. IPAP, however, provides a means to provide ventilatory support and increased tidal volumes.

Although CPAP is indicated for those patients with obstructive breathing disorders during sleep, bi-level therapy is used to treat patients with complex SRBDs, like hypoventilation disorders or Cheyne–Stokes respiration, and those who have difficulty tolerating high CPAP pressures. Providing a lower EPAP allows the patient to exhale more easily without having to push as hard against the incoming positive pressure. Conversely, providing an increased IPAP allows the patient to inhale larger volumes of air with greater ease.

Bi-level PAP therapy is often used for patients with central respiratory sleep disorders. Central sleep apnea is different from obstructive sleep apnea in that patients with central sleep apnea do not attempt to breathe. Central apneas are not caused by an obstruction; rather, they are caused by either **hypocapnea** (decreased CO_2 levels), which would communicate to the brain that a breath is not necessary, or a blunted **hypoxic respiratory drive** because of **hyperoxemia** (increased arterial oxygen levels). For most people, the central chemoreceptors respond to high carbon dioxide levels and drive the urge to breathe so they can rid their bodies of excess carbon dioxide. This is known as the **hypercapneic respiratory drive**. When carbon dioxide levels are high (**hypercapnea**), a patient with a hypercapneic drive will breathe heavily. When CO_2 levels are low, that patient will breathe less or not at all. Alternatively, some patients—especially those with lung disease (because of the normally high levels of carbon dioxide they become tolerant to)—may be reliant on a hypoxic respiratory drive. This is driven by the peripheral chemoreceptors and responds to levels of oxygen in the blood. When a patient with a hypoxic respiratory drive has elevated levels of oxygen, it will decrease the urge to breathe, causing central apneas.

Whichever the cause, because CPAP therapy only acts as a splint to address airway obstruction, it will not be effective at addressing these complex sleep-related breathing disturbances. Because bi-level therapy offers a means of assisting ventilation, it is a more appropriate treatment option for complex sleep breathing disorders like hypoventilation and Cheyne–Stokes respiration, which are characterized by varying tidal volumes and minute ventilations. Bi-level PAP therapy can provide ventilatory support by increasing the inspiratory pressure, which allows the patient to inhale larger volumes of air with greater ease.

Various forms of bi-level therapies are currently available to address more complex SRBDs. These include **adaptive support ventilation (ASV)** and **average volume assured pressure support (AVAPS)**. These will be described in more detail later in the chapter.

PAP Equipment

The initiation of PAP therapy requires several pieces of equipment, including a patient interface, a PAP device, and tubing to connect the interface to the device. Most PAP units come standard with a humidifier to improve comfort and compliance. These features will be discussed.

Interface Selection

Many different types, styles, and sizes of interfaces are available for use with PAP therapy. A large number of patients are able to use a standard **nasal mask** that covers the nose and sits between the upper lip and bridge of the nose (see **Figure 10-3**). **Full face masks** are available for those patients who have difficulty breathing through their nose or keeping their mouth closed while asleep. Patients with untreated OSA frequently open their mouths wide during sleep in an attempt to increase the opening of the upper airway. If the mouth is open while wearing a nasal mask, the air flows into the nose and then directly out of the mouth, making it difficult to inhale. The full face mask corrects this by covering both the nose and the mouth (see **Figure 10-4**). A **nasal pillow interface** rests at the end of the patient's nares and looks similar to a large oxygen cannula

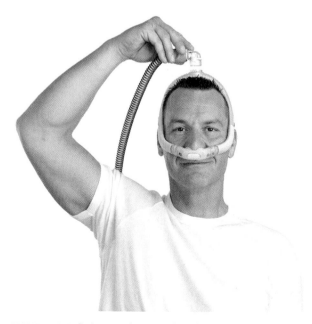

FIGURE 10-3 Patient wearing a nasal mask.
Courtesy of ResMed.

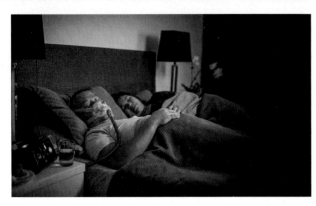

FIGURE 10-4 Patient wearing a full face mask.
Courtesy of ResMed.

(see **Figure 10-5**). This interface covers less of the face and is often chosen for patients who are claustrophobic or bothered by a mask. Other considerations in choosing an interface include facial hair, nasal or facial abnormalities, and field of vision. Deciding on an appropriate interface for a patient takes patience and becomes easier after gaining experience in working with and managing patients on PAP therapy.

When fitting an interface, the technologist must use the sizing gauzes that are supplied by the manufacturer. Once the correct size has been determined, the mask should be placed lightly against the patient's skin, exactly as the patient would wear it at night. The straps are then put into place around the patient's head and tightened to a level that is comfortable for the patient. The mask should not be overtightened. Most masks are equipped to create a seal against the patient's skin while fitted loosely against the face. If overtightened, the mask seal will fold and crinkle, causing air leakage. Overtightening the mask can also be extremely uncomfortable for the patient, often leading to headaches and skin irritations.

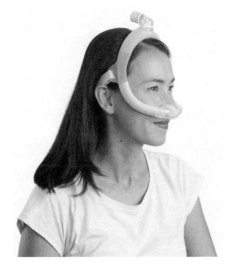

FIGURE 10-5 Patient wearing a nasal pillow mask.
Courtesy of ResMed.

PAP Devices

PAP devices provide positive airway pressure to the airway to treat various SRBDs. As noted previously, pressures are measured in centimeters of water (cm H_2O). PAP levels can be verified by a device called a *water column manometer*. The manometer is filled to a specified point with water, and the air from the PAP machine pushes the water to a certain level. Increased PAP levels push the water higher. Hence, a water column manometer is a true mechanical measure of PAP pressure.

PAP units designed for diagnostic use in the sleep lab often have capabilities that far exceed those of home units. Diagnostic units typically include options for remote monitoring and controlling, live output data for recording on the polysomnograph, leak measurements, and the ability to switch modes among CPAP, bi-level PAP, and **auto positive airway pressure (auto PAP)**. CPAP mode delivers a constant positive pressure, whereas bi-level mode allows settings for separate IPAP and EPAP pressures. If IPAP and EPAP pressures were set at the same level, then the machine would essentially be delivering CPAP therapy. Auto PAP mode automatically adjusts CPAP as needed, based on detected airflow and vibrations from the upper airway. If the system detects vibrations in the upper airway from snoring or a decrease or absence of airflow, then the pressure increases. After a period of time without detected vibrations or changes in airflow, the pressure decreases.

Bi-level units include settings for backup respiratory rates and timing of the respiratory cycle. A timed bi-level mode does not detect the changes in patient respirations but switches between IPAP and EPAP on a specific time base as defined by the user. This method of bi-level PAP delivery is extremely uncomfortable for most patients, and it is typically reserved only for severe patients who require controlled ventilation. A spontaneous bi-level mode automatically shifts between IPAP and EPAP when it detects a change in the patient's respirations. A third option available on many bi-level machines is a spontaneous mode with a timed backup. This allows the patient to determine the change of respirations but with the safety of a timed backup in case the patient does not breathe on his or her own.

As noted previously, advanced forms of bi-level therapies have been developed to address more complex SRBDs. ASV is a positive pressure mode of ventilation that can automatically adjust respiratory rate, tidal volume, and inspiratory time based on the patient's requirements. It collected information on a breath-by-breath basis and adjusts pressure support to optimize a patient's breathing pattern. ASV machines are used to treat central sleep apnea, mixed sleep apnea, and Cheynes–Stokes respiration, an abnormal waxing and waning breathing with central apneic events. The unit uses an algorithm that detects significant reductions or pauses in breathing and provides positive pressure, between the minimum and maximum pressure support settings, to maintain the patient's breathing. Despite its success, a recent study reported that ASV may be harmful to patients with chronic heart failure who have significantly reduced left ventricular ejection fractions. Therefore, confirmation of cardiovascular status by the physician is recommended before ASV therapy is prescribed.

AVAPS is a positive pressure mode of ventilation that automatically adapts the pressure support (IPAP) a patient needs to maintain an average tidal volume. AVAPS uses an algorithm to estimate tidal volume at each breath, compares it to the target volume, and adjusts IPAP accordingly. These units are commonly used to treat patients with complex SRBDs such as obesity hypoventilation syndrome and chronic obstructive pulmonary disease. The prescribed settings would include the target tidal volume and IPAP limits.

Home units are typically much simpler and easier to use. The pressure on these units cannot be changed without an interface device or a combination of key entries on the machine. Many home PAP devices include memory cards, data storage, or Wi-Fi capabilities with downloadable data, for use at patient follow-ups. There are various manufacturers of CPAP and bi-level machines, and many have developed features for improved patient comfort. For example, many have pressure reliefs at the end of inhalation and the beginning of exhalation to allow for a more comfortable transition. Many patients find this option much more comfortable and tolerable.

When choosing an appropriate machine for a patient to use at home, the available features and the cost of the machine should be considered. One type of machine may be appropriate for one patient but not another.

Humidification

An important feature added to most PAP units is humidification. A common side effect of PAP therapy is nasal and upper airway dryness. Humidification helps alleviate this complaint. Adjustments in humidity levels and temperature can be tailored to improve patient comfort. Many PAP machines have integrated heated humidifiers, whereas others use external humidifiers. When heated humidification is used, water sometimes pools inside the hose when the room air temperature is significantly cooler than the hose temperature. This can block the passage of air. This issue is commonly addressed by wrapping the tubing with an insulated hose cover.

Adverse Effects

Although PAP therapy is noninvasive, several adverse effects are common to users. Nasal dryness is one of the most common side effects and can be addressed with increasing humidity and temperature settings as noted previously. In addition, many patients simply have difficulty tolerating the air pressure that is delivered. One of the most effective methods of addressing this issue involves coaching patients through the experience, helping them relax while using the therapy and talking through their concerns. Facial soreness at various pressure points can also occur, most commonly from overtightening or improper mask fit. This is most appropriately addressed by confirming that the correct size interface is being used and readjusting the head straps for comfort. If the problem persists, a different style interface should be considered.

PAP Titration

Most patients begin the sleep study process with a diagnostic polysomnogram. If the results of this test afford the diagnosis of sleep disordered breathing, then a PAP titration is almost always indicated. The word *titration* refers to the gradual process of adjusting the strength or dose of a medication or treatment until an acceptable or optimal treatment level is achieved. Therefore, a PAP titration involves gradually adjusting the PAP levels during a patient's sleep until the upper-airway obstruction or breathing disorder is effectively corrected.

The hookup procedure for a PAP titration study mirrors that of the diagnostic study with one exception: The two airflow sensors used in a PSG are replaced with a PAP mask for the titration. The montage selected for these two studies are nearly identical, usually with the addition of a PAP pressure channel and PAP flow channel. The PAP flow is detected by the PAP machine rather than, or in addition to, a thermistor, thermocouple, or pressure transducer.

During the hookup process, the technologist should take the time to properly fit the patient with an appropriate mask that the patient will feel comfortable using. Proper mask fitting can greatly improve a patient's tolerance of therapy. In addition, the *AASM Clinical Guidelines for the Manual Tritration of Positive Airway Pressure in Patients with Obstructive Sleep Apnea*[1] recommends that all patients receive education, hands-on demonstration of the equipment, and **acclimatization** before the first night of PAP titration. Specifically, the technologist should educate patients about their sleep disorders and the rationale behind the use of PAP therapy to treat it. They should give patients the opportunity to handle the equipment, make self-adjustments, and ask questions.

The level of patient education can have large and lasting effects for a patient when he or she is deciding whether or not to comply with treatment. Sleep technologists serve an important role in improving both compliance and tolerance to PAP therapy by educating their patients about the effects of untreated sleep-related breathing disorders and the potential benefits of using PAP therapy. PAP therapy should be introduced at the lowest pressure setting, and time should be allowed for the patient to acclimate. The technologist should coach the patient through the initial application, instructing him or her to breathe in and out, keeping the mouth closed if possible. The technologist should be patient and provide positive reinforcement. This can have a great influence on whether the patient can successfully complete the titration study and whether they will be compliant with therapy.

PAP **desensitization** involves the use of techniques to assist those patients who continue to have difficulty acclimating to the therapy. These techniques can be performed in the sleep clinic or the home environment and are meant to expose patients to the therapy in shorter increments and more gradually to help them better tolerate it. The success of desensitization relies on repeated positive reinforcement and giving the patient more control of the therapy—for example, giving patients the ability to hold the mask against their face and the opportunity to pull the mask away if the therapy gets too overwhelming. Also, pressure adjustments are accomplished gradually, encouraging the patient along the way. The desensitization procedure is considered successful if the patient is able to tolerate 8 cm H_2O for approximately 15 minutes.

Once the patient is tolerant of the therapy, the titration procedure can begin. The overall aim of the titration study is to adjust the therapeutic pressures while the patient is asleep to eliminate sleep-disordered breathing events. There are some differences in CPAP and bi-level titration protocols that will be discussed here. It is important that the technologist reviews the patient record and confirms the physician's study order on file to determine which protocol should be implemented and any additional orders or instructions that are given.

CPAP Titration Protocols

According to the *AASM Clinical Guidelines* for treating patients with obstructive sleep apnea,[1] the recommended minimum starting CPAP should be 4 cm H_2O for adult patients. The following sections summarize the AASM guidelines for a CPAP titration. Note that sleep centers can customize protocols based on these guidelines. Sleep technologists should ensure that they follow lab-specific protocols.

Increasing CPAP

During a CPAP titration study, pressure is used as a splint to maintain the patency of the upper airway. Pressures should be titrated upward in ≥1 cm increments over at least 5-minute periods of time in response to the following breathing events:

- Two or more obstructive apneas
- Three or more hypopneas
- Five or more respiratory effort–related arousals (RERAs)
- Three or more minutes of loud snoring

The AASM recommends that this protocol be continued throughout the testing period until the technologist has observed at least 30 consecutive minutes without breathing events. At this point, it is recommended that the technologist maintain the therapeutic pressure for the remainder of the study period or until he or she notes additional breathing events that would prompt a return to the protocol. The technologist should always note the reasons for increasing CPAP and the time at which the increase occurred. The recommended maximum CPAP pressure is 20 cm H_2O for patients 12 years of age or older.

According to the AASM clinical guidelines for the manual titration of PAP therapy,[1] an optimal titration is defined as:

- A **respiratory disturbance index (RDI)** of less than five events for a period of 15 minutes
- $SpO_2 > 90\%$
- Fewer than five electroencephalogram (EEG) arousals per hour in supine rapid eye movement (REM)
- Snoring eliminated

The ideal titration will reach these goals while maintaining a high level of patient tolerance.

Patients with SRBDs may exhibit associated events with the respiratory disturbances that can include limb movements or EEG arousals. When titrating PAP therapy, the sleep technologist should watch for and make note of these events, because they may indicate more subtle flow limitation and the need for higher treatment levels. Some respiratory events may be difficult to visually detect on a 30-second epoch. Most digital systems include features to help with this. The review mode allows the technologist to look back to previously recorded pages in the sleep study without interrupting the recording of live data. Many digital systems also include multiple time-based views that allow the technologist to view the EEGs, electrooculograms (EOGs), and other parameters at the standard 30 seconds per page while viewing the respiratory channels at longer time bases. This allows the technologist to more easily see long, subtle hypopneas and the presence of abnormal breathing patterns.

Decreasing CPAP

Occasionally, a technologist may need to decrease CPAP during a titration. CPAP decreases are often necessary at the beginning portion of the study if the patient is unable to tolerate the initial upward titration or awakens during the night feeling overwhelmed with the pressure. Increasing the CPAP pressure too quickly can cause changes in the patient's drive to breathe and can lead to central apneas. Therefore, a series of unexpected central apneas during a titration procedure, especially on a patient who has no history of central

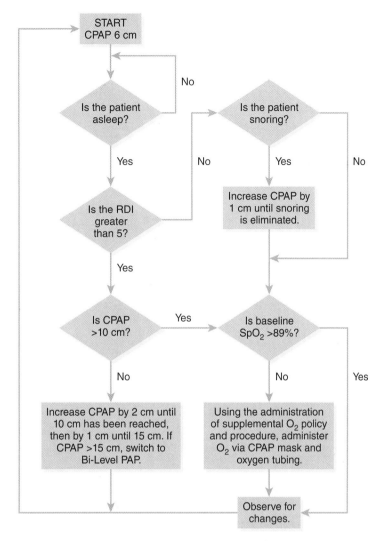

FIGURE 10-6 Sample CPAP protocol.

Data from: Principles of Polysomnography, Sleep Management Services, 2002.

events, may warrant a decrease back to the previous successful pressure. The technologist should always note the reason for decreasing CPAP pressure and the time at which the decrease occurred.

Sleep centers may customize titration protocols under the direction of the medical director. The protocols should, however, be consistent with clinical practice guidelines.

Figure 10-6 shows a sample CPAP titration.

Bi-Level Titration Protocols

When preparing for a bi-level titration, the technologist should be especially careful in mask selection. Because patients on bi-level PAP often require high treatment levels, the technologist should select a mask that can handle high pressures with minimal leakage.

According to the *AASM Clinical Guidelines*,[1] the recommended minimum starting IPAP should be 8 cm H_2O, whereas EPAP should be set at 4 cm H_2O. If a patient is uncomfortable or intolerant of high CPAP

above 14 cm H_2O, then the mode may be switched over from CPAP to bi-level. In this case, it is recommended that the EPAP be set at the CPAP whereby apneic events were eliminated and the IPAP set 4 cm H_2O above that. The recommended minimum IPAP–EPAP differential is 4 cm H_2O, while the maximum differential is 10 cm H_2O.

The titration of bi-level therapy should include upward titration of the IPAP *and* EPAP by at least 1 cm H_2O for apneic events and upward titration of the IPAP pressure *only* by at least 1 cm H_2O in response to hypopnea, RERAs, or snoring. IPAP can also be increased to correct for hypoxemia that persists despite a patent airway. It is recommended that the technologist maintain each pressure setting for at least 5 minutes and continue to follow this protocol until a 30-minute period is noted without the presence of breathing events. At this point, the technologist should maintain the therapeutic pressure for the remainder of the study period or until he or she notes additional breathing events that would prompt a return to the protocol.

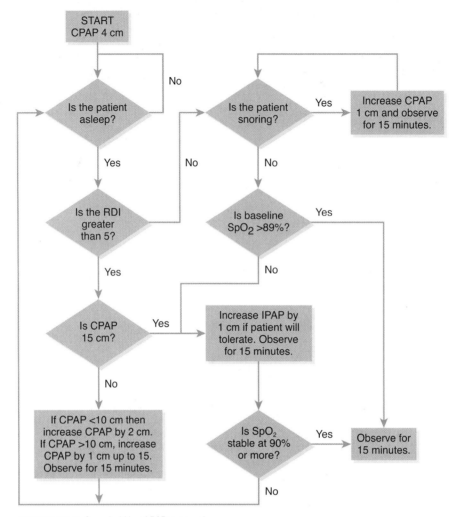

FIGURE 10-7 Sample bi-level PAP protocol.

If treatment-emergent central apneas are observed, a decrease in IPAP or a switch to spontaneously timed mode with backup rate may be helpful. The recommended maximum IPAP pressure is 30 cm H_2O for patients 12 years of age and older. An optimal bi-level titration is defined the same as for a CPAP titration.

Figure 10-7 contains a sample flowchart of how bi-level PAP titrations are performed at some labs.

Split-Night Studies

A **split-night sleep study** begins as a diagnostic polysomnogram and concludes with a CPAP titration if certain requirements are met. One advantage of a split-night study versus separate diagnostic and therapeutic studies is that the patient spends only one night in the lab. This is especially beneficial for patients who have difficulty affording two separate studies. It may also be beneficial for severe patients who need treatment quickly. A split-night study may also help in cases where the sleep lab is full and the patient needs to be seen quickly.

Split-night studies are now always advantageous, however. Decreasing the time spent performing the diagnostic portion of the study may lead to a misdiagnosis. Further, decreasing the titration portion of the study may greatly hinder the physician's ability to accurately determine the optimal PAP level. Also, the **first night effect** can decrease the amount and quality of sleep during both the diagnostic and treatment portions of the study, and the technologist may simply not have enough time to accomplish the goals of the study.

When performing a split-night study, the technologist is required to carefully count the number of apneas and hypopneas during the diagnostic portion of the study to ensure that the patient qualifies for a PAP study. Most health insurance plans require an **apnea–hypopnea index (AHI)** of at least 30 events per hour over a period of at least 2 hours of sleep before they will approve the switch to a PAP titration. Figure 10-8 contains a sample flowchart for performing split-night studies.

Supplemental O_2

Supplemental oxygen is often used in the sleep lab to address **hypoxemia**. Technologists should check the baseline oxygen saturation at the beginning of the night by using a pulse oximeter (SpO_2). A patient with a low baseline SpO_2 while awake often needs supplemental O_2

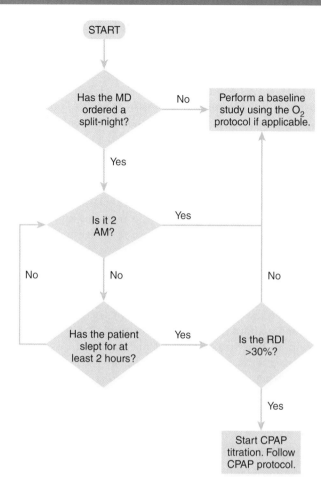

FIGURE 10-8 Sample split-night protocol.

during the night. Thus, if a patient demonstrates decreased SpO_2 levels, the technologist should notify the physician to make him or her aware and obtain an order for supplemental O_2. For patients with SRBDs that demonstrate decreased SpO_2 levels during the study, it is most often recommended to correct the respiratory events via PAP therapy first. Once the SRBD is addressed, if oxygen desaturation persists, then supplemental oxygen may be indicated. In this case, supplemental O_2 can be introduced into the PAP circuit by connecting oxygen tubing to one of the small outlet holes on the PAP interface. Initiation and titration of supplemental O_2 should always be accomplished according to lab protocols. **Figure 10-9** contains a sample O_2 titration protocol.

Post PAP Titration

After completing a CPAP titration, the technologist should discuss the experience with the patient. The patient's perception of the success of the therapy is important and should be noted by the technologist, especially if the patient feels he or she would not use it at home. In some cases, patients believe they sleep poorly using the therapy, when in fact, they sleep well. When discussing the study with the patient in the morning, the technologist must be careful to not make treatment recommendations to the patient. This type of discussion should be accomplished with the ordering physician. At the end of the study, the technologist should provide the patient with educational materials such as brochures and flyers that can remind the patient of the things they discussed in the study.

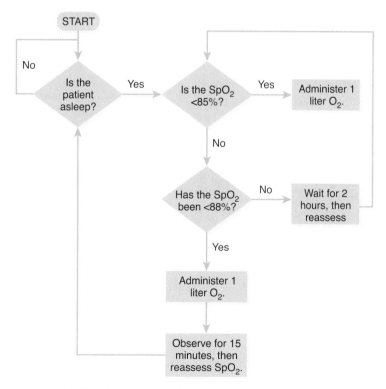

FIGURE 10-9 Sample supplemental O_2 protocol.

Data from: Sleep Management Services, South Jordan, UT. (2002). Principles of Polysomnography.

Certain key data are calculated at each PAP level during the scoring process to enable the interpreting physician to easily determine the appropriate treatment level. These data usually include the respiratory disturbance index, the mean and minimum oxygen saturation (SpO_2), the EEG arousal index, the amount of time spent asleep and in REM at each treatment level, and how these values relate to body position. The physician considers these data when selecting the most appropriate therapeutic pressure setting to prescribe.

After the physician prescribes PAP at an appropriate mode and level, the patient is set up at home with a device that is set to the prescribed pressure by a durable medical equipment (DME) company. The patient is fitted with a mask, which the insurance company will replace every few months as needed. The patient is then followed up with periodically by the DME company, the physician, and the sleep lab to ensure the patient is continuing treatment and that the treatment continues to be effective. Most medical insurance plans will pay for one follow-up sleep study per year to allow the patient to be retitrated if certain symptoms persist. Support groups such as AWAKE (Alert, Well, and Keeping Energetic) can help PAP therapy patients in a group setting with mask issues, insurance issues, compliance, and patient education.

Chapter Summary

Positive airway pressure is the preferred treatment for SRBDs. PAP provides additional air pressure through the nose or mouth (or both) to act as a mechanical splint to hold the upper airway open or supplement ventilation, thus improving sleep quality.

Common side effects of PAP include air leakage, facial discomfort from the mask, dryness of the nose and throat, and feelings of anxiety for claustrophobic patients. Many of these side effects can be corrected by proper mask selection and fitting. A technologist who properly fits a patient's mask can greatly increase the likelihood that he or she will comply with treatment.

Many PAP masks, machines, and humidifiers are available. Technologists should become well versed in these devices so they can effectively help their patients.

Standard titration guidelines are valuable resources and help to direct titration procedures. Sleep labs can customize their PAP protocols, but it is the responsibility of the technologist to be familiar with and apply the lab protocols. Technologists should know when to increase or decrease the pressure and when to switch to bi-level PAP or add supplemental O_2. CPAP therapy involves the application of a consistent positive pressure to the upper airway. The goals of treatment are to correct obstructive breathing events, including apneas, hypopneas, and snores, as well as associated events such as EEG arousals and oxygen desaturations. Bi-level therapy consists of a higher pressure during inhalation (IPAP) and a lower pressure during exhalation (EPAP). Bi-level PAP can help patients who are noncompliant with high CPAP pressures or those who have complex SRBDs. Separate bi-level PAP protocols are needed in the lab and should be used by the technologists.

Split-night studies consist of a diagnostic period lasting at least 2 hours followed by a CPAP titration. These are ordered when a patient needs to be treated quickly or cannot afford two studies. Split studies are advantageous for those reasons but are not commonly used because they do not allow as much time to fully titrate.

If the patient's obstructions are corrected but the SpO_2 is still low, supplemental O_2 may need to be added. This should be done according to lab protocol.

Chapter 10 Questions

Please consider the following questions as they relate to the material in this chapter.

1. Why is CPAP necessary for many patients?
2. How tightly should a CPAP mask be placed against the face?
3. What are some of the options available in CPAP machines?
4. What are the goals of a CPAP titration?
5. When is it appropriate to switch to bi-level PAP?
6. Why is a physician's order required for adding supplemental O_2?

Footnote

1. American Academy of Sleep Medicine. (2012). *AASM Clinical Guidelines for the Manual Titration of Positive Airway Pressure in Patients with Obstructive Sleep Apnea.* Available at http://www.aasmnet.org/Resources/clinicalguidelines/040210.pdf

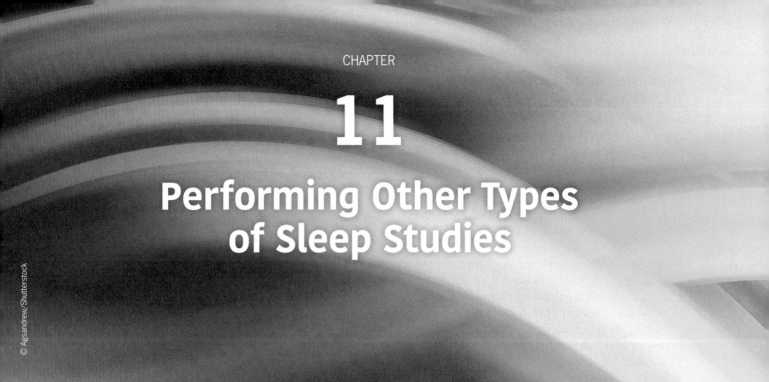

11

Performing Other Types of Sleep Studies

© Agsandrew/Shutterstock

CHAPTER OUTLINE

Multiple Sleep Latency Test
Maintenance of Wakefulness Test
REM Behavior-Disorder Study
Nocturnal Seizure Study
Ambulatory Sleep Studies
Other Diagnostic Testing
Chapter Summary

LEARNING OBJECTIVES

1. Learn about the indications for the MSLT and MWT.
2. Learn how to perform an MSLT and MWT.
3. Understand the importance of an MWT.
4. Learn about other diagnostic studies used in sleep testing.
5. Understand how various diagnostic tools can supplement sleep testing.

KEY TERMS

multiple sleep latency test (MSLT)
hypersomnolence
sleep onset
mean sleep latency
sleep onset REM period (SOREM)
maintenance of wakefulness test (MWT)
unequivocal sleep

REM behavior-disorder study
nocturnal seizure study
ambulatory sleep study
home sleep test (HST)
first night effect
gastric reflux
pH probe
esophageal balloon
arterial blood gas (ABG)

Multiple Sleep Latency Test

A **multiple sleep latency test (MSLT)** is a diagnostic sleep study that consists of a series of five daytime nap opportunities following an overnight diagnostic polysomnogram. It is used to help diagnose narcolepsy and provide information regarding excessive daytime sleepiness and **hypersomnolence**.

An overnight diagnostic study is performed the night before the MSLT primarily to rule out sleep disorders such as obstructive sleep apnea and periodic limb movement disorder, which may contribute to excessive daytime sleepiness and other narcoleptic-like symptoms. Once these other primary sleep disorders are ruled out and after a "normal" overnight polysomnogram consisting of at least 6 hours of sleep, the MSLT testing proceeds.

Significant events during sleep are of less interest during an MSLT than are the amount of time it takes for a patient to fall asleep and the sleep stages the patient achieves. With sleep staging as the primary point of interest in an MSLT, the leg electromyograms (EMGs), oxygen saturation (SpO$_2$), body position, and respiratory channels included for the overnight study are removed. The following channels are recorded during a multiple sleep latency test:

- F3–M2
- F4–M1
- C3–M2
- C4–M1
- O1–M2
- O2–M1
- E1–M2
- E2–M2
- Chin 1
- Chin 2
- electrocardiogram (ECG)

According to the AASM *Practice Parameters*,[1] the first MSLT nap should begin 1.5 to 3 hours after the lights on time noted on the overnight diagnostic study. In between lights on for the overnight study and lights off for the first nap, the patient should remain awake and as alert as possible. For example, the patient should not be allowed to lie down in bed but should be encouraged to walk around the lab, sit in a chair, read, eat breakfast, and so on.

The testing protocol for an MSLT is highly specific and must be followed closely to improve the validity of the study. During each nap, the patient is given 20 minutes after lights out to try to fall asleep. The patient should try to fall asleep rather than try to remain awake during this time. If the patient does not fall asleep during the first 20 minutes of the recording, the nap attempt is concluded. The patient is moved out of the bed and instructed to remain awake until the next nap opportunity. If the patient falls asleep during the nap opportunity, the nap is concluded exactly 15 minutes after

sleep onset. **Sleep onset** is defined as the beginning of the first epoch of sleep. If the patient achieves only one epoch of sleep and then awakens, the nap is still terminated 15 minutes after the first epoch of sleep or sleep onset. The technologist should carefully note the sleep stages achieved during the nap attempts, especially rapid eye movement (REM) sleep. Sleep latencies and REM latencies are of particular interest in an MSLT. As with an overnight sleep study, amplifier calibrations, impedance checks, and physiologic calibrations should be performed at the beginning and end of each nap. Each nap opportunity begins 2 hours after the beginning of the previous nap until five naps are achieved.

To increase the validity of an MSLT, the patient must remain awake between nap opportunities. The technologist must be vigilant about observing the patient during this time. The patient should not lie down or sit in the bed in between naps. Instead, the patient should sit in a chair, stand, or walk around the lab. In addition, patients must not consume caffeine, alcohol, or other drugs that may affect the ability to initiate or maintain sleep. The exception to this protocol is the patient who takes prescription medication on a regular basis; the sleep physician should be aware of it, and it should be documented in the patient record. If a patient consumes caffeine between naps, the technologist should instruct him or her not to do so and document the instruction. If the patient does fall asleep in between naps, the technologist should awaken the patient and document it accordingly. Although this may affect the results of the testing, a patient falling asleep in between naps is not reason to discontinue the test. Some testing facilities include drug screening as part of their MSLT protocol. Exercise and smoking should be avoided completely if possible for at least 30 minutes before a nap opportunity.

The MSLT report should include the start and end times and sleep latency (amount of time from lights out to the first epoch of sleep) of each nap opportunity as well as the **mean sleep latency** (arithmetic mean of all nap opportunities) and the number of nap opportunities that included an episode of REM sleep, which is often referred to as a **sleep onset REM period (SOREM)**. If the patient does not sleep during a nap opportunity, the sleep latency is recorded as 20 minutes. Mean sleep latency values less than 8 minutes and the presence of two or more SOREMs during the MSLT can be diagnostic for narcolepsy. The data from the MSLT is assessed in conjunction with the patient history, the sleep logs collected, and the previous night's overnight polysomnogram to come to a diagnosis and indicate treatment options.

Maintenance of Wakefulness Test

A **maintenance of wakefulness test (MWT)** is a unique diagnostic sleep study performed during the daytime that is used to test a patient's ability to remain awake in monotonous situations. The MWT is often performed on airline pilots, heavy-machine operators, and truck drivers, who may be a hazard to others if they are unable to remain awake while on the job. It is also used on patients previously diagnosed with a primary sleep disorder to document that they are treated optimally. Many clinicians believe that this is a better test of excessive daytime sleepiness than the MSLT because it tests a patient's ability to remain awake rather than their ability to fall asleep.

The MWT montage is identical to that of the MSLT and includes the same channels previously listed. The recommended MWT protocol includes four daytime trials lasting 40 minutes in duration. Unlike the MSLT, it is not a standard that the test be preceded by an overnight polysomnogram, although some sleep physicians prefer to order the testing in that way. The first MWT trial should begin around 9 A.M. According to the AASM's *Practice Parameters*,[1] each MWT trial must begin by placing the patient in bed, seated with the back and head supported by a bedrest. The room should be dimly lit with a light source equivalent to a 7.5-watt night light positioned slightly behind the subject's head.

Like an MSLT, amplifier calibrations, impedance checks, and physiologic calibrations should be performed at the beginning and end of each trial. The patient is then instructed to "Please sit still and remain awake for as long as possible. Look directly ahead of you and do not look directly at the light." The patient is also asked not to use extraordinary measures to maintain wakefulness. Each trial begins 2 hours after the beginning of the previous one. Each MWT trail is terminated after the 40-minute duration or if the patient achieves **unequivocal sleep**, which is defined as three consecutive epochs of stage N1 sleep or one epoch of any other stage of sleep.

Similar to the MSLT, the patient must remain awake between MWT trials. The use of tobacco, caffeine, and medications by the patient before and during MWT should be decided on by the sleep clinician and communicated to the technologist before the MWT. In addition, exercise and smoking should be avoided completely if possible for at least 30 minutes before each MWT trial. Some testing facilities include a drug screening as part of their MWT protocol.

The MWT report should include start and stop times for each trial, sleep latency, total sleep time, stages of sleep achieved for each trial, and the mean sleep latency (the arithmetic mean of the four trials).

REM Behavior-Disorder Study

A **REM behavior-disorder study** is a diagnostic sleep study used to diagnose REM behavior disorder. A patient with a REM behavior disorder often acts out dreams and makes other body or limb movements during REM sleep. Therefore, a sleep study with the purpose of diagnosing REM behavior disorder includes the standard derivations with the addition of arm EMG leads, a video camera (preferably digital) with recording capabilities, and audio monitoring with recording. Arm EMG leads should be placed on the forearm to detect arm and hand movements. Additional electroencephalogram (EEG) channels may be included during a REM behavior-disorder study to rule out nocturnal seizures. A technologist performing a REM behavior-disorder study should pay careful attention to the patient during REM sleep and note muscle movements and changes or lack of changes in chin EMG muscle tone.

Nocturnal Seizure Study

Nocturnal seizure studies utilize the standard diagnostic polysomnogram (PSG) montage with the addition of additional EEG electrodes and video and audio recording (preferably digital video). These studies typically do not warrant the recording of arm EMG activity unless the physician specifically orders it. Various different seizure montages can be used. A sample seizure montage follows.

- Fp1–F3
- F3–C3
- C3–P3
- P3–O1
- Fp2–F4
- F4–C4
- C4–P4
- P4–O2
- E1–M2
- E2–M2
- Chin 1
- Chin 2
- ECG

Like REM behavior disorders, nocturnal seizures are difficult to diagnose in one night and may require multiple sleep studies.

Ambulatory Sleep Studies

Ambulatory sleep studies have become more popular to keep up with the demand for sleep testing and to reduce costs. Ambulatory sleep testing is accomplished with portable equipment, usually using limited channels, in a setting outside the sleep clinic. **Home sleep testing (HST)** is the most common type of ambulatory sleep test. It is performed in the patient's home and is used primarily to identify patients with a high pretest probability of obstructive sleep apnea. Home sleep-testing devices allow the collection of anywhere from three to seven channels of data and most often include the collection of airflow, respiratory effort, ECG, and oxygen saturation via SpO_2. Ambulatory sleep studies can be attended by a technologist or unattended.

Advantages of HST

HST allows the ability to record a patient's sleep in the same setting in which he or she normally sleeps. This may decrease the severity of the **first night effect**. The first night effect describes the effects that anxiety of sleep testing and sleeping in a different environment can have on a patient's sleep study. First night effect often causes patients to have a decreased sleep efficiency and increased EEG arousals and awakenings. In addition, HST is less costly than in-lab sleep testing and often requires a shorter waiting period. This can offer a good alternative to a 2- to 3-month waiting period that may exist in some area sleep-testing facilities. HST can also be used as a screening instrument for those strongly suspected of having obstructive sleep apnea. If the patient tests positive, further testing can be performed.

Disadvantages of HST

Although testing in the home environment has its benefits, there are also factors that are not ideal. First, most HST devices are not equipped to collect all of the data that are standard for a diagnostic polysomnogram. Instead, they allow collection of a limited number of channels that must be selected by the ordering physician based on the patient's history and presenting symptoms. In most cases, this does not include the collection of brain wave data. As a result, determining sleep staging is not possible and abnormalities in sleep architecture would not be revealed. Second, HST is thought to underdiagnose patients with sleep-related breathing disorders, especially if they are mild to moderate in severity. This may lead to a false-negative result, leaving a patient undiagnosed and untreated. HST is also not recommended for patients who have certain medical conditions such as chronic obstructive pulmonary disease, congestive heart failure, or neuromuscular disorders.

Ambulatory sleep studies that are unattended require that the patient perform the setup themselves. Specifically, the technologist instructs the patient how to apply the sensors and use the device and then sends the patient home to perform the study alone. If the patient were to perform the setup incorrectly or if a sensor falls off during the night, the quality of the study would be poor and likely not conclusive. Finally, the home environment may be a source of poor sleep habits or distractions that prevent the patient from sleeping well. These can include disruptions from children, pets, digital devices, or the bed partner.

At the conclusion of an HST or any ambulatory sleep testing, the information collected is downloaded, reviewed, and interpreted. The sleep physician will then determine next steps, which may include further testing or initiation of treatment.

Other Diagnostic Testing

The diagnostic tests discussed in this section can supplement the information gathered from the sleep study:

- pH testing
- Esophageal-pressure studies
- Arterial blood gases (ABGs)

Many obstructive sleep apnea (OSA) patients also have **gastric reflux** (gastroesophageal reflux disease, or GERD), in which stomach acids move upward into the esophagus during the night. This is of interest in polysomnography because the acids not only cause heartburn, which can disturb a patient's sleep, but also can lead to increased upper-airway obstruction and apnea. If GERD is suspected to play a role in a sleep-related breathing disorder, a **pH probe** can be included as part of the study. A pH probe is inserted through the nose, down into the esophagus, and left to sit right above the lower esophageal sphincter. In this location, a probe can detect changes in acidity that are indicative of acid-reflux events. This information can then be assessed in correlation to respiratory events.

Esophageal balloons are used in esophageal-pressure studies primarily to detect increased respiratory effort associated with upper-airway resistance. An esophageal-pressure study is an overnight diagnostic sleep study that uses the standard PSG montage with the addition of an esophageal balloon. Esophageal balloon catheters are inserted through the nose and down into the esophagus where they can detect extremely subtle changes in respiratory effort. They are highly accurate in recording minute changes in upper-airway patency. However, they are invasive and uncomfortable for patients, and they can lead to sleep disturbances. This type of study is primarily used in clinical research.

Another diagnostic procedure that may be performed in sleep labs is the **arterial blood gas (ABG)** test. Respiratory therapists perform ABGs by drawing a sample of blood from the patient's artery and storing it in a glass syringe. The patient should be relaxed at this time and should not have performed any aerobic exercises before the draw. The respiratory therapist records the fraction of inspired oxygen, the patient's temperature, what artery the blood was drawn from, and the ventilator settings if applicable. The sample is immediately stored in an ice slurry to rapidly cool the sample. Then the sample is analyzed by a computer as soon as possible. Normal ABG values are shown in **Table 11-1**.

Hospital-based sleep labs with easy access to respiratory therapists can perform ABG tests on sleep patients. This provides the physician and technologist with detailed gas levels in the patient's blood, which is especially useful for decisions about the use of

Table 11-1
Arterial Blood Gas Measurements

Gas Measure	Description	Normal Levels
SaO_2	The percentage of hemoglobin that is saturated with oxygen. This provides an actual measurement of oxygen saturation, whereas the SpO_2 is an estimated measure.	95–100%
PCO_2	The actual measurement of carbon dioxide levels in the blood	35–45 mmHg
pO_2	The actual measurement of oxygen levels in the blood (the amount of oxygen rather than the percentage of saturation)	80–100 mmHg
pH	The acidity level of the blood. A decreased pH is usually the result of a high CO_2, which leads to more acidity in the blood.	7.35–7.45
BE	Base excess. This is the amount of acid required to return the blood to normal pH levels.	–2.0–+2.0 mmol/L
HB	The actual amount of hemoglobin in the blood. A low level may indicate anemia.	12–16 g/dL
HCO_3	Bicarbonate level, or *carboxy*. Smokers often have a high HCO_3.	22–26 mEq/L

supplemental oxygen. Sleep labs performing ABG tests on their patients should have detailed written protocols regarding the results of these tests.

Chapter Summary

Although a majority of sleep studies are baseline diagnostic PSGs or continuous positive airway pressure titrations, other types of sleep studies also can be performed. The multiple sleep latency test (MSLT) consists of a series of short daytime naps and is used primarily to help diagnose narcolepsy and determine the level of excessive daytime sleepiness. An overnight diagnostic sleep study is performed before the MSLT to rule out sleep disorders such as OSA that may cause the patient to exhibit certain narcoleptic symptoms. The naps begin 2 hours apart from each other. During the naps, the patient is given 20 minutes to fall asleep. Results are based on mean sleep latency and number of sleep onset REM periods (SOREMs).

The maintenance of wakefulness test (MWT) is used to asses a patient's ability to stay awake. The MWT consists of a series of tests in which the patient attempts to remain awake while relaxing in a dimly lit room. This test is most beneficial in determining the ability of truck drivers, airline pilots, and others to stay awake under difficult circumstances.

The REM behavior-disorder study is used to diagnose REM behavior disorders. It is similar to a diagnostic PSG but with additional limb leads and occasionally a full EEG montage to rule out nocturnal seizures. Video recording is used, and digital video integrated with the polysomnograph is preferred.

Nocturnal seizure disorder studies are used to diagnose nocturnal seizures, and consist of a diagnostic baseline PSG montage with the inclusion of additional EEG electrodes. Arm leads may be used if desired, and video recording is required. Digital video integrated with the polysomnograph is preferred.

Ambulatory sleep studies are performed outside the sleep lab environment. Home sleep testing may decrease the instance of first night effect but face the challenge of distractions from home and poor-quality recordings. In-home sleep studies may be attended by a technologist or unattended.

Other diagnostic procedures are occasionally performed in the sleep lab, including diagnostic tools that can assist the physician such as esophageal balloons, pH probes, and arterial blood gases.

Case Study

A patient had an overnight polysomnogram followed by an MSLT study. The overnight study revealed normal sleep with no evidence of sleep disorders. The following table outlines the results of MSLT.

1. **Calculate the sleep latency for each nap.**
2. **Calculate the mean sleep latency.**
3. **How many SOREM periods were achieved?**
4. **Do these findings likely indicate narcolepsy?**

(Continues)

Case Study

(continued)

	NAP 1	NAP 2	NAP 3	NAP 4	NAP 5
			MSLT Results		
START TIME	7:00 AM	9:00 AM	11:00 AM	1:00 PM	3:00 PM
END TIME	7:23 AM	9:28 AM	11:18 AM	1:25 PM	3:20 PM
SLEEP ONSET	7:08 AM	9:13 AM	11:03 AM	1:10 PM	NO SLEEP
REM ONSET	7:15 AM	NO REM	NO REM	NO REM	NO SLEEP

Chapter 11 Questions

Please consider the following questions as they relate to the material in this chapter.

1. How long is a patient given to fall asleep during an MSLT nap?
2. When is an MWT performed? When is an MWT more beneficial than an MSLT?
3. How is the montage for a REM behavior-disorder study different from a baseline polysomnogram?
4. Why is video recording required during a nocturnal seizure disorder study?
5. What are some benefits and drawbacks to ambulatory sleep studies?

Footnote

1. American Academy of Sleep Medicine (2005). *Practice Parameters for Clinical Use of the Multiple Sleep Latency Test and the Maintenance of Wakefulness Test.*

CHAPTER

12
Sleep Staging

© Agsandrew/Shutterstock

CHAPTER OUTLINE

LEARNING OBJECTIVES

1. Describe a brief history of sleep staging and event scoring.
2. Learn the classification of sleep stages as outlined by the AASM.
3. Identify specific characteristic waveforms.
4. Identify sleep stages and the significance of each.

KEY TERMS

rapid eye movement
   (REM) sleep
delta sleep
nonrapid eye movement
   (NREM) sleep
electroencephalogram
   (EEG)
alpha waves
theta waves
low-amplitude,
   mixed-frequency
   (LAMF) activity
sleep spindles
K-complex
slow waves

stage W
electrooculogram (EOG)
slow eye movements (SEMs)
electromyogram (EMG)
stage N1
vertex sharp waves
   (V waves)
sleep onset
sleep state misperception
stage N2
stage N3
stage R
muscle atonia
alpha intrusion

Note: The staging rules discussed in this chapter are for scoring adult sleep studies. Rules for scoring sleep stages in pediatric studies can be found in Chapter 16.

Rechtschaffen and Kales

In 1967, Allan Rechtschaffen and Anthony Kales (R&K) revolutionized the sleep industry by publishing *A Manual of Standardized Terminology, Techniques and Scoring System for Sleep Stages of Human Subjects*.[1] This manual set the standard for scoring sleep stages. These standards were upheld for 40 years, a time when the sleep industry grew to a level far greater than expected. Under those guidelines, sleep consisted of the stages wake, 1, 2, 3, 4, and **rapid eye movement (REM) sleep**. Stages 3 and 4 together made up a state of slow-wave sleep called **delta sleep**, and stages 1–4 combined to form the **nonrapid eye movement (NREM) sleep** stages.

After much research, development, and growth in sleep medicine, it became necessary to create a new standard for scoring. The new standard of scoring and recording sleep parameters was officially introduced by the American Academy of Sleep Medicine (AASM) in 2007, and these practices became required for accreditation in mid-2008. In 2013, the AASM updated these rules in the *AASM Manual for the Scoring of Sleep and Associated Events, Second Edition*.[2] The staging rules in this chapter are reflective of the rules presented by the American Academy of Sleep Medicine *AASM Manual for the Scoring of Sleep and Associated Events, Version 2.4*.

EEG Waveforms

The following characteristic **electroencephalogram (EEG)** waveforms have been identified and are used in polysomnography to help determine sleep stages.

Alpha Waves

Alpha waves (see **Figure 12-1**) are fast-frequency EEG waves (8–13 Hz) that are seen primarily in the occipital channels during eye closure with relaxed wakefulness. Alpha activity is also often associated with EEG arousals.

Theta Waves

Theta waves (see **Figure 12-2**) are **low-amplitude, mixed-frequency (LAMF) activities** associated with sleep. Theta activity has a frequency range between 4 and 7 Hz. As we fall into sleep, brain wave activity

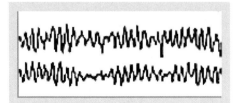

FIGURE 12-1 Alpha waves.

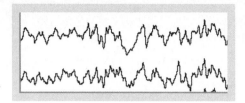

FIGURE 12-2 Theta waves.

slows from the alpha frequency range to the theta frequency range. Theta activity makes up the background activity of stages N1, N2, and REM.

Sleep Spindles

Sleep spindles (see **Figure 12-3**) are brief bursts of high-frequency (11–16 Hz) activity, most often appearing in the central EEG channels. Sleep spindles are usually associated with stage N2 sleep. There are no amplitude criteria to score a sleep spindle, but the duration of the burst must be at least 0.5 seconds. Sleep spindles and K-complexes are often associated with the blockage of sensory input from external stimuli.

K-Complex

A **K-complex** (see **Figure 12-4**) is a unique waveform characterized by a sharp upward pen deflection (indicating a negative voltage) followed by a slower downward pen deflection (positive voltage). These

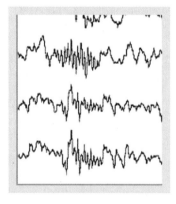

FIGURE 12-3 Sleep spindles.

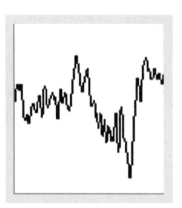

FIGURE 12-4 K-complex.

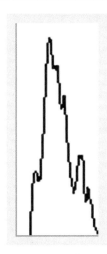

FIGURE 12-5 Slow waves.

waveforms have no amplitude requirement but last at least 0.5 seconds in duration. K-complexes are mostly associated with stage N2 sleep and are often immediately followed by sleep spindles.

Slow Waves

Slow waves (see **Figure 12-5**), formerly known as *delta waves*, are low-frequency, high-amplitude waves seen primarily in the frontal regions of the brain. These are associated with stage N3 sleep. Slow waves are between 0.5 and 2 Hz and have a peak-to-peak amplitude criterion of at least 75 µV.

The remainder of this chapter discusses these and other waveforms and how they help us identify sleep stages. Although more than one sleep stage may occur in a single epoch, each 30-second epoch must be assigned to a single sleep stage. The stage that has more than 50% of the epoch is the stage that is assigned.

Learning to identify sleep stages is like learning a new language. Competence is gained with practice and experience. This chapter provides various examples to illustrate the relevant waveforms and scoring criteria. Note, however, that the sample epochs in this chapter are not sequential or from the same patient and therefore should be assessed individually. On an actual sleep study, scoring is accomplished over sequential epochs, and sleep stages transition from one stage to the next.

Stage W

On a sleep study, **stage W** is scored when the majority of an epoch demonstrates that the patient is awake. During wakefulness, the patient may be physically active or inactive. In active patients, movement artifact occurs because of muscle or body movements, and much or all of the epoch may be obscured by the movements. Because the patient is active, the eyes remain open and are characterized by REMs as the patient observes his or her environment.

Rapid eye movements appear as fast, conjugate, irregular, and sharply peaked waveforms in the **electrooculogram (EOG)** channels.

In relaxed wakefulness, the patient is often still. When the eyes are open, blinking occurs. Eye blinks are characterized by fast, conjugate, vertical waveforms in the EOG channels. These eye blinks should not be confused with rapid eye movements often seen in stages W and R. When the eyes are closed, alpha activity often appears in the occipital channels, and **slow eye movements (SEMs)** can often be observed in the EOG channels. SEMs are observed as regular, sinusoidal, and conjugate waveforms. Stage W is also accompanied by high-amplitude chin **electromyogram (EMG)** activity.

Figure 12-6 shows an example of stage W. Note the alpha activity throughout the EEG channels and the high-amplitude chin EMG activity. Approximately 10 seconds of this epoch (the highlighted section) is composed of body movements and eye blinks. During the latter half of the epoch, SEMs are seen, indicating that the patient is awake with eyes closed.

During the first 20 seconds of the epoch shown in **Figure 12-7**, the patient is in a state of relaxed wakefulness. The chin EMG amplitude is high, the occipital EEGs show alpha activity, and the EOG channels demonstrate slow eye movements. This epoch is scored as stage W.

In the sample shown in **Figure 12-8**, the patient is awake with his eyes closed for the first 20 seconds. The enlarged sample shows the resulting alpha waves in the occipital channels. During the final 10 seconds of the epoch, the patient opens his eyes and the alpha waves disappear. Note the REMs in the EOG channels after the eyes are opened. This epoch is scored as stage W.

In the sample shown in **Figure 12-9**, the patient is awake with his eyes open and blinking during the first 15 seconds. During the final 15 seconds, the patient moves. Note the movement artifact seen in the EEGs, EOGs, and chin EMG channel. This epoch is scored as stage W.

In **Figure 12-10**, the patient is awake and active throughout the entire epoch. The body movements obscure the tracings in nearly all of the channels with movement artifact.

In the sample shown in **Figure 12-11**, the patient is in a state of relaxed wakefulness with eyes closed. Alpha waves are prevalent in the occipital channels throughout the entire epoch. This epoch is scored as stage W.

In the sample shown in **Figure 12-12**, the patient is awake, relaxing with eyes closed throughout the epoch. Alpha waves persist in the occipital channels, as shown in the enlarged section. This epoch is scored as stage W.

In the sample shown in **Figure 12-13**, the patient is awake with eyes closed. Alpha waves appear in the occipital channels, and SEMs are seen in the EOG channels. This epoch is scored as stage W.

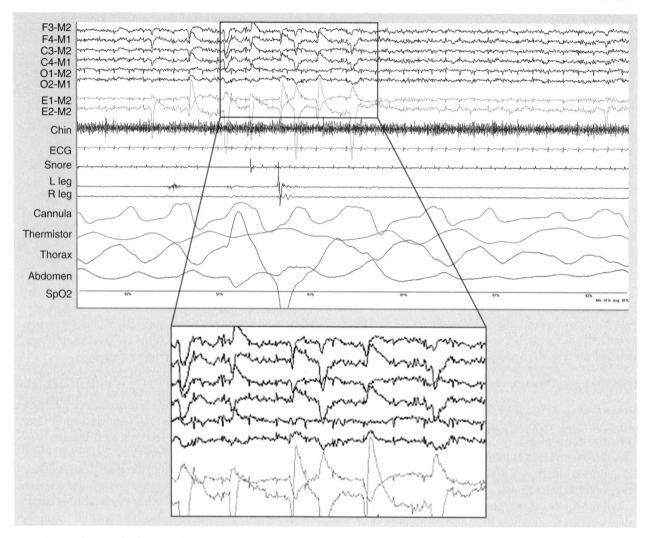

FIGURE 12-6 An example of stage wake.

In the epoch shown in **Figure 12-14**, the patient is in stage N1 during the first 13 seconds. Then the patient wakes up, as indicated by the increase in amplitude in the chin EMG and the shift in frequency in the EEG channels to alpha activity. The patient remains awake for the rest of the epoch. Because more than half of the epoch is wake, the entire epoch is scored as stage wake.

In the epoch shown in **Figure 12-15**, the patient is awake for the first 20 seconds. Note the movement artifact in the EEG, EOG, and chin EMG channels during the first half of the epoch. In the enlarged section, alpha activity is seen, indicating relaxed wakefulness. During the final 10 seconds, the patient falls asleep, as noted by the attenuation of alpha activity in the occipital channels and its replacement by slower-frequency theta activity. Even though the patient did fall asleep for a short time, the entire epoch is scored as stage W because the patient was awake for more than half of the epoch.

Stage N1

Stage N1 sleep is characterized by a relatively LAMF EEG pattern, with waveforms in the theta frequency range (4–7 Hz). During stage N1, SEMs are normally seen in the EOG channels, and the amplitude of the chin EMG is usually slightly decreased from that seen in wake. On occasion, and often during transition to stage N1 sleep, the central EEG channels may exhibit **vertex sharp waves (V waves)**. V waves are fast, high-voltage waveforms with a frequency of less than 0.5 seconds.

Sleep onset is defined as the first epoch of sleep. N1 is usually the first stage of sleep entered from wakefulness in most individuals. The onset of stage N1 from relaxed wakefulness is characterized by a slowing of EEG activity. Specifically, alpha activity of 8–13 Hz is replaced by 4–7 Hz theta activity. Concurrently, the chin EMG amplitude decreases slightly. SEMs seen during relaxed wakefulness continue into stage N1 and may become more pronounced.

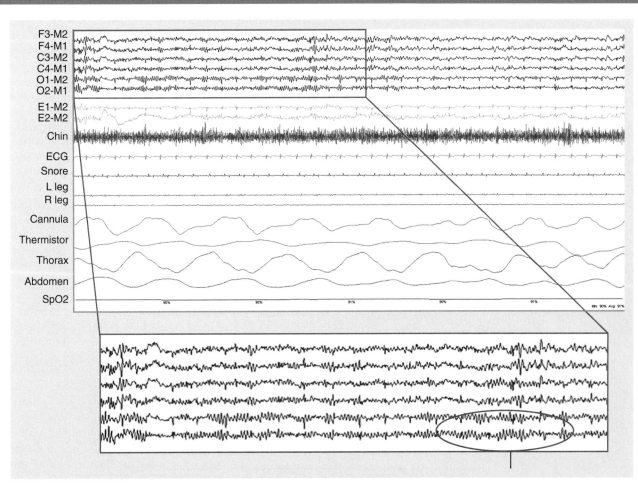

FIGURE 12-7 For the first 20 seconds of this epoch, the patient is in a state of relaxed wakefulness.

Stage N1 is often called a *transitional stage* of sleep because it is meant to connect wake to the deeper stages of sleep. During N1, the senses are not completely blocked, the patient can often still hear noises in the room and may even perceive him- or herself as still awake. Individuals with normal sleep staging do not spend a great deal of time in N1 sleep. In normal healthy adults, N1 sleep constitutes just 5–10% of total sleep time.

Increased N1 is often the result of frequent awakenings and EEG arousals. Patients who drift in and out of stage N1 during much of the night will often perceive that they did not sleep at all, an experience termed **sleep state misperception**.

The sample shown in **Figure 12-16** depicts an EEG pattern of both alpha and theta activity. Theta activity makes up the initial 3–4 seconds of the EEG. This is quickly replaced by alpha activity, which continues for approximately 10 seconds. The enlarged section shows a transition from alpha to theta activity. Theta activity then continues for the remainder of the epoch. Because

the EEG demonstrates theta activity for more than half of the epoch, the entire epoch is scored as stage N1.

In the sample shown in **Figure 12-17**, the EEG pattern shows alpha wave activity for some 10 seconds. However, most of the epoch consists of LAMF activity. This epoch is scored as stage N1.

In the enlarged section in **Figure 12-18**, a low-voltage, mixed-frequency theta pattern can be seen. This pattern exists throughout most of the epoch. In the absence of sleep spindles, K-complexes, and REMs, this epoch meets the criteria for stage N1 sleep.

In the sample shown in **Figure 12-19**, the beginning portion of the epoch shows LAMF EEG activity and SEMs. Toward the end of the epoch, spindlelike activity appears in the EEG channels, indicating the patient may start to transition to N2 sleep. However, because the majority of the epoch is characterized by LAMF activity and SEMs, the epoch is scored as stage N1.

The enlarged section in **Figure 12-20** shows a close-up of the SEMs associated with N1 sleep.

In **Figure 12-21**, the patient is on continuous positive airway pressure (CPAP) in stage N1. Note the LAMF

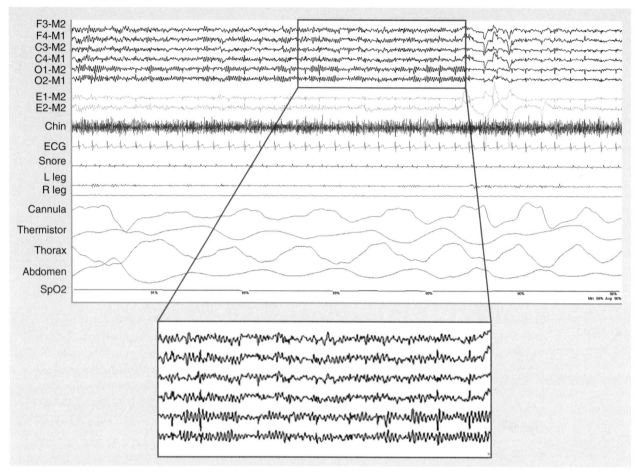

FIGURE 12-8 The patient is awake with his eyes closed for the first 20 seconds. During the final 10 seconds of the epoch, the patient opens his eyes.

EEG activity, the moderate to high chin EMG amplitude, and the presence of SEMs.

In **Figure 12-22**, the patient exhibits a low-voltage, mixed-frequency EEG pattern throughout the entire epoch without the presence of sleep spindles or K-complexes. The chin EMG is of moderate to high amplitude and there are no REMs. The epoch is scored as stage N1.

Stage N2

Stage N2 makes up approximately 50% of total sleep time in normal healthy adults. It is characterized by a LAMF background EEG activity with the presence of sleep spindles and K-complexes in the central EEG channels. During N2 sleep, the chin EMG amplitude decreases from that noted in stage N1, and the SEMs that were seen in stages W and N1 normally disappear.

N2 begins at the first set of sleep spindles or the first K-complex that occurs unassociated with an EEG arousal. Sleep spindles and K-complexes mark

the points at which the senses begin to be blocked. These waveforms may appear in N3 sleep as well, but N2 is nearly absent of slow waves. Stage N2 continues until the transition to N3, R, or wake. N2 transitions to stage N1 only after an EEG arousal, a major body movement, or an awakening.

In the epoch shown in **Figure 12-23**, the EEG demonstrates a background LAMF activity with K-complexes and sleep spindles seen intermittently (seen in the enlargements). Note the lower chin EMG amplitude and the absence of SEMs in the EOG channels. The epoch is scored as N2 sleep.

In the sample shown in **Figure 12-24**, a large K-complex appears some 7 seconds into the epoch and is prominent against the background LAMF EEG activity. Note the absence of SEMs and moderate chin EMG amplitude. This epoch is scored as stage N2 sleep.

In the sample shown in **Figure 12-25**, the central and frontal EEGs exhibit several K-complexes as seen in the enlarged sections. These waveforms are noted against a background of theta activity. Again, note the absence of

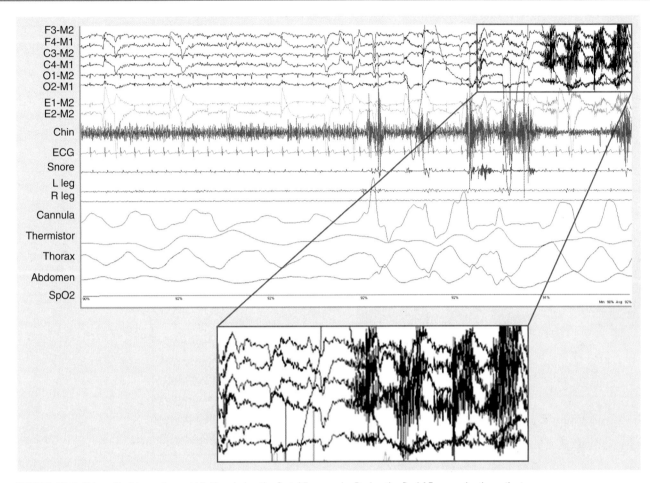

FIGURE 12-9 This patient is awake and blinking during the first 15 seconds. During the final 15 seconds, the patient moves.

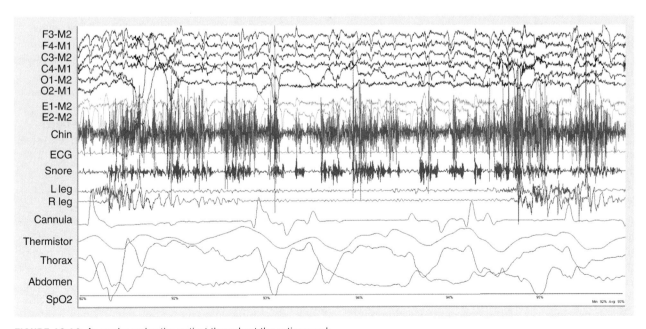

FIGURE 12-10 An awake and active patient throughout the entire epoch.

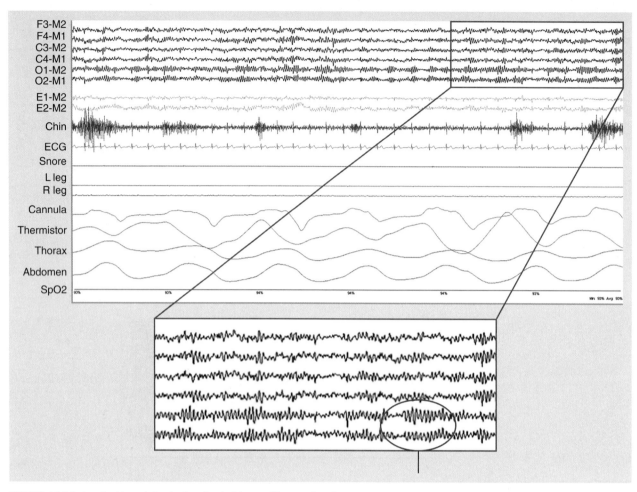

FIGURE 12-11 A patient in a state of relaxed wakefulness with eyes closed.

SEMs and moderate chin EMG amplitude. This epoch is scored as stage N2.

The EEG channels in the sample shown in **Figure 12-26** exhibit K-complexes and spindles with an absence of slow waves. The chin EMG amplitude is moderate, and no SEMs are seen. This epoch is scored as N2.

In the sample shown in **Figure 12-27**, theta activity occurs throughout the majority of the epoch with K-complexes and sleep spindles seen. The enlarged section shows a K-complex immediately followed by a sleep spindle. During the final 5 seconds of the epoch, the EEG pattern transitions to alpha activity, indicating that the patient has awakened. Note the return of SEMS and the increase in amplitude in the chin EMG. However, because the majority of the epoch meets criteria, the epoch is scored as N2.

The EEGs shown in **Figure 12-28** exhibit sleep spindles and K-complexes in the absence or near absence of slow waves. SEMs are absent, and a moderate chin EMG amplitude is seen. This epoch is scored as stage N2.

The sample shown in **Figure 12-29** has few dominant waveforms. However, a K-complex at the beginning of the epoch indicates that this should be scored as N2.

The epoch shown in **Figure 12-30** could easily be mistaken for N1. The SEMs and the low-voltage, mixed-frequency theta pattern would ordinarily indicate N1; however, the high-voltage waveform approximately 10 seconds into the epoch is longer than 0.5 seconds, indicating that it is not a vertex sharp wave. The shape of it is more like a K-complex, indicating stage N2 sleep. This sample is at the beginning of N2, during which SEMs may occasionally persist. This can also be a result of certain medications.

The epoch shown in **Figure 12-31** is yet another example of a LAMF background EEG pattern with sleep spindles and K-complexes, indicating N2.

The epoch shown in **Figure 12-32** portrays background theta activity with sleep spindles and K-complexes. Note a few slow waves in this epoch, although not enough to meet the criteria for scoring stage N3, so this epoch is scored as stage N2.

Stage N3

Stage N3 is made up of deep sleep and associated with high-amplitude slow waves. Slow waves have a minimum amplitude criterion of 75 µV and a frequency range

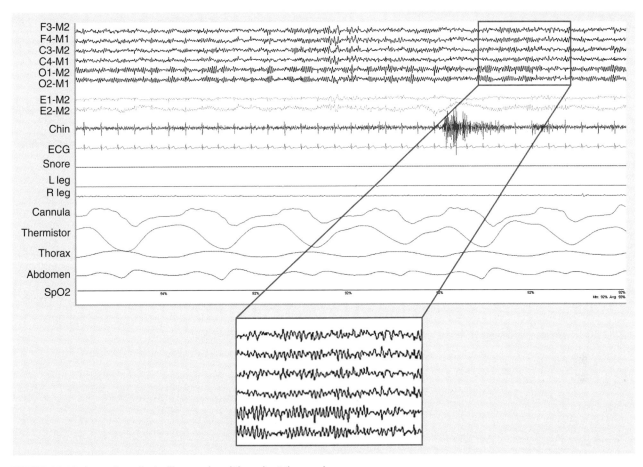

FIGURE 12-12 An awake patient with eyes closed throughout the epoch.

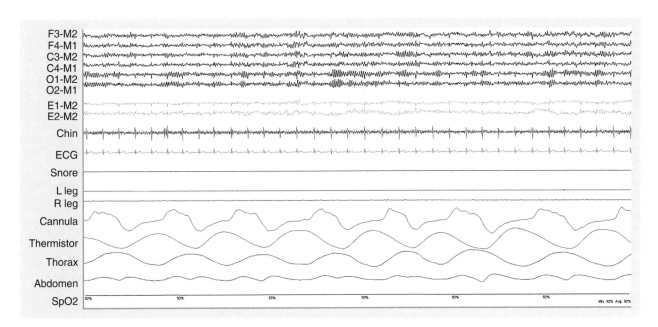

FIGURE 12-13 Another awake patient with eyes closed.

between 0.5 Hz and 2 Hz. They are primarily seen in the frontal EEG channels but can often be seen in the central regions as well. Stage N3 is now inclusive of previous stages 3 and 4 under the old R&K scoring rules.

An epoch is scored as stage N3 when at least 20% of the epoch consists of EEG slow waves. Sleep spindles and K-complexes may appear in stage N3 sleep. The chin EMG amplitude during N3 sleep may vary but is

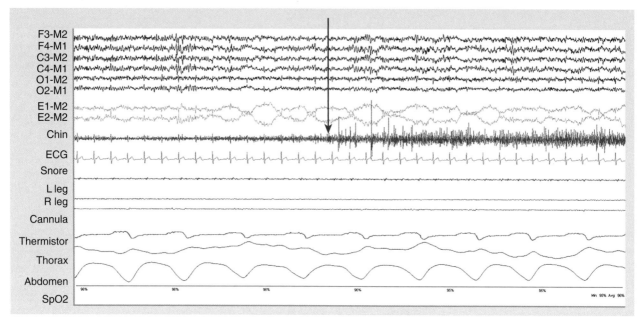

FIGURE 12-14 A patient is in stage N1 during the first 13 seconds, after which the patient wakes up.

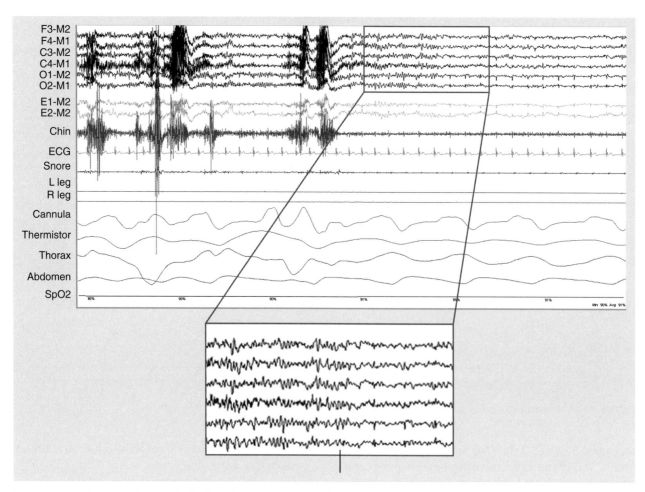

FIGURE 12-15 The patient is awake for the first 20 seconds and then falls asleep.

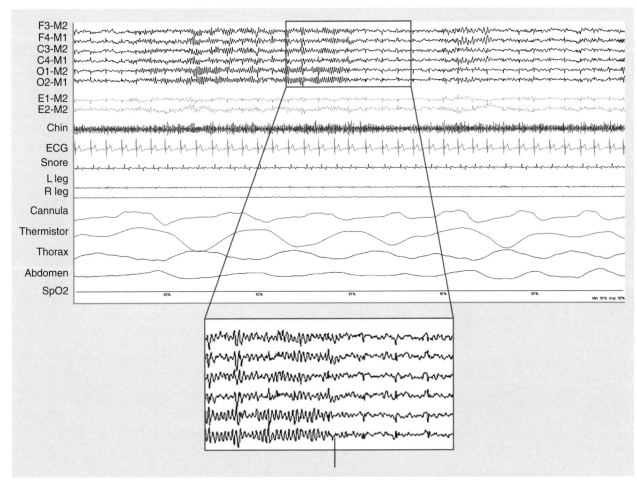

FIGURE 12-16 A patient is awake for just under half the epoch; it is deemed stage N1.

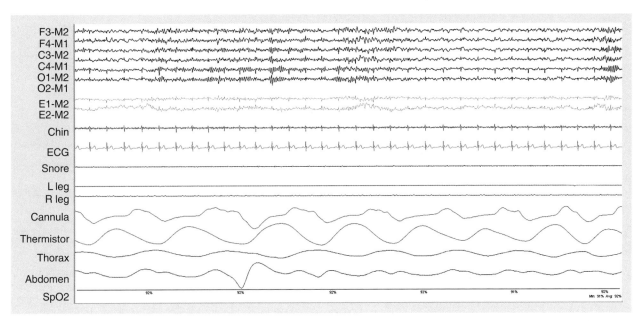

FIGURE 12-17 A patient in stage N1 during nearly all of the epoch.

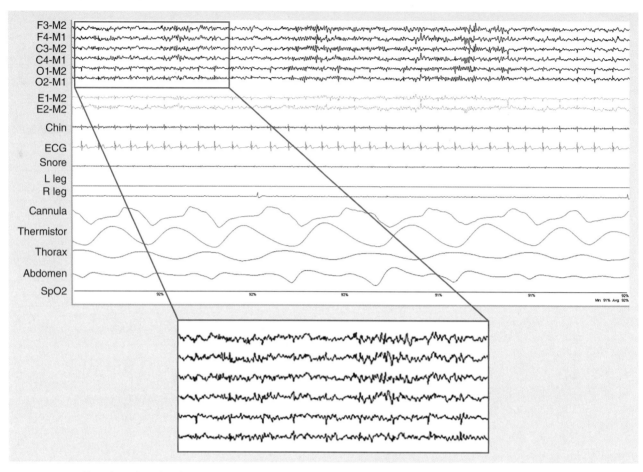

FIGURE 12-18 The enlarged section shows a low-voltage, mixed-frequency theta pattern.

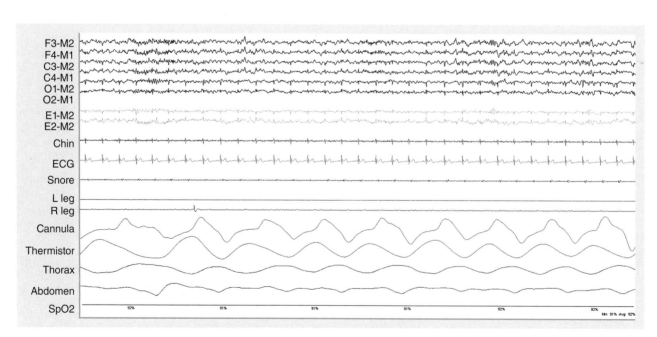

FIGURE 12-19 A patient with LAMF activity throughout most of the epoch, indicating stage N1.

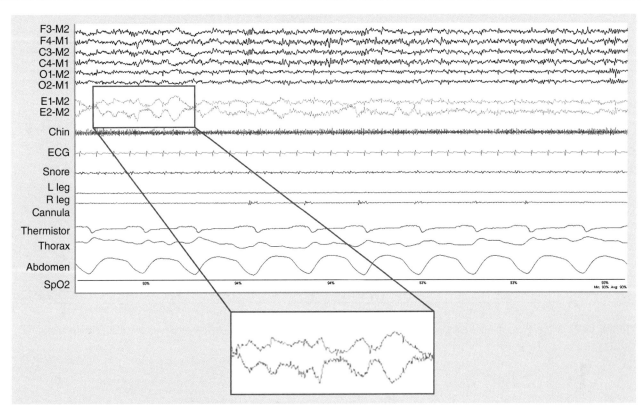

FIGURE 12-20 An enlarged section showing a close-up of SEMs.

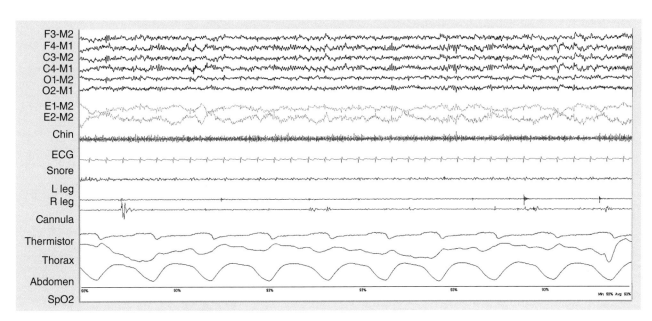

FIGURE 12-21 A patient on CPAP in stage N1.

often low. In addition, eye movements are not typically seen during N3 sleep. However, because slow waves have such high amplitude, these waveforms can be seen in the EOG channels and are often mistaken for eye movements.

Deep sleep is the period in which human growth hormone is released, so N3 sleep is a period of physical restoration and tissue repair. It is typically difficult to awaken a patient from stage N3. N3 sleep is most often seen during the first third of the night and in steadily

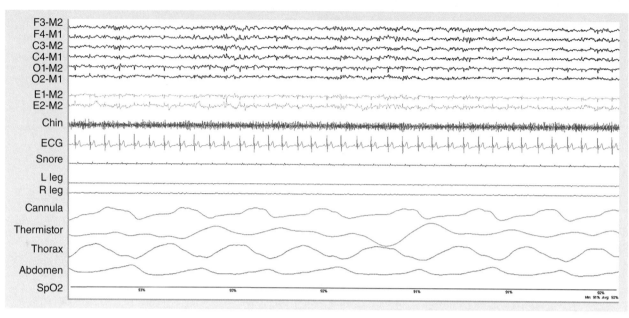

FIGURE 12-22 A low-voltage, mixed-frequency EEG pattern throughout an epoch and moderate to high-amplitude chin EMG, signifying stage N1.

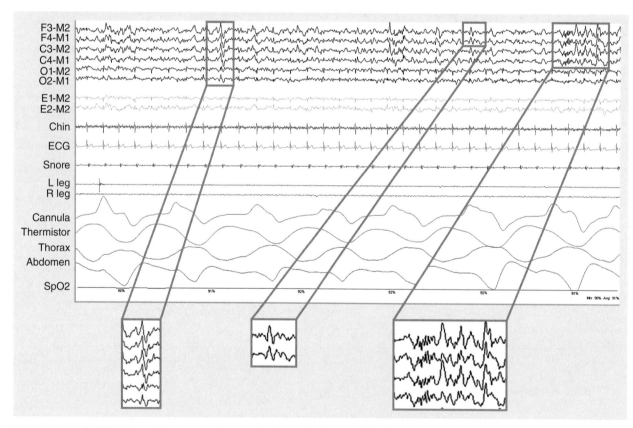

FIGURE 12-23 LAMF activity with K-complexes and spindles in a patient in stage N2 sleep.

shorter periods as the night progresses. In normal healthy adults, N3 constitutes approximately 20–25% of total sleep time. This increases among infants, children, and adolescents but tends to decrease with age. By the time a person enters late adulthood, N3 sleep may be completely absent. A decrease in N3 sleep may also be a result of frequent EEG arousals or awakenings, which are often caused by a disorder such as

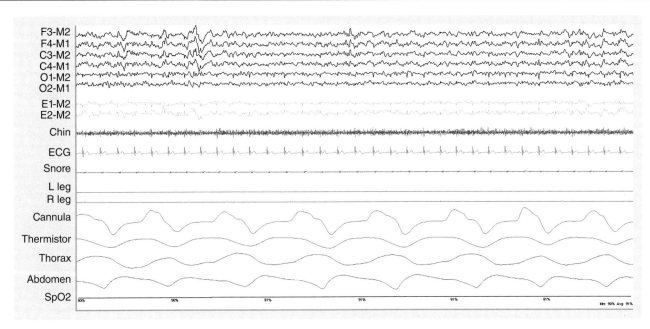

FIGURE 12-24 A prominent K-complex on a background of theta activity, indicating stage N2 sleep.

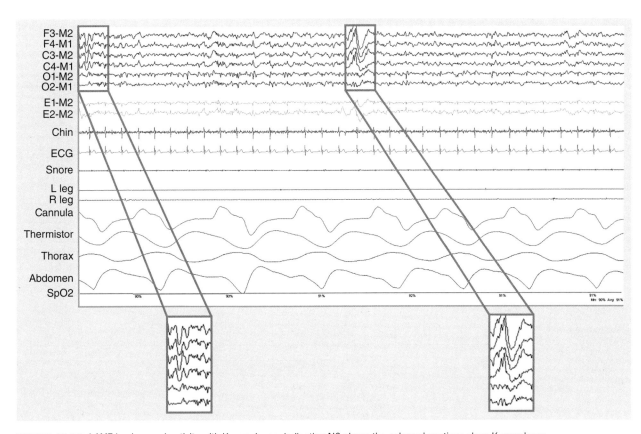

FIGURE 12-25 LAMF background activity with K-complexes, indicating N2 sleep; the enlarged sections show K-complexes.

obstructive sleep apnea (OSA) or periodic limb movements disorder.

In the sample in **Figure 12-33**, slow waves are present throughout much of the epoch. The enlarged section shows slow waves that are especially high amplitude and low in frequency. This epoch is scored as stage N3.

The sample in **Figure 12-34** shows an epoch in which the slow waves are not as high amplitude as in the

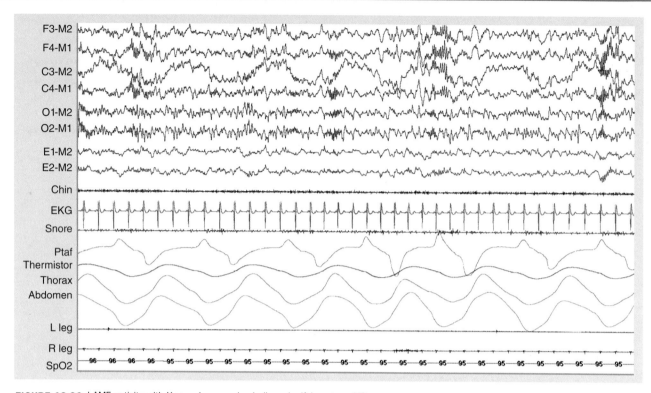

FIGURE 12-26 LAMF activity with K-complexes and spindles, signifying stage N2.

Figure by Lisa M. Endee; produced from a sleep study provided to Stony Brook University School of Health Technology and Management's Polysomnographic Technology Program by Dr. Kala Sury.

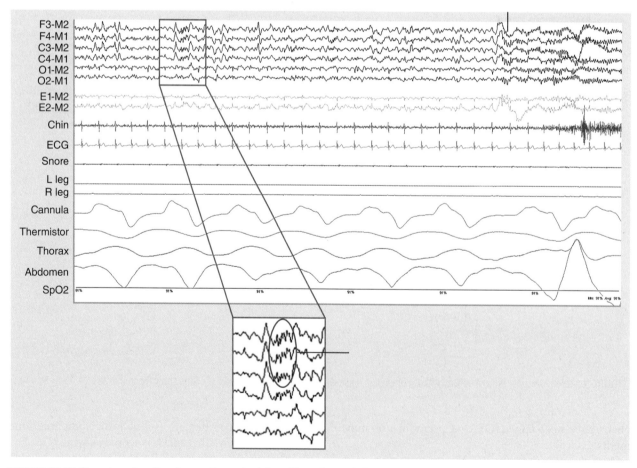

FIGURE 12-27 The enlarged section shows a K-complex followed by a sleep spindle on an epoch meeting criteria for N2 sleep.

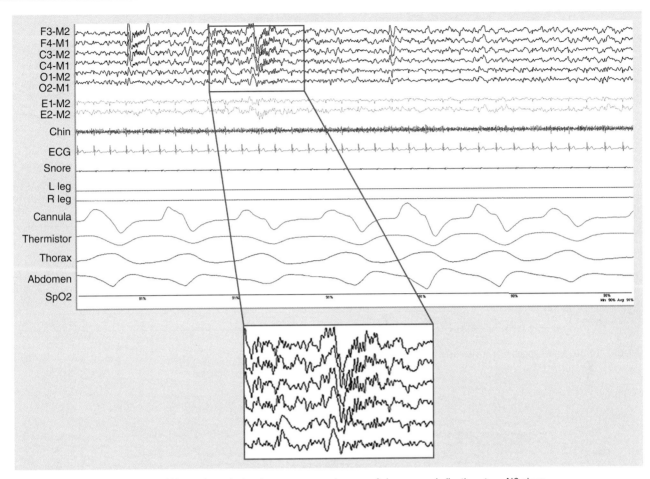

FIGURE 12-28 Sleep spindles and K-complexes in the absence or near absence of slow waves, indicating stage N2 sleep.

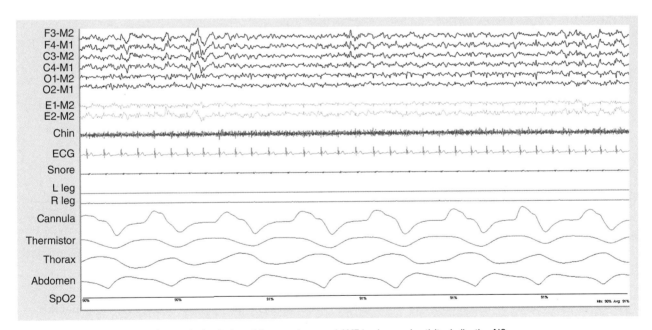

FIGURE 12-29 A K-complex exists at the beginning of the epoch over a LAMF background activity, indicating N2.

previous example but still meet the 75 µV criterion for N3 sleep.

The sample in **Figure 12-35** shows another epoch of N3 sleep in which slow waves make up most of the

epoch. Note the low-amplitude chin EMG that is characteristic of deep sleep.

As seen in the epoch shown in **Figure 12-36**, slow waves are occasionally of such high amplitude that they

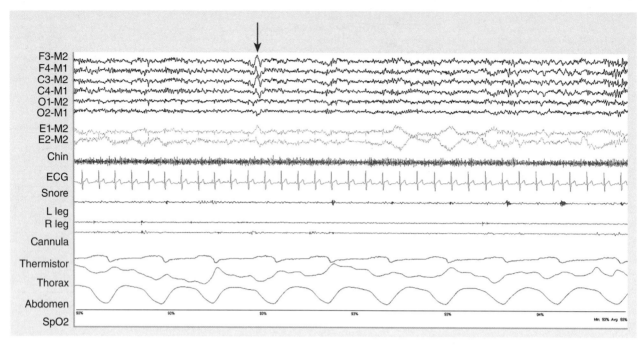

FIGURE 12-30 An N2 epoch that could easily be mistaken for N1.

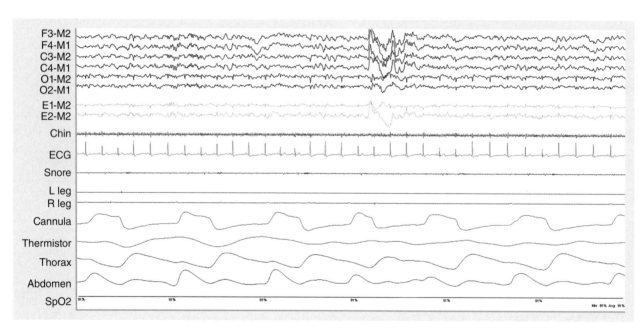

FIGURE 12-31 Sleep spindles and K-complexes over a background LAMF activity, indicating N2.

reach above the normal channel parameters. This epoch meets the criteria for stage N3.

The epoch shown in **Figure 12-37** just meets the 20% slow-wave criterion for N3 sleep. If not carefully reviewed, this epoch might be mistaken as N2.

The middle 15 seconds of the epoch shown in **Figure 12-38** is nearly completely composed of slow waves, qualifying it for stage N3. Note the low-amplitude chin EMG that is characteristic of deep sleep and the slow waves intruding into the EOG channels.

The epoch shown in **Figure 12-39** appears to qualify for N3, but it contains a slow-wave artifact that may be causing the EEGs to appear higher amplitude and lower frequency than normal. The technician should cool the patient, correct the artifact, and then determine the sleep stage.

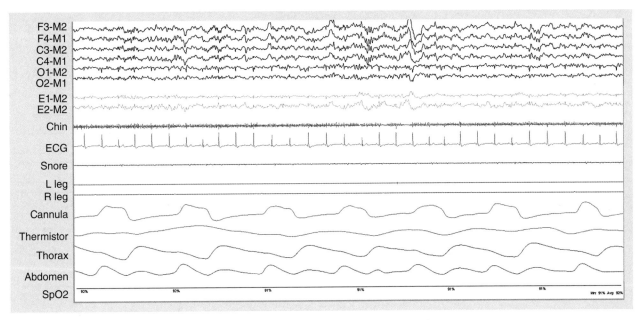

FIGURE 12-32 Sleep spindles and K-complexes indicating N2, although some slow waves are also present.

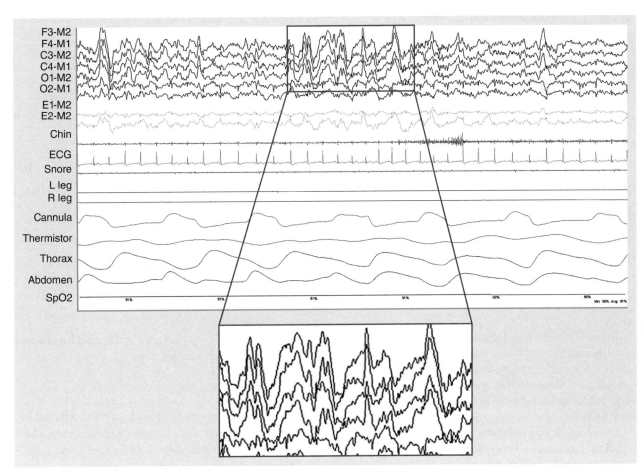

FIGURE 12-33 Stage N3; the enlarged section shows especially high-amplitude and low-frequency slow waves.

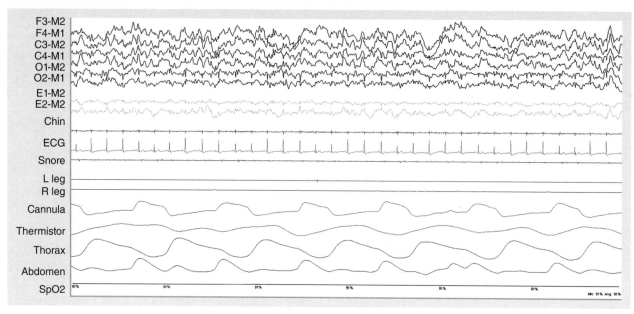

FIGURE 12-34 Slow-wave EEG activity and low amplitude chin EMG, indicating N3.

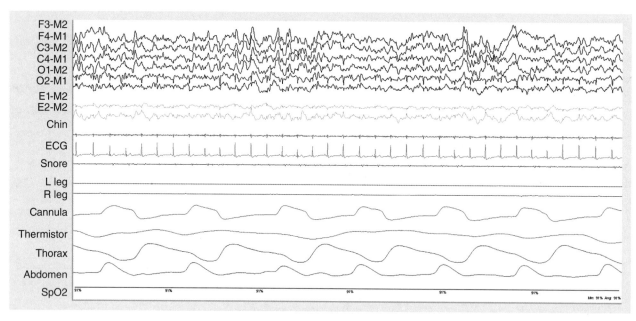

FIGURE 12-35 An epoch of N3 in which slow waves make up most of the epoch.

The epoch shown in **Figure 12-40** contains sleep spindles and K-complexes. However, the K-complexes also meet the criteria for slow waves. There are enough slow waves in this epoch to qualify as stage N3, despite the presence of K-complexes and sleep spindles.

The epoch shown in **Figure 12-41** is mostly composed of slow waves seen in the frontal and central EEG channels. Note the snore activity seen in the snore channel and the EKG artifact seen in the right leg channel. This epoch meets criteria for stage N3.

Stage R

Stage R, rapid eye movement sleep, is characterized by a background LAMF activity in the EEG channels, the presence of REMs in the EOGs, and a chin EMG amplitude that is at its lowest point of the night.

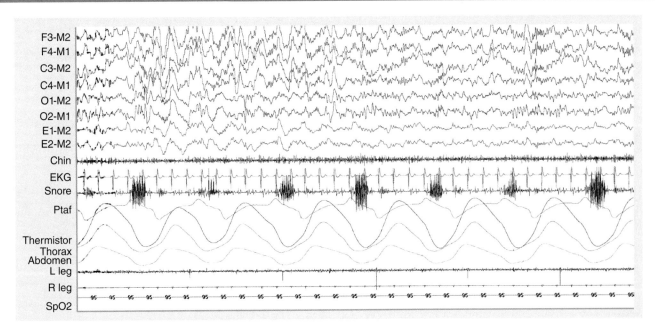

FIGURE 12-36 High-amplitude slow waves, signifying N3 sleep.

Figure by Lisa M. Endee; produced from a sleep study provided to Stony Brook University School of Health Technology and Management's Polysomnographic Technology Program by Dr. Kala Sury.

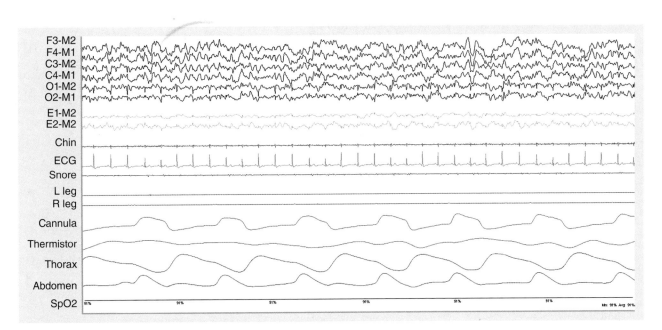

FIGURE 12-37 This epoch has just enough slow waves to qualify for N3.

Stage R has fascinated observers for centuries. It is during REM sleep that dreaming occurs. Although there is still much to learn about the role of dreams, we now understand that stage R sleep is highly beneficial in creating long-term memories and restoring wakefulness and alertness. The onset of stage R typically occurs 60–120 minutes after sleep onset and once during each sleep cycle. The duration of stage R tends to be short at the beginning of the sleep period and increasingly longer as the night progresses. Most stage R occurs in the final third of the night.

The body's core temperature and respiratory pattern are less regular during stage R sleep. As a result, the body temperature drops and the respiratory pattern tends to be slightly variable. Further, during stage R, large muscle activity is usually absent, except for extremely fast muscle twitches. Because **muscle atonia** occurs during stage R, respiratory disturbances such as

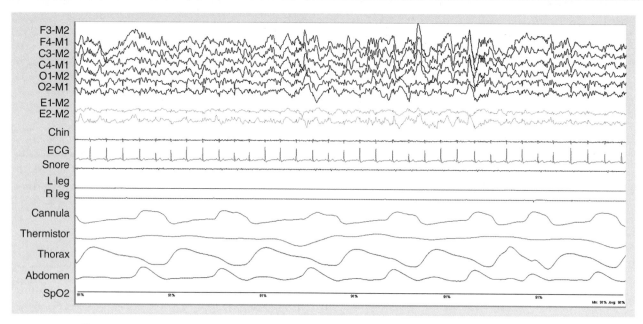

FIGURE 12-38 The middle 15 seconds of this epoch portray a burst of slow-wave activity, meeting criteria for stage N3.

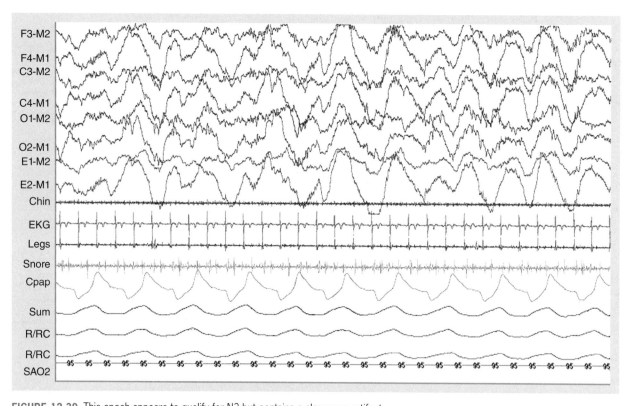

FIGURE 12-39 This epoch appears to qualify for N3 but contains a slow-wave artifact.

Figure by Lisa M. Endee; produced from a sleep study provided to Stony Brook University School of Health Technology and Management's Polysomnographic Technology Program by Dr. Kala Sury.

apnea, hypopnea, and snoring tend to be more prevalent and severe during this stage.

Stage R makes up approximately 20–25% of the total sleep time. The total time spent in stage R sleep tends to remain about the same throughout the lifetime, although disorders such as OSA may cause alterations.

Specifically, frequent arousals tend to cause increases in the lighter stages of sleep (N1 and N2) while sacrificing the deeper ones (N3, R).

The EEGs during stage R are characterized by a low-voltage, mixed-frequency pattern similar to those during N1. However, the chin EMG amplitude

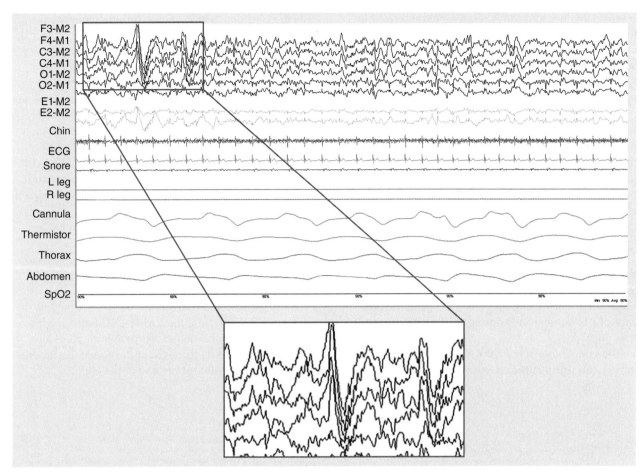

FIGURE 12-40 Sleep spindles and K-complexes but with enough slow waves in this epoch to meet criteria for stage N3.

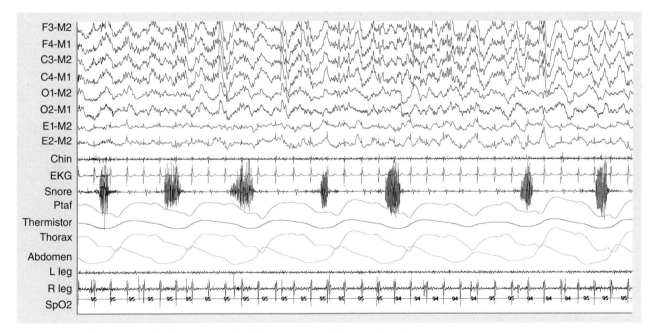

FIGURE 12-41 Slow waves in the frontal and central EEG channels, qualifying as stage N3.

Figure by Lisa M. Endee; produced from a sleep study provided to Stony Brook University School of Health Technology and Management's Polysomnographic Technology Program by Dr. Kala Sury.

is especially low, and the EOGs are characterized by REMs rather than SEMs. The EEGs during stage R may also demonstrate sawtooth waves—a series of pointed waves in the 2–6 Hz range seen in the central EEG channels. These waveforms usually precede rapid eye movements.

After an epoch of stage R, the ensuing epochs remain scored as stage R in the absence of spindles, K-complexes, EEG arousals, or slow waves, as long as the chin EMG amplitude remains decreased.

Stage R ends when there is a transition to wake or N3, when the chin EMG increases in amplitude, when an EEG arousal or major body movement occurs and the following period qualifies as another stage, or when sleep spindles or K-complexes occur.

The epoch shown in **Figure 12-42** shows stage R sleep. Note the background low-voltage, mixed-frequency EEG pattern (enlargement), the low chin EMG amplitude throughout the epoch, and the presence of REMs, especially during the final 10 seconds of the epoch.

The sample shown in **Figure 12-43** shows rapid eye movements during the first few seconds of the epoch.

The EEGs present a low-voltage, mixed-frequency pattern. The chin EMG is decreased. This epoch is scored as stage R.

The enlarged section in **Figure 12-44** shows sawtooth waves often seen during stage R sleep. Rapid eye movements and low chin EMG amplitude are also seen during this epoch.

The sample shown in **Figure 12-45**, demonstrates a LAMF background EEG pattern with sawtooth waves visible at the beginning of the epoch. The chin EMG amplitude is low and there is a high amplitude sharply peaked rapid eye movement seen. This epoch is staged as R.

In the sample shown in **Figure 12-46**, the patient is in stage R throughout the epoch. There is a low-voltage, mixed-frequency pattern in the EEGs, rapid eye movements in the EOGs, and a low-amplitude chin EMG.

In the sample shown in **Figure 12-47**, the patient is in stage R sleep. Note the LAMF EEG pattern without the presence of K complexes or spindles and low-amplitude chin EMG throughout the epoch. Rapid eye movements are visible at the end of the epoch.

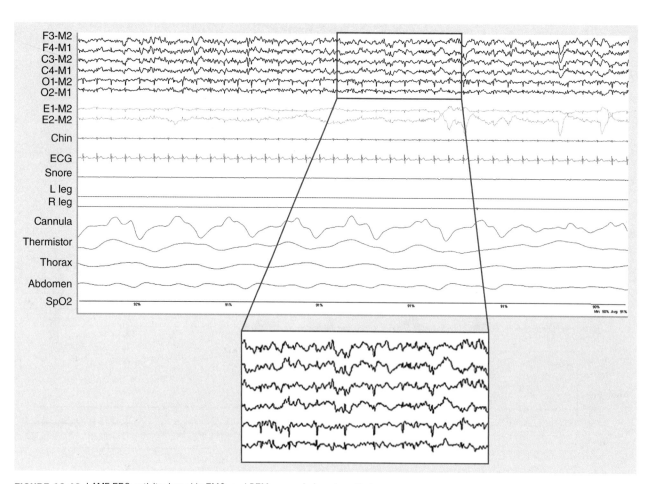

FIGURE 12-42 LAMF EEG activity, low chin EMG, and REMs seen during stage R sleep.

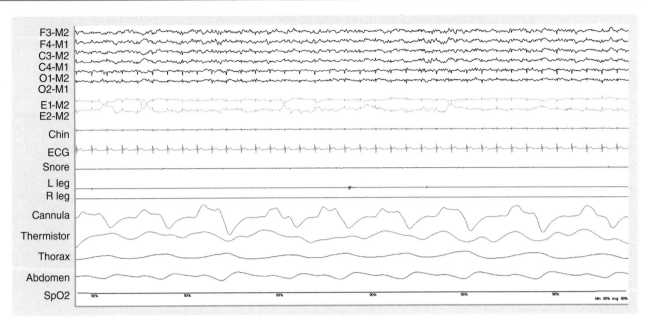

FIGURE 12-43 Stage R sleep: REMs during the first few seconds of the epoch, low-voltage, mixed-frequency EEGs, and a decreased chin EMG.

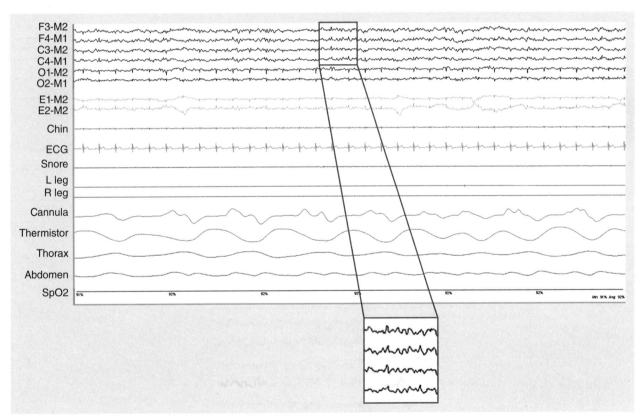

FIGURE 12-44 The enlarged section shows sawtooth waves often seen during stage R sleep.

The epoch in **Figure 12-48** shows another example of stage R sleep. The EEGs show a low-voltage, mixed-frequency activity, the chin EMG is decreased, and the EOGs show REMs.

The epoch in **Figure 12-49** shows an example of **alpha intrusion** during stage R. In some individuals, alpha activity can occasionally intrude into the EEG in stage R. However, the alpha frequency seen in

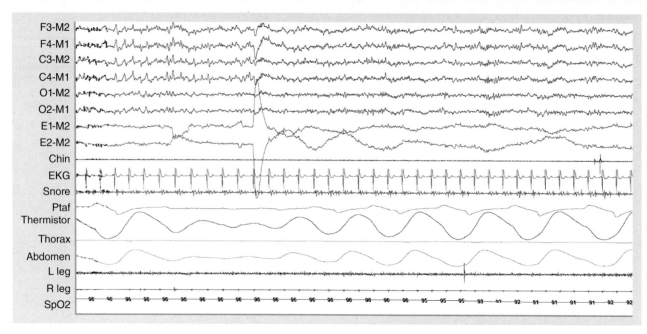

FIGURE 12-45 Low amplitude, mixed frequency activity with sawtooth waves, REMs, and low-amplitude chin EMG, signifying stage R.

Figure by Lisa M. Endee; produced from a sleep study provided to Stony Brook University School of Health Technology and Management's Polysomnographic Technology Program by Dr. Kala Sury.

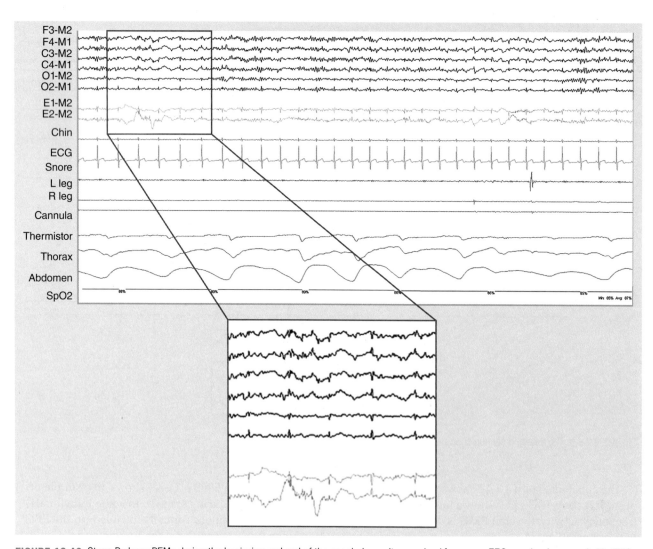

FIGURE 12-46 Stage R sleep: REMs during the beginning and end of the epoch, low-voltage, mixed-frequency EEGs, and a decreased chin EMG.

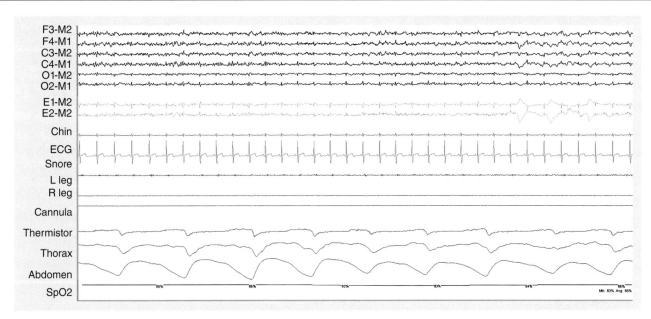

FIGURE 12-47 Stage R sleep: low-voltage, mixed-frequency EEGs, decreased chin EMG throughout the epoch, and REMs seen at the end of the epoch.

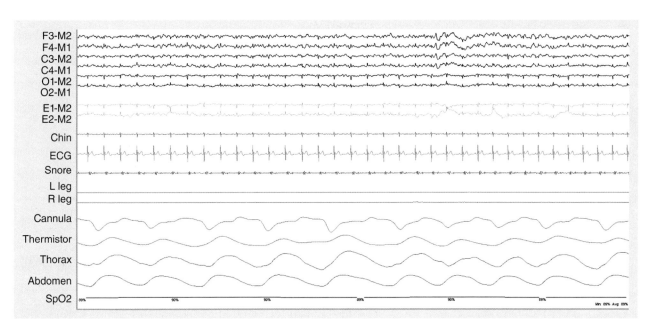

FIGURE 12-48 Another example of stage R sleep.

stage R sleep is often 1–2 Hz slower than alpha seen in relaxed wakefulness.

In the sample shown in **Figure 12-50**, the patient is in stage R throughout the epoch. Again, note the low-voltage, mixed-frequency EEG activity, decreased chin EMG, and REMs.

The sample shown in **Figure 12-51** portrays another epoch of stage R, with alpha intrusion during the first 5 seconds of the epoch. Note the decreased chin EMG. REMs are not seen during this epoch of stage R.

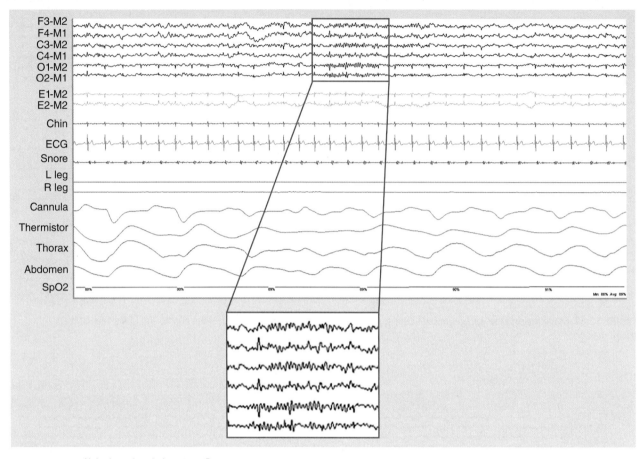

FIGURE 12-49 Alpha intrusion during stage R.

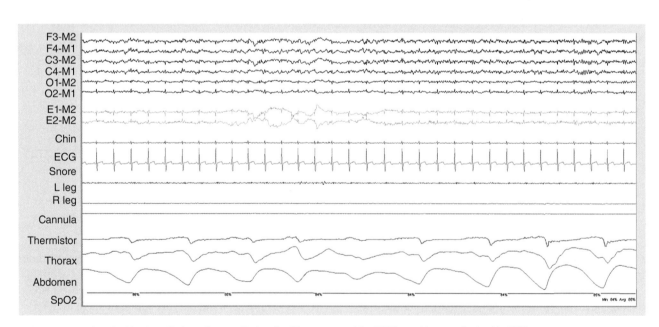

FIGURE 12-50 A patient in stage R sleep; low amplitude mixed frequency activity, REMs, and low amplitude chin EMG.

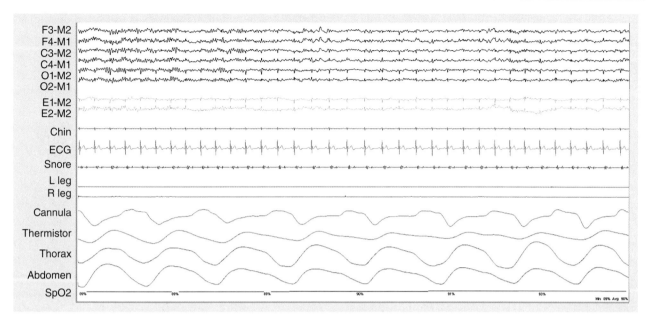

FIGURE 12-51 Alpha intrusion during the first 5 seconds of the epoch during stage R.

Chapter Summary

The first step in learning how to score a sleep study is to learn how to stage it. Rechtschaffen and Kales were among the first to standardize sleep staging in 1967. Their rules for staging and scoring sleep events were in effect for 40 years. In 2007, the American Academy of Sleep Medicine introduced a new standard of sleep staging and sleep event scoring; updates followed in 2013.

The first step to understanding sleep staging is to be able to identify certain characteristic EEG waveforms. Alpha waves are seen primarily in the occipital channels and are in the 8–13 Hz range. Theta activity is a low-amplitude, mixed-frequency waveform that has a frequency range between 4 and 7 Hz and is the background rhythm seen during stages N1, N2, and R. Sleep spindles are bursts of fast EEG activity ranging from 11–16 Hz but most often in the 12–14 Hz range, seen primarily in the central leads. K-complexes are sharp negative waveforms with an upward pen deflection followed by a slower positive component. Sleep spindles often follow K-complexes. Slow waves are in the 0.5–2 Hz range and have amplitudes of at least 75 µV.

Stage W, or wake, is scored when the patient is awake. Alert wakefulness with body movements is characterized on the polysomnograph by disrupted signals and movement artifact from the muscle activity. Relaxed wakefulness with the eyes open is characterized by eye blinks and fast EEG activity. Relaxed wakefulness with the eyes closed is characterized primarily by alpha activity in the occipital channels. The chin EMG amplitude is high during wakefulness.

Sleep onset occurs when a patient transitions from stage W to any stage of sleep, although the first stage of sleep is usually N1. Stage N1 is considered a transitional stage of sleep in which patients can often still hear and sense external stimuli. The transition to N1 sleep is characterized by a slowing of the EEG pattern into the theta frequency range. The EEGs present a low-voltage, mixed-frequency pattern with no sleep spindles, K-complexes, or slow waves. The chin EMG decreases in amplitude slightly at sleep onset, and the EOGs often present slow eye movements.

Stage N2 is the first stage in which the senses are blocked. Approximately 50% of the total sleep time is spent in N2. N2 is characterized by a background LAMF EEG pattern with the presence of K-complexes and sleep spindles in the central EEG leads.

Stage N3 makes up approximately 20–25% of the night in young healthy adults. N3 sleep is prevalent among infants and children, decreases dramatically with age, and may be completely absent by late adulthood. Stage N3 is characterized by the presence of slow waves in the frontal EEG channels. To qualify for N3 sleep, at least 20% of the epoch, or 6 seconds, must be composed of slow waves. It is during N3 sleep that tissue repair and growth occur.

Stage R, or REM sleep, also constitutes approximately 20–25% of the night in healthy young adults; however, stage R tends to remain fairly constant throughout the lifetime. Most dreaming occurs during stage R, as does the storage of long-term memories and the restoration of wakefulness and alertness.

Stage R is characterized by three main criteria: low-voltage, mixed-frequency EEG, rapid eye movements, and low chin EMG amplitude. The EEGs may also contain occasional strings of sawtooth waves. During stage R, muscle atonia occurs. Other than occasional brief muscle twitches, the body is paralyzed during stage R while the brain is highly active.

Case Examples

Identify the stage of sleep seen in the following epochs.

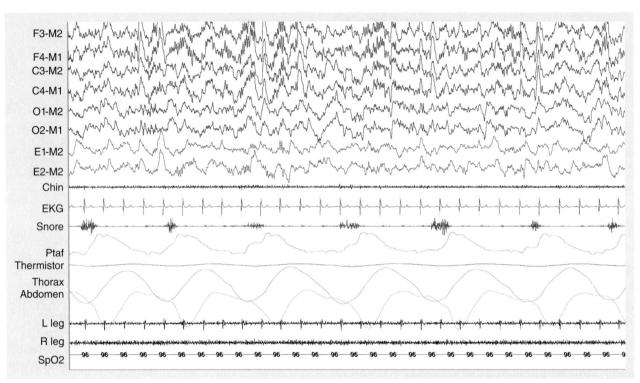

FIGURE 12-52 Epoch A.

Figure by Lisa M. Endee; produced from a sleep study provided to Stony Brook University School of Health Technology and Management's Polysomnographic Technology Program by Dr. Kala Sury.

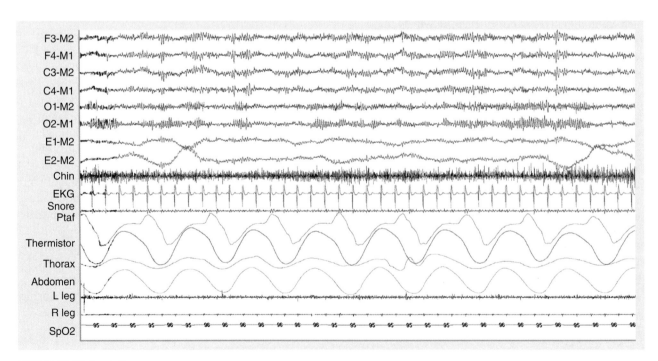

FIGURE 12-53 Epoch B.

Figure by Lisa M. Endee; produced from a sleep study provided to Stony Brook University School of Health Technology and Management's Polysomnographic Technology Program by Dr. Kala Sury.

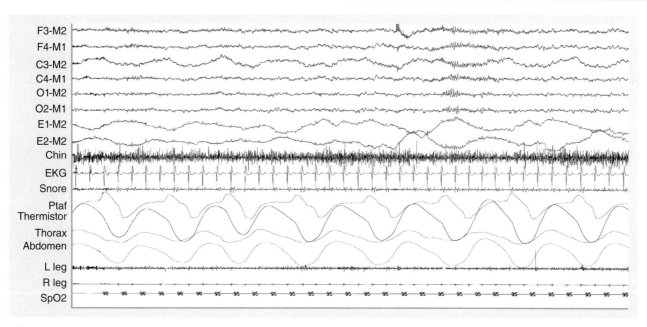

FIGURE 12-54 Epoch C.

Figure by Lisa M. Endee; produced from a sleep study provided to Stony Brook University School of Health Technology and Management's Polysomnographic Technology Program by Dr. Kala Sury.

Chapter 12 Questions

Please consider the following questions as they relate to the material in this chapter.

1. What is a K-complex? What sleep stage does it help identify?
2. What are some characteristic features of stage N1?
3. Approximately what percentage of the total sleep time is spent in stage N2?
4. How does stage N3 change as we age?
5. What are some significant features of stage R?

Footnotes

1. Rechtschaffen, A., Kales, A., et al. (1968). *A manual of standardized terminology, techniques and scoring system of sleep stages in human subjects.*
2. American Academy of Sleep Medicine. (2017). *AASM Manual for the Scoring of Sleep and Associated Events, Second Edition,* version 2.4.

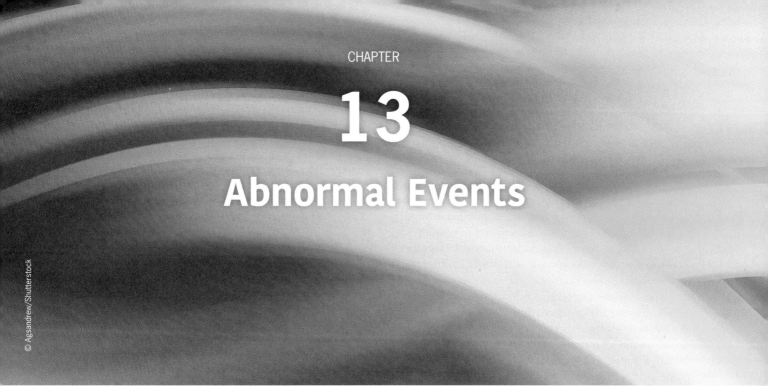

© Agsandrew/Shutterstock

CHAPTER OUTLINE

LEARNING OBJECTIVES

1. Identify sleep-related events.
2. Know the scoring rules for sleep-related events.
3. Understand the significance of specific sleep-related events.

KEY TERMS

EEG arousal
microarousal
EEG arousal index
movement arousal
beta waves
beta spindles
chronic pain
fibromyalgia
Parkinson's disease
epileptiform discharges
epilepsy
nocturnal seizure
American Society of
    Electroneurodiagnostic
    Technologists
leg movement
limb movement index
periodic limb movements
periodic limb
    movement index
restless leg movements
sleep start
phasic leg EMG activity

REM extremity movement
bruxism
obstructive apnea
obstructive apnea
    index (OAI)
paradoxical breathing
hypopnea
apnea–hypopnea
    index (AHI)
central apnea (CA)
congestive heart
    failure (CHF)
central apnea index
central sleep apnea
mixed apnea
Cheyne–Stokes
    breathing (CSB)
snoring
primary snoring
respiratory effort–related
    arousal (RERA)
respiratory disturbance
    index (RDI)

Note: The event rules discussed in this chapter are based on the adult scoring criteria from the *AASM Manual for Scoring Sleep and Associated Events*.[1] Rules for scoring events in pediatric studies can be found in Chapter 16.

EEG Arousals

An **EEG arousal** is defined as a shift in frequency in the electroencephalogram (EEG) activity during sleep that lasts at least 3 seconds. To be scored, an EEG arousal must be preceded by at least 10 seconds of uninterrupted sleep and can occur during an epoch staged as wake or any other sleep stage. A shift in EEG frequency for less than 3 seconds is referred to as a **microarousal** but does not meet criteria to be scored as an arousal.

Occasional EEG arousals during sleep are normal. However, sometimes patients with sleep disorders have more frequent arousals that are associated with a shift to a lighter stage of sleep or a brief awakening. When a sleep study is scored for significant events, EEG arousals are marked. An **EEG arousal index** is calculated on the sleep report, which represents the average number of EEG arousals per hour of sleep. Like other event indexes, it is calculated by dividing the total number of events by the total sleep time in hours. An arousal index of less than 5 is usually considered within normal ranges; an index higher than 5 may suggest that other sleep events such as apneas, hypopneas, or limb movements are causing a sleep disturbance. Frequent EEG arousals are also significant in that they can lead to excessive daytime sleepiness.

The EEG frequency shift required to score an arousal can include alpha, theta, or frequencies greater than 16 Hz but excludes spindles. Alpha activity is frequently seen. EEG arousals are often associated with an increase in chin electromyogram (EMG) amplitude, indicating a rise in muscle tone. An associated increase in chin EMG amplitude must be present for at least 1 second to score an arousal during stage R. Stages of NREM are not required to have this concurrent increase in chin tone, although it is often noted. EEG arousals can also be associated with a body movement such as a leg kick. These are often referred to as **movement arousals**. The next several figures present examples of EEG arousals.

Figure 13-1 shows a brief EEG arousal. The enlarged section emphasizes the frequency shift to alpha activity.

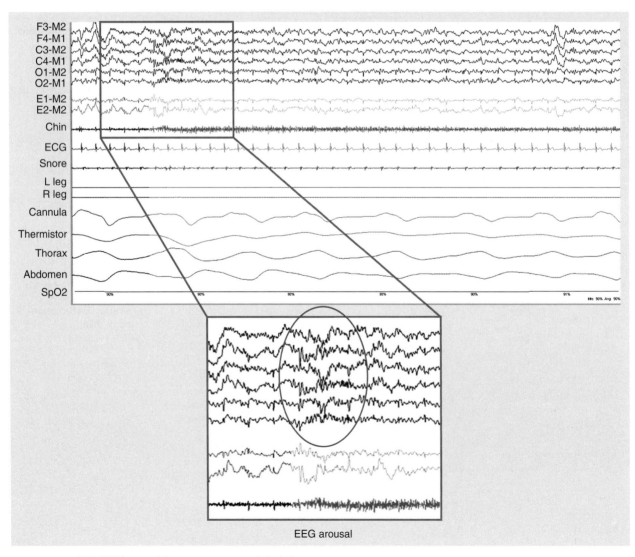

EEG arousal

FIGURE 13-1 A brief EEG arousal that appears to occur in isolation.

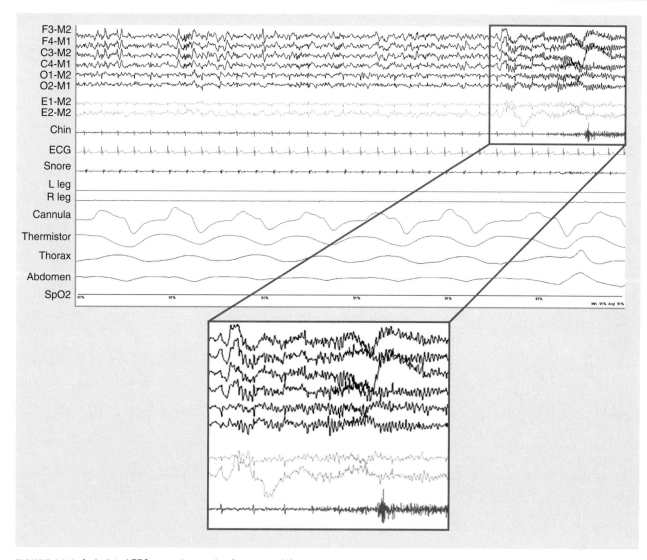

FIGURE 13-2 An isolated EEG arousal occurring from stage N2 sleep.

This arousal appears to occur in isolation and is not associated with any other event. The arousal is short-lived and followed by a quick return to sleep.

In **Figure 13-2**, an EEG arousal is noted at the end of the epoch of N2 sleep (enlargement). Note the frequency shift from theta to alpha accompanied by rapid eye movement (REM) and an increase in chin EMG activity.

In the sample in **Figure 13-3**, the EEG arousal is associated with a leg movement at the beginning of the epoch. The leg movement occurs just before the beginning of the arousal, which suggests it may be the cause of the arousal.

In **Figure 13-4**, the EEG arousal is seen as a burst of alpha activity (circled area) and is the result of a hypopnea. EEG arousals often occur at the end of respiratory events as the patient attempts to regain his or her breath.

The sample in **Figure 13-5** demonstrates an EEG arousal as noted by a shift to alpha activity. Note the accompanying increase in chin EMG and leg movement.

Beta Spindles

With frequencies greater than 14 Hz, **beta waves** are normally associated with waking consciousness when the brain is actively engaged. **Beta spindles** are fast, distinct bursts of EEG waves that can be seen during sleep in select patients. Beta spindles look similar to the sleep spindles seen in stage N2 but are higher frequency and usually higher amplitude and may persist into any stage of sleep. Specifically, although sleep spindles normally occur at frequencies between 12–14 Hz, beta spindles will occur at frequencies above this. Beta spindles are most often present in patients taking certain classes of drugs including benzodiazepines and barbiturates, as well as patients who experience **chronic pain**. They are also seen in patients with **fibromyalgia** and **Parkinson's disease**. EEG arousals may also span into the beta frequency range.

The following figures show examples of beta spindles. The paper speeds are varied in these examples to show details of these high-frequency waveforms.

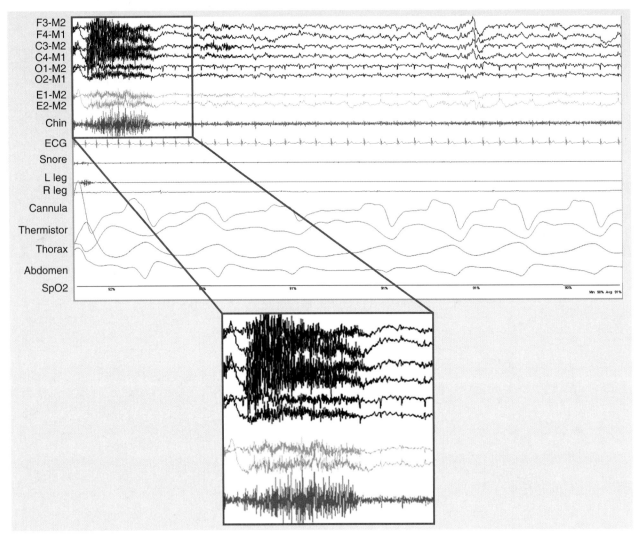

FIGURE 13-3 An EEG arousal associated with leg movement at the beginning of an epoch.

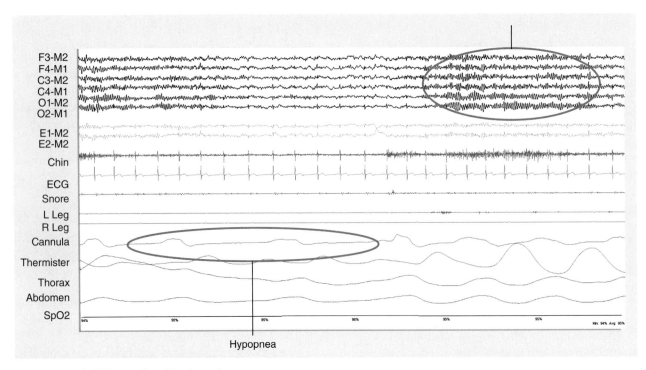

FIGURE 13-4 An EEG arousal resulting from a hypopnea.

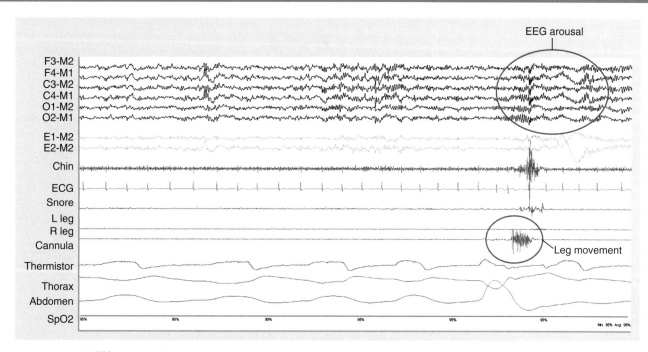

FIGURE 13-5 An EEG arousal with accompanying increase in chin EMG and leg movement.

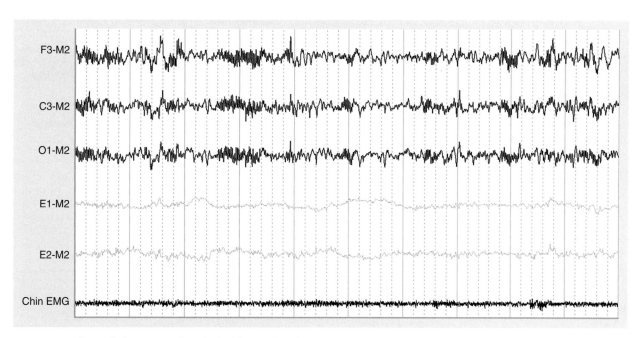

FIGURE 13-6 Beta spindles at approximately the 10-second mark.

In **Figure 13-6**, the patient has beta spindles at approximately the 10-second mark. Each solid green line represents 3 seconds. **Figure 13-7** shows the same example at a faster paper speed, 10 seconds per page. Each solid green line represents 1 second. This allows the scorer to count the individual waves to determine if these are sleep spindles or beta spindles. With the paper speed at 10 seconds/page (30 mm/sec), we can see that the frequency of these spindles is 15 Hz, putting them into the beta frequency range.

In **Figure 13-8** the paper speed is at 30 seconds/page (10 mm/sec). Again, it can be difficult to validate the frequency at this speed. The example in **Figure 13-9** shows the same sample at a faster paper speed, 10 seconds/page (30 mm/sec). Note again that these waveforms have frequencies above the typical spindling frequency of 12–14 Hz.

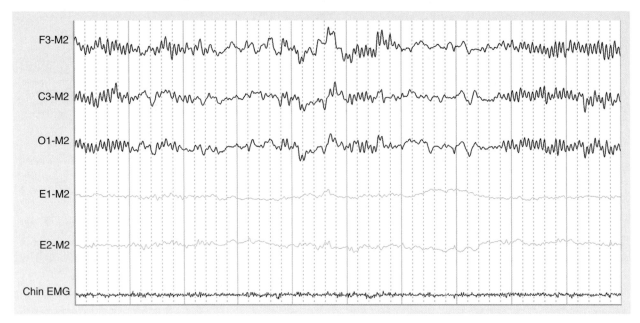

FIGURE 13-7 The same example as in Figure 13-6 shown at 10 seconds per page. The frequency of these spindles are 15 Hz, which qualifies them as beta spindles.

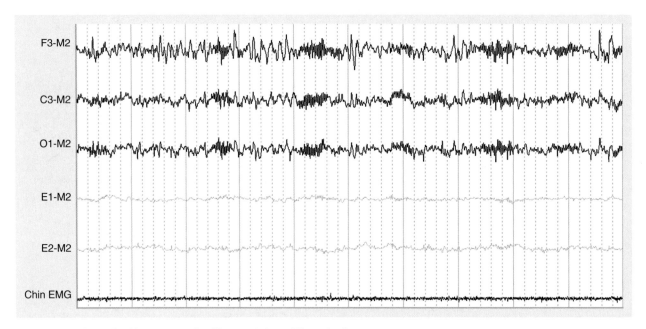

FIGURE 13-8 A sample with paper speed at 30 seconds/page (10 mm/sec).

Nocturnal Seizures

A seizure is a sudden, uncontrolled electrical misfire in the brain. It is characterized by hypersynchronous **epileptiform discharges** that may be accompanied by changes in consciousness or muscle movements. Seizure activity may be manifested simply as a slight mind alteration or may include large-scale convulsions. Various types of seizure activity can range from mild to severe. Patients with recurring seizures are diagnosed with **epilepsy**, or seizure disorder.

Epileptic activity that occurs during sleep is called a **nocturnal seizure**. Nocturnal seizures may be generalized (occurring in all parts of the brain) or focal (occurring in one part of the brain). However, because nocturnal seizures often occur without obvious body movements, they may go unrecognized by the patient or family members.

The connection between epilepsy and sleep is complex. One of the most common triggers for seizure activity in those with epilepsy is sleep deprivation. In addition, seizure activity seems to be influenced by

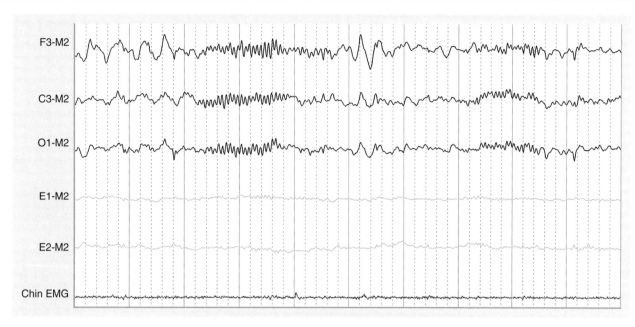

FIGURE 13-9 The same example as in Figure 13-8 at 10 seconds/page (30 mm/sec).

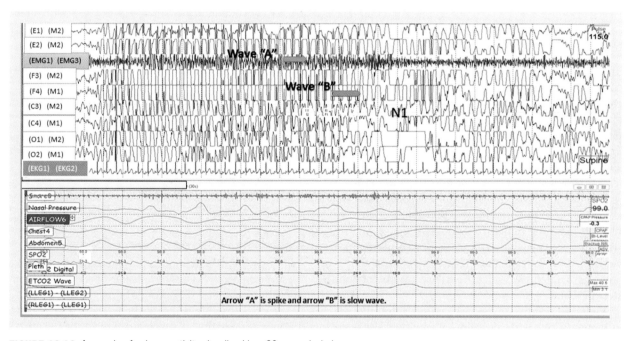

FIGURE 13-10 A sample of seizure activity visualized in a 30-second window.
Courtesy of Sameh Morkous, MD, FAAP, FAAN.

changes in the electrical activity in the brain when transitioning between different stages of sleep.

A physician who suspects a nocturnal seizure disorder may order a sleep study with a seizure montage, which includes a standard polysomnogram (PSG) montage with additional EEG electrodes to detect activity in all parts of the brain. In most cases, a bipolar montage is used in which each channel portrays two active electrode locations (e.g., F3–C3). Sample seizure montages are provided in Chapter 9.

The EEG during seizure activity is characterized by a generalized high-amplitude spike and slow-wave activity that usually begins and ends abruptly. Seizure activity occurring during a standard sleep study often appears as a rapid, high-amplitude spike wave pattern. To visualize and confirm the characteristic spike and slow-wave pattern, it is beneficial to view the activity in a 10-second epoch window. **Figure 13-10** depicts a 30-second window of a standard sleep study in which seizure activity is noted

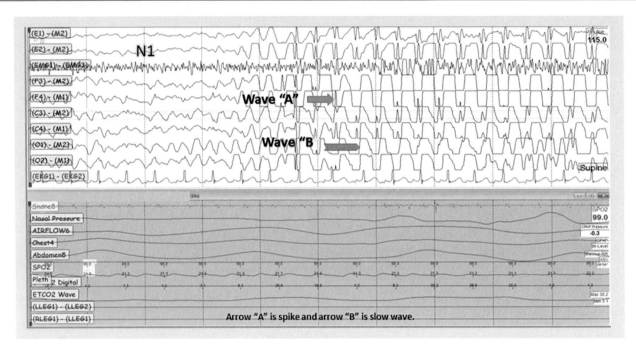

FIGURE 13-11 The same activity as in Figure 13-10 in a 10-second window.
Courtesy of Sameh Morkous, MD, FAAP, FAAN.

during the latter half of the epoch. Note the abrupt start of a generalized fast-wave activity. **Figure 13-11** provides a 10-second window of this same activity. Note how the waveform pattern can be more easily distinguished in this window. Specifically, high-amplitude spike waves are noted to be followed by slower waveforms.

An expanded EEG montage offers the ability to localize the activity. For example, if the spike wave activity is highest in amplitude in the frontal channels, it is localized to the frontal lobe of the brain. The seizure activity may be accompanied by respiratory events or body movements. Frequently, central apnea can be associated with seizure activity both before and after the event.

Nocturnal seizure studies also include video and audio monitoring with recording capabilities. The technologist must observe the patient closely if a seizure is suspected. The technologist is responsible for ensuring the patient's safety and following all facility protocols for observed seizure activity.

Polysomnograms collected with expanded seizure montages should be reviewed by an experienced EEG technologist or a physician familiar with reading EEGs. The many different types of seizure activity are beyond the scope of this text. However, books and resources from the **American Society of Electroneurodiagnostic Technologists** and other EEG resources should be studied for further information on this topic, especially if a technologist is employed in a neurology-based sleep testing facility.

The following types of seizures are discussed in *Principles and Practice of Sleep Medicine*, 5th edition[2]:

- Classified seizures
- Unusual behavioral seizures
- Episodic nocturnal wanderings
- Nocturnal paroxysmal dystonia
- Pure tonic seizures
- Autonomic and diencephalic seizures
- Electrical status epilepticus of sleep

Leg Movements

A **leg movement** is defined in polysomnography as a burst of EMG activity in the anterior tibialis muscle for a duration of at least 0.5 seconds but no longer than 10 seconds. The amplitude must be at least 8 μV above the amplitude of the leg movements recorded during the resting period. The scoring of the leg movement starts at the point in which the amplitude reaches 8 μV above the resting EMG and ends at the point in which the amplitude is no more than 2 μV above the resting point.

Having separate EMG channels for each leg is strongly preferred. In this case, two electrodes should be placed 2 to 3 cm apart on the anterior tibialis of each leg. If not enough channels are available, then one leg EMG channel can be used to identify muscle activity in both legs by placing one electrode on each leg and referencing them together. In this scenario, however, it is not possible to determine where leg muscle activity originates.

Leg movements may be associated with events such as respiratory events or EEG arousals or with disorders such as restless legs syndrome or periodic limb movement disorder (PLMD). Leg movements are not scored if they occur within a period of 0.5 seconds of the beginning to 0.5 seconds of the end of an apnea, hypopnea, or respiratory event-related arousal. In addition, leg movements that occur on both legs but are separated by less than 5 seconds are scored as a single leg movement.

The following statistics regarding leg movements are usually included in the final scored report:

- Total number of leg movements
- Total number of leg movements associated with EEG arousals
- Total **limb movement index** (total number of limb movements per hour of sleep)
- Limb movement index associated with EEG arousals
- Total number of **periodic limb movements**
- The **periodic limb movement index** (total number of periodic leg movements per hour of sleep)

Leg movements are categorized as follows:

- *Periodic limb movements in sleep (PLMs)* occur in a relatively high percentage of patients in the sleep lab. Limb movements are classified as periodic if there are at least four leg movements that meet the duration and amplitude requirements listed previously that occur between 5 and 90 seconds apart. A PLM index is calculated, which represents the average number of limb movements per hour of sleep.
- **Restless leg movements** occur while the patient is awake and typically last at least 5 seconds.

These movements are not scored on the PSG. Patients who suffer from restless leg syndrome often describe feeling an uncomfortable, creepy-crawly or numbing sensation in the lower portion of the legs.

- **Sleep starts** are sudden, quick jerking motions in the legs that commonly occur during the transition from wake to sleep. They do not occur in periodic episodes and often include larger body movements called *generalized hypnic myoclonus*. Sleep starts are sometimes caused by sleep onset dreaming that provokes fear or surprise.
- **Phasic leg EMG activity** consists of low-amplitude, brief leg jerks that typically last 0.1 to 0.5 seconds. These movements are common in patients with PLMD but do not meet the duration criteria to be scored as a leg movement.
- **REM extremity movements** are movements that occur during rapid eye movement sleep. These movements occur in most REM periods but are brief and not usually associated with any other nocturnal events. They are considered somewhat normal even though complete muscle atonia is a characteristic of REM.

The next few figures show examples of leg movements. In **Figure 13-12**, both legs move at the 20-second mark of the epoch. These leg movements are associated with an EEG arousal as noted by the shift in frequency in the EEG and the increase in chin EMG amplitude.

In the sample in **Figure 13-13**, a leg movement in the left leg is not associated with an EEG arousal.

Figure 13-14 shows a brief leg twitch that lasts less than 0.5 seconds. In this case, this muscle activity is not scored as a leg movement.

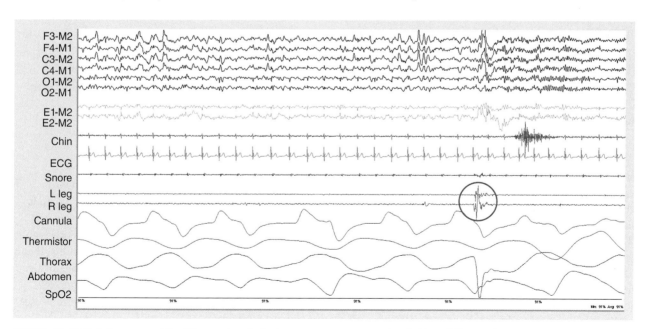

FIGURE 13-12 Both legs move at the 20-second mark; the leg movements are associated with an EEG arousal.

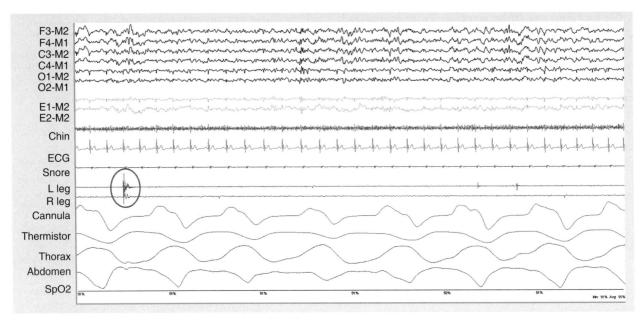

FIGURE 13-13 The leg movement in the left leg is not associated with an EEG arousal.

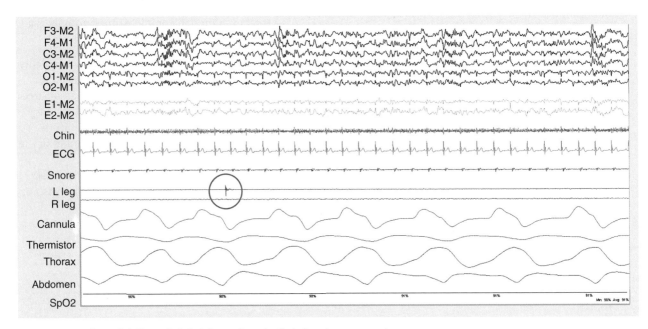

FIGURE 13-14 A very brief leg twitch that does not meet criteria for a leg movement.

The sample in **Figure 13-15** shows movements in the left and right legs occurring at less than 5 seconds apart. As a result, they are scored as a single leg movement. Note that these leg movements are associated with an EEG arousal as noted by the shift in frequency in the EEG and the increase in chin EMG amplitude.

The sample in **Figure 13-16** is compressed to show 300 seconds of recording on one page. During the first 150 seconds, five leg movements occur (circled). Because these movements are associated with respiratory events—occurring during the period of 0.5 seconds before to 0.5 seconds after the event—they should not be scored as leg movements.

Bruxism

The word **bruxism** is derived from the Greek word *brugmos*, which means "gnashing of teeth." Bruxism is characterized by a sustained clenching of the jaw or a repetitive grinding of the teeth during sleep. Although it is most prevalent in adolescents and young adults, it can be seen in all ages. It can occur during any stage of sleep but occurs most commonly during stage N1 and N2. Bruxism usually diminishes with age, but in some cases it can last a lifetime.

As part of the physiologic calibrations, the patient is asked to clench and grind the teeth, mimicking the

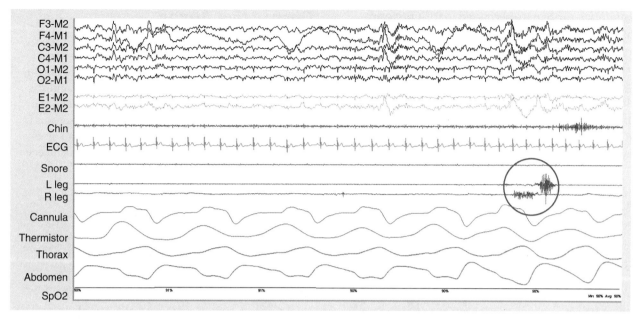

FIGURE 13-15 Movements in the left and right legs occurring less than 5 seconds apart count as one leg movement.

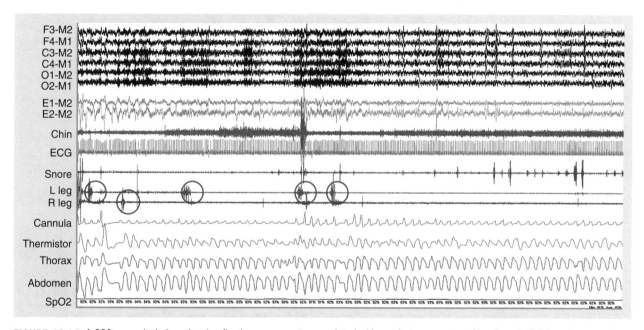

FIGURE 13-16 A 300-second window showing five leg movements associated with respiratory events making them ineligible to be scored as periodic limb movements.

high-amplitude, high-frequency signal seen in the EEGs, electrooculograms (EOGs), and chin EMGs during episodes of bruxism. Scoring criteria for bruxism include visualization of at least three brief elevations of chin or masseter EMG activity that last 0.25–2 seconds in sequence or sustained elevations of chin or masseter EMG activity lasting more than 2 seconds.

Episodes of teeth grinding during sleep are accompanied by highly characteristic audible sounds that are commonly described as grating. As such, the recording technician should note if teeth grinding is heard over the audio monitor. Diagnosis of bruxism also includes at least two audible episodes of tooth grinding.

Sometimes, a snore artifact that intrudes into the chin EMG channel may be confused with bruxism. To distinguish between the two, it is useful to compare the activity seen in the snore channel with the chin EMG. Bruxism tends to be more visible in the chin EMG channel, whereas snoring will be higher in amplitude in the snore channel.

Sleep physicians often refer patients with bruxism to a qualified dentist who can assess the patient's dentition and make recommendations. The most common treatment for bruxism involves using a specially designed mouth guard that helps protect the teeth and prevents grinding. Although certain vitamins and even Botox (*botulinum* toxin) have been used to treat bruxism, there is currently no known cure.

The next few figures show examples of sleep-related bruxism during a polysomnogram. In **Figure 13-17** through **13-19**, the patient clenches the jaw several times. The jaw clenching is associated with bursts of increased amplitude chin EMG that last at least 0.25–2 seconds. In addition, note how the activity is associated with muscle artifact in the EEG, EOG, and snore channels.

Obstructive Apnea

An **obstructive apnea** is defined as at least a 90% reduction in airflow from pre-event baseline for at least 10 seconds, with continued respiratory effort in the chest or abdomen (or both). During a diagnostic polysomnogram, apneic events should be identified with the use of an oronasal thermal airflow sensor. If the thermal sensor is not functioning, then an alternative apnea sensor (e.g., nasal pressure transducer)

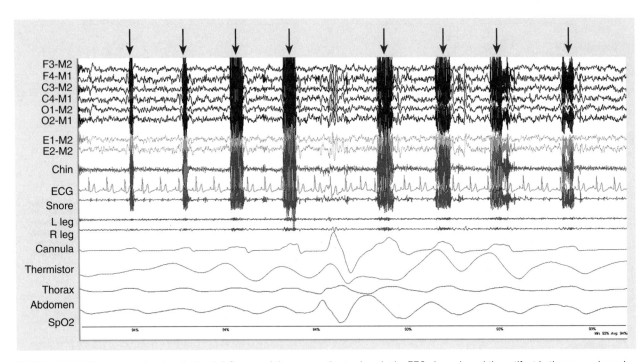

FIGURE 13-17 The patient clenches the jaw briefly several times; note the tracings in the EEG channels and the artifact in the snore channel.

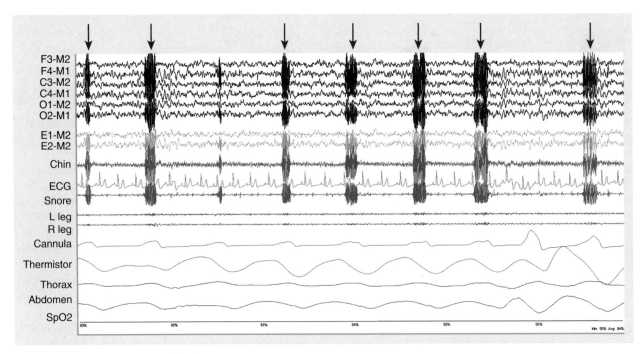

FIGURE 13-18 Several episodes of bruxism.

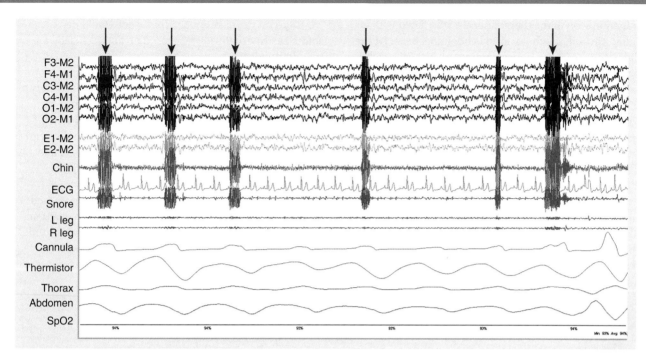

FIGURE 13-19 Several periods of bruxism, causing artifact in the EEG, EOG, and snore channels.

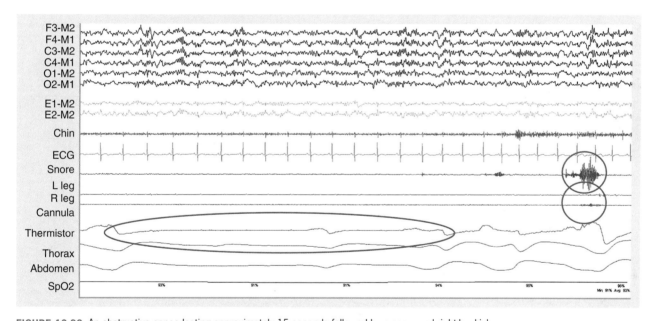

FIGURE 13-20 An obstructive apnea lasting approximately 15 seconds followed by a snore and right-leg kicks.

may be used. During a positive airway pressure (PAP) titration study, apneas are identified through the PAP device's flow sensor. Oxygen desaturations or EEG arousals frequently occur with obstructive apneas. At the end of an apnea, it is also common to see leg jerks, snores, body movements, or full awakenings. Often during an obstructive event, the respiratory effort will decrease slightly. However, if the effort is absent, it is not an obstructive event.

An obstructive apnea (OA) is a single respiratory event. The sleep study report will include the total numbers of OAs as well as the **obstructive apnea index (OAI)**,

which is the number of obstructive apneas per hour of sleep. *Obstructive sleep apnea*, meanwhile, refers to the sleep disorder of obstructive sleep apnea, a diagnosis that only a physician can make.

Respiratory events are most frequently scored in window widths between 120 and 300 seconds. This view allows the events to be more easily visualized, especially those that are of longer duration. The next several figures show examples of obstructive apneas. The sample in **Figure 13-20** depicts a 30-second window of a diagnostic PSG with an obstructive apnea lasting approximately 15 seconds. This is evident by the significant flow reduction seen in the thermal sensor associated with continued effort in the thoracic and abdominal belts. At the end of the apnea, the patient snores and kicks the right leg. Note the increased chin EMG amplitude corresponding with the end of the respiratory event.

Figure 13-21 shows another 30-second window portraying an obstructive apnea that lasts approximately 10–15 seconds. Again, airflow as seen in the thermal device is almost absent while the respiratory effort persists. At the end of the event, the patient snores and kicks.

In the 30-second window shown in **Figure 13-22**, the patient has an obstructive apnea during the final 20 seconds of the epoch and into the next epoch. The event should be scored from the initial cessation of airflow in this epoch to the point at which airflow

resumes on the next epoch. This event would be more easily visualized and scored on an increased window width.

Figure 13-23 portrays a 60-second window (two consecutive epochs) of a diagnostic sleep study to better visualize respiratory events. Note the two obstructive apneic events. These are evident by the cessation of airflow seen in the thermal sensor accompanied by continued effort in the thoracic and abdominal effort channels. In addition, the effort channels demonstrate opposite phase effort movements, or **paradoxical breathing**, indicating increased work of breathing. At the termination of each event an EEG arousal is seen, along with an increased amplitude chin EMG and snoring. Note also the desaturations associated with each event.

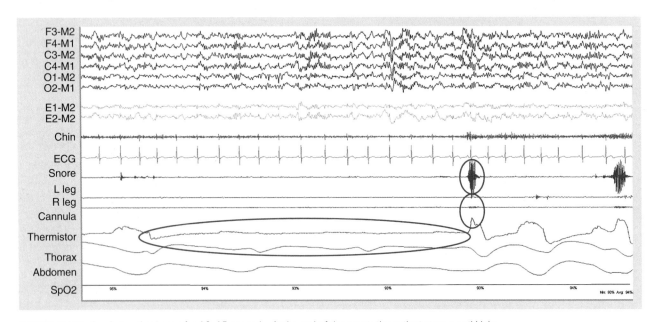

FIGURE 13-21 An obstructive apnea for 10–15 seconds. At the end of the event, the patient snores and kicks.

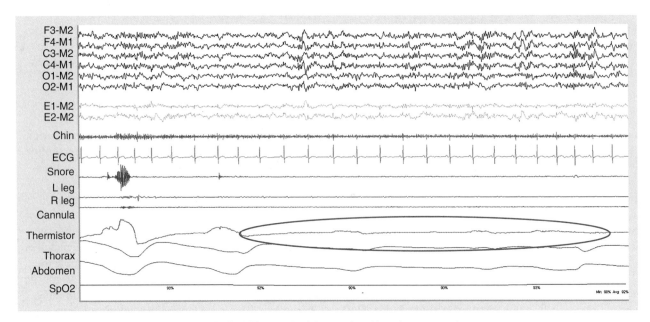

FIGURE 13-22 An obstructive apnea during the final 20 seconds of the epoch and into the next epoch.

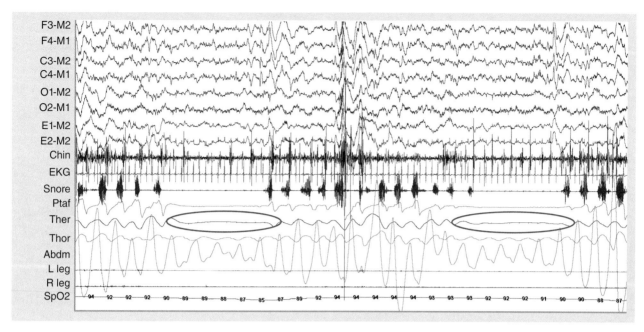

FIGURE 13-23 A 60-second window showing two obstructive apneas.

Figure by Lisa M. Endee; produced from a sleep study provided to Stony Brook University School of Health Technology and Management's Polysomnographic Technology Program by Dr. Kala Sury.

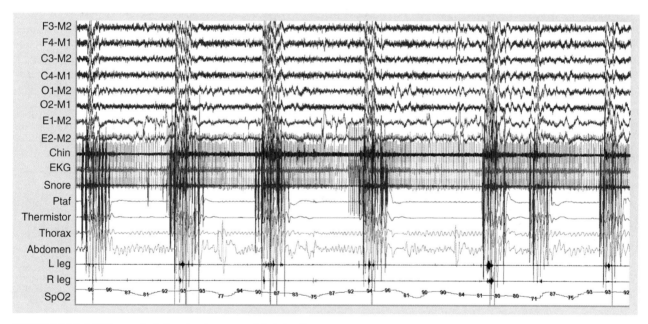

FIGURE 13-24 A 300-second window showing sequential obstructive apneas.

Figure by Lisa M. Endee; produced from a sleep study provided to Stony Brook University School of Health Technology and Management's Polysomnographic Technology Program by Dr. Kala Sury.

The paper speed in the sample in **Figure 13-24** has been increased to 300 seconds/page to show several minutes of respiratory patterns. With this view, we are able to see that the patient is having repeated consecutive obstructive apneas as noted by the cessation of airflow in the thermal sensor and persistent respiratory effort. The events last between 10 and 50 seconds and are associated with significant desaturations and obvious EEG arousals. Between apneas, the patient takes only a few deep breaths and then obstructs again.

In the 30-second epoch in **Figure 13-25**, a long obstructive apnea is noted during stage R sleep that

extends beyond the end of the epoch. This event is associated with paradoxical breathing and alpha intrusion into the occipital EEG channels.

Hypopnea

A **hypopnea** is defined as a reduction in airflow by at least 30% of the pre-event baseline for at least 10 seconds. During a diagnostic polysomnogram, hypopneic events should be identified with the use of a nasal pressure transducer. If the signal from the nasal transducer is not functioning, then a thermal sensor may be used. Like

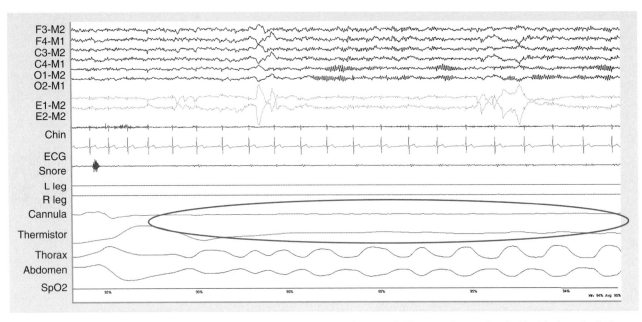

FIGURE 13-25 A long apnea during stage R sleep extending beyond the end of the epoch. The event is associated with alpha intrusion in the occipital EEGs.

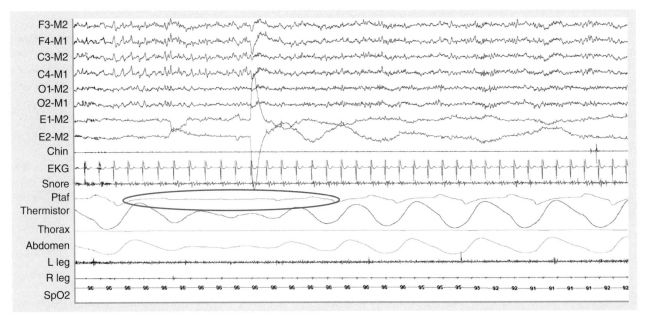

FIGURE 13-26 A 10- to 15-second hypopnea.

Figure by Lisa M. Endee; produced from a sleep study provided to Stony Brook University School of Health Technology and Management's Polysomnographic Technology Program by Dr. Kala Sury.

apneas, during a PAP titration study, hypopneas are identified through the PAP device flow sensor. To score a hypopneic event, in addition to the reduction in airflow by 30%, it must be associated with either an EEG arousal or an oxygen desaturation of at least 3% (4% if using the alternative Medicare guideline). If the airflow is noted to be reduced by more than 90%, then the event is considered an apnea. Further, if any portion of the event qualifies as an apnea, then the event is scored as an apnea. Hypopneas can be associated with the same side effects and related events as apneic events.

On a sleep study report, total number of hypopneic events are reported. In addition, the number of apneas and hypopneas are totaled and used to calculate an **apnea–hypopnea index (AHI)**. The AHI describes the number of apneic and hypopneic events noted per hour of sleep. This number is the most frequently used statistic to classify the severity of the various sleep-related breathing disorders. Normal values for AHI in adults range from 0–4 events per hour of sleep, with mild, moderate, and severe ranges at 5–15, 16–29, and >30, respectively.

The following figures show examples of hypopneic events as seen on a polysomnogram.

The sample in **Figure 13-26** shows a 10- to 15-second hypopnea. The event is shown in a 30-second window during stage R. Note the >30% reduction in airflow in the pressure transducer (pressure transducer airflow [PTAF] channel) and the persistence of respiratory effort as the airflow decreases in volume. The event is also associated with a 5% oxygen desaturation, meeting the criteria for scoring it as a hypopnea.

Figure 13-27 portrays a 60-second window that includes two respiratory events. For each event, a greater than 30% reduction in airflow is seen in the PTAF channel that lasts approximately 15 seconds. To score a hypopnea, the required reduction in airflow must be associated with an oxygen desaturation of at least 3% or an EEG arousal or both. In the second event shown, the patient desaturates from 94% to 91%, meeting the 3% desaturation criteria

and qualifying as a hypopnea. However, in the first event, oxygen levels fall from 94% to 92% and thus do not meet the desaturation criteria. For this event to be scored as a hypopnea, the technologist would need to view the 30-second window to determine if an EEG arousal is present at the termination of the event.

In Figure 13-28, a slight decrease in airflow is detected in the pressure cannula. Because the event lasts less than 10 seconds, it is not scored as a hypopnea.

In the sample shown in Figure 13-29, the patient has a 10-second hypopnea that is followed by an EEG arousal and a leg movement. The leg movement is not scored because it occurs at the end of a respiratory event.

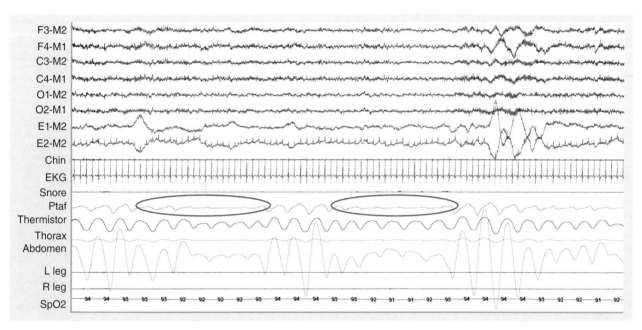

FIGURE 13-27 A 60-second window with hypopneic events.

Figure by Lisa M. Endee; produced from a sleep study provided to Stony Brook University School of Health Technology and Management's Polysomnographic Technology Program by Dr. Kala Sury.

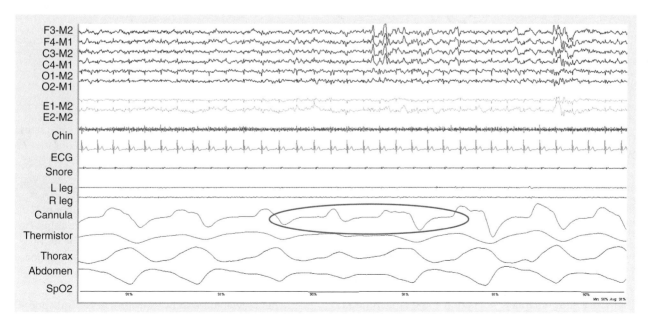

FIGURE 13-28 A slight decrease in airflow.

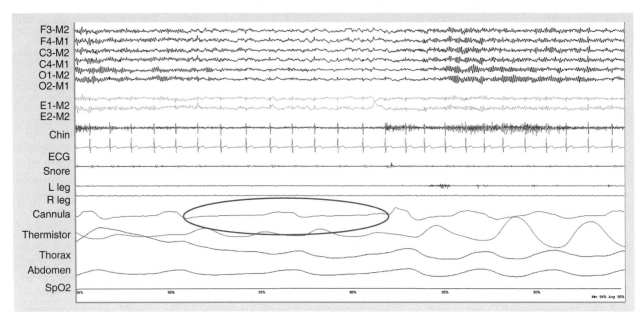

FIGURE 13-29 A 10-second hypopnea followed by an EEG arousal and a leg movement.

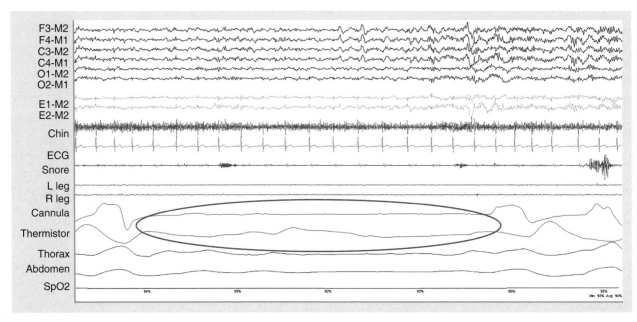

FIGURE 13-30 An apnea with no respiratory effort throughout the event (central apnea) lasting about 15 seconds.

Central Apnea

A **central apnea (CA)** is the cessation of airflow with an absence of respiratory effort. It is identified by the presence of at least a 90% decrease in airflow for at least 10 seconds and the lack of respiratory effort throughout the entire event. As noted previously, during a diagnostic polysomnogram, apneic events should be identified with the use of an oronasal thermal airflow sensor. If the thermal sensor is not functioning, then an alternative apnea sensor (e.g., nasal pressure transducer) may be used.

During a central apnea, the thoracic and abdominal respiratory effort channels will flatten at the same time as the airflow ceases. This indicates that there is no attempt by the patient to breathe. At the end of the central apneic event, the airflow and effort return simultaneously. Central apneas are less common than obstructive apneas or hypopneas and are most often seen at sleep onset, during continuous positive airway pressure (CPAP) titrations, and in the elderly or patient with certain medical disorders such as **congestive heart failure (CHF)**. A CA is scored on the polysomnogram, and the number of central apneas are totaled on the report. This number is used to calculate the **central apnea index**, or the number of central apneas per hour of sleep. **Central sleep apnea** refers to a sleep-related breathing disorder that only a physician can diagnose.

The next few figures show examples of central apneas.

Figure 13-30 displays an apnea that is noted by the significant reduction in airflow in the thermistor channel for approximately 15 seconds. Respiratory effort is lacking throughout the event, thus meeting criteria for a central apnea. Note the EEG arousal noted at the termination of the event.

In the sample shown in **Figure 13-31**, a 10-second central apnea is seen as the airflow and effort stop and begin at the same times. An EEG arousal can be seen at the end of the event.

In **Figure 13-32**, a central apnea is immediately followed by an EEG arousal and a leg movement as the patient begins to breathe again. Because the leg movement occurs at the end of a respiratory event, it will not be scored. Note the absence of effort associated with greater than 90% reduction in airflow in the thermal channel.

In the beginning of the epoch shown in **Figure 13-33**, alpha activity, slow eye movements, and increased chin EMG indicate an EEG arousal has occurred. As the EEG transitions back to sleep, a central apnea is seen. Note the cessation of airflow in the thermistor channel associated with lack of respiratory effort. This respiratory event proceeds into the subsequent epoch.

In the sample shown in **Figure 13-34**, a 180-window width is used to visualize sequential central apneic events occurring during a PAP titration. For each event, there is >90% reduction in the CPAP flow channel associated with lack of respiratory effort. The events are approximately 20 seconds and accompanied by desaturations down to 90–91%.

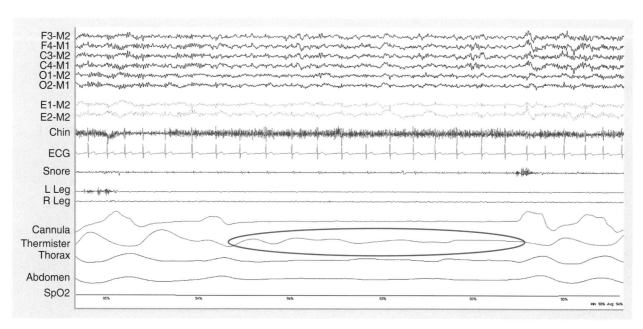

FIGURE 13-31 A 10-second central apnea.

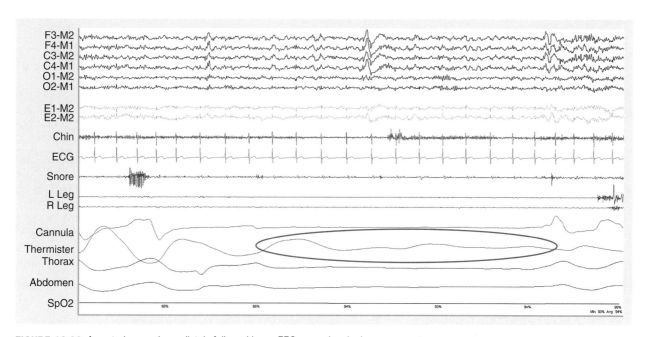

FIGURE 13-32 A central apnea immediately followed by an EEG arousal and a leg movement.

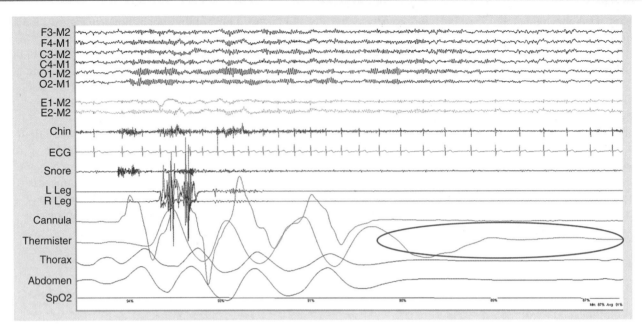

FIGURE 13-33 A central apnea occurring with transition from wake to sleep.

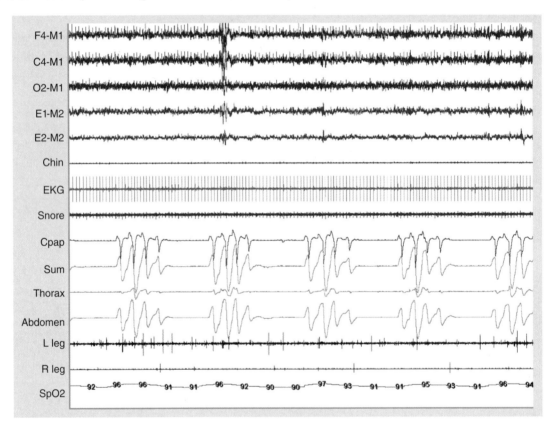

FIGURE 13-34 A 180-second window demonstrating central apneic events.

Figure by Lisa M. Endee; produced from a sleep study provided to Stony Brook University School of Health Technology and Management's Polysomnographic Technology Program by Dr. Kala Sury.

Mixed Apnea

A **mixed apnea** is characterized by a 90% or greater decrease in airflow for at least 10 seconds associated with a lack of respiratory effort during the initial phase and a return of respiratory effort during the latter phase. In essence, a mixed apnea is a combination of a central apnea and an obstructive apnea. Currently, there are no duration criteria for each of the central and obstructive components, only that the total duration of the event is at least 10 seconds. Similar to obstructive and central apneas, mixed apneic events should be identified with the use of an oronasal thermal airflow sensor. If the thermal sensor is not functioning, then an alternative apnea sensor (e.g., nasal pressure transducer) may be used.

The following figures show examples of mixed apneas.

In **Figure 13-35**, the patient has a mixed apnea that lasts approximately 15 seconds. During the first 5 seconds there is no respiratory effort, indicating a central component. Then the effort returns before the airflow returns, indicating an obstructive component. Note the pattern of paradoxical breathing in the obstructive portion of the apnea.

In the sample in **Figure 13-36**, the patient has a mixed apnea lasting approximately 10–15 seconds. Effort is absent during the first portion of the event and then returns in the latter portion. Note the pattern of paradoxical breathing in the obstructive portion of the apnea. At the end of the event, the patient has an EEG arousal and a leg movement in each leg. The leg movements are not scored because they occur at the end of a respiratory event.

Figure 13-37 demonstrates a mixed apnea lasting nearly the entire length of the epoch. Note the lack of effort during the first portion of the event with a return

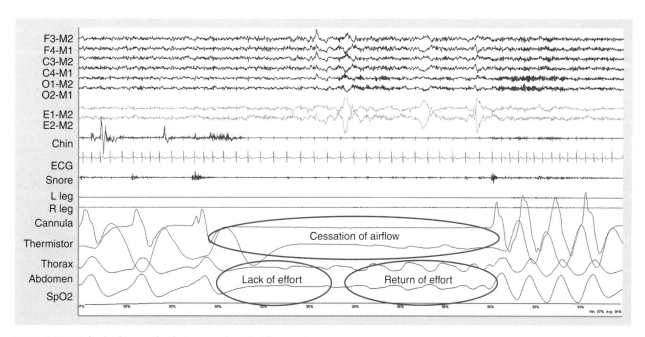

FIGURE 13-35 A mixed apnea that lasts approximately 15 seconds.

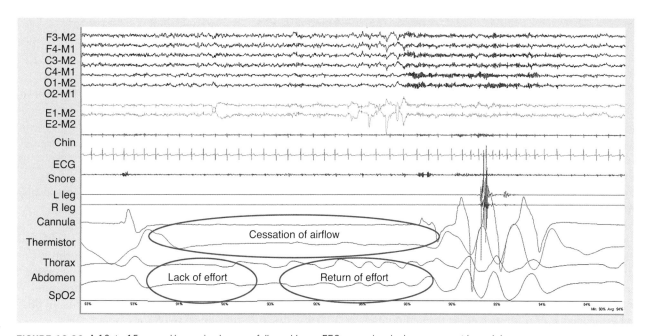

FIGURE 13-36 A 10- to 15-second-long mixed apnea, followed by an EEG arousal and a leg movement in each leg.

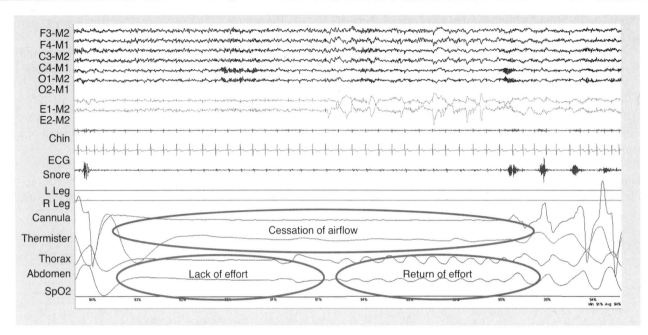

FIGURE 13-37 A mixed apnea during stage R sleep associated with an EEG arousal.

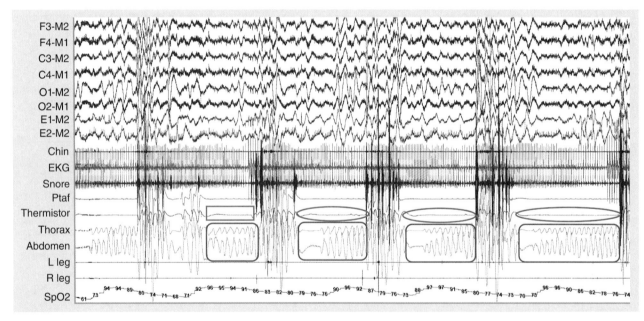

FIGURE 13-38 A 240-second window with obstructive and mixed apneic events.

Figure by Lisa M. Endee; produced from a sleep study provided to Stony Brook University School of Health Technology and Management's Polysomnographic Technology Program by Dr. Kala Sury.

of paradoxical effort in the latter half. This apnea occurs during stage R sleep and is associated with an EEG arousal at its termination.

Obstructive and mixed events can be compared in the 240-second window seen in **Figure 13-38**. In this figure, the event outlined in a square meets the criteria for an obstructive apnea as noted by the absence of flow in the thermal channel for approximately 20 seconds and associated with continued effort throughout the event (red outline below). The subsequent events (ovals) meet criteria for mixed apneas. These events also demonstrate absence of flow in the thermal channel for greater than 10 seconds, but they are associated with absence of effort during the beginning phase of the event with return of effort during the latter portion (red boxes below). Note the significant desaturations associated with both types of respiratory events. In this case, desaturations down to 68% are noted.

Cheyne–Stokes Breathing

Cheyne–Stokes breathing (CSB) is characterized by a repetitive waning and waxing pattern in airflow volume with intermittent central apneas or hypopneas. This breathing pattern is seen in approximately 50% of patients with CHF but often goes unrecognized[3] in this population. It can also be seen in patients with renal failure, a previous history of stroke, and those taking opioid medications. CSB is believed to result from an unstable control of ventilation, a prolonged circulation time, and a diminished capacity for buffering of blood gases.

Usually, the breathing pattern associated with Cheyne–Stokes is extremely difficult to detect on a 30-second epoch, but it becomes more apparent when visualizing in larger window widths (e.g., a 300-second window). Occurrence of a pattern of consecutive central apneas or hypopneas should prompt further assessment for this breathing pattern.

The criteria for scoring Cheyne–Stokes breathing include the presence of three or more consecutive cycles of the waxing–waning pattern (often called a *crescendo–decrescendo pattern*) with either central apneas or central hypopneas, and a full cycle length of at least 40 seconds. Also, there must be at least five central apneas or hypopneas per hour of sleep during the night, during at least 2 hours of recording time. **Figure 13-39** illustrates the distinctive pattern of breathing seen in CSB.

Snoring

Snoring is the most frequent respiratory disturbance during sleep. In rare cases, snoring can be considered benign. However, because snoring is caused by a partial obstruction in the upper airway, it is often a sign of a sleep-related breathing disorder.

Snoring can disturb the sleep of the snorer and the bed partner. Often snoring is also accompanied by other signs of sleep-related breathing disorders such as pauses in breathing, gasping, frequent arousals, and restless sleep.

Many treatments are available for benign snoring, which is often referred to as **primary snoring**. These include over-the-counter treatments such as mouth guards, snore strips, throat lubricants, and specialized pillows. Treatment of patients with snoring associated with obstructive sleep apnea most frequently includes the use of PAP therapy or an oral appliance.

Snoring appears on the polysomnogram as brief increases in amplitude in the snore channel. This is sometimes seen as an artifact in the chin EMG channel. In some cases, if the snoring is very heavy, it can be seen in the EEG channels as well. In most cases, individual snore events are not marked on a sleep study. However, many of the newer sleep scoring software technologies include modules that automatically pick up these events. In these cases, the snore events can be totaled and included in the PSG report. In all cases, it is important for technologists to document the presence of snoring on their reports.

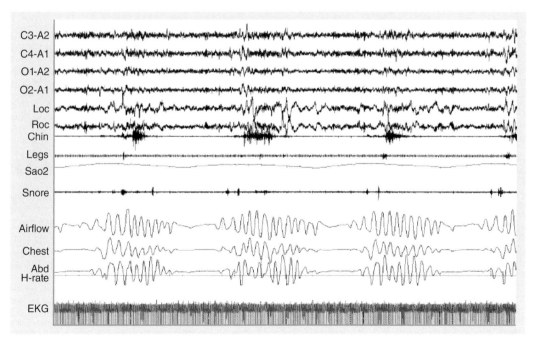

FIGURE 13-39 A 180-second window portraying a Cheyne–Stokes breathing pattern.

The next few figures show examples of snoring on a polysomnogram. In the sample shown in **Figure 13-40**, the patient, currently in stage N2 sleep, has one small snore at the end of the epoch. In the sample shown in **Figure 13-41**, persistent snoring is noted with every breath. These snores are not associated with EEG arousals.

The sample in **Figure 13-42** shows a 300-second epoch in which the patient has snoring associated with

variability in airflow. The sample in **Figure 13-43** shows another 300-second epoch in which the patient is snoring with every breath.

In **Figure 13-44**, the patient has only a few distinct light snores. In the 30-second epoch in **Figure 13-45**, the patient is on CPAP therapy and is snoring lightly. Because snoring indicates that airflow limitation exists, the CPAP level will need to be increased slightly to correct this.

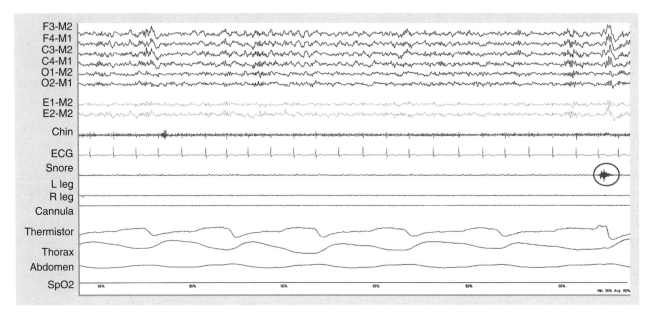

FIGURE 13-40 One small snore at the end of the epoch.

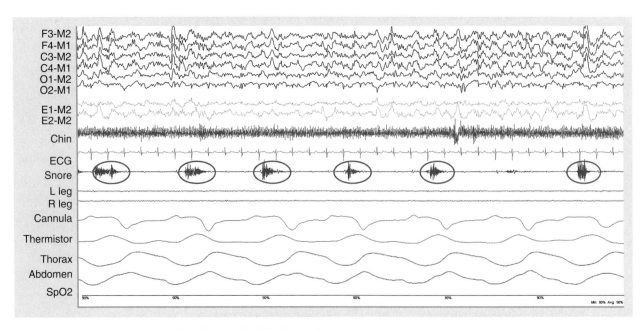

FIGURE 13-41 Persistent snoring with nearly every breath in the epoch.

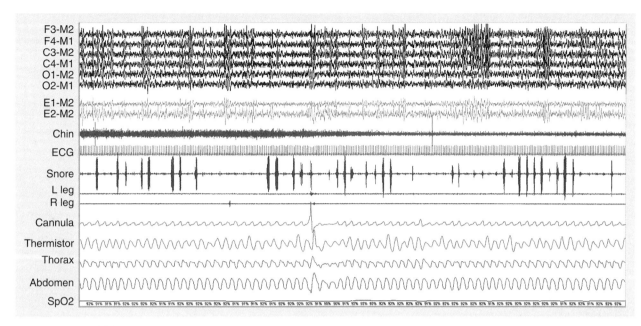

FIGURE 13-42 A 300-second epoch in which the patient is snoring heavily.

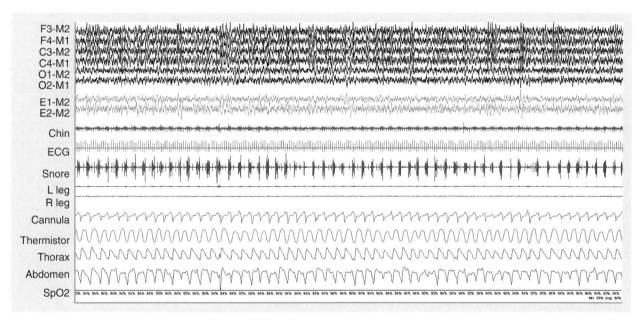

FIGURE 13-43 A 300-second epoch in which the patient is snoring with every breath.

Respiratory Effort–Related Arousals

Respiratory effort–related arousals (RERAs) are arousals that are associated with a sequence of breaths lasting at least 10 seconds that exhibit decreased airflow of <30% or are associated with increasing respiratory effort. RERAs are significant because there are many patients whose mild upper-airway obstructions cause disturbances to their sleep, although they are not severe enough to classify as apneas or hypopneas. The EEG arousals associated with these events have consequences on daytime function and overall health and safety.

Scoring RERAs in a sleep study is optional and may vary with the lab protocol and physician preferences. If scored, RERAs are counted, and the total number is used to calculate a RERA index (the number of RERAs that occur each hour of sleep). The RERA index is added to the AHI to determine the **respiratory disturbance index (RDI)**. Although the AHI includes apneas and hypopneas, the RDI includes apneas, hypopneas, and RERAs.

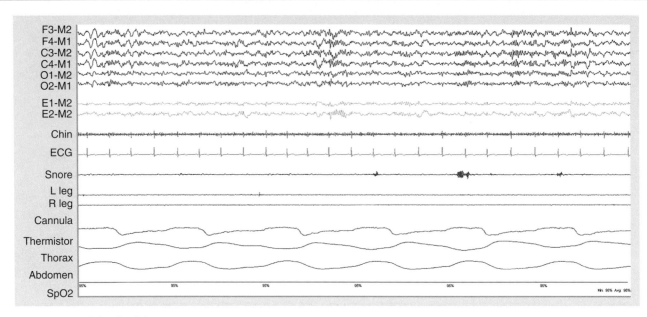

FIGURE 13-44 Only a few light snores.

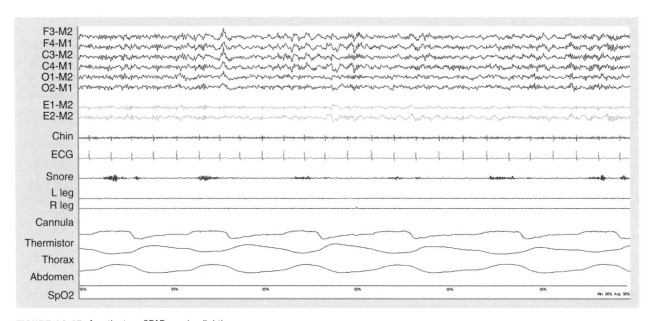

FIGURE 13-45 A patient on CPAP snoring lightly.

Chapter Summary

Scoring sleep events on a polysomnogram requires the use of American Academy of Sleep Medicine scoring parameters and careful review of the sleep study record. An EEG arousal is a shift in EEG frequency lasting at least 3 seconds. EEG arousals are similar to brief awakenings and are often associated with other sleep events. Increased EEG arousals can greatly disturb a patient's sleep and can lead to excessive daytime sleepiness.

Beta spindles are characterized by rapid (14–16 Hz) and usually high-amplitude EEG waves intruding into

sleep. Beta spindles are usually the result of certain medications but can also be caused by chronic pain.

Nocturnal seizures may occasionally be seen during a sleep study. The technologist should be able to recognize the appearance of generalized seizure activity in the EEG. Sleep labs should have protocols in place for when seizure activity is identified.

Leg movements are seen as brief increases in amplitude in the leg EMG channels of at least 8 μV over the baseline recording. To be scored, leg movements must be between 0.5 and 5 seconds in length and cannot be associated with an apnea or a hypopnea. There are several different types of leg movements. Periodic limb movements in sleep are common and can cause disruptions to a patient's sleep.

Bruxism is characterized by grinding of the teeth or clenching of the jaw during sleep. This is most common among adolescents; its occurrence decreases with age. Bruxism can damage the teeth and create pain in the jaw and headaches. Bruxism is most often treated with a mouth guard.

Obstructive apneas are respiratory events in which there is a complete or near complete (at least 90% decrease) cessation of airflow despite the effort to breathe. On the polysomnogram, obstructive apneic events must last at least 10 seconds and be associated with at least a 90% drop in amplitude in the thermal airflow channel. Respiratory effort remains present throughout the duration of the event.

Breathing events that have less than a 90% reduction in flow can be assessed for meeting criteria for a hypopnea. A hypopneic event is defined as at least a 30% decrease in airflow as seen in the nasal pressure channel. In addition, the reduction in flow must be associated with either a 3% oxygen desaturation or an EEG arousal. Similar to obstructive apneas, hypopneas must last at least 10 seconds.

A central apnea is a complete cessation of airflow (at least a 90% decrease in airflow amplitude) caused by a lack of effort to breathe. On the polysomnogram, central events must be at least 10 seconds, be accompanied by at least a 90% drop in airflow, and exhibit a complete cessation of respiratory effort throughout the event.

A mixed apnea is an apnea that contains both central and obstructive components. Specifically, the beginning portion of a mixed apnea is absent of respiratory effort while effort returns in the latter portion of the event.

In the sleep study report, the total number of apneas and hypopneas are used to calculate the apnea hypopnea index (AHI). This value provides the number of events that were observed per hour of sleep and indicates the severity of the sleep-related breathing disorder.

Cheyne–Stokes breathing is a waxing–waning breathing pattern that includes central apneas and hypopneas. It is most often seen in patients with underlying neurologic or cardiac disease. The breathing pattern usually requires a faster paper speed to detect.

Snoring is perhaps the most common respiratory-related sleep event. When snoring is isolated and not associated with any other event, it may be benign. However, because snoring is a partial obstruction of the upper airway, it is often associated with obstructive apneas and hypopneas. Several treatments are available for snoring.

Respiratory effort–related arousals (RERAs) are EEG arousals that are associated with slight decreases in airflow or increases in respiratory effort. RERAs are included in the respiratory disturbance index (RDI).

Case Study

What type of significant event is seen in the 240-second window shown in **Figure 13-46**?

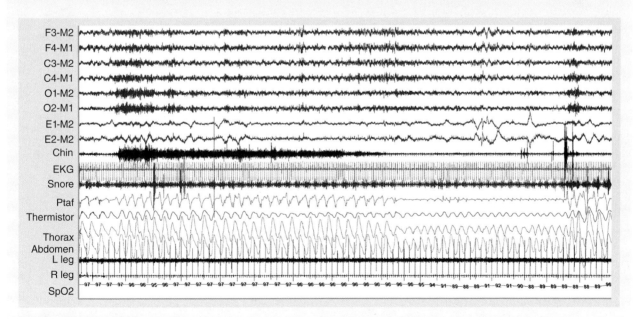

FIGURE 13-46 Case Study.

Figure by Lisa M. Endee; produced from a sleep study provided to Stony Brook University School of Health Technology and Management's Polysomnographic Technology Program by Dr. Kala Sury.

Chapter 13 Questions

Please consider the following questions as they relate to the material in this chapter.

1. What is the required duration for EEG arousals?
2. Why are leg movements significant?
3. What is bruxism and how is it identified?
4. What are the different types of apneas and how do the scoring criteria for these differ from one another?
5. What is Cheyne–Stokes breathing and why it is significant?
6. What is a RERA and what are the potential consequences of frequent RERAs?

Footnotes

1. American Academy of Sleep Medicine. (2017). *AASM Manual for the Scoring of Sleep and Associated Events*, version 2.4. Darien, IL: Author.
2. Kryger, M. H., Roth, T., & Dement, W. C, (2011). *Principles and practice of sleep medicine*, 5th ed. New York: Elsevier.
3. Ingbir, M., Freimark, D., Motro, M., & Adler, Y. (2002). The incidence, pathophysiology, treatment and prognosis of Cheyne–Stokes breathing disorder in patients with congestive heart failure. *Herz*, *27*(2), 107–112.

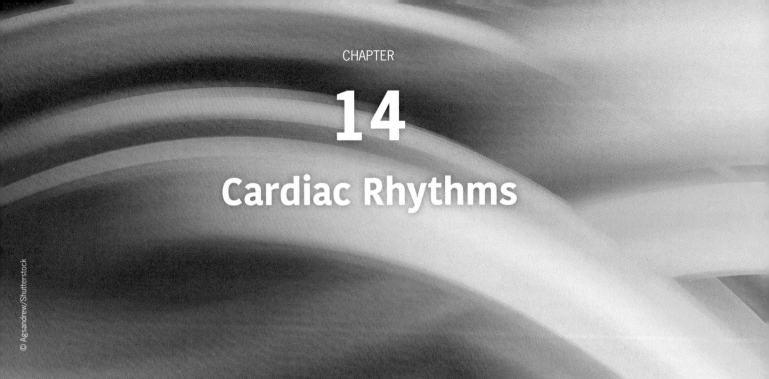

14
Cardiac Rhythms

© Agsandrew/Shutterstock

CHAPTER OUTLINE

Reading ECG Tracings
Normal ECG Ranges
Sinus Rhythms
Atrial Rhythms
Junctional Rhythms
Ventricular Rhythms
Escape Rhythms
AV Blocks
Chapter Summary

LEARNING OBJECTIVES

1. Learn the importance of recognizing cardiac rhythms.
2. Understand how the electrical pathway of the heart affects ECG tracings.
3. Recognize a normal cardiac rhythm.
4. Know normal ECG rates and intervals.
5. Identify abnormal cardiac rhythms.
6. Know the proper responses to specific abnormal cardiac rhythms.

KEY TERMS

electrocardiogram (ECG)
arrhythmia
sinoatrial (SA) node
internodal pathways
atrioventricular (AV) node
atria
ventricles
AV bundle
bundle branches
Purkinje fibers
P wave
QRS complex
T wave
PR interval
ST segment
QT interval
RR interval
rhythm
rate
normal sinus rhythm (NSR)
sinus arrhythmia
sinus bradycardia
ectopy
myocardial infarction (MI)
sinus tachycardia
premature atrial complex (PAC)
compensatory pause

atrial flutter
fibrillation
atrial fibrillation
premature junctional contractions (PJCs)
supraventricular tachycardia (SVT)
premature ventricular contraction (PVC)
bigeminy
trigeminy
couplet
ventricular tachycardia (V tach)
ventricular fibrillation (V fib)
ventricular standstill
asystole
junctional escape rhythm
ventricular escape rhythm
AV block
first-degree AV block
second-degree AV block type 1
second-degree AV block type 2
third-degree (complete) AV block

Reading ECG Tracings

An **electrocardiogram (ECG)** (sometimes written EKG) is a recording of the electrical activity of the heart. Every sleep technologist should know how to read an ECG tracing and be able to recognize deviations from a normal sinus rhythm, also called **arrhythmias**. Further, because arrhythmias are increasingly likely in patients with sleep-related breathing disorders (e.g., obstructive sleep apnea or OSA) and thus not uncommon to encounter during a sleep study, technologists must be familiar with their facility protocols in responding to arrhythmias when they occur.

The first step to understanding the ECG is to understand the anatomy, mechanics, and flow of blood through the heart. **Figure 14-1** illustrates the external cardiac anatomy. It depicts the four main chambers of the heart, which include the right and left atria and ventricles, as well as the right and left coronary arteries, which feed the heart tissue. **Figure 14-2** illustrates the flow of blood into the heart and through the different chambers. Specifically, deoxygenated blood enters the heart through the superior and inferior vena cava and is dumped into the right atrium. As the heart beats, the blood is pumped through the tricuspid valve and into the right ventricle. From here, the right ventricle pumps the blood through the pulmonary valve and into the pulmonary artery. The pulmonary artery delivers blood to the lungs for gas exchange and oxygenation. The pulmonary veins carry blood back into the heart, entering the left atrium. The oxygenated blood is then pumped from the left atrium, through the mitral

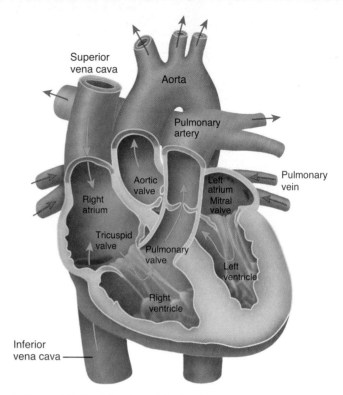

FIGURE 14-2 Blood flow through the heart.

valve, into the left ventricle. Finally, blood is pumped from the left ventricle through the aortic valve and into the aorta to be delivered to the body. The valves within the heart serve to prevent the backward flow of blood.

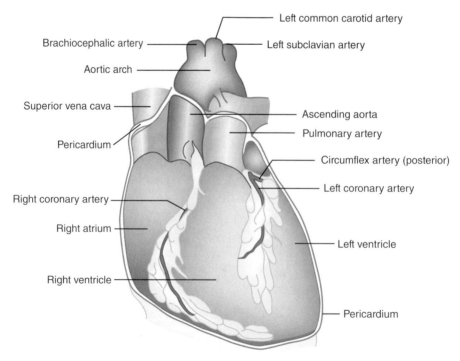

FIGURE 14-1 External cardiac anatomy.

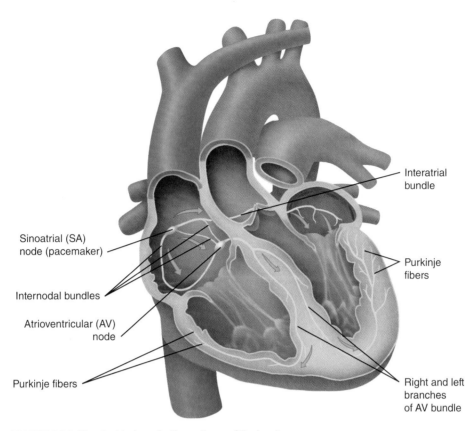

FIGURE 14-3 The electrical conduction pathway of the heart.

The heart beats because of electrical impulses generated at the **sinoatrial (SA) node**. This structure is commonly referred to as the *pacemaker* of the heart. **Figure 14-3** depicts the heart's electrical conduction pathway. Each impulse generated by the SA node moves through the **internodal pathways** to the **atrioventricular (AV) node**, which conducts electrical impulses from the **atria** to the **ventricles**. At the AV node, the impulse is slightly delayed, which allows the atria to empty before the ventricles contract. The electrical impulse then travels through the **AV bundle**, down the left and right **bundle branches** of the **Purkinje fibers**, and through the ventricle. The electrical impulses generate muscle contractions in the various areas of the heart that pump blood through the chambers, into the lungs, and out to the rest of the body.

The ECG tracing consists of a series of waveforms that depict the electrical activity in the heart. One complete cardiac cycle includes both a contraction and a relaxation of the heart muscle.

A diagnostic ECG includes the collection of data from a full 12-lead hookup. However, for a sleep study, typically only one monitoring channel is collected through the use of two active electrodes. Some facilities will include an additional electrode as a backup. The proper placement of the electrodes is shown in **Figure 14-4**. Specifically, one is placed just under the right collar bone

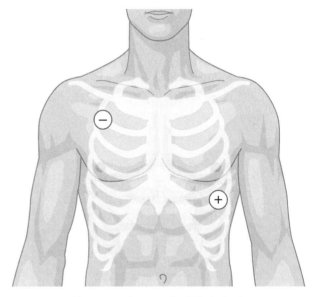

FIGURE 14-4 The proper placement for ECG electrodes.

and the other low on the left rib cage. With this orientation, a bipolar lead II channel is collected.

The ECG consists of four basic waveforms (see **Figure 14-5**): the **P wave**, the **QRS complex**, the **T wave**, and the U wave. In many cases, the U wave is not visible or easily discernible. The shape and interval of these

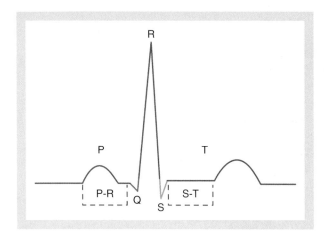

FIGURE 14-5 An ECG waveform.

Table 14-1
Cardiac Activity and Associated Waveforms

ECG Waveform	Cardiac Activity
Space before P wave	Impulse from sinus node
P wave	Atrial contraction
PR interval	Atrial depolarization
QRS complex	Ventricular contraction
ST segment	Early ventricular repolarization
T wave	Ventricular repolarization
QT interval	Ventricular activity

waveforms are carefully reviewed. Intervals include the **PR interval**, **ST segment**, and **QT interval**. The length of the QRS complex is also reviewed as an important time interval in the ECG. The significance of these waveforms and time intervals is shown in **Table 14-1** and will be discussed in the following sections.

Normal ECG Ranges

The following are normal ECG ranges:

PR interval: 0.12–0.20 seconds
QRS complex: 0.04–0.10 seconds
QT interval: 0.36–0.44 seconds

The normal resting heart rate for a healthy adult is 60–100 beats per minute (bpm). The rate can be calculated by counting the number of R waves per minute because it is the most easily recognizable part of the ECG waveform. Alternately, the rate can be estimated by counting the number of beats during 6 seconds and multiplying by 10.

ECGs are typically examined on grid paper. The grid includes small and large boxes for ease of measurement. Each small box on the grid paper is equal to 0.04 seconds, and five small boxes are included in one large box, which is equal to 0.20 seconds in duration. Further, five large boxes make up 1 second. In the sample in **Figure 14-6**, a large box is outlined in red at the bottom of the grid paper. In this example, note that 20 large horizontal boxes make the strip 4 seconds long. Because there are five QRS complexes in this strip, the heart rate is estimated at 75 beats per minute. When calculating the ECG rate, it is preferred to use at least a 6-second sample because shorter strips can skew the results. Ten-second strips are preferred.

Another method of calculating the heart rate is by analyzing the distance between two R waves (the **RR interval**). Because each large square on the grid paper is 0.20 seconds in duration, we know there are 300 large squares per minute. Using the ECG in **Figure 14-6**, the distance between the R waves is approximately four large squares. Dividing 300 by the number of squares between R waves—in this case, four—results in a rate of 75 bpm.

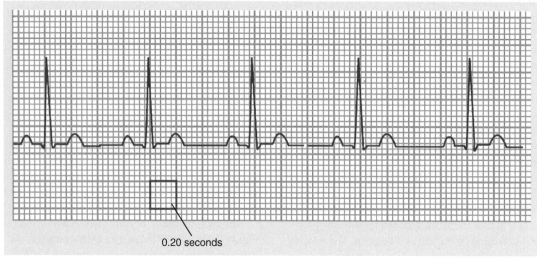

0.20 seconds

FIGURE 14-6 An ECG rhythm strip on grid paper.

When reviewing an ECG strip such as the one shown in **Figure 14-6**, there are many aspects to analyze. First is the rhythm. The technician should look to see if the **rhythm** is regular or if it varies from beat to beat. Second, the technician should determine the ventricular **rate** by looking at the R waves and using one of the calculation methods described previously. Third, the technician should determine the atrial rate by counting the P waves and using the same calculation methods. There should be a P wave for every QRS complex. Next, the technician should visually inspect the QRS complexes to determine whether they are narrow or wide. Finally, the technician should calculate the duration of the PR intervals. Using these methods can help determine if an ECG arrhythmia is present. The significance of these variables will be discussed in the sections to follow.

Sinus Rhythms
Normal Sinus Rhythm

A **normal sinus rhythm (NSR)** is characterized by a normal rate and regular rhythm (no beat-to-beat variability) with normal intervals.

Rate: 60–100 bpm
Rhythm: Regular
QRS complex: <0.10 seconds
P waves: Uniform and upright in appearance
PR interval: 0.12–0.20 seconds

The strip in **Figure 14-7** shows an ECG with an NSR. Note that the QRS complexes are consistently equidistant from each other. This indicates that the rhythm is regular. The rate is calculated at 70 bpm, which is within the normal range. In addition, the P waves are uniform and upright, and the PR interval and QRS complexes are within the normal measurement ranges as outlined.

Sinus Arrhythmia

A **sinus arrhythmia** describes an irregular rhythm that originates in the SA node. The rate can be within or outside the normal range. In a *respiratory* sinus arrhythmia, the heart rate changes in a cycling fashion with the patient's breathing. Specifically, the rate increases during inspiration and deceases during exhalation. Sinus arrhythmia is common in young, healthy adults, and children and, in most cases, is benign.

Rate: Usually 60–100 bpm, but may vary
Rhythm: Irregular
QRS complex: <0.10 seconds
P waves: Uniform and upright in appearance
PR interval: 0.12–0.20 seconds

In the sample shown in **Figure 14-8**, the heart rate is estimated to be approximately 80 bpm and falls within the normal range. However, although the PR interval remains consistent from beat to beat and there is a P wave for every QRS, the distance from one P wave to the next changes with nearly every cycle, indicating that the underlying rhythm is irregular. This rhythm is thus classified as a *sinus arrhythmia*.

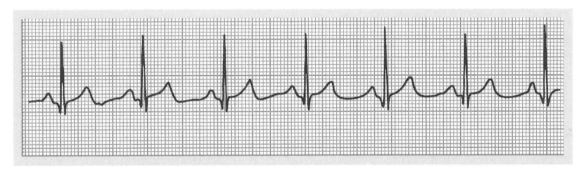

FIGURE 14-7 An ECG with a normal sinus rhythm.

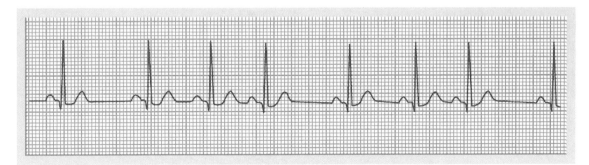

FIGURE 14-8 In this sample, the rate falls within normal ranges, but the rhythm is irregular.

Sinus Bradycardia

Sinus bradycardia is another arrhythmia originating from a sinoatrial mechanism. It is characterized by a slow heart rate. Although the underlying rhythm is regular and the intervals are normal, the rate remains less than 60 beats per minute. When scoring sleep studies, sinus bradycardia during sleep is defined as a sustained heart rate of less than 40 beats per minute.[1]

Rate: <60 bpm
Rhythm: Regular
QRS complex: <0.10 seconds
P waves: Uniform and upright in appearance
PR interval: 0.12–0.20 seconds

In the sample shown in **Figure 14-9**, the ECG appears to be a normal sinus rhythm with no **ectopy**. However, the calculated rate is estimated to be 40 beats per minute, which is below the normal range and meets the criteria of sinus bradycardia. Sinus bradycardia is considered normal in conditioned athletes but may be seen in patients on certain medications, with thyroid disease, or after a **myocardial infarction (MI)** (heart attack).

Sinus Tachycardia

Sinus tachycardia is an arrhythmia characterized by a fast heart rate and, like bradycardia, originates from a sinoatrial mechanism. To meet the criteria for a sinus tachycardia, the heart rate must be faster than 90 bpm. This rhythm is regular, and all other features are within the normal range. When scoring sleep studies, sinus tachycardia during sleep is defined as a sustained heart rate of greater than 90 beats per minute for adults.[1]

Rate: >100 bpm
Rhythm: Regular
QRS complex: <0.10 seconds
P waves: Uniform and upright in appearance
PR interval: 0.12–0.20 seconds

The ECG shown in **Figure 14-10** reveals a normal heart rhythm with a rate of approximately 120 bpm. Sinus tachycardia can indicate decreased oxygen levels, or it may be the result of anxiety, pain, or stress.

Atrial Rhythms

Premature Atrial Complexes (PACs)

A **premature atrial complex (PAC)** is an irregular heart beat that originates from an area within the atria outside of the sinoatrial node. The beat occurs earlier than expected and is characterized by an abnormally shaped P wave and a normal, narrow QRS complex. After the occurrence of a PAC, a **compensatory pause** is often seen before the next normal heart beat.

Rate: Usually normal, but depends on underlying rhythm
Rhythm: Irregular because of PAC
QRS interval: Usually <0.10 seconds but may be prolonged
P waves: P wave shape of the early beat differs from sinus P waves

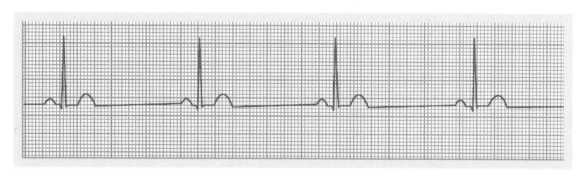

FIGURE 14-9 This ECG appears to be a normal sinus rhythm with no ectopy, but when the rate is calculated it reveals sinus bradycardia.

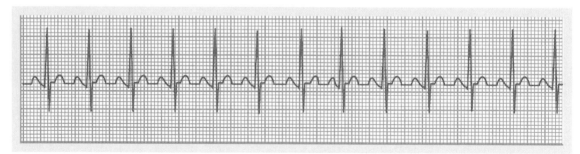

FIGURE 14-10 An ECG with sinus tachycardia.

PR interval: Varies from 0.12 to 0.20 seconds when the pacemaker site is near the SA node to 0.12 seconds when the pacemaker site is nearer the AV node

Figure 14-11 depicts a normal sinus rhythm with the occurrence of a PAC. In this example, the rate is estimated to be approximately 75 bpm, and the underlying rhythm is regular with the exception of the fifth beat. Note that this abnormal beat occurs before expected and the shape of its P wave appears different than all other normal beats. Despite the difference in morphology of the P wave, the QRS complex appears narrow and identical in shape to the other beats, indicating that the conduction of the signal through the ventricles has not been affected. In addition, the abnormal beat is followed by a compensatory pause before the normal rhythm resumes. These features all fit the criteria for a PAC.

In most cases, PACs are benign and carry no health risks. For a small population, however, they may indicate a related heart condition. PACs are more likely to occur in people who smoke or ingest a lot of caffeine, have high blood pressure, or suffer from excessive stress.

Atrial Flutter

Atrial flutter is an ectopic rhythm that occurs when the electrical signal travels in an abnormal circular motion within the atria. This causes the atrial muscle contractions to be much faster than and out of sync with the ventricles. In some cases, the atrial rate can be as high as 350 bpm even as the ventricular rate remains within normal range. This rhythm is often regular and characterized by fast and distinct sawtooth (flutter) waves instead of the normally shaped P waves. The QRS complexes seen in atrial flutter usually remain narrow but in some cases can be wide if the flutter waves are superimposed on the QRS waveform.

Rate: Atrial rate 250–350 bpm; ventricular rate variable
Rhythm: Atrial rhythm regular; ventricular rhythm usually regular, but may be irregular
QRS complex: Usually < 0.10 seconds, but may be widened if flutter waves are buried in the QRS complex
P waves: Sawtoothed "flutter" waves
PR interval: Not measurable

The sample in **Figure 14-12** shows a rhythm strip depicting atrial flutter. Note the distinct sawtooth pattern and regular rhythm. In this example, the ventricular rate is approximately 150 bpm while the atrial rate is more than double that. Atrial flutter becomes more dangerous with faster ventricular rates. Certain medical conditions increase the risk of atrial flutter, including high blood pressure, alcoholism, heart failure, and previous MI. In addition, this rhythm is often associated with mitral or tricuspid disorders, digitalis or quinidine toxicity, and electrolyte abnormalities.

Atrial Fibrillation

Fibrillation is defined as unorganized activity. **Atrial fibrillation** is characterized by an irregular rhythm with unorganized "quivering" activity in the atria. Similar to atrial flutter, the atrial rate in this rhythm is often extremely high. However, unlike atrial flutter, the

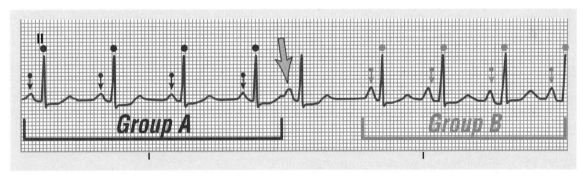

FIGURE 14-11 An ECG with a PAC.
From Arrhythmia Recognition: The Art of Interpretation, Second Edition, courtesy of Tomas B. Garcia, MD.

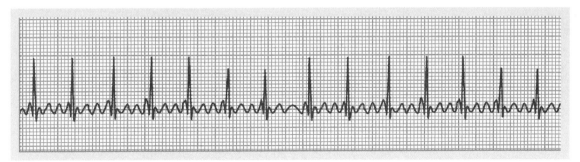

FIGURE 14-12 A rhythm strip with an atrial flutter.

P waves in atrial fibrillation are of variable shapes and the ventricular rate is highly irregular. When fibrillation occurs, atrial contraction, which normally aids in pumping blood into the ventricles, is absent. As a result, blood tends to pool in the atrial chambers, increasing the risk for blood clotting and stroke.

Rate: Atrial rate usually >350; ventricular rate may be slow, normal, or fast
Rhythm: Atrial and ventricular highly irregular
QRS complex: Usually <0.10 seconds
P waves: No identifiable P waves
PR interval: Absent

The P waves in the sample shown in **Figure 14-13** are extremely fast and of variable shape because of fibrillation occurring in the atria. Note also the irregularity of the rhythm. Atrial fibrillation can occur as a result of a primary electrical abnormality or be related to an underlying cardiac issue, including heart disease, previous MI, coronary artery disease, or congestive heart failure (CHF). Signs and symptoms of decreased cardiac output may also be present.

Junctional Rhythms
Premature Junctional Contractions (PJCs)

Premature junctional contractions (PJCs) are abnormal heart beats that originate in the AV junction and occur before the next expected P wave. PJCs are identified by inverted or abnormal P waves and a short PR interval. The QRS complex will be of normal shape and interval, and the rhythm will be irregular because of the premature beat.

Rate: Underlying rate; may be slow
Rhythm: Irregular because of PJC
QRS complex: Normal <0.10 seconds
P waves: Present before, during, or after QRS; may be inverted
PR interval: Absent or short

Figure 14-14 portrays a normal sinus rhythm with the occurrence of a PJC. Note that the fourth beat occurs prematurely, includes an inverted P wave, and has a QRS complex that is normal in shape and duration. PJCs can occur as a result of stress or excessive caffeine, nicotine, or alcohol use. However, they are not often seen in patients with healthy heart tissue. More often, PJCs occur in those with underlying heart disease.

Supraventricular Tachycardia (SVT)

Supraventricular tachycardia (SVT) is an abnormally fast heart rhythm that originates from an impulse that is generated above the ventricles and therefore within the atria or AV node. The rhythm is fast, regular, and has normal QRS complexes. P waves are often difficult to see because of the fast rate. SVT often occurs

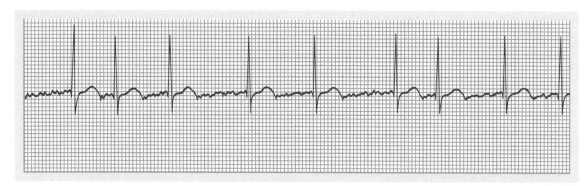

FIGURE 14-13 Extremely fast P waves indicate atrial fibrillation.

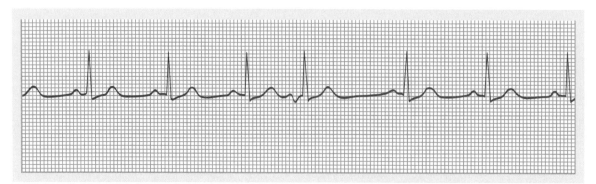

FIGURE 14-14 A normal sinus rhythm with a PJC.

suddenly and can last a few minutes to a several days. Symptoms can include palpitations, shortness of breath, and dizziness, although some patients will have no symptoms at all.

Rate: 150–250
Rhythm: Regular
QRS complex: Normal <0.10 seconds
P waves: Mixed with T wave
PR interval: Normal but difficult to measure

Figure 14-15 demonstrates the appearance of an SVT. Note the fast, regular rhythm of approximately 170 bpm with narrow complex QRS. SVT may be related to stress and exertion or occur because of an abnormal electrical conduction pathway or underlying illness such as heart, lung, or thyroid disease. SVT is treated with various methods, depending on frequency and symptoms.

Ventricular Rhythms
Premature Ventricular Contractions (PVCs)

Premature ventricular contractions (PVCs) are abnormal heart beats that originate in one of the ventricles and occur before the next expected beat. PVCs are identified by a wide, bizarre QRS complex. Because the impulse originates in the ventricle, there is no P wave present. A compensatory pause is often seen after the occurrence of a PVC.

Rate: Atrial and ventricular rates depend on the underlying rhythm.
Rhythm: Irregular because of PVC
QRS complex: >0.10 seconds; wide and bizarre. T wave may be in the opposite direction of the QRS complex.
P waves: Absent
PR interval: None with the PVC because the ectopic beat originates in the ventricles

The sample shown in **Figure 14-16** contains a rhythm strip that includes a PVC. Note the underlying normal sinus rhythm with one beat that is premature, lacks a P wave, and is wide and bizarre looking.

Multiple PVCs that occur in groups or patterns are classified as follows.

- Unifocal PVCs: Originate from the same location and therefore look the same as each other
- Multifocal PVCs: Different origins and therefore appear different from each other
- **Bigeminy**: A PVC every other beat
- **Trigeminy**: A PVC every third beat
- **Couplet**: Two PVCs in a row
- Ventricular tachycardia: Three or more PVCs in a row

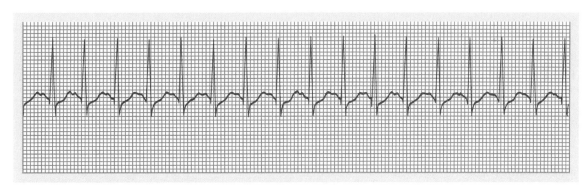

FIGURE 14-15 Supraventricular tachycardia (SVT).

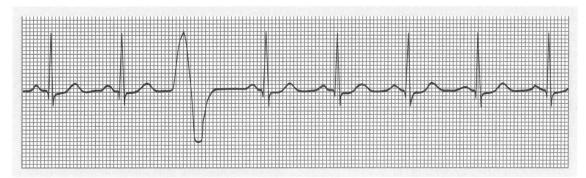

FIGURE 14-16 A normal sinus rhythm with a PVC.

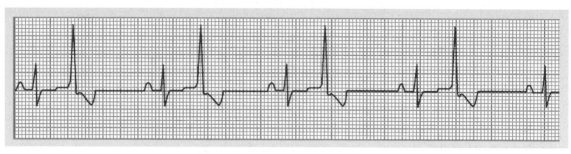

FIGURE 14-17 Bigeminy.

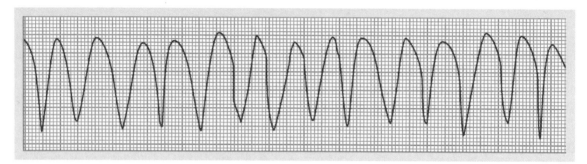

FIGURE 14-18 Ventricular tachycardia.

The sample shown in **Figure 14-17** contains a rhythm strip that demonstrates bigeminy. Note the occurrence of multiple wide complex PVCs that occur every other beat.

Isolated PVCs may occur in healthy individuals, however. When they occur more frequently, it may be a sign of an underlying problem. PVCs can be associated with stress, anxiety, certain medications, and the use of alcohol, caffeine, or tobacco products. In addition, they increase in frequency in patients with high blood pressure and heart disease and under conditions of hypoxia. Because OSA is often associated with marked desaturations, PVCs may be seen during the overnight sleep study and in conjunction with respiratory events.

Ventricular Tachycardia

Ventricular tachycardia (V tach) is characterized by the presence of three or more PVCs in a row at a rate greater than 100 bpm. This rhythm usually occurs as a result of electrical disturbances, ischemia, and cardiac disease. V tach is often associated with such symptoms as chest pain, hypotension, shortness of breath, and loss of consciousness and is considered a medical emergency requiring intervention. If not addressed, V tach will eventually degrade to ventricular fibrillation.

Rate: Atrial rate not discernible; ventricular rate 100–250 bpm
Rhythm: Atrial not discernible; ventricular essentially regular
QRS interval: >0.10 seconds; wide and bizarre
P waves: Absent
PR interval: Not discernible

The sample in **Figure 14-18** demonstrates ventricular tachycardia. Note that every beat is a PVC, the rhythm is regular, and the rate approximately 140 bpm. Sustained ventricular tachycardia is considered emergent; left untreated, it will progress to a deteriorating rhythm.

Ventricular Fibrillation

Ventricular fibrillation (V fib) is an extremely severe arrhythmia that is fatal unless life support is initiated. In this rhythm, there is rapid and irregular ventricular activity that causes the heart to quiver rather than contract in a productive way. As a result, there is a sudden loss of cardiac output. On the ECG, there are no discernible waveforms during ventricular fibrillation.

Rate: Cannot be determined
Rhythm: Rapid and chaotic
QRS complex: Not discernible
P waves: Not discernible
PR interval: Not measurable

During ventricular fibrillation, the only signals seen in the ECG are those of a quivering heart (see **Figure 14-19**). V fib has numerous causes, including acute MI, blunt force trauma, pulmonary embolism, hypothermia, stroke, and OSA. If this rhythm is identified, immediate action should be taken, including calling 911, performing CPR, and preparing for defibrillation.

Ventricular Standstill (Asystole)

Ventricular standstill (also known as **asystole**) refers to the absence of electrical and mechanical activity of the heart. Asystole is a lethal arrhythmia because there is no cardiac

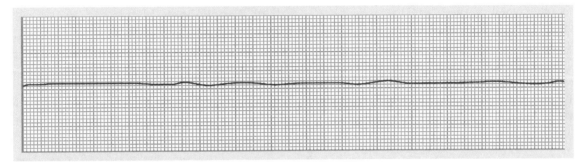

FIGURE 14-19 An ECG showing ventricular fibrillation.

FIGURE 14-20 An ECG showing asystole.

output present. This rhythm most often occurs after a deterioration of nonperfusing ventricular rhythms. The ECG signal during asystole is a flat line (see **Figure 14-20**). Immediate action must be taken when this rhythm is seen, including calling 911 and performing CPR. When scoring sleep studies, asystole is scored when there is a cardiac pause of more than 3 seconds in duration.[1]

Rate: Cannot be determined
Rhythm: Atrial may be discernible, ventricular indiscernible
QRS complex: None
P waves: Usually not discernible
PR interval: Not measurable

Escape Rhythms

Junctional and ventricular escape rhythms are self-generating electrical rhythms that occur when the rate of discharge of the SA node falls below a certain rate. Under normal pacing conditions, these rhythms are suppressed by the rapid impulses from the SA node. However, escape rhythms are protective mechanisms meant to take over the role of the pacemaker should the SA node fail. In a **junctional escape rhythm**, the rate will range from 40 to 60 bpm, and the P waves can occur before, during, or after the QRS complex and may be inverted. The QRS complex will appear of normal width and morphology. In contrast, a **ventricular escape rhythm** will have an underlying regular rate of 20–40 bpm and have no P waves, and the QRS will be wide and bizarre.

Junctional

Rate: 40–60
Rhythm: Regular
QRS complex: Normal <0.10 seconds
P waves: Present before, during, or after QRS; may be inverted
PR interval: Not measurable

Ventricular

Rate: 20–40
Rhythm: Regular
QRS complex: >0.10 seconds; wide, bizarre
P waves: Absent
PR interval: not measurable

AV Blocks

First-Degree AV Block

An **AV block** is an impairment in the conduction of the electrical impulses from the atria to the ventricles. In **first-degree AV block**, the time it takes for the impulse to travel from the atria into the ventricles is delayed. As a result, the rate and rhythm are normal but the PR interval is prolonged.

Rate: Normal
Rhythm: Normal
QRS complex: <0.10 seconds
P waves: Normal in size and configuration
PR interval: Prolonged (>0.20 seconds), but constant

Figure 14-21 demonstrates a first-degree heart block. Note that the rate and rhythm are normal, but the distance between the P waves and the following QRS complexes are longer than normal. First-degree AV block can occur as a result of AV node abnormalities or medications. Intervention for a first-degree AV block is not usually necessary.

Second-Degree AV Block Type 1 (Wenckebach, Mobitz 1)

A second-degree AV block is characterized by occasional nonconducted P waves that result in a QRS complex that is skipped. Second-degree AV blocks are classified as either type 1 or type 2.

Second-degree AV block type 1 occurs when the PR interval gradually increases until the QRS complex is missed.

Rate: Atrial rate is greater than ventricular rate, but both are usually within normal limits
Rhythm: Atrial regular, ventricular irregular
QRS: <0.10 seconds but is dropped periodically

P waves: Normal in size and configuration
PR interval: Lengthens with each cycle until a P wave appears without a QRS

Figure 14-22 demonstrates a rhythm strip with second-degree AV block type 1. Note that the length of the PR interval gradually increases until there is a dropped QRS complex (fourth P wave). Patients with Mobitz 1 are usually asymptomatic and do not require treatment. Those who have symptoms may require an implantable pacemaker.

Second-Degree AV Block Type 2 (Non-Wenckebach, Mobitz 2)

Second-degree AV block type 2 occurs when there is an abnormality in the bundle of His or Purkinje fibers that conduct impulses through the ventricles. As a result, in this rhythm, the conduction block occurs after the AV node, and the PR interval is normal. Instead, P waves occur at a regular rate, and occasionally there is a dropped QRS complex (see Figure 14-23).

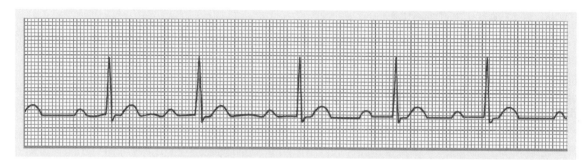

FIGURE 14-21 An ECG showing a first-degree AV block.

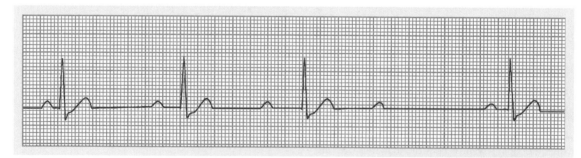

FIGURE 14-22 An ECG showing a second-degree AV block type I.

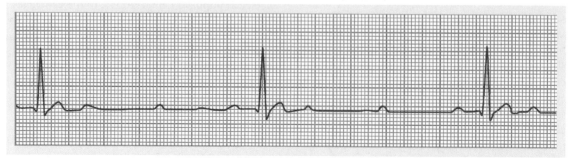

FIGURE 14-23 An ECG showing a second-degree AV block type II.

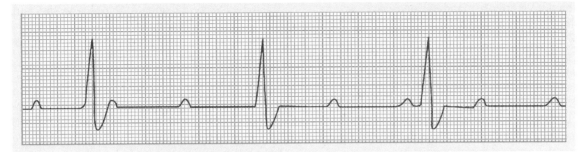

FIGURE 14-24 An ECG showing a third-degree AV block.

Rate: Atrial rate is greater than ventricular rate

Rhythm: Atrial regular, ventricular irregular

QRS complex: >0.10 seconds but is dropped periodically

P waves: Normal in size and configuration

PR interval: May be within normal limits or prolonged but is constant for each QRS

Second-degree AV block type 2 risks deteriorating to a complete heart block. For this reason, a pacemaker is indicated in patients in which this rhythm is identified.

Third-Degree (Complete) AV Block

Third-degree (complete) AV block occurs because the AV node fails to conduct impulses from the atria to the ventricles. As a result, while the SA node continues to pace the atria, junctional or ventricular escape rhythms will take over pacing the ventricles. This creates a complete lack of association between the electrical activity of the atria and the ventricles; in essence, the P waves and the QRS complexes occur independently. Because junctional and ventricular escape rhythms are slower than normal heart rates, the ventricular rate can range from 20 to 40 bpm. This can result in symptoms of dizziness, shortness of breath, and chest pain.

Rate: Atria rate is normal, ventricular rate slow

Rhythm: Atrial regular, ventricular regular

QRS complex: May be narrow or wide, depending on the location of the escape pacemaker

P waves: Normal in size and configuration

PR interval: None because there is no relationship between the P waves and the QRS complexes.

Figure 14-24 shows a third-degree AV block. Note the dissociation between the P waves and QRS complexes. In this example, the atrial rate is approximately 80 bpm, while the ventricular rate is 30 bpm. Third-degree AV block is dangerous because at any time the ventricular escape rhythm can fail and cardiac arrest can occur. Patients with this rhythm are treated with an implantable pacemaker. If this rhythm is seen during a sleep study, the technician should activate the emergency response system immediately.

Chapter Summary

An important aspect of patient safety in the sleep-testing facility is the ability to interpret ECG tracings. Every sleep technologist needs to understand basic cardiac rhythms and be able to respond appropriately.

A normal, healthy adult heart beats approximately 60–100 times per minute. This varies according to an individual's size and health. The heart beats as a result of an electrical impulse that travels from the SA node through the internodal pathways to the AV node and down through the ventricles. The resulting ECG waveform seen on a polysomnograph consists of a P wave, a QRS complex, and a T wave. The rate, rhythm, width, and distance between the waves are all taken into account when reading the ECG tracing.

A normal sinus rhythm has a rate of approximately 60–100 beats per minute, a PR interval of 0.12–0.20 seconds, and a QRS complex lasting less than 0.10 seconds. The P waves and the QRS complex are uniform and upright. A sinus arrhythmia is similar, but the rhythm is irregular from beat to beat. During sleep, sinus bradycardia is scored when the rate is less than 40 beats per minute, whereas sinus tachycardia refers to a rate faster than 90 beats per minute.

Premature atrial complexes (PACs) are characterized by an irregular rhythm that is the result of an early P wave. An atrial flutter shows fast flutter waves for P waves. Atrial fibrillation is a more dangerous rhythm that shows especially fast unorganized activity in the P waves.

Premature junctional contractions (PJCs) are identified by inverted or abnormal P waves and a short PR interval. The QRS complex will be of normal shape and interval, and the rhythm will be irregular because of the premature beat.

Supraventricular tachycardia (SVT) is an abnormally fast heart rhythm that often starts and ends abruptly. The rhythm is fast, regular, and has normal QRS complexes.

Premature ventricular contractions (PVCs) are characterized by wide, bizarre-looking QRS complexes that start early. PVCs are categorized by the frequency of these contractions and the points of origin. Ventricular tachycardia (V tach) is the occurrence of three or more PVCs in a row and a rate above 100 bpm. Ventricular fibrillation (V fib) is an extremely severe ventricular rhythm with no discernible QRS complexes: The ventricles quiver but are not able to effectively contract to pump blood. Ventricular standstill, or asystole, occurs when the heart fails to exhibit electrical or mechanical activity.

Escape rhythms can take over the role of the pacemaker should the SA node fail. A junctional escape rhythm will pace the heart at rate between 40 and 60 bpm whereas a ventricular escape rhythm is slower at 20–40 bpm.

AV blocks represent a block between the atria and the ventricles. First-degree AV block has a prolonged PR interval. Second-degree AV block type 1 shows a gradual increase in PR intervals until a QRS complex is skipped. Second-degree AV block type 2 is characterized by dropped QRS complexes without warning. In third-degree AV block, there is no apparent association between the QRS complexes and the P waves.

Patients with sleep-related breathing disorders are more likely to experience cardiac arrhythmias, especially when significant apnea and hypoxemia is present. Sleep technologists must be able to identify abnormal cardiac rhythms, understand which ones require immediate action, and be trained in basic life support. This level of competence is directly related to patient safety.

Case Study

The following images are taken from overnight diagnostic sleep studies.

1. **What type of arrhythmia is seen in Figure 14-25?**

2. **What type of arrhythmia is seen in Figure 14-26?**

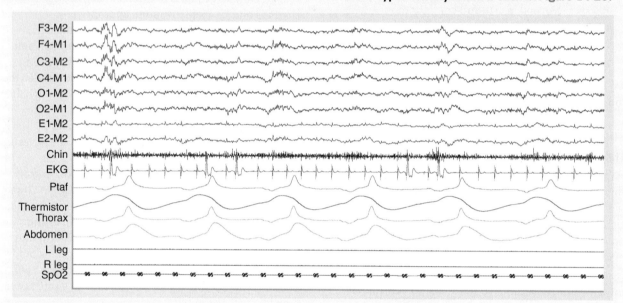

FIGURE 14-25 Case Study 1.

Figure by Lisa M. Endee; produced from a sleep study provided to Stony Brook University School of Health Technology and Management's Polysomnographic Technology Program by Dr. Kala Sury.

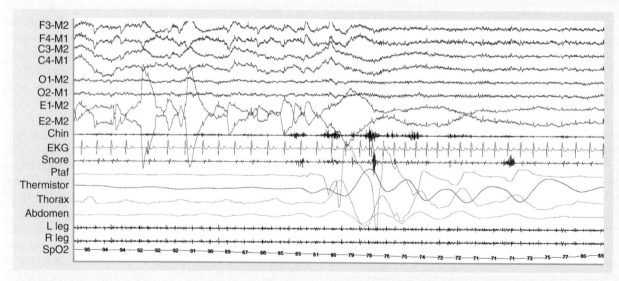

FIGURE 14-26 Case Study 2.

Figure by Lisa M. Endee; produced from a sleep study provided to Stony Brook University School of Health Technology and Management's Polysomnographic Technology Program by Dr. Kala Sury.

Chapter 14 Questions

Please consider the following questions as they relate to the material in this chapter.

1. Why must a sleep technician be able to recognize cardiac rhythms?
2. What does an ECG tracing represent? What can we tell by looking at an ECG tracing?
3. What is a normal PR interval?
4. What are the characteristics of a PAC?
5. What is it called when every other beat is a PVC?
6. How do the different types of AV blocks differ from each other?

Footnote

1. American Academy of Sleep Medicine (2017). *The AASM Manual for the Scoring of Sleep and Associated Events*, version 2.4. Darien, IL.

© Agsandrew/Shutterstock

CHAPTER OUTLINE

Sleep Study Times, Formulas, and Calculations
Types of Sleep Reports
Sample Sleep Reports
Scoring Notes
Chapter Summary

LEARNING OBJECTIVES

1. Learn how to generate a report and verify all calculations.
2. Discuss the types of sleep reports available.
3. Understand the data in a sleep report, including graphical data.
4. Be able to write detailed, accurate scoring notes.

KEY TERMS

sleep study report
total recording time (TRT)
total sleep time (TST)
sleep efficiency (SE)
total awake time (TWT)
sleep onset
sleep latency (SL)
wake after sleep
   onset (WASO)
apnea hypopnea index (AHI)
respiratory disturbance
   index (RDI)

periodic limb movement
   (PLM) index
arousal index (Arl)
diagnostic (baseline)
   polysomnograph report
hypnogram
titration report
split night report
HST report
technologist notes

Sleep Study Times, Formulas, and Calculations

After the sleep technologist analyzes and scores a sleep study, a report is generated. The **sleep study report** compiles all sleep-staging and significant events into summary form. The data can be presented in various layouts that include graphs, tables, and pie charts. Report templates that include the recommended American Academy of Sleep Medicine (AASM) reporting variables are made available by most sleep software companies on the market. However, the sleep center medical director and interpreting physicians may choose to customize the facility's reports with additional information.

The sample reports in this chapter show various layouts with statistical information from sleep studies. Although digital systems generate calculations automatically, it is crucial for sleep technologists to understand and be able to verify the data. The scoring technologist should also know how to create report templates using the data-acquisition software in the lab. **Table 15-1** contains statistical categories often used in sleep reports, along with their definitions.

Table 15-1
Statistical Categories Used in Sleep Reports

Term	Definition
Lights out	Indicates the time that the study has officially begun and when the patient first attempts to fall asleep. Before lights out, the lights, television, and other devices should be turned off. Impedance checks, amplifier calibrations, and physiologic calibrations are all completed before lights out.
Lights on	Indicates the official end of the study or the time when the technician enters the room to wake the patient. Posttest calibrations are performed after lights on.
Total recording time (TRT)	Total time in minutes from lights out to lights on. This is calculated by subtracting lights out time from lights on time or subtracting the lights out epoch from the lights on epoch and dividing by 2. TRT = Lights on time − Lights out time
Total sleep time (TST)	Total time spent asleep. This can be calculated by adding the time spent in each sleep stage or by subtracting the total wake time from the total recording time. TST = TRT − TWT OR TST= TRT − SL − WASO
Sleep efficiency (SE)	Percentage of total recording time the patient was asleep. SE = TST/TRT × 100 Normal sleep efficiency for sleep testing >85%.
Total awake time (TWT)	Total amount of time spent awake during the study. TWT = TRT − TST
Sleep onset	Time at which sleep first occurs after lights out. This is defined as the first epoch of sleep, regardless of the stage. It is usually marked by the first epoch of stage N1.
Sleep latency (SL)	Amount of time in minutes from lights out to sleep onset. This calculation is especially important in multiple sleep latency test (MSLT) reports. In an MSLT, the mean, median, and mode sleep latencies are often calculated. SL= (First epoch of sleep − Lights out epoch)/2 Normal sleep latency for sleep testing is less than 30 minutes.
Mean sleep latency	The average sleep latency over all five naps of an MSLT. Mean SL= (SL of nap 1 + SL of nap 2 + SL of nap 3 + SL of nap 4 + SL of nap 5)/5 Normal values are >10 minutes
Median sleep latency	When viewing the sleep latencies from the naps in an MSLT in numerical order, the median sleep latency is the middle number. For example, if the sleep latencies from the naps in an MSLT were 2, 3, 4, 8, and 8 minutes, then the median sleep latency is 4 minutes.
Mode sleep latency	When viewing the sleep latencies from MSLT naps, the mode sleep latency is the number that occurs the most number of times. For example, if the sleep latencies for five MSLT naps were 2, 3, 4, 8, and 8 minutes, the mode sleep latency is 8 because it occurs more frequently than the other numbers.
Wake after sleep onset (WASO)	Total time in minutes spent awake after the first epoch of sleep. WASO = TRT − TST − Sleep latency

Term	Definition
Stage R onset	First epoch of stage R.
Stage R latency	Amount of time in minutes from sleep onset to stage R onset. R latency = (R onset epoch – SL epoch)/2 Normal R latency-60 = 120 minutes
% stage R	Percentage of total sleep time spent in REM sleep. For normal sleepers, the % stage R should be approximately 25%. Percentages for other stages of sleep are calculated in the same way, but norms may vary according to age and other factors. % stage R = (Total REM time/TST) × 100
Apnea hypopnea index (AHI)	Total number of apneas and hypopneas per hour of sleep. AHI = (No. of apneas + No. of Hypopneas)/TST in hours Normal 0–4, mild 5–15, moderate 16–29, severe 30+
Respiratory disturbance index (RDI)	Total number of apneas, hypopneas, and respiratory effort–related arousals (RERAs) per hour of sleep. RDI = (No. of Apneas + No. of Hypopneas + No. of RERAs)/TST in hours Normal 0–4, mild 5–15, moderate 16–29, severe 30+
Periodic limb movement (PLM) index	Total number of limb movements that are part of a PLM sequence per hour of sleep. PLM index = Total number of PLMs/TST in hours
Arousal index (ArI)	Total number of EEG arousals per hour of sleep. ArI = No. of EEG arousals/TST in hours

Types of Sleep Reports

As mentioned, various types of sleep study reports serve to summarize the data collected. All reports will include the patient's name and date of birth or age and the date the study was performed. Often, the patient's height and weight are also included. It is recommended that the AASM manual[1] be used as a guide for data that must be included in the different reports. Most sleep study software includes report layouts that are customizable in the presentation of vital statistics and data collected. Preferably, the information should be outlined in a simple, concise manner that is easily understood. Tables are often used to display the study data with normal values provided as a reference. In addition, having a section for technologist notes can be useful to communicate any unique information from the study that may not be reflected in the numbers.

Diagnostic Reports

A **diagnostic (baseline) polysomnograph report** summarizes all of the sleep-staging and significant events scored on the sleep study. This report is used to help the interpreting physician determine an accurate diagnosis based on the information obtained in the overnight sleep study. Information included in the report may include, but is not limited to, the following:

- Basic study information such as lab name, referring physician, interpreting physician, and study date
- Patient demographics such as name, age, date of birth, height, weight, body mass index, gender,

and score on screening tools such as the Epworth Sleepiness Scale, Berlin Questionnaire, or others
- Study time summary, including lights off time, lights on time, TRT, and so on
- Sleep time summary, including total sleep time, sleep efficiency, sleep latency, stage R latency, number of awakenings, WASO, time in stage N1, time in stage N2, time in stage N3, time in stage R, total nonrapid eye movement (NREM) time, and percentage of total sleep time spent in each stage of sleep
- Respiratory summary, including total number of obstructive apneas, number of hypopneas, number of central apneas, number of mixed apneas, and indexes for each. The indexes are often divided by sleep stages and body positions. RERAs may be included as well.
- Electroencephalogram (EEG) arousal summary, including total number of arousals, arousal index, and the total number and index of each type of arousal (categorized into spontaneous arousals, those associated with respiratory events, and those associated with leg movements)
- Limb movement summary, including total limb movements, PLMs, and limb movements associated with other events such as respiratory disturbances
- Electrocardiogram (ECG) summary, including mean, maximum, and minimum heart rate during rapid eye movement (REM), nonrapid eye movement (NREM), and wake
- Oxygen-saturation summary, including number of oxygen desaturations, mean SpO_2, and lowest oxygen desaturation

Note that the current AASM guideline[1] for scoring hypopneic respiratory events includes two options that differ only in the percentage of oxygen desaturation. Both hypopnea criteria include a drop in signal excursion greater than or equal to 30% in the nasal pressure transducer for at least 10 seconds. In addition to these two criteria, the recommended guideline (1A) includes the occurrence of a ≥3% desaturation or an EEG arousal. The acceptable alternative guideline (1B) includes the occurrence of a ≥4% desaturation. This alternative was adopted to comply with Medicare guidelines for the diagnosis of obstructive sleep apnea (OSA). As a result of the variable use of these two options, diagnostic reports should declare which guideline (1A or 1B) was used in generating the data on the report. This can have implications on reimbursement for therapy when Medicare guidelines are upheld.

Diagnostic reports typically include a **hypnogram**, a graphical display that portrays an overview of the entire night on one page. The sleep hypnogram usually includes stages of sleep, arousals, respiratory events, leg movements, body position, saturation, and heart rate. Visualizing these events in this way is helpful in making associations between events that may not be as easily understood by looking at the numbers alone. For example, the data may show that the AHI is higher during REM sleep than during NREM. However, the hypnogram may show that the patient happened to be in the supine position during most of the REM periods, and it may be that the positional component is more of a factor in this patient than the staging component. The hypnogram allows the viewer to compare all data during specific time frames.

Titration Reports

A **titration report** includes much of the same data as diagnostic reports with the addition of comparing the patient's sleep with and without treatment with positive airway pressure (PAP) therapy. Titration reports reveal the range of pressures used during the night when each pressure was initiated and the duration of time spent at each. Often, a PAP table is included that helps readers visualize the therapeutic trial. PAP tables divide the data by the time period in which each PAP level was tried. Data provided at each stratified time period can include total sleep time, R time, NREM time, sleep efficiency, total arousals, low oxygen saturation, PLM index, and number and index of obstructive apneas, hypopneas, central apneas, and mixed apneas. In addition, the PAP table will reveal the calculated AHI at each PAP level that was attempted during the study. This information is extremely valuable in helping the interpreting physician make a proper treatment recommendation for the patient. The titration report also typically includes information about the type, style, and size of the mask used; the mode of PAP therapy used (continuous positive airway pressure [CPAP] or bi-level, for example); the humidification settings used; and other accessories such as chin straps or head gear.

Split Night Reports

A **split night report** contains much of the information available in the diagnostic and titration reports. As a result, the report is useful for making a sleep-disorder diagnosis as well as for determining appropriate PAP pressure requirements. In addition, split night study reports provide a pretreatment and posttreatment comparison. Visualizing the data in this way provides a confirmation of the effectiveness of the therapy and helps guide treatment recommendations.

Home Sleep-Testing Reports

Home sleep-testing (HST) devices now allow sleep studies to be accomplished outside the laboratory facility. The devices offer a limited number of channels and are customizable (to some extent) on the data to be collected. In addition, data from the device can be downloaded, reviewed, and presented in a report form. Because HST is often limited in the data that can be collected, the reports are often more concise and limited in the information they provide. Similar to the other reports discussed, the **HST report** will include the patient name, date of birth, date of the study, and the referring physician. The number and choice of channels used will determine the other information available on the report. For example, a patient suspected of having OSA may undergo a home sleep test that is set up to collect data on airflow, oxygen saturation, and respiratory effort. The report associated with this test will include information about the respiratory events noted, desaturations that occurred, and the AHI that is calculated. HST reports must also declare which hypopnea rule was used to identify events and calculate report statistics. Unlike diagnostic, titration, and split night reports, most home sleep-testing reports do not provide information on sleep staging. HST reports are interpreted using the same AHI severity guidelines used in for diagnostic reports. In some cases, the information collected during the HST may warrant a follow-up in lab study.

Sample Sleep Reports

Figures 15-1 through **15-4** contain sample reports from two sleep studies. The names and other vital information in these reports are not real. The first sleep report is from a diagnostic sleep study performed on a 45-year-old female. The results of this study showed moderate OSA, so she returned for a CPAP titration. The second sample report is from the same patient's CPAP titration. Comparing the results of the two studies reveals that the obstructions were mostly corrected with CPAP; as a result this patient was able to stay asleep, achieve more REM sleep, and maintain better blood oxygen levels while on CPAP than without it. A sample HST report is shown in **Figure 15-5**. Although limited in detail as compared to the in-lab report, respiratory event data reveal an AHI in the severe category.

Diagnostic Sleep Report

Patient:	Jane Doe	Date of Service:	2/18/2008
Date of Birth:	12/1/1962	Place of Service:	Sleep Lab
Referring Physician:	Dr. Sleep, MD	Interpreting Physician:	Dr. Sleep, MD

Patient History: Jane Doe is a 45-year-old Female who is 65 inches tall, weighs 195 pounds and has a BMI of 32.4. Sleep Complaints include drowsiness, fatigue, snoring, morning headaches, and witnessed apnea. Current-known medical history includes hypertension, diabetes, CHF, seasonal allergies, and sinus problems. Known current medications include Lexapro and Diovan, which were taken on the day of the test. The patient does not smoke. Patient had 7 hours of sleep the previous night and indicated that this was not adequate. The patient consumed 1 caffeinated and 0 alcoholic beverages on the day of the test. The patient did not take a nap on the day of the test. Epworth Sleepiness Scale = 11, which indicates moderate daytime sleepiness.

Symptoms Consistent with OSA

Protocol: This sleep study included recording and monitoring of EEG, EOG, EMG, ECG, respiratory effort and flow, snoring, pulse oximetry, and position. Video recordings were obtained as needed.   A qualified sleep technologist continuously monitored the patient throughout the night. Data was digitally stored and tabulated using Sandman software. Sleep staging and respiratory events were scored manually using AASM standards.

Test Information:

Lights Out:	9:47:29 PM	Lights On:	5:18:16 AM	Pre-B/P:	131/80	Post-B/P:	138/88

PSG

Sleep Architecture

Total Study Time:	450.8 minutes		REM Latency:	108.0 minutes
Total Sleep Time:	361.8 minutes		Sleep Efficiency:	80.3% — Normal: >90%
Sleep Latency:	12.0 minutes		Awake after Sleep:	77.0 minutes — Decreased Sleep Efficiency

			Normal
Stage 1:	5.4%	19.5 minutes	5%-10%
Stage 2:	57.4%	207.5 minutes	55%-62%
Stage 3+4:	11.9%	43.0 minutes	5%-20%
Stage REM:	25.4%	92.0 minutes	21%-25%

Respiratory Events

Obstructive Apneas:	10	Apnea / Hypopnea Index:	18.9	Normal: <5 per hour / sleep
Hypopneas:	97	N-REM Event Index:	9.8	Increased AHI
Central Apneas:	7	REM Event Index:	45.7	
Mixed Apneas:	0	Supine Event Index:	24.9	AHI Elevated During REM
Total Events:	114	REM / Supine Index:	61.8	

SpO₂ Statistics

SpO$_2$ Baseline:	94.3 %	SpO$_2$ Minimum:	81.0 %	Decreased Oxygen Saturation
Time below 90%:	12.5 min.	# of Desaturations:	123	

PLMS Events

# of PLMS:	73	PLMS Index:	12.1 per hour / sleep

Arousal Statistics

PLMS Arousals:	11	PLMS Arousal Index:	1.8	
Resp. Arousals:	9	Resp. Arousal Index:	1.5	*Increased Number of Leg Movements*
Snore Arousals:	0	Snore Arousal Index:	0.0	
Spontaneous Arsls:	24	Spontaneous Arsl. Index:	4.0	
Total Arousals:	44	Total Arousal Index:	7.3	

FIGURE 15-1 PSG report page 1.

Scoring Notes

An important feature of the sleep study report is the **technologist notes** section. The notes section provides the scoring technologist with an opportunity to highlight certain areas of the study or critical information that may help diagnose or treat the patient. For example, if cardiac changes are noted during the study, the notes section can be used to bring attention to those findings (e.g., "EKG changes noted during epochs 65–68"). This section may be included as part of the report, or it can be a separate sheet intended only for the physician.

The format of the scoring notes depends on the needs of the physician and sleep-testing facility. However, in general, scoring notes often include the following information:

- Type of study
- Subjective interpretation of the results of the study
- Sleep architecture

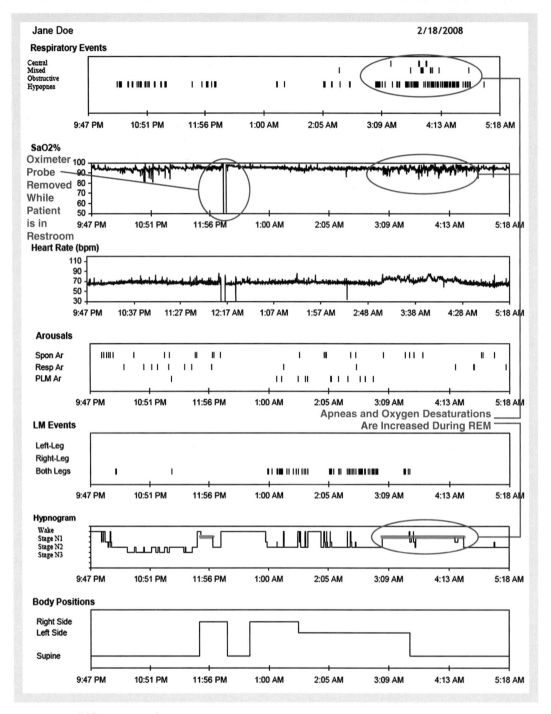

FIGURE 15-2 PSG report page 2.

- Prevalence and severity of events
- Association of events to other findings
- Cardiac rhythms
- Anything noteworthy from the patient's history and questionnaires

Type of Study

The scoring notes are often introduced by stating the type of study, whether it is a baseline diagnostic study, a CPAP titration, or another type. This helps the physician verify the information listed in the study.

Results of Study

Depending on the facility needs, the scoring technologist may be asked to provide a subjective summary of the results of the study based on what was observed during the testing. For example, the technologist can document that the "sleep study data show frequent obstructive apneic events with moderate to severe snoring and oxygen desaturation." This alerts the physician to the significant findings. This feature should not be confused with the interpretation and diagnosis, which is only accomplished by the interpreting physician.

CPAP Titration Report

Patient:	Jane Doe	Date of Service:	2/26/2008
Date of Birth:	12/1/1962	Place of Service:	Sleep Lab
Referring Physician:	Dr. Sleep	Interpreting Physician:	Dr. Sleep

Patient History: Jane Doe is a 45 year-old Female who underwent a PSG on 2/18/2008 that revealed an overall AHI of 18.9 events per hour and a REM AHI of 45.7 events per hour with a minimum oxygen saturation of 81.0%. Sleep architecture was abnormal with an increase in Wake. Sleep onset was early with a latency of 12 minutes and REM onset was normal with a latency of 108 minutes.

Jane Doe is a 45 year-old Female who is 65 inches tall, weighs 195 pounds and has a BMI of 32.4. Sleep Complaints include drowsiness, fatigue, snoring, morning headaches, and witnessed apnea. Current known medical history includes hypertension, diabetes, CHF, seasonal allergies, and sinus problems. Known current medications include Lexapro and Diovan, which were taken on the day of the test. The patient does not smoke. Patient had 7 hours of sleep the previous night and indicated that this was not adequate. The patient consumed 1 caffeinated and 0 alcoholic beverages on the day of the test. The patient did not take a nap on the day of the test. Epworth Sleepiness Scale = 11, which indicates moderate daytime sleepiness.

Protocol: This sleep study included recording and monitoring of EEG, EOG, EMG, ECG, respiratory effort and flow, snoring, pulse oximetry, and position. Video recordings were obtained as needed. A qualified sleep technologist continuously monitored the patient throughout the night. Data was digitally stored and tabulated using Sandman software. Sleep staging and respiratory events were scored manually using AASM standards. CPAP pressure was increased per Sleep Healers protocol.

Test Information:

Lights Out:	10:07:47 PM	Lights On:	4:40:24 AM	Pre-B/P:	123/77	Post-B/P:	120/68

Sleep Architecture

Total Study Time:	392.6 minutes			REM Latency:	220.0 minutes	
Total Sleep Time:	321.0 minutes			Awake after Sleep:	35.7 minutes	
Sleep Latency:	35.9 minutes			Sleep Efficiency:	81.8%	Normal: >90%
				Normal		
Stage 1:	4.4%	14.00 minutes		5%-10%		
Stage 2:	58.1%	186.50 minutes		55%-62%		
Stage 3+4:	24.0%	77.0 minutes		5%-20%		
Stage REM:	13.6%	43.5 minutes		21%-25%		

Respiratory Events

Obstructive Apneas:	0	Apnea / Hypopnea Index:	0.2	Normal: <5 per hour / sleep	
Hypopneas:	1	N-REM Event Index:	0.2		
Central Apneas:	0	REM Event Index:	0.0	**AHI Within**	
Mixed Apneas:	0	Supine Event Index:	0.2	**Normal Ranges**	
Total Events:	1	REM / Supine Index:	0.0		

SpO₂ Statistics

SpO$_2$ Baseline:	95.1 %	SpO$_2$ Minimum:	90.0 %	
Time below 90%:	4.4 min.	# of Desaturations:	4	**SpO$_2$ Within Normal Ranges**

PLMS Events

# of PLMS:	2	PLMS Index:	0.4 per hour / sleep

Arousal Statistics

PLMS Arousals:	2	Leg Movements	PLMS Arousal Index:	0.4
Resp. Arousals:	0	Within Normal	Resp. Arousal Index:	0.0
Snore Arousals:	0	Ranges	Snore Arousal Index:	0.0
Spontaneous Arsls:	15		Spontaneous Arsl. Index:	2.8
Total Arousals:	17		Total Arousal Index:	3.2

FIGURE 15-3 CPAP report page 1.

Sleep Architecture

The scoring technologist can also detail significant changes to sleep architecture that were noted. For example, if the patient spent 15% of the night in stage N1, it could be noted that there was a mild increase in stage N1 sleep. This change could be further correlated with frequent arousals or respiratory events if applicable. Decreases in stage R or stage N3, as is often noted in sleep-disordered breathing patients, should be highlighted here as well. Other noteworthy data may include increased or decreased sleep or REM latencies. These can indicate a problem with the patient's ability to initiate or maintain sleep.

Events

A detailed description of the prevalence and severity of sleep-related events during the night is another important finding to highlight. When describing the events,

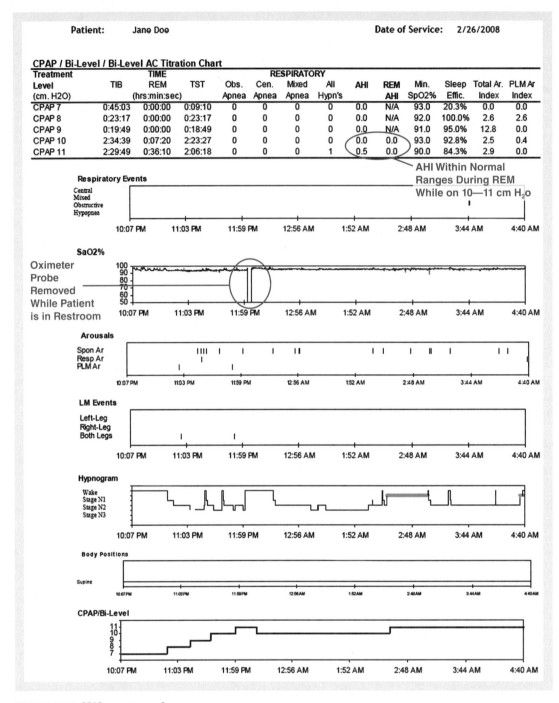

FIGURE 15-4 CPAP report page 2.

the scoring technologist should be detailed and accurate and include the frequency and type of events (e.g., "frequent obstructive apneas" rather than "apneas"). He or she should also detail when these events occurred (e.g., "Respiratory events were more frequent while patient was in the supine position than in other positions"). The scorer's notes should include details about limb movements to let the physician know what type of limb movements the patient is having. Although limb movements associated with respiratory events are not typically scored, the scorer can make note of them because this information can be useful for the physician's interpretation.

Association of Events

The scoring technologist should also make note of how significant events appear to be associated with each other. For example, if the patient has frequent EEG arousals, it would be important for the physician to know why the patient has these arousals. If these arousals occur at the end of an apneic event, that should be stated—for example, "EEG arousals were mostly associated with respiratory events."

ApneaLink - Report of 02/12/2013 15:15

Treating physician

Referral to

Patient data

First name:	Cheyne Stokes	Patient ID:
Last name:	Example	DOB: 01/12/1958
Street:		Height: 170.18 cm
City, ST, Zip:		Weight: 92.41 kg
Phone:		BMI: 31.9 kg/m^2

Recording

Data:	21/01/2009
Start:	21:13.
End:	05:56.
Duration:	8 h 43 min

Evaluation

Start:	21:23.
End:	05:54.
Duration:	7 h 55 min

AHI*

Normal range | Suspected pathological breathing disorder

Result (33)

*See clinical guide for abbreviations and resthed standard parameters

Analysis   (Flow evaluation period: 7 hr 55 min / SpO2 evaluation period: 8 h 32 min)

Indices		Normal	Result	
AHI*:	32.9	< 5/h	Average breaths per minute [bpm]:	14.45
RI*:	33.8	< 5	Breaths:	6857
Apnea index:	20.6	< 5/h	Apneas:	163
UAI:	0		Unclassifled apneas:	0 (0%)
OAI:	5.6		Obstructive apneas:	44 (27%)
CAI:	14.9		Central apneas:	118 (72%)
MAI:	0.1		Mixed apneas:	1 (1%)
Hypopnea index:	12.3	< 5/h	Hypopneas:	97
% Flow lim. Br. without Sn (FL):	12	< Approx. 60	Flow lim. Br. without Sn (FL):	792
% Flow lim. Br. with Sn (FS):	0	< Approx. 40	Flow lim. Br. with Sn (FS):	3
			Snoring events:	66
ODI Oxygen Desaturation Index*:	33.5	< 5/h	No. of desaturations:	286
Average saturation:	91	94%–98%	Saturation <= 90% :	234 min (46%)
Lowest desaturation:	7.2	-	Saturation <= 85% :	77 min (15%)
Lowest saturation:	72	90%–98%	Saturation <= 80% :	7 min (1%)
Baseline saturation:	90	%		
Minimum pulse:	59	> 40 bpm		
Maximum pulse:	71	< 90 bpm		
Average pulse:	62	bpm		
Proportion of probable CS epochs:	70	0%		

Analysis status: Analyzed automatically

Analysis parameters used (Default)

Apnea [20%; 10%; 80%; 1.0%; 20%; 60%; 8%]: Hypopnea [70%; 10%; 100%; 1.0%]: Snorng [6.0%; 0.3s; 3.5s; 0.5s]: Desaturation [4.0%]: CSR[0.50]

Comments

FIGURE 15-5 Sample HST report.

Comprehensive reporting, ResMed. Retrieved from https://www.capecodhealth.org/app/files/public/4864/apnealink-air-product-brochure.pdf

Cardiac Rhythms

ECG arrhythmias are yet another important finding to be highlighted in the report. Because the cardiac event summary on many sleep study reports is often limited to minimum, maximum, and average heart rate, any abnormalities in rhythm should be detailed in the narrative summary. The frequency of any significant event as well as any associated findings should be noted and detailed. In addition, the technologist should reference the epoch for an event so that the interpreting physician can review the waveforms. For example, the scoring technologist may write "2-lead ECG presented frequent unifocal PVCs associated with hypopneic respiratory events as observed on epochs 119–125."

Patient History and Questionnaires

The scoring technologist is responsible for carefully reviewing the patient history and questionnaires for anything noteworthy or of significance to the physician. This should include a brief medical history of the patient and notes about anything that may affect the patient's ability to initiate or maintain quality sleep or that may lead to excessive daytime sleepiness. In the questionnaires, the technologist should look for and note medications taken before the test, any unusual activities such as napping the day of the test, and post-test answers as to the subjective quality and duration of sleep during the study.

The scoring technologist's primary responsibility is to compile the data into a concise summary for the physician. Ultimately, this should include all pertinent history and physical information and important observations and significant events noted on the study.

Chapter Summary

The final and perhaps most important responsibility in scoring a sleep study is to generate a summary report. This report should include all sleep-related data and significant information about the patient gathered before, during, and after the study. The report contains several different sections, each of which includes specific clinical data. Sleep study reports should be inclusive of the data recommended by the AASM.

Several different types of sleep reports are available, usually determined by the type of study performed. These reports include baseline or diagnostic reports, titration reports, split night reports, and MSLT reports, among others. Titration reports are similar to diagnostic reports but include a PAP table dividing the data by treatment level. Other information about the PAP equipment and pressures is also included. The style and layout of each report can vary according to the specific needs of the physician and lab.

Most sleep reports contain information about sleep study times, including lights out time, lights on time, sleep-onset time, total recording time, total sleep time, and the like. Certain calculations are derived from these times, including the percentage of the TST spent in each sleep stage, and event indexes.

An important aspect of the scored report is the scoring technologist's notes. Scoring notes include all subjective information not seen within the numbers, tables, and graphs of the report, or information that may be more easily understood in narrative format. The scoring technologist should make detailed, accurate notes regarding anything significant that was seen while scoring the study, reviewing the report, or reading the patient history and questionnaires.

Case Study

A patient's sleep report includes the data shown in **Table 15-2**.

Based on the information in **Table 15-2**, calculate the following sleep parameters:

1. **total recording time (TRT)**
2. **sleep latency (SL)**
3. **total sleep time (TST)**
4. **sleep efficiency (SE)**
5. **percentage stage R**

Table 15-2
Case Study Sleep Report Data

Lights Out	Epoch 25
Lights On	Epoch 875
First Epoch of Sleep	Epoch 45
First Epoch of Stage R	Epoch 225
Total Stage R Time	100 min
WASO	25 minutes

Chapter 15 Questions

Please consider the following questions as they relate to the material in this chapter.

1. How is the total recording time calculated?
2. What is the difference between the mean, median, and mode sleep latencies of MSLT naps? Why are these data kept?
3. If a patient has 20 apneas and 10 hypopneas during 360 minutes of total sleep time, what is the AHI?
4. What is included in a titration report that is not included in a diagnostic baseline study report?
5. Why is it important to keep detailed scoring notes? What types of information should the scorer note?

Footnote

1. American Academy of Sleep Medicine. (2017). *The AASM Manual for the Scoring of Sleep and Associated Events*, version 2.4. Darien, IL: Author.

CHAPTER

16
Pediatric Sleep Medicine

© Agsandrew/Shutterstock

CHAPTER OUTLINE

Significance of Pediatric Sleep Medicine
Special Considerations
Pediatric Patient Hookup
Pediatric Sleep Recordings
Scoring Pediatric Sleep Studies
Chapter Summary

LEARNING OBJECTIVES

1. Understand the need for pediatric sleep medicine.
2. Discuss the challenges of performing a pediatric sleep study.
3. Learn how the hookup process is different for pediatrics.
4. Discuss the differences in scoring rules in pediatric studies.

KEY TERMS

pediatric sleep medicine
transcutaneous CO_2
end-tidal CO_2
dominant posterior rhythm
periodic breathing

Significance of Pediatric Sleep Medicine

Proper sleep is essential to the growth and development of infants, children, and adolescents. The National Sleep Foundation (NSF) recommends that children between ages 6 and 17 years obtain at least 9 hours of sleep per night.[1] However, according to the NSF's Sleep in the Modern Family poll,[2] a large proportion of our youth are falling short of this recommendation. Specifically, 31% of children ages 6 to 11 years, 71% of 12- to 14-year-olds, and 90% of those 15 to 17 years old are getting less than 9 hours of sleep per night. The NSF study also revealed a significant decline in sleep quantity and quality with increasing age. Further, 89% of parents and 75% of children have at least one electronic device in their bedrooms, a factor that has been associated with decreases in sleep quantity and quality.

Practitioners in **pediatric sleep medicine** work with children up to18 years of age. Pediatric sleep medicine has helped reveal many potentially negative effects of inadequate sleep in children. These include, but are not limited to, drowsiness, hyperactivity, difficulty concentrating, decreased physical development and growth, obesity, and illness. Further, sleep deprivation in children can be the results of behavioral or social-emotional factors, or primary sleep disorders, like obstructive sleep apnea (OSA). It is estimated that between 25% and 50% of children will experience a sleep disturbance during childhood, 1% to 5% suffer from OSA, and 5% to 50% will experience a parasomnia.[3] Because growth and development are critical in children, poor sleep can often have more far-reaching consequences in this age group.

Special Considerations

Performing a sleep study on a child or an infant requires special considerations that may not be required with an adult. For example, a parent or guardian must be present when any procedure is being performed on a minor. In the case of a sleep study, this means that the facility must provide the parent or guardian with a bed or chair to sleep in for the duration of the testing.

To maintain safety, it is important to consider the environment where the testing will take place. Safety measures should include using outlet covers and ensuring that all cables and equipment are out of the patient's reach. Viewing the environment from a child's height can offer additional perspective on potential safety issues.

In addition, the testing environment should be made to be inviting to children of all ages. Entering a new environment and having to undergo a "test" can seem frightening for a child. Many facilities decorate with brightly colored paints and interesting decals in an effort to make the sleep room look more comfortable. Some pediatric sleep labs have rooms specifically designed for boys or girls. Because pediatric patients come in all ages and sizes, a variety of bed sizes and styles may need to be available. This may include cribs, toddler beds, and full-size beds. Many facilities are prepared with children's videos and games to entertain their patients and help to distract the child during the long setup process.

At the Pediatric Sleep Institute in Plano, Texas, each room is designed to be convenient not only for working with infants but also for entertaining toddlers and small children. Each room has a different theme: a space room, a jungle room, and an under-the-sea room. The walls are left a neutral color for teenage patients, but they have the option of displaying a variety of toys for the younger patients. The stain-resistant love seat on the other side of the room converts to a bed for the parents, and the headboards are soft for children who head bang or move around frequently during the night. Diagnostic equipment and cameras are hidden from view. The lab is also equipped with cribs, which are ordinarily stored in a separate room but can be rolled into the patient room when an infant patient arrives. A small chalkboard in each room allows the technician to write a welcome note with each patient's name (see **Figure 16-1**). In addition, the sleep technologist uses a variety of tools to keep the children happy during the hookup, such as toys, stuffed animals, and videos. Technologists maintain a cheerful, friendly, positive attitude at all times to make the experience pleasant for children and their parents. These extras can make a difference

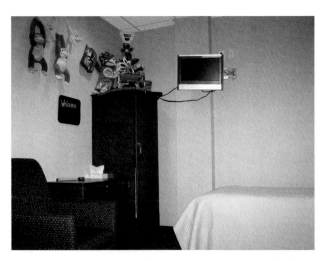

FIGURE 16-1 Designing and decorating a pediatric sleep lab often requires additional thought and care. The room seen here is at the Pediatric Sleep Institute in Plano, Texas. Its jungle theme helps entertain and relax young patients.

in reducing fear and anxiety for a child who must undergo sleep testing.

In addition to environmental and safety considerations, the sleep technologist working with pediatric patients should recognize normal developmental milestones and understand that there are significant differences in sleep needs, patterns, behaviors, and architecture across the ages. For example, infants require 14–16 hours of sleep per 24 hours and sleep just as much during the day as during the overnight period. In contrast, school-age children have a more regular sleep schedule, need approximately 10–12 hours of sleep per night, and should have mostly eliminated napping during the day. Also, toddlers undergo an important developmental milestone when transitioning from a crib to a bed and learning to fall asleep on their own. Similarly, teenagers undergo a delay or shift in circadian rhythm that makes it difficult to fall asleep at their previously scheduled bed times.

Pediatric Patient Hookup

The electroencephalogram (EEG) electrode locations for pediatric patients are found by using the international 10/20 electrode system for placement in the same way it is used in adult patients. In younger pediatric patients, the measurements for electrooculogram (EOG) and electromyogram (EMG) electrodes may be adjusted to accommodate smaller facial features. Specifically, EOG electrodes are often placed 0.5 cm from the eye rather than the 1 cm measurement used for adults, and chin EMG electrodes are often placed 1 cm from the inferior edge of the mandible rather than 2 cm. Also noteworthy is that because infants have short necks, snore sensors are often replaced with snore microphones on the chest. Leg electrodes are usually not used in the infant population. Collodion should never be used on infants or young children. **Figure 16-2** shows an example of a pediatric sleep study hookup.

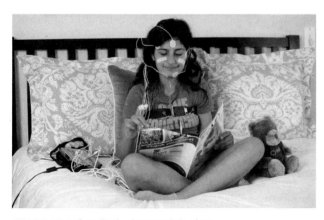

FIGURE 16-2 A pediatric sleep study hook-up.
Courtesy of Hackensack Sleep and Pulmonary Center.

To ensure that small children do not tug on electrode wires, Coban or a similar elastic-type wrap can be used to hold the wires in place. Although quite useful, this may cause additional sweating, which may lead to sweat artifact in the EEGs. An alternative strategy is to wait until the patient is asleep to perform the setup and attach electrode wires. This option may be beneficial in toddler age children who will not tolerate the setup process.

Smaller respiratory effort bands and airflow sensors are available for use on pediatric patients. Straps such as stretchy holsters for the ankles may be used in place of standard EMG electrodes in pediatric patients to help decrease the likelihood these sensors will detach during the night. To increase the tolerance of nasal oral sensors, some technologists tape together the thermal device and the nasal pressure cannula. This makes it a bit easier to place as well.

Pediatric sleep testing also includes the addition of **transcutaneous CO$_2$** or **end-tidal CO$_2$** monitoring. Transcutaneous CO$_2$ monitoring uses a heated sensor placed on the skin to read the CO$_2$ level in the blood, whereas end-tidal CO$_2$ monitoring uses a nasal–oral cannula to detect the CO$_2$ level in the patient's expired air. Both options provide an accurate account of the pediatric patient's ventilatory status, more so than SaO$_2$. Pediatric sleep labs are also faced with the challenge of stocking a variety of pediatric-sized continuous positive airway pressure masks.

Pediatric Sleep Recordings

There are inherent differences in the sleep of children as compared to adults. In general, children have higher-amplitude EEG waveforms compared to adults, and these tend to decrease with age. Infant sleep includes a great deal of extremely high-amplitude slow-wave activity in the EEGs. To ensure that entire waveforms are visible within the channel parameters, pediatric EEGs are typically viewed with a sensitivity level of 7 μV/mm. Also, normal sleep architecture varies significantly based on age, with children having higher percentages of slow-wave (delta) sleep and little N1 sleep. For example, in infants, 50% of sleep is spent in nonrapid eye movement (NREM) sleep, specifically stage N3, while the other 50% is spent in stage R. In contrast, teenagers have architecture more similar to adults with approximately 25% of sleep spent in stage R and 75% in NREM.

Other nuances are noteworthy. Normal heart rate and respiratory rates are faster in pediatric patients than in adult patients and can vary significantly with age. The American Heart Association's normal heart and respiratory rate guidelines for children are included in **Figure 16-3**. Also, arousals in children can be more subtle than those in adult patients, and children—especially young children—tend to have a higher arousal threshold.

Heart rate		
Normal heart rate by age (beats/minute) Reference: PALS guidelines, 2015		
Age	Awake rate	Sleeping rate
Neonate (< 28 d)	100–205	90–160
Infant (1 mo–1 y)	100–190	90–160
Toddler (1–2 y)	98–140	80–120
Preschool (3–5 y)	80–120	65–100
School-age (6–11 y)	75–118	58–90
Adolescent (12–15 y)	60–100	50–90

Respiratory rate	
Normal respiratory rate by age (breaths/minute) Reference: PALS guidelines, 2015	
Age	Normal respiratory rate
Infants (< 1 y)	30–53
Toddler (1–2 y)	22–37
Preschool (3–5 y)	20–28
School-age (6–11 y)	18–25
Adolescent (12–15 y)	12–20

FIGURE 16-3 The American Heart Association pediatric guidelines for normal heart rate and respiratory rate.
Developed by Dr. Chris Novak and Dr. Peter Gill for PedsCases.com

Scoring Pediatric Sleep Studies

Pediatric sleep studies are scored in a similar manner as with adult studies. Specifically, an epoch-by-epoch approach is used, and each 30-second epoch is assigned to a single sleep stage. In addition to sleep staging, sleep-related events are scored, including respiratory events, limb movements, and EEG arousals. Scoring criteria used for identifying arousals and limb movements are identical to those used in adult patients. However, some of the criteria for staging and identification of respiratory events differ. These differences are outlined in the following sections.

Sleep-Staging Rules

The AASM provides two different sleep-staging guidelines for the pediatric population. The first set is meant to be used to score the sleep of infants 0–2 months postterm. Because many of the characteristic waveforms seen in adult sleep have not yet developed, infant sleep staging is limited to stage wake (W), stage N (NREM), and stage R (REM) sleep. These stages are identified by characteristics noted in the EEG, EOG, and chin EMG as well as behavioral observations and respiratory pattern. In stage W, the eyes are generally open and blinking, the EEG portrays a low-voltage irregular or mixed pattern, the chin EMG is higher in amplitude, and an irregular pattern of respiration is seen. In stage N, the eyes are closed with little movement, the EEG portrays a high-voltage slow-wave activity, trace alternant (bursts of delta activity alternating with theta) or mixed pattern, the chin EMG is low in amplitude, and there is a regular pattern of respiration. Finally, in stage R, the eyes are closed with rapid eye movements noted, the EEG portrays a low-voltage irregular or mixed pattern, the chin EMG is low in amplitude, and the respiratory pattern is irregular. **Figure 16-4** portrays the characteristic EEG patterns seen in infant sleep.

After 2 months postterm, the pediatric staging rules are used. These guidelines are mostly similar to those of adults but with several nuances. First, during relaxed wakefulness, rather than alpha activity as seen in adults, pediatric patients portray a **dominant posterior rhythm**. This EEG pattern is slightly slower (4–7 Hz) than typical alpha frequencies (8–13 Hz). As the patient advances in age, the pattern tends to increase in frequency until normal alpha frequencies are seen in most by 9 years of age (see **Figure 16-5**).

In addition, pediatric scoring guidelines include a stage N that can be chosen for nonrapid eye movement sleep that is unidentifiable as a specific stage of NREM. The development of characteristic EEG waveforms such as K-complexes and sleep spindles can vary from patient to patient. Sleep spindles typically develop by age 4–6 weeks and are seen in nearly all children by 2–3 months of age. K-complexes are sometimes not seen until age 4–6 months. Therefore, stage N is scored for epochs identifiable as NREM sleep but in which there are no recognizable sleep spindles, K-complexes, or slow waves. Once sleep spindles, K-complexes, and slow waves are recognizable, the stages are scored the same as in adults. For further details about scoring sleep stages among pediatric patients, refer to the *AASM Manual for the Scoring of Sleep and Associated Events*, second edition.[4]

Respiratory Event Rules

The rules for scoring respiratory events in pediatric patients are different than those used for adults. Pediatric respiratory rules should be used for all children ages 2 months to 13 years. For children 14–18 years old, the medical director or interpreting physician can choose between using the pediatric or adult guidelines.

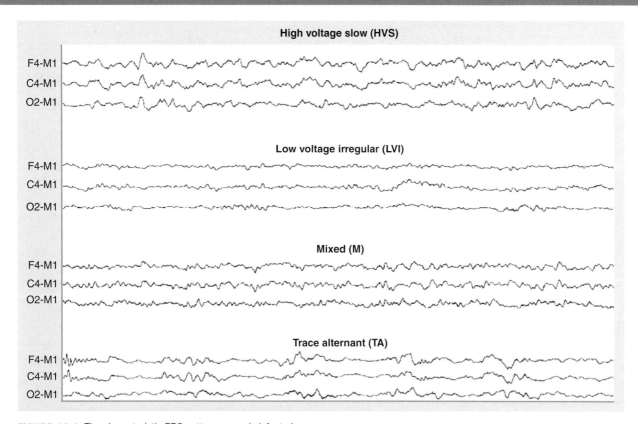

FIGURE 16-4 The characteristic EEG patterns seen in infant sleep.

Accessed from the American Academy of Sleep Medicine. AASM Manual for the Scoring of Sleep and Associated Events. Rules Terminology and Technical Specifications. Version 2.5 (2018).

Age	Frequency (Hz)
2–5 months	3–4
6–11 months	4–5
1–2 years	5–7
3 years and beyond	8–13

FIGURE 16-5 Dominant posterior rhythm seen in pediatric sleep across the ages.

Under pediatric rules, obstructive apneas are scored if there is at least a 90% decrease of airflow for at least two breaths and a continuation of respiratory effort. Mixed apneas are scored if there is an absence of airflow (>90% reduction) for at least two breaths that begins with a central component and ends with an obstructive one. There are three separate conditions in which central apneas are scored in pediatric patients. The first is if there is at least a 90% decrease of airflow and no effort for at least two breaths associated with either an arousal or an O_2 desaturation of at least 3%. The second condition is if there is a 90% decrease of airflow with complete cessation of respiratory effort for at least 20 seconds. The third situation in which a central apnea may be scored is if a 90% decrease of airflow with no effort is noted for

at least two breaths and associated with a heart rate of less than 50 bpm for 5 seconds. A heart rate in an infant of less than 60 bpm for 15 seconds would also satisfy this rule. **Periodic breathing** is scored if there are at least three central apneas lasting at least 3 seconds each, with no more than 20 seconds of normal breathing between the central apneas (see **Figure 16-6**). This breathing pattern is most common in infants in which ventilatory control is not yet fully developed.

A hypopnea is scored in pediatric patients if the airflow volume decreases by at least 30% for at least two breaths and there is an associated EEG arousal, awakening, or oxygen desaturation of at least 3%. A respiratory effort–related arousal is scored if there is an EEG arousal associated with increased respiratory effort, flow limitation, snoring, or an elevation in PCO_2 above the pre-event baseline that lasts at least two breaths duration.

The monitoring of capnography as a standard in pediatric patients allows the scoring of hypoventilation. Hypoventilation is scored when more than 25% of the child's total sleep time is spent with the PCO_2 above 50 mm Hg.

For further information or detailed scoring rules regarding respiratory events in pediatric patients, refer to the *AASM Manual for the Scoring of Sleep and Associated Events*, second edition.[4]

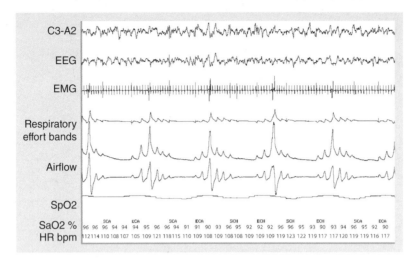

FIGURE 16-6 Periodic breathing observed in an infant patient.

Image courtesy of Dr. Sadasivam Suresh, Department of Respiratory & Sleep Medicine, Queensland Children's Hospital, Brisbane, Australia.

Chapter Summary

Poor sleep can have far-reaching consequences in children. Age-related and developmental changes across the pediatric population, however, make assessment and management of sleep-related issues particularly complex.

Sleep disorders and behavioral issues surrounding sleep are prevalent among pediatric patients. Pediatric polysomnography is a rising specialty within the field. There is an increasing need for technologists with competency and skill both in testing procedures and scoring of records. The processes of recording, scoring, and interpreting sleep studies in infants, toddlers, children, and adolescents present many challenges not seen in adult studies.

Sleep labs performing pediatric sleep studies are challenged with creating an atmosphere that is safe and aesthetically pleasing to young children but not offensive to adolescents. Sleep technologists performing studies on children are faced with the challenge of entertaining a child while performing a quality hookup.

Although the hookup is generally the same for pediatric patients as for adults, a few minor differences exist. For example, because of children's smaller head sizes, the chin EMG leads are placed closer to each other than they are in adults. Also, the EOG leads are placed closer to the eyes in pediatric patients than they are in adults.

Smaller wires and electrodes may be chosen to accommodate the child's size. Finally, because capnography is standard for a pediatric sleep study, the technologist must perform either transcutaneous or end-tidal CO_2 monitoring and integrate it into the study.

Pediatric sleep studies are scored in a manner similar to adult studies; however, some of the rules are different. The AASM provides two different sleep-staging guidelines for the pediatric population. The first set is used for infants 0–2 months postterm and includes stages wake (W), N (NREM), and R (REM) sleep. After 2 months postterm, the pediatric staging rules are used. Because children less than 6–9 months of age may not have developed sleep spindles, K-complexes, or slow waves, the staging rules include a stage N (NREM) for those epochs that are unidentifiable as a particular NREM stage.

In children, apneas and hypopneas are required to be at least two breaths in duration rather than 10 seconds, and periodic breathing is scored when several central apneas are recorded in a short period of time. Finally, the monitoring of capnography as a standard in pediatric patients allows the scoring of hypoventilation.

Early identification and management of sleep issues in the pediatric population can greatly improve sleep, development, and overall health.

Case Study

Arriving for his overnight shift, the sleep technologist reviews his assigned sleep study cases and sees that he will be performing a baseline sleep study on a 4-year-old child.

- What can the technologist do to better prepare for this patient?
- What accommodations or environmental changes can the technologist make to ensure the patient's safety and help make him or her feel less anxious?
- What age-specific details should the technologist consider in his strategy for a successful setup process?
- What changes will the technologist make in the placement of electrodes or sensors?

Chapter 16 Questions

Please consider the following questions as they relate to the material in this chapter.

1. Why is pediatric sleep medicine important?
2. What are some challenges in designing a pediatric sleep lab?
3. How is a pediatric patient hookup different than an adult hookup?
4. Why is the EEG sensitivity setting different in pediatric studies than in adult studies?
5. What scoring rules are changed when scoring a pediatric study?

Footnotes

1. National Sleep Foundation (2015). Sleep duration recommendations. Accessed at https://www.sleepfoundation.org/sites/default/files/2018-10/NSF_sleep_duration_recommendations_chart.png
2. National Sleep Foundation (2014). Sleep in America® poll: Sleep in the modern family. Accessed at https://www.sleepfoundation.org/professionals/sleep-america-polls/2014-sleep-modern-family
3. Carter, K. A., Hathaway, N. E., & Lettieri, C. F. (2014). Common sleep disorders in children. *American Family Physician*, 89(5).
4. American Academy of Sleep Medicine (2017). *AASM manual for the scoring of sleep and associated events. Rules terminology and technical specifications*, Version 2.4. Darien, IL: Author.

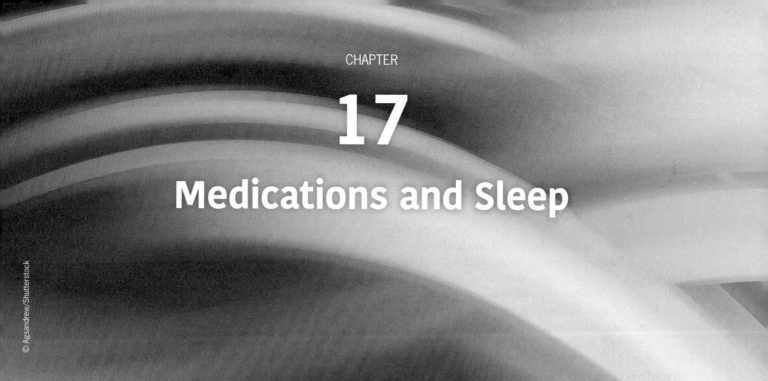

CHAPTER

17

Medications and Sleep

© Agsandrew/Shutterstock

CHAPTER OUTLINE

Drug Effects on Sleep
Analgesics
Antidepressants
Antihistamines
Antiepileptic Medications
Cardiovascular Medications
Sedative–Hypnotic Medications
Orexin Receptor Antagonists
Stimulants
Alcohol
Sleep Aids: Selection and Safety
Chapter Summary

LEARNING OBJECTIVES

1. Understand how certain classes of medications can impact sleep quality and architecture.
2. Understand how substances like alcohol and caffeine can impact sleep.
3. Learn about how commonly prescribed sleep aids are selected and the safety issues that must be considered.
4. Learn about some over-the-counter sleep aids on the market.

KEY TERMS

Opioids
anti-inflammatories
nonsteroidal anti-
    inflammatory
    drugs (NSAIDs)
ataxic breathing
tricyclic antidepressant
    (TCA)
selective serotonin
    reuptake inhibitor (SSRI)
monoamine oxidase
    inhibitors (MAOI)
antihistamines
antiepileptic drug (AED)
antiarrhythmic
beta blocker
antihypertensive
ACE inhibitor

calcium channel blocker
diuretic
sedative–hypnotic
    medication
barbiturate
benzodiazepine
nonbenzodiazepine
orexin receptor antagonist
sleep-onset insomnia
sleep-maintenance
    insomnia
onset of action
duration of action
half-life
over-the-counter
    (OTC) sleep aid
melatonin

Drug Effects on Sleep

Many commonly prescribed medications can effect sleep by causing sleepiness or insomnia, reducing sleep quality, or changing sleep architecture. In fact, one of the most commonly reported side effects of both prescribed and over-the-counter (OTC) medications is sleepiness. Various neurotransmitters—including dopamine, serotonin, histamine, and acetylcholine—play a role in the regulation of sleep and alertness.[1] Medications that have an effect on these chemicals can have sedating or alerting side effects and hence may cause sleepiness or insomnia. Because a great number of drugs on the market can impact sleep, this chapter will discuss these effects by medication class. The latter part of the chapter will be used to discuss prescribed and OTC sleep aids, how they are selected, and the safety implications that must be considered before use.

Analgesics

Analgesics include three classes of drugs used to alleviate pain: **opioids**, **anti-inflammatories**, and **nonsteroidal anti-inflammatory drugs (NSAIDs)**. In general, the anti-inflammatory medications have the potential to improve sleep quantity or quality by relieving pain that can disrupt sleep. For example, Motrin or Tylenol may be recommended to a patient with back pain or arthritis who has difficulty sleeping because of pain.

Opioids activate the mu receptors in the brain that produce analgesia, euphoria, respiratory depression, sedation, and decreased gastrointestinal motility. Opioids represent an important group of drugs that can significantly affect sleep. With acute use, they are associated with sedation, but chronic use can lead to the development of insomnia. Opioid medications have the potential to significantly decrease deep sleep and stage R sleep while increasing stage N1 (light sleep). This results in considerably less restorative sleep and daytime sleepiness. In addition, because they suppress respiration, opioids decrease respiratory rate and tidal volume and increase the likelihood of central apneic events and **ataxic breathing**.[2] Further, the decrease in muscle tone associated with this drug increases the risk of upper-airway collapse and obstructive sleep apnea (OSA). Opioid medications have a long list of adverse effects, including respiratory arrest, constipation, orthostatic hypotension, urinary retention, nausea, vomiting, and dysphoria.[1–4] This medication category is significantly associated with abuse because tolerance and dependence develop quickly.

Antidepressants

Antidepressants are medications designed to treat depression. There are three uniquely different agents that are used to treat depression: **tricyclic antidepressants (TCAs)**, **selective serotonin reuptake inhibitors (SSRIs)**, and **monoamine oxidase inhibitors (MAOIs)**. Occasionally, a physician will prescribe an antidepressant at lower doses to treat insomnia. If the sleep disturbance is secondary to anxiety or depression, then an antidepressant could be useful in addressing both conditions. However, in many cases, tolerance develops to the sedating effects of the antidepressant. The three antidepressant classes are discussed below.

Tricyclic Antidepressants (TCAs)

Tricyclic antidepressants work by inhibiting the reuptake of norepinephrine and serotonin. TCAs have sedating properties and thus are associated with reduced sleep latency and increased total sleep time and sleep efficiency. Sleep architecture changes include increased stage N2 and N3 sleep, with significant reductions in REM. In addition, TCAs may worsen leg movements during sleep and other sleep disorders such as REM behavior disorder.[1,3,4]

Selective Serotonin Reuptake Inhibitors (SSRIs)

Selective serotonin reuptake inhibitors have a greater selectivity and act specifically to maintain higher levels of serotonin in the brain. When serotonin is increased, mood is elevated. These medications tend to be better tolerated as antidepressants. However, SSRIs have a significant impact on sleep quality and architecture. They are associated with increased sleep fragmentation, wake after sleep onset (WASO), stage N1 sleep, and decreased total sleep time, sleep efficiency, and stage R sleep. In some cases, the reductions in REM can be as much as 30%.[1,3,4] In addition, SSRIs can exacerbate other sleep disorders such as REM behavior disorder or periodic limb movement disorder. Poor nighttime sleep often leads to excessive daytime sleepiness in patients taking these medications. Finally, the occurrence of slow eye movements persisting past stage N1 and into other stages of NREM sleep is an interesting characteristic often noted in patients taking SSRIs.[4] This phenomenon is frequently referred to as "Prozac eyes."

Monoamine Oxidase Inhibitors (MAOIs)

Monoamine oxidase inhibitors differ from TCAs and SSRIs by their side effects and are typically reserved for patients who do not respond well to either TCAs or SSRIs. MAOIs have a broad range of effects on sleep quality and architecture and vary between individual medications.

In general, almost all antidepressants have some impact on sleep quality and architecture. Most increase the latency to stage R sleep and decrease the percentage of total sleep time (TST) spent in REM. In addition, abrupt withdrawal from these medications can result in sleep disturbance and significant REM rebound. This can often be associated with nightmares. General side effects of antidepressants include drowsiness, dizziness, daytime cognitive and performance deficits, headache, tremor or agitation, dry mouth, or nausea.[1–4]

Antihistamines

Antihistamines block the release of histamine, which is an inflammation-producing substance produced from white blood cells that occurs with an injury or an allergic reaction. Antihistamines are labeled for the relief of cold and allergy symptoms and for motion sickness. A marked side effect of this group of medications is sedation and drowsiness. As a result, many people reach for this medication class as a self-prescribed sleep aid. These medications are associated with decreased sleep latency and improved sleep continuity. However, antihistamines are not labeled for use as sleep aids and have a myriad of other side effects, including dry mouth, altered mental state, confusion, and urinary retention.[1–4] Older adults can also experience parasomnias, posing safety risks. For this reason, patients should be always cautioned against using these medications as sleep aids.

Antiepileptic Medications

Antiseizure medications, or **antiepileptic drugs (AEDs)**, work by inhibiting central nervous system (CNS) activity or by enhancing gamma-aminobutyric acid (GABA) activity. Numerous medications are available in this category, and many are selective for particular types of seizure activity. Traditional antiepileptics have been tested extensively, and their efficacy has been well established. However, they tend to be less tolerated than the newer antiepileptic medications on the market that have been developed to be safer with fewer side effects. Common side effects of seizure medications include dizziness, double vision, headache, sedation, cognitive impairment, and gastrointestinal issues.[1–4] These medications tend to decrease sleep latency and awakenings and increase TST. Traditional AEDs have variable effects on sleep architecture, including increasing stage N3 and reducing REM sleep.[1,3,4]

Cardiovascular Medications

Cardiovascular drugs are some of the most widely prescribed medications today. Because of the documented association between OSA and cardiovascular diseases, many patients referred for sleep studies are taking prescription cardiovascular medications. These medications can have a variety of effects on a patient's sleep.

Antiarrhythmics and **beta blockers** are cardiac medications used to treat abnormal heart rhythms and hypertension. These medications can cause nighttime sleep difficulties, insomnia, and nightmares. In addition, they are associated with decreases in stage R sleep. **Antihypertensives** are commonly prescribed cardiovascular drugs designed to decrease blood pressure. These medications can include **ACE inhibitors**, **calcium channel blockers**, and **diuretics**. Angiotensin-converting-enzyme (ACE) inhibitors act by reducing salt and water retention and inhibiting vascular constriction. They have been associated with nighttime coughing, which can disturb sleep and cause daytime sleepiness. Calcium channel blockers promote smooth muscle relaxation in the blood vessels. They are associated with drowsiness and can increase the likelihood of gastroesophageal reflux disease, which can also disturb nighttime sleep.[2] Finally, diuretics work by decreasing fluid volume within the blood vessels. In doing so, they create an excess of urine and the frequent urge to urinate, which can greatly disturb the sleep period. In addition, some patients on diuretics experience leg cramps, yet another factor that can interrupt sleep.

Sedative–Hypnotic Medications

Sedative–hypnotic medications are used to treat anxiety, insomnia, and seizure disorders. These medications depress the central nervous system; they are typically used at lower doses to relieve anxiety and at higher doses to promote sleep. This drug class can be further subdivided into three groups: **barbiturates**, **benzodiazepines**, and **nonbenzodiazepines**. We will discuss these in the next several sections.

Barbiturates

Barbiturates are nonselective CNS depressants that work by directly mimicking the actions of GABA and producing effects that range from mild sedation to general anesthesia. This class of medication has been used for many years to promote sleep, suppress seizure activity, and produce various levels of sedation. However, barbiturates are associated with a myriad of adverse effects, including significant respiratory depression, severe sedation, slowed bodily functions, slurred speech, difficulty concentrating, increased collapsibility of the upper airway, aspiration, coma, and death.[1–4] Further, these medications have a high abuse potential because tolerance and dependence can develop quickly. Interestingly, development of drug tolerance does not reduce suppression of respiratory drive.[2] Because of the significant adverse effects associated with their use, barbiturates have largely been phased out as sleep aids.

In general, barbiturates increase total sleep time by significantly reducing sleep latency and WASO time, effectively improving the quality of sleep. These medications tend to reduce stage N1, N3, and R sleep while significantly increasing stage N2 sleep.[1,3,4]

Benzodiazepines

Benzodiazepines work by intensifying the effects of GABA, an action that reduces neuronal excitability throughout the nervous system and causes muscle relaxation. These effects make this medication class useful for reducing anxiety. In addition, because of the sedating effects at higher doses, benzodiazepines can also be used as short-term sleep aids. Finally, certain benzodiazepines are used to treat seizure disorders.

In general, benzodiazepines increase total sleep time by reducing sleep latency and WASO, effectively improving the quality and efficiency of sleep. These medications tend to increase stage N2 sleep and the fast-frequency spindle activity seen in this stage. Some benzodiazepines may produce significant reductions in stages N3 and R when used at higher doses. These drugs can also increase the likelihood of sleep-disordered breathing, hypoventilation, and leg movements during sleep.[1,3,4]

Side effects of benzodiazepine medications include daytime sleepiness, light-headedness, headaches, difficulty concentrating, and incoordination. Some studies have demonstrated significant residual daytime effects, including impaired driving the morning and afternoon after administration.[5] In some cases, they can be associated with anterograde amnesia and paradoxical effects.[2] Rebound insomnia can be experienced during the first night after discontinuing the drug.[1,3,4] As a result of these significant side effects, these medications have been largely replaced as sleep aids with better alternatives.

Nonbenzodiazepine Receptor Agonists

Nonbenzodiazepine receptor agonists act on the GABA receptor complex to promote sedation. This class of drug was developed primarily as an alternative to traditional benzodiazepines for the treatment of insomnia. The medications in this class are generally well tolerated with fewer side effects than benzodiazepines, although caution should be used when prescribing them to older patients.[6] Daytime drowsiness and dizziness are the most commonly reported adverse effects. The effects on sleep quality and architecture parallel those seen with traditional benzodiazepines.

In general, this class of medication increases TST by reducing sleep latency and WASO time, effectively improving the quality of sleep and sleep efficiency. In addition, they are associated with increases in stage N2 sleep and in some mild reductions in N3 and R.[1,3,4] The selection and safety considerations of these medications will be discussed later in the chapter.

Orexin Receptor Antagonists

Orexins are neuropeptides located in the hypothalamus that activate neurons to produce consolidated periods of wakefulness. **Orexin receptor antagonists** are a newer class of medications developed for the treatment of insomnia. These medications generally decrease sleep latency and increase sleep quality. Effects on sleep architecture include decreased REM latency and increased stage R time and density. Side effects include residual daytime effects, including impaired performance and drowsiness. Currently, there is no evidence of rebound or withdrawal effects.[1,3,4]

Stimulants

Stimulants are a class of psychoactive drugs that produce enhanced alertness, wakefulness, and locomotion. Common stimulants include caffeine, nicotine, and amphetamines. Depending on the dosage and the time of day taken, they can have a significant impact on sleep. Specifically, they are associated with reductions in sleep quality and stage N3 and REM sleep. Daytime sleepiness often occurs because of poor nighttime sleep.

Stimulants are also associated with increases in blood pressure, heart rate, and respiratory rates as well as a multitude of adverse effects, including anxiety, irritability, headaches, dizziness, tremors, insomnia, disturbing dream content, and hallucinations or paranoia in some cases. This class of drug is also known for the development of tolerance and dependence.

Alcohol

Alcohol is one of the most frequently used substances to help promote sleep. However, contrary to common thought, although alcohol may reduce sleep latency, it actually increases sleep fragmentation and decreases overall sleep quality. In addition, alcohol is associated with suppressed REM sleep, significantly reduced stage N3 sleep, and the increased likelihood of obstructive apneic events and periodic limb movements during sleep.[1,3,4] Finally, alcohol can trigger acid reflux during the night and increase the urge to urinate, both adding to the disruption of sleep quality. In patients who use alcohol nightly to sleep, the abrupt withdrawal often results in dramatic REM rebound, nightmares, and insomnia.[1,3,4] These symptoms make it more likely that the patient will relapse. In addition, the deleterious effects on REM and deep sleep are often permanent even after abstinence.

Sleep Aids: Selection and Safety
Prescription Sleep Aids

Prescription sleep aids are indicated for the short-term treatment of sleep-onset insomnia, sleep-maintenance insomnia, or both. **Sleep-onset insomnia** refers to having difficulty falling asleep, and **sleep-maintenance insomnia** refers to having difficulty staying asleep throughout the night.

In selecting a sleep aid, the sleep physician should consider which of these symptoms the patient experiences, as well as the **onset of action** and the

duration of action of the medication options. A medication's onset of action refers to the amount of time it takes for the drug to take effect. The duration of action is the length of time that the medication remains effective in the body. A medication's **half-life** refers to the time it takes for half of the dose to be metabolized by the body and eliminated from the bloodstream. For example, a drug with a half-life of 6 hours will be 50% less effective after 6 hours, and its effects will slowly decrease after that point. Duration of action can be influenced by various factors, including advancing age, pregnancy, and having comorbidities such as liver, kidney, or metabolic disorders that can slow the breakdown or elimination of the medications from the body. For example, caffeine, which normally has a half-life of 5 hours in normal health adults, can have stimulating effects for as long as 15–20 hours in older adults and pregnant women.

For a patient who experiences sleep-onset insomnia, a sleep aid with a faster onset of action and shorter half-life should be sufficient to treat the issue. This is the case because the medication will take action quickly to help the patient fall asleep but will be rapidly eliminated by the body so the patient has fewer residual daytime effects. Conversely, a patient who wakes up frequently during the night and has difficulty falling back to sleep will need a sleep aid with a longer half-life so that the effects are maintained throughout the sleeping period. When this type of sleep aid is selected, the patient may experience residual effects into the daytime period.

Before sleep aids are prescribed, the physician should have a clear understanding of the patient's sleep patterns and have ruled out any underlying conditions or primary sleep disorders. Some sleep disorders—OSA for example—can be made worse with sleep aids. In addition, the patient should be provided with detailed education about the proper use of the medication and its potential side effects.

Side effects of common sleeping aids include dizziness or feeling light-headed, headaches, prolonged drowsiness, and detriments in performance, cognition, or daytime memory.[1-4] These can have safety implications on daytime function and driving ability. Some sleep aids, when used in older adults, have contributed to falls or injuries. Zolpidem has been reported to be responsible for more than 20% of all ER visits for adverse drug effects in older adults, causing agitation, falls, and delirium.[6]

Being on sleep aids for longer periods carries the potential for abuse, tolerance, and dependence. In addition, significant withdrawal effects may be seen when the drug is discontinued.

In summary, physicians must consider many factors when prescribing sleep aids. First, treatment should always be based on diagnosis and not on complaint. This means that primary sleep disorders or underlying pathology should be ruled out before providing treatment with medications. Next, medications should be chosen wisely using information about the patient's sleep patterns, medical history, and the dynamics of the drug options. In addition, side effects of these medications and the safety implications should be considered. Lastly, physicians should recognize that variation in medication effects may occur based on risk factors for prolonged or enhanced effects such as advanced age and comorbidities (see **Tables 17-1** to **17-5**).

Over-the-Counter Sleep Aids

In recent years, **over-the-counter (OTC) sleep aids** have become popular and effective in initiating sleep. Common ingredients include melatonin, valerian, and tryptophan. Although these drugs are marketed as safe, they should only be considered after consulting with a physician. Many of these supplements have not been approved by the Food and Drug Administration, lack consistency in dose per tablet, and have variable effects on sleep. Misuse and abuse of these drugs is common. In addition, withdrawal from these medications can result in difficulty initiating and maintaining sleep.

Table 17-1
Drug Effects on Sleep

	Benzodiazepines	Nonbenzodiazepines	Tricyclics	SSRIs	SNRIs*	Antihistamines
Sleep latency	–	–		+	+	–
Total sleep time	+	+	+	–	–	+
Sleep efficiency	+	+		–	–	
Wake after sleep onset	–	–	–	+	+	
Stage N1	+	–			+	+
Stage N2	+	+	+			+

(Continues)

Table 17-1
Drug Effects on Sleep (*Continued*)

Stage N3	−	−	+	−		+
Stage R	−	−	−	−	−	−
Arousals	−			+		
Restless legs		+	+	+		
Periodic limb movements			+	+	+	
Daytime sleepiness	+		+	+	+	
Eye movements in NREM				+		
REM behavior disorder				+		
Obstructive sleep apnea	+					

*Serotonin-norepinephrine reuptake inhibitors.

Table 17-2
Common Medication Stems[1–4]

Word Stem	Drug Class	Word Stem	Drug Class
-andr-	Androgens	-irudin	Anticoagulants
-ase	Enzymes	-lol	Beta blockers
-azepam	Antianxiety	-mycin	Antibiotics
-bactam	Beta-lactamase inhibitors	-olone	Steroids
-bamate	Tranquilizers and antiepileptics	-oxacin	Antibiotics
-barb	Barbituric acids	-pamil	Coronary vasodilators
-butazone	Anti-inflammatory analgesics	-parin	Heparin derivatives
-caine	Local analgesics	-peridol	Antipsychotics
-cillin	Penicillins	-pred	Prednisone derivatives
-conazole	Antifungals	-pril	Antihypertensives (ACE inhibitors)
-cort	Cortisones	-profen	Anti-inflammatories
-curium	Neuromuscular blocking agents	-setron	Serotonin receptor antagonists
-cycline	Tetracycline antibiotics	-statin	Antihyperlipidemics
-dralazine	Antihypertensives	-terol	Bronchodilators
-estr-	Estrogens	-thiazide	Diuretics
-fibrate	Antihyperlipidemics	-tocin	Oxytocin derivatives
-flurane	Inhalation anesthetics	-trexate	Antimetabolites
-gest-	Progesterins	-triptyline	Antidepressants
-ipine	Calcium channel blockers	-zosin	Alpha blockers
-ipramine	Antidepressants		

Table 17-3
Medication Classes Associated with Insomnia[1–4]

Anti-epileptics
Beta blockers
Bronchodilators
Decongestants
Diuretics
Steroids
Selective serotonin reuptake inhibitors (SSRIs)
Stimulants

Melatonin

Melatonin is a natural hormone that helps regulate our sleep–wake cycle. It is produced by the pineal gland; its secretion is stimulated by darkness and suppressed by environmental light. When taken artificially, it can reset the circadian clock and cause sedating effects. These effects make it useful to alleviate sleep-onset and sleep-maintenance insomnia as well as jet lag. Studies have shown 2-mg sustained release formulations to be associated with improvements in sleep latency, quality, and morning alertness.[7] There are few reported side effects of melatonin, especially at low doses, but higher doses have been associated with headache and nightmares. Table 17-5 provides examples of medications by class. Table 17-2 shows commonly used medication word

Table 17-4
Common Sleep Aids[1–4]

Medication Name	Medication Class	Use
Estazolam	Benzodiazepine	Sleep-onset insomnia Sleep-maintenance insomnia
Eszopiclone (Lunesta)	Nonbenzodiazepine (sedative–hypnotic)	Sleep-onset insomnia Sleep-maintenance insomnia
Ramelteon (Rozerem)	Nonbenzodiazepine (sedative–hypnotic)	Sleep-onset insomnia
Temazepam (Restoril)	Benzodiazepine	Sleep-onset insomnia Sleep-maintenance insomnia
Zaleplon (Sonata)	Nonbenzodiazepine (sedative–hypnotic)	Sleep-onset insomnia
Zolpidem (Ambien)	Nonbenzodiazepine (sedative–hypnotic)	Sleep-onset insomnia
Zolpidem extended release (Ambien CR)	Nonbenzodiazepine (sedative–hypnotic)	Sleep-onset insomnia Sleep-maintenance insomnia
Suvorexant (Belsomra)	Orexin receptor antagonist	Sleep-onset insomnia Sleep-maintenance insomnia

Table 17-5
Medications by Class[1–4]

Medication Class	Medication Name: Generic (Brand)	Medication Class	Medication Name: Generic (Brand)
Antiarrhythmic	amiodarone (Cordarone) procainamide (Pronestyl)	Non benzodiazepine receptor agonist	zaleplon (Sonata) zolpidem (Ambien)
Antiepileptic	carbamazepine (Tegretol) gabapentin (Neurontin)	Nonsteroidal anti-inflammatory drug (NSAID)	aspirin (Bayer, St. Joseph) ibuprofen (Advil, Motrin, Midol, Nuprin)
Antihistamine	diphenhydramine (Benadryl) loratadine (Claritin)	Opioid	hydrocodone (Hysingla, Zohydro ER) hydrocodone/acetaminophen (Vicodin) methadone (Dolophine, Methadose)

(Continues)

Table 17-5
Medications by Class[1–4] (Continued)

Antihypertensive	Furosemide (Lasix) Diltiazem (Cardizem)	Orexin receptor antagonist	suvorexant (Belsomra)
Barbiturate	pentobarbital (Nembutal) secobarbital (Seconal)	Selective serotonin reuptake inhibitor (SSRI)	fluoxetine (Prozac) paroxetine (Paxil, Pexeva) sertraline (Zoloft)
Benzodiazepine	clonazepam (Klonopinl) diazepam (Valium) lorazepam (Ativan)	Stimulant	dextroamphetamine (Dexedrine) dextroamphetamine/amphetamine (Adderall) methylphenidate (Ritalin, Concerta)
Beta blocker	atenolol (Tenormin) metoprolol (Lopressor, Toprol-XL) propranolol (Inderal LA, InnoPran XL)	Tricyclic antidepressant (TCA)	nortriptyline (Pamelor) protriptyline (Vivactil)
Monoamine oxidase inhibitor (MAOI)	isocarboxazid (Marplan) phenelzine (Nardil)		

stems and their meanings. Table 17-1 summarizes the common drug classes and their impact on sleep.8 Table 17-3 lists common medication classes that are associated with insomnia. Table 17-4 provides examples of common sleep aids, their medication class, and use.

Chapter Summary

Many commonly prescribed medications can cause sleepiness or insomnia, reduce sleep quality, or change sleep architecture. Medications used as sleep aids should be used with caution and after careful consideration of patient history.

Opioid medications decrease respiratory rate and tidal volume, and they increase the likelihood of central apneic events. In addition, decreases in muscle tone increase the risk of collapse of the upper airway and obstructive sleep apnea.

Tricyclic antidepressants are associated with increased total sleep time, sleep efficiency, and stages N2 and N3 sleep. In contrast, SSRIs are associated with decreases in total sleep time and sleep efficiency. Both medications tend to decrease the percentage of TST spent in REM and worsen leg movements and other sleep disorders.

A marked side effect of antihistamine medications is sedation and drowsiness. As a result, many people reach for this medication class as a self-prescribed sleep aid. However, because of the associated side effects, patients should be cautioned against using these drugs outside their indicated use.

Epileptic medications have variable effects on sleep architecture, including increasing total sleep time and stage N3, while reducing REM sleep. In contrast, cardiac medications can cause nighttime sleep difficulties, insomnia, and nightmares.

Sedative–hypnotic medications include barbiturates, benzodiazepines, and nonbenzodiazepines. Barbiturates are associated with significant adverse effects and abuse and have largely been phased out as sleep aids. Benzodiazepines are used to treat anxiety and sleep-onset and sleep-maintenance insomnia. In general, they are associated with increased total sleep time and quality of sleep. However, many produce significant reductions in stage N3 and R and can increase the likelihood of sleep-disordered breathing, hypoventilation, and leg movements during sleep. Nonbenzodiazepines were developed as an alternative to traditional benzodiazepines for the treatment of insomnia and have been associated with fewer side effects and better tolerance. Drugs of this kind are currently used widely as sleep aids.

Stimulants are associated with increased blood pressure, heart rate, and respiratory rate and can decrease the quantity and quality of sleep. Although alcohol may reduce sleep latency, it actually increases sleep fragmentation and decreases overall sleep quality.

Sleep aids are indicated for the short term treatment of sleep-onset insomnia, sleep-maintenance insomnia, or both. Selection is based on onset and duration of action as well as on safety considerations. In addition, it is important to fully understand a patient's sleep patterns and rule out any underlying conditions or primary sleep disorders before considering the use of a sleep aid. Supplemental melatonin can be useful to alleviate sleep-onset and sleep-maintenance insomnia as well as jet lag.

Chapter 17 Questions

Please consider the following questions as they relate to the material in this chapter.

1. What are the effects of certain classes of drugs on sleep?
2. Discuss some of the adverse effects common to various categories of medications.
3. How do alcohol and caffeine impact sleep?
4. What are the important considerations for the selection and use of sleep aids?

Footnotes

1. Mattice, C., Brooks, R., & Lee-Chiong, T. L. (2012). *Fundamentals of sleep technology*, 2nd ed. Philadelphia: Lippincott Williams & Wilkins.
2. Rosenjack Burchum, J., & Rosenthal, L. (2016). *Lehne's pharmacology for nursing care*, 9th ed. St. Louis, MO: W.B. Saunders.
3. Kryger, M. H., Roth, T., & Dement, W. C. (2016). *Principles and practices of sleep medicine*, 6th ed. St Louis, MO: Elsevier Saunders.
4. Roux, F. J., & Kryger, M. H. (2010). Medication effects on sleep. *Clinics in Chest Medicine, 31*, 397–405.
5. Verster, J. C., Veldhuijzen, D. S., & Volkerts, E. R. (2004). Residual effects of sleep medication on driving ability. *Sleep Medicine Reviews, 8*(4), 309–325.
6. Hampton, L. M., Daubresse, M., Chang, H. Y., Alexander, G. C., & Budnitz, D. S. (2014). Emergency department visits by adults for psychiatric medication adverse events. *JAMA Psychiatry, 71*(9), 1006–1014.
7. Culpepper, L., & Wingertzahn, M. A. (2015). Over-the-counter agents for the treatment of occasional disturbed sleep or transient insomnia: A systematic review of efficacy and safety. *The Primary Care Companion for CNS Disorders, 17*(6), 10.4088/PCC.15r01798. doi:10.4088/PCC.15r01798
8. Spriggs, W. (2003). *Principles of Polysomnography*. Sleep Management Services.

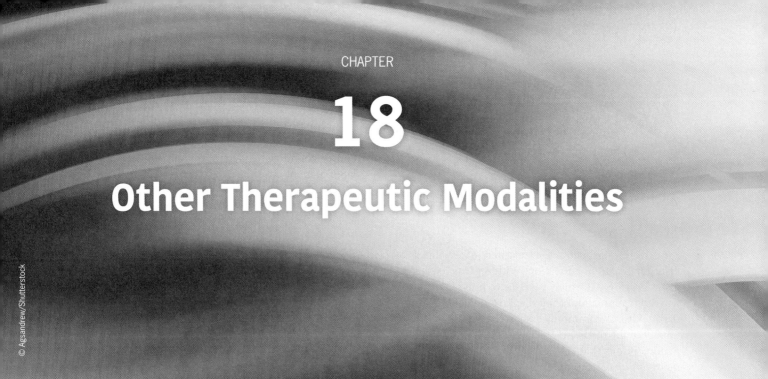

CHAPTER

18

Other Therapeutic Modalities

© Agsandrew/Shutterstock

CHAPTER OUTLINE

Treatment of Sleep Disorders
Education
Chronotherapy
Phototherapy
Cognitive Behavioral Therapy
Positional Therapy
Nutritional Counseling and Weight Loss
Pharmacological Treatments
Oral Appliance Therapy
Rapid Maxillary Expansion
Hypoglossal Nerve Stimulation
Nasal Surgery
Adenotonsillectomy
Somnoplasty
Uvuloplasty
Maxillomandibular Advancement
Tracheostomy
Other Surgical Procedures
Chapter Summary

KEY TERMS

sleep hygiene
chronotherapy
phototherapy
bright light therapy (BLT)
Cognitive Behavioral
  Therapy (CBT)
sleep-restriction therapy
stimulus control
paradoxical intention
cognitive control
biofeedback
positional therapy
bariatric surgery
oral appliances
retrognathia
rapid maxillary
  expansion (RME)

hypoglossal nerve stimulation
otolaryngologist
adenotonsillectomy
adenotonsillar hypertrophy
somnoplasty
uvuloplasty
laser-assisted uvuloplasty
  (LAUP)
uvulopalatopharyngoplasty
  (UPPP)
maxillomandibular
  advancement (MMA)
tracheostomy
genioglossus advancement
hyoid suspension

LEARNING OBJECTIVES

1. Learn about the various therapeutic modalities used in the treatment of sleep disorders.
2. Understand how patient education and cognitive behavioral therapy techniques can be valuable to treatment success.
3. Discuss the indications for both surgical and nonsurgical treatment options.
4. Describe some of the common surgical procedures used in the treatment of snoring and obstructive sleep apnea.

Treatment of Sleep Disorders

Various therapies are used to manage sleep disorders. In Chapter 10, we discussed basic and advanced positive airway pressure (PAP) therapies to treat sleep-disordered breathing. This chapter will cover other therapeutic options available for treating sleep-related breathing disorders (SRBDs) as well as the numerous other primary sleep disorders currently recognized.

Education

An important aspect in the treatment of any illness or disorder is patient education. With regards to sleep disorders, it is extremely valuable to provide patients with education about their diagnosed sleep disorders, the symptoms commonly associated with them, the impact of the disorders if left untreated, and the therapeutic options that are available. Further, many treatment options are complex and require that a patient be provided with a full understanding of the rationale, proper use, and side effects of therapy to help improve compliance.

It is never a wasted effort to spend time educating patients about proper sleep habits. **Sleep hygiene** is a term used to refer to the practice of good sleep habits with the aim of protecting sleep health. These practices include following a regular sleep–wake schedule, developing a relaxing bedtime routine, and avoiding alerting substances and activities before bedtimes. Sleep hygiene techniques are discussed in detail in Chapter 1. At times, education about good sleep habits and the importance of these practices to overall health may be the most relevant first-line treatment, especially for a patient whose main sleep issues involve dysfunction in this area. Other times, sleep education can be added as an adjunctive therapy to supplement other treatment modalities.

In addition to sleep hygiene recommendations, it can be useful to educate patients about avoiding practices that can make various sleep disorders worse. For example, patients with sleep apnea should be cautioned to avoid alcohol and sedatives. It is also important to review the list of medications that a patient may be taking to identify ones that may be problematic to his or her sleep issue.

Chronotherapy

Chronotherapy is a therapeutic modality used to treat various circadian rhythm disorders. The technique aims to reset the internal biological clock to the desired time for sleep by systematically and gradually delaying or advancing bedtimes and rise times. This treatment has been particularly successful when implemented on patients with delayed sleep phase syndrome (DSPS). In these cases, patients are directed to advance bedtimes incrementally over a period of several weeks. For example, a patient with DSPS who normally falls asleep at 4 A.M. would be directed to gradually move bedtimes earlier over time until they are able to achieve sleep at times more consistent with social settings.

Chronotherapy is often used in conjunction with other treatments, like sleep education, phototherapy, and/or cognitive behavioral therapy. In the case of the DSPS patient described above, he/she would also be instructed to avoid bright light exposure in the evenings and maintain a dark, quiet bedroom during sleep and a well-lit room upon awakening.

Phototherapy

Phototherapy, also called **bright light therapy (BLT)**, is a treatment that uses purposeful exposure to natural daylight or specific wavelengths of light using lamps or light boxes (see **Figure 18-1**) to treat various medical conditions, including skin disorders, jaundice, some types of cancers, and sleep and mood disorders. As a treatment for sleep disorders, BLT is often used to help reset the circadian rhythm. The timing, strength, and duration of light exposure are critical components of this treatment option. For example, light exposure in the evening is often recommended for patients with advanced sleep phase disorder. These patients have difficulty staying awake until normal bed times. Exposure to evening light has stimulating effects, counteracts their urge to sleep, and helps them achieve normal bed times. In essence, it phase delays their circadian rhythm. Conversely, bright light exposure after the body temperature minimum or in the morning can act to advance the sleep–wake cycle, something that would be beneficial to a patient with DSPS. Phototherapy can also be beneficial to people with shift work sleep disorder or jet lag. Phototherapy can be associated with headaches, fatigue, insomnia, hyperactivity, and irritability.

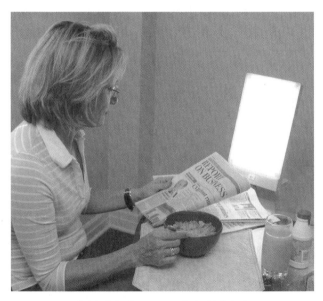

FIGURE 18-1 Bright light therapy supplied with light boxes.
Northern Light Technologies, Retrieved from https://northernlighttechnologies.com/wp-content/uploads/2011/11/TRAVelite-life2.jpg

Cognitive Behavioral Therapy

Cognitive Behavioral Therapy (CBT) is a psychological intervention that focuses on changing cognitive distortions and behaviors and improving skills for emotional regulation and coping. CBT is used to manage a wide range of issues, including insomnia. When used as a therapy for insomnia, it aims to identify poor sleep habits and misconceptions about sleep that perpetuate the disorder, and it uses specific techniques to facilitate change. CBT strategies can include **sleep-restriction therapy**, **stimulus control**, **paradoxical intention**, relaxation, **cognitive control**, and **biofeedback**.[1]

Sleep restriction aims to consolidate sleep by decreasing the amount of time spent in bed. In patients with insomnia, much of this time is spent awake. Sleep restriction involves working with a clinician to set an "allowed time in bed," which is determined by the average total sleep time from 2 weeks of sleep logs. Consideration is given to when the patient needs to wake in the morning, and the bed time is set by counting backward from the desired wake time. The patient is instructed to strictly follow the determined schedule for at least 2 weeks, to avoid napping, and to practice good sleep hygiene. The therapy is largely effective because it increases sleepiness and the likelihood that the patient will fall asleep. In addition, it establishes a strict sleep–wake schedule and trains the brain to associate the bed with sleep.

Stimulus control involves looking at the patient's sleep habits and identifying actions that may be prohibiting sleep. This therapy includes patient education about proper sleep hygiene practices, especially those designed to strengthen the association of the bed for sleep. These include creating a comfortable sleep environment and hiding the clock from view.

Paradoxical intention is valuable for those patients who are strongly preoccupied with sleep and sleep loss. It aims to reduce performance anxiety and the associated concern with difficulty falling asleep by changing the focus to passively trying to stay awake. This often removes the preoccupation with sleeping and allows sleep to come naturally.

Relaxation approaches include meditation, imagery, and muscle relaxation to help calm the body and mind. This is often paired with biofeedback strategies, which teach the patient how to observe their muscle tension and heart rate and adjust them using learned relaxation techniques.

Cognitive control therapy aims to calm an overactive mind and remove it from the bedroom environment. It includes changing attitudes and beliefs about sleep and teaching strategies and building skills to "lay the day to rest." For example, a patient who has negative thoughts like "I am never going to be able to sleep well" is taught to replace those beliefs with thoughts like "If I stop

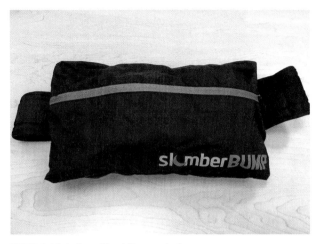

FIGURE 18-2 A positional therapy device.
Used with permission from slumberBUMP, https://www.slumberbump.com/

worrying so much and focus on positive solutions, I can learn to sleep well."

Positional Therapy

Positional therapy can be useful as an adjunctive treatment for obstructive sleep apnea (OSA) when there is a strong positional correlation to apneic or hypopneic events. It can also be used as a secondary treatment option when other therapies have failed. In many patients with OSA, respiratory events occur more frequently and to a more severe degree when the patient is sleeping in a specific position. Most often, this "positional OSA" is noted as most severe in the supine position. The goal of positional therapy is to prevent the patient from sleeping in the supine position, thus minimizing respiratory events.

Various positional therapy strategies are available, including the traditional "tennis ball method," a self-made construction of sewing a tennis ball to a sleep shirt, and the more advanced commercial waistband with air-filled balloons (see **Figure 18-2**). A 2015 study examining the effectiveness of positional therapy strategies found that all methods seem equally effective, with reported short-term success rates around 68%. However, long-term use is not as positive, with 65% of patients abandoning the therapy.[2]

Nutritional Counseling and Weight Loss

Nutritional counseling is an important adjunctive therapeutic intervention for the management of OSA when weight is considered a contributing factor. Obesity is an important risk factor for OSA, with the prevalence of OSA in obese patients almost twice that of adults of normal weight. Studies have shown that patients who achieve a 10% weight loss can see more than a 20% improvement in the severity of their

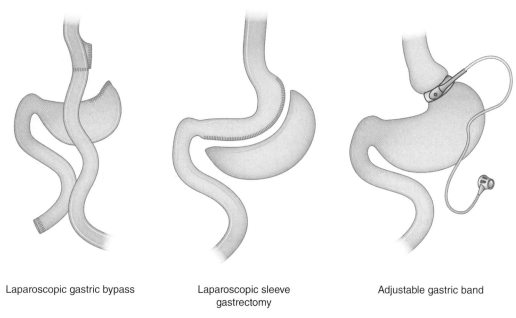

Laparoscopic gastric bypass   Laparoscopic sleeve gastrectomy   Adjustable gastric band

FIGURE 18-3 Three different bariatric procedures used to reduce the size of the stomach.

OSA.[3] Recommended weight-loss therapies include low-calorie diets, nutritional or lifestyle counseling, diabetes education, and cognitive behavioral programs.

More recently, **bariatric surgery** has gained popularity as a weight-loss option. Bariatric procedures reduce the size of the stomach, making it harder to eat as much food. **Figure 18-3** portrays three different bariatric procedures currently used. These surgeries are associated with a large range of risks and adverse effects, including anesthesia-related risks, infection, chronic nausea and vomiting, inability to eat certain foods, low blood sugar, and malnutrition. Many of the recent trials assessing weight loss and OSA have demonstrated that patients experience dramatic weight reduction and significant reductions in the apnea–hypopnea index (AHI). However, despite this, most patients continued to have at least moderate OSA.[3]

Pharmacological Treatments

Generally speaking, pharmacological treatments for sleep disorders are usually reserved for when after other therapeutic options have been tried. For example, for patients with chronic insomnia, first-line treatment often includes education and attempts at improving sleep hygiene. It can also incorporate various constructs of Cognitive Behavioral Therapy. If these treatment options prove to be unsuccessful, then the physician may choose to prescribe a short-term sleep aid to help break the cycle of insomnia. This would require close follow-up and eventual weaning from the medication.

Medications can also be used to treat sleep disorders in conjunction with other therapeutics. For example, for patients being treated with PAP therapy for an SRBD, the physician may prescribe steroidal nasal sprays to address nasal inflammation, which can make using PAP therapy more difficult.

Narcolepsy and periodic limb movement disorder (PLMD) are examples of two sleep disorders in which pharmacologic treatment is indicated. Treatment of narcolepsy includes nonmedication and medication-based components. Education about sleep hygiene, maintaining a routine sleep–wake schedule, and scheduled naps are important to managing the disorder. However, many of the symptoms are controlled with the use of stimulants such as methylphenidate or modafinil and selective serotonin reuptake inhibitors to suppress REM sleep and alleviate the symptoms of cataplexy, hypnagogic hallucinations, and sleep paralysis. More recently, sodium oxybate (Xyrem), has gained popularity after it was demonstrated to be highly effective at improving daytime sleepiness, reducing cataplectic attacks, and improving nighttime sleep.[4]

After other primary causes are ruled out, restless leg syndrome and PLMD are often treated with dopamine or GABA agonists or anticonvulsant agents to reduce muscle contractions and movements. According to the 2012 update to the *Practice Parameters for the Treatment of Restless Legs Syndrome and Periodic Limb Movement Disorder in Adults*,[5] the standard recommendation is for the use of either pramipexole or ropinirole. Levodopa and gabapentin are also considered acceptable treatments with a high level of evidence for success.

Oral Appliance Therapy

Oral appliances are dental devices that are commonly offered as an alternative therapy for those patients diagnosed with mild to moderate OSA and are not compliant with the use of continuous positive airway pressure (CPAP). These devices are worn during sleep and act to pull the lower jaw forward. By stabilizing the mandible, tongue, and pharyngeal structures in this forward position, the oral appliance can create a more patent airway (see **Figure 18-4**). Oral appliance therapy is considered most effective in nonobese patients with **retrognathia**.

Various types and brands of oral appliance therapies differ in design, material, flexibility, and adjustability. More recently, there are options that allow in-lab titration of protrusion, which can increase efficiency and expedite treatment. The selection of device usually includes consideration of the patient's history, state of dentition, oral anatomy, and severity of diagnosis. The use of oral appliance therapy can be associated with excessive salivation, shifting of the teeth, gum soreness, or temporomandibular joint pain.

The American Academy of Sleep Medicine's clinical guidelines[6] for use of oral appliance therapy emphasize that diagnosis and medical evaluation should precede consideration of this therapeutic option and that the appliance fitting and selection should be performed by an experienced and credentialed dentist. In addition, the guidelines recommend periodic evaluation by the dentist and follow-up sleep studies when applicable to document the resolution of clinical symptoms and the normalization of the AHI and O_2 saturation during sleep.

Rapid Maxillary Expansion

Rapid maxillary expansion (RME) includes the use of an oral appliance to gradually increase the width of the hard palate. This device and procedure is most often used in children to improve the patency of the airway, a treatment that can significantly reduce or eliminate OSA. Often referred to as a *butterfly brace*, the appliance is created and inserted by a credentialed orthodontist. It slides over the rear teeth and is held in place by metal brackets. It includes an expansion screw that the parents are instructed to turn in varying intervals (e.g., one to two turns per day) over the course of several weeks to months (see **Figure 18-5**). The adjustments increase the pressure applied to the teeth and palate and act to expand and reduce the arch of the palate. This increases the size of the nasal cavity and allows more air to enter into the throat and lungs. Once the ideal expansion has been achieved, a retainer is often used to maintain the shape of the palate. Braces may also be used to straighten the teeth and create a wider and more aesthetically pleasing smile.

RME is best performed in children early in their growth and development before the palate fuses. In addition, the child must have molars on which to secure the device and be able to tolerate the brace and adjustments. Most often, RME is performed on patients between 6 and 12 years old. Side effects of the device can include mild pain or discomfort, sore tongue or gums, temporary excess in salivation, and difficulty with speech.[7]

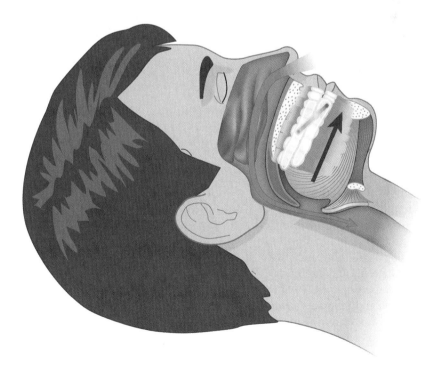

FIGURE 18-4 An oral appliance.

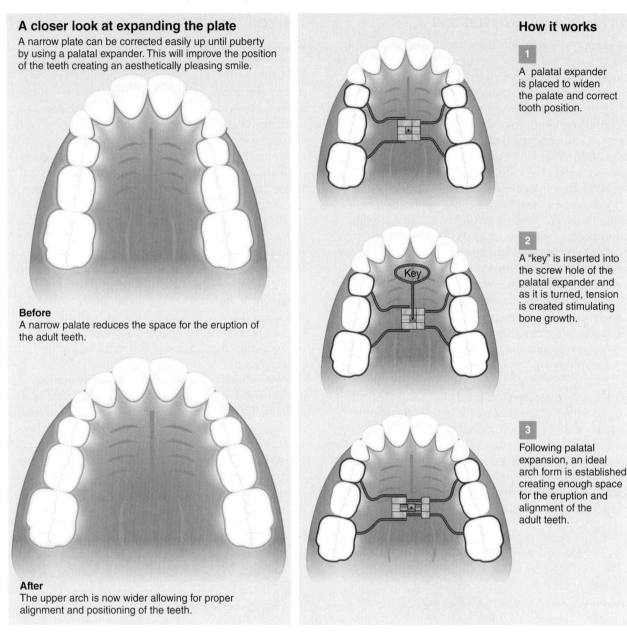

A closer look at expanding the plate

A narrow plate can be corrected easily up until puberty by using a palatal expander. This will improve the position of the teeth creating an aesthetically pleasing smile.

Before
A narrow palate reduces the space for the eruption of the adult teeth.

After
The upper arch is now wider allowing for proper alignment and positioning of the teeth.

How it works

1
A palatal expander is placed to widen the palate and correct tooth position.

2
A "key" is inserted into the screw hole of the palatal expander and as it is turned, tension is created stimulating bone growth.

3
Following palatal expansion, an ideal arch form is established creating enough space for the eruption and alignment of the adult teeth.

FIGURE 18-5 A closer look at how a palatal expander works.

Hypoglossal Nerve Stimulation

Hypoglossal nerve stimulation was recently developed as an alternative therapy for patients with OSA. It includes an implantable pulse-generating device that is surgically implanted under the clavicle, a stimulation electrode placed on the hypoglossal nerve, and a sensing lead placed between the external and intercostal muscles (see **Figure 18-6**). When turned on, the device measures the breathing pattern and generates an electrical signal that stimulates the tongue during inspiration. The hypoglossal stimulation acts to prevent muscle relaxation and collapse of the airway. In a clinical trial consisting of 126 patients with OSA, a 68% reduction in

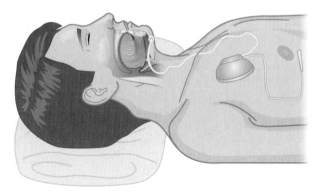

FIGURE 18-6 A hypoglossal nerve stimulator device.

AHI was reported with the use of the stimulator, along with improvements in daytime functional outcomes.[8]

The hypoglossal nerve stimulator is usually turned on 1 month after it is implanted, and the settings are then adjusted. The patient is provided with a remote control and instructed to turn the device on at night before going to sleep. Reported side effects are minor, and include mild pain at incision and transient tongue weakness or soreness.

Nasal Surgery

Patients who suffer from SRBDs and whose history includes having a deviated septum, nasal injury, or nasal polyps should be evaluated by an **otolaryngologist**, or an ear, nose and throat specialist. These issues can cause mild to severe restriction of air flow, increase the likelihood of airway collapse, and make treatment of SRBDs more difficult. Surgical correction of these issues has been shown to improve symptoms of SRBDs and compliance with CPAP therapy. Nasal surgical procedures include septoplasty to straighten a deviated septum and turbinate reduction. The risks of nasal surgical procedures can include bleeding, infection, perforation, an impaired sense of taste and smell, and various levels of pain.

Adenotonsillectomy

Adenotonsillectomy is the surgical removal of the adenoidal and tonsillar tissues and is the most common major surgical procedure performed on children. This procedure is often used as the first-line treatment of moderate to severe OSA in children over 2 years old who have enlarged adenoids and tonsils, or **adenotonsillar hypertrophy**.[9]

Adenotonsillectomy can be performed using a variety of techniques including surgical removal/sutures, electrocautery, and coblation, which uses a gentle radiofrequency energy to shrink tissue. Children undergoing adenotonsillectomy may experience bleeding, fever, nausea and/or vomiting, and throat and/or ear pain for up to two weeks post-surgery. In rare cases, patients may experience transient laryngospasm or mild desaturation requiring supplemental oxygen. Improvements in symptoms, behavior, cognition, and AHI are mostly positive following adenotonsillectomy, but vary considerably, with reported success rates ranging from 27 to 80 percent.[10]

Somnoplasty

Somnoplasty is offered as a treatment option to relieve nasal obstruction or diminish snoring. This minimally invasive surgical procedure is performed using a needle probe under local anesthesia in a physician's office. Somnoplasty uses temperature-controlled radiofrequency technology to reduce and tighten the tissue of the nasal turbinates, palate, or tongue. After the procedure, the tissue undergoes healing, contraction, and stiffening over the course of the next 6–8 weeks. Patients undergoing somnoplasty may experience swelling or some discomfort, but the procedure is generally well tolerated. Somnoplasty is associated with an approximate 70% reduction in report of snoring via bed partner report.[11] This treatment modality is not indicated for the treatment of sleep-related breathing disorders.

Uvuloplasty

Uvuloplasty is a surgical procedure performed to remove either parts of or the entire uvula. This treatment option aims to reduce or eliminate snoring. It is performed as an outpatient procedure with a local anesthetic. Most often, a laser is used at the rear of the mouth to scar and tighten the uvula. It some cases, some of the soft palate is also treated (**laser-assisted uvuloplasty [LAUP]**). LAUP may require as many as five treatments and may be difficult to perform on a patient who has a strong gag reflex. Most patients who undergo uvuloplasty experience a sore throat that can last up to 10 days. Other risks include infection and bleeding. A 2007 study found that LAUP reduced snoring in 88% of patients.[12] This procedure is not routinely recommended as a treatment for sleep apnea.

Uvulopalatopharyngoplasty (UPPP) is an invasive procedure in which the tonsils, uvula, and part of the soft palate are surgically removed in an effort to enlarge and stabilize the airway (see **Figure 18-7**). The UPPP procedure is sometimes recommended as an alternative treatment option for patients with OSA who are unable to tolerate treatment with CPAP. However, reports of effectiveness are variable, with success rates ranging from 35% to 95.2%.[13] A 2009 study found that of 63 patients with OSA, only 24% achieved a surgical cure

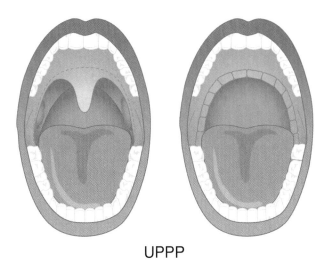

UPPP

FIGURE 18-7 The uvulopalatopharyngoplasty procedure.

and only 33% achieved a postsurgical AHI of less than 10.[14] The UPPP procedure requires the use of a general anesthetic and is associated with significant pain. Its many side effects include airway swelling, bleeding, velopalatine insufficiency, palatal–nasopharyngeal stenosis, difficulty swallowing, and tongue numbness.

Maxillomandibular Advancement

Maxillomandibular advancement (MMA) is considered a a treatment option for patients with moderate to severe OSA with mandibular retrognathism (backward displacement of the jaw) who have failed to use CPAP or oral appliance therapy. MMA is a major anatomical surgical procedure performed in a hospital or surgery center under general anesthesia. The procedure involves cutting into the bones of the upper and lower jaws and advancing the midface, palate and mandible forward. The use of small titanium plates, screws, braces, and rubber bands preserves the integrity of the bite (see **Figure 18-8**).

The MMA procedure effectively enlarges the size of the upper airway, significantly reducing the likelihood of airway obstruction. Success rates—defined as having a postoperative AHI of less than 20 and an AHI reduction of more than 50%—are reported to range from 80% to 100%. A 2012 study reported that 43% of patients were cured of their OSA, achieving postoperative AHIs of less than 5.[15]

The risks of the MMA procedure include bleeding, hematoma, infection, and failure of the bone to heal. Postoperatively, patients may experience pain, swelling, and temporary numbness of the lower lip and chin. After undergoing an MMA, patients must endure having their jaws wired closed for a period of time to allow healing and a limited diet of soft foods and liquids for several weeks after the procedure. Most patients report that changes in facial appearance occur and are quite positive.

Tracheostomy

A **tracheostomy** is an invasive procedure used in rare and emergency situations to address airway obstruction or to facilitate long-term mechanical ventilation or airway secretion clearance. Because this procedure completely bypasses the upper airway, it is a highly effective treatment for severe OSA when CPAP or other alternative therapies are refused, ineffective, or not tolerated. During a surgical tracheostomy, a surgeon creates an incision directly into the trachea in the lower portion of the neck and inserts a tracheostomy tube. The tube is secured around the patient's neck with a collar and ties (see **Figure 18-9**). When used to treat OSA, the tracheostomy tube can be plugged during the day, allowing the patient to breathe and speak normally. Before going to sleep, the patient removes the cap, allowing the patient to breathe past any obstruction occurring in the upper airway.

The tracheostomy procedure can be associated with bleeding, infection, aspiration of secretions, damage to the larynx or trachea, and impaired swallowing and vocal function. In addition, patients with a tracheostomy experience a major change in their quality of life. Careful and regular care of the site, including changing and cleaning of the tube, is labor intensive but extremely important at preventing infection and complications.

Other Surgical Procedures

Other surgical procedures used to treat OSA include **genioglossus advancement** and **hyoid suspension**, both aimed to increase the size of the upper airway. Genioglossus advancement involves cutting into the lower jaw and moving the major tongue attachment forward. This prevents the tongue from falling backward during sleep, increasing the size of the airway and preventing obstruction. Hyoid suspension

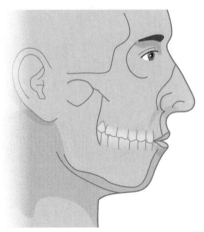
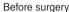
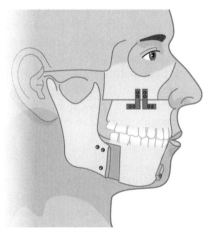

Before surgery   After surgery

FIGURE 18-8 The maxillomandibular advancement procedure.

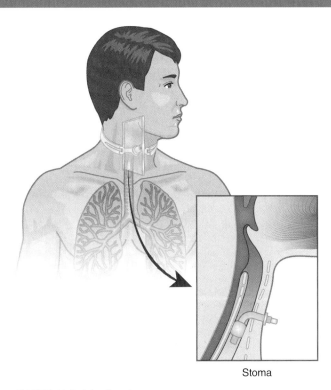

Stoma

FIGURE 18-9 A tracheostomy.

involves pulling the hyoid bone and the muscles attached to the tongue and airway forward. These procedures have variable efficacies. A 2015 study found that genioglossus advancement had a 53% success rate, which corresponded to a patient having a postprocedure AHI of less than 20 with at least a 50% reduction in value.[16] A 2016 study found that patients undergoing isolated hyoid suspension demonstrated a decrease in AHI by 38.3%.[17]

Chapter Summary

Various therapies are used to manage sleep disorders. It is never a wasted effort to spend time educating patients about proper sleep hygiene. Education about good sleep habits and the importance of these practices to overall health may be a relevant first-line treatment. Other times, sleep education can be added to supplement other treatment modalities.

Chronotherapy and phototherapy are therapeutic modalities used to treat various circadian rhythm disorders by helping to advance or delay the internal biological sleep–wake rhythm. Cognitive Behavioral Therapy includes strategies such as sleep restriction, stimulus control, paradoxical intention, relaxation, and biofeedback.

Positional therapy is useful as an adjunctive treatment for obstructive sleep apnea when there is a strong positional correlation to respiratory events. Various positional therapy strategies are available with similar degrees of effectiveness.

When weight is considered a contributing factor, nutritional counseling can be an important adjunctive therapeutic intervention for the management of OSA. Bariatric procedures reduce the size of the stomach and make it harder to eat as much food. They have gained popularity as a weight-loss option.

Pharmacologic treatment is often indicated for the treatment of narcolepsy and periodic limb movement disorder. Symptoms of narcolepsy are most often managed with stimulants and sodium oxybate, and leg movements are controlled with dopamine or GABA agonists or anticonvulsant agents.

Oral appliances are worn during sleep to stabilize the mandible, tongue, and pharyngeal structures in a forward position, creating a more patent airway. These devices are commonly offered as an alternative therapy to patients with mild to moderate obstructive sleep apnea who are not compliant with the use of CPAP.

Rapid maxillary expansion is most often used in children with OSA to improve the patency of the airway. It includes the use of an oral appliance to gradually increase the width of the hard palate.

Hypoglossal nerve stimulation was developed as an alternative therapy for patients with OSA. It is an implantable device that acts to stimulate the hypoglossal nerve during inspiration to prevent the tongue from falling back and obstructing the airway.

Nasal surgical procedures include septoplasty to straighten a deviated septum and turbinate reduction. Adenotonsillectomy is used as a first-line treatment of moderate to severe OSA in children over 2 years old with enlarged tonsils or adenoids. It involves removing the adenoidal and tonsillar tissues and is the most common major surgical procedure performed on children.

Somnoplasty uses temperature-controlled radiofrequency technology to reduce and tighten the tissue of the nasal turbinates, palate, or tongue. Uvuloplasty is a surgical procedure performed to remove either parts of or the entire uvula. These treatments aim to reduce or eliminate snoring. Uvulopalatopharyngoplasty is an invasive procedure in which the tonsils, uvula, and part of the soft palate are removed in an effort to enlarge the upper airway in patients with OSA.

Maxillomandibular advancement is a major surgical procedure that involves cutting into the bones of the upper and lower jaws and advancing the midface, palate, and mandible forward. It is most often used in OSA patients with recessed jaws with the aim of creating a more open upper airway.

Tracheostomy is a highly effective treatment for patients with severe OSA who refuse or cannot tolerate CPAP or other alternative therapies. The procedure involves placing a tracheostomy tube that completely bypasses the upper airway. It is highly invasive and requires long-term care.

Case Study

The medical director of a sleep-disorders center asks you for advice on options for managing a 34-year-old woman with chronic insomnia. She explains that the patient complains of "not being able to shut her mind off at night" and has been experiencing trouble sleeping for the past 2 years. Her sleep logs show an irregular sleep–wake schedule and increased sleep latencies. The patient is otherwise healthy and of normal body mass index. She is not taking any prescribed medications but does report using over-the-counter sleep aids when needed.

What therapies are relevant for this patient?

Chapter 18 Questions

1. What are some common nonsurgical treatments used to treat sleep disorders?
2. How can patient education and Cognitive Behavioral Therapy techniques impact treatment success?
3. Describe the indications and rationale for oral appliance therapy.
4. What is uvuloplasty and how is it used in treating sleep disorders?
5. How is rapid maxillary expansion accomplished? What are the goals of treatment?
6. Name some of the common surgical procedures used to treat obstructive sleep apnea.

Footnotes

1. Gasperetti, C. E., Dolsen, M. R., & Harvey, A. G. (2017). Cognitive Behavioral Therapy for sleep disorders. In *The science of cognitive behavioral therapy* (pp. 381–403). Cambridge, MA: Academic Press.
2. de Vries, G. E., Hoekema, A., Doff, M. H., Kerstjens, H. A., Meijer, P. M., van der Hoeven, J. H., & Wijkstra, P. J. (2015). Usage of positional therapy in adults with obstructive sleep apnea. *Journal of Clinical Sleep Medicine, 11*(2), 131–137.
3. Romero-Corral, A., Caples, S. M., Lopez-Jimenez, F., & Somers, V. K. (2010). Interactions between obesity and obstructive sleep apnea: Implications for treatment. *Chest, 137*(3), 711–719.
4. Bhattarai, J., & Sumerall, S. (2017). Current and future treatment options for narcolepsy: A review. *Sleep Science, 10*(1), 19.
5. Aurora, R. N., Kristo, D. A., Bista, S. R., Rowley, J. A., Zak, R. S., Casey, K. R., . . . & Rosenberg, R. S. (2014). The treatment of restless legs syndrome and periodic limb movement disorder in adults—An update for 2012: Practice parameters with an evidence-based systematic review and meta-analyses: An American Academy of Sleep Medicine clinical practice guideline. *Focus, 12*(1), 99–121.
6. Ramar, K., Dort, L. C., Katz, S. G., Lettieri, C. J., Harrod, C. G., Thomas, S. M., & Chervin, R. D. (2015). Clinical practice guideline for the treatment of obstructive sleep apnea and snoring with oral appliance therapy: An update for 2015. *Journal of Clinical Sleep Medicine, 11*(7), 773–827.
7. Camacho, M., Chang, E. T., Song, S. A., Abdullatif, J., Zaghi, S., Pirelli, P., . . . & Guilleminault, C. (2017). Rapid maxillary expansion for pediatric obstructive sleep apnea: A systematic review and meta-analysis. *The Laryngoscope, 127*(7), 1712–1719.
8. Kezirian, E. J., Goding Jr, G. S., Malhotra, A., O'donoghue, F. J., Zammit, G., Wheatley, J. R., . . . & Maddison, K. J. (2014). Hypoglossal nerve stimulation improves obstructive sleep apnea: 12-month outcomes. *Journal of Sleep Research, 23*(1), 77–83.
9. Mitchell, R. B., Archer, S. M., Ishman, S. L., et al. (2019). Clinical practice guideline: Tonsillectomy in children (update). *Otolaryngology—Head and Neck Surgery,* 160:S1–S42.
10. Friedman, M., Wilson, M., Lin, H. C., & Chang, H. W. (2009). Updated systematic review of tonsillectomy and adenoidectomy for treatment of pediatric obstructive sleep apnea/hypopnea syndrome. *Otolaryngology—Head and Neck Surgery,* 140:800.
11. Cartwright, R., Venkatesan, T. K., Caldarelli, D., & Diaz, F. (2000). Treatments for snoring: A comparison of somnoplasty and an oral appliance. *The Laryngoscope, 110*(10), 1680–1683.
12. Klozar, J., Plzák, J., Zábrodský, M., & Betka, J. (2007). Effectiveness and side effects of one-stage laser-assisted uvuloplasty in primary rhonchopathy. *Journal for Oto-Rhino-Laryngology, Head and Neck Surgery, 69*(5), 316–321.
13. Stuck, B. A., Ravesloot, M. J., Eschenhagen, T., de Vet, H. C. W., & Sommer, J. U. (2018, October). Uvulopalatopharyngoplasty with or without tonsillectomy in the treatment of adult obstructive sleep apnea–A systematic review. *Sleep Medicine, 50,* 152–165.
14. Khan, A., Ramar, K., Maddirala, S., Friedman, O., Pallanch, J. F., & Olson, E. J. (2009, September). Uvulopalatopharyngoplasty in the management of obstructive sleep apnea: The Mayo Clinic experience. *Mayo Clinic Proceedings, 84*(9), 795–800.
15. Blumen, M. B., Vezina, J. P., Pigot, J. L., & Chabolle, F. (2012). Maxillomandibular advancement for obstructive sleep apnea syndrome. *Operative Techniques in Otolaryngology—Head and Neck Surgery, 23*(1), 60–66.
16. KuŞÇu, O., Süslü, A. E., Özer, S., Günaydın, R. Ö., Öğretmenoğlu, O., & Önerci, M. (2015). Sole effect of genioglossus advancement on apnea hypopnea index of patients with obstructive sleep apnea. *Acta Oto-Laryngologica, 135*(8), 835–839.
17. Song, S. A., Wei, J. M., Buttram, J., Tolisano, A. M., Chang, E. T., Liu, S. Y. C., . . . & Camacho, M. (2016). Hyoid surgery alone for obstructive sleep apnea: A systematic review and meta-analysis. *The Laryngoscope, 126*(7), 1702–1708.

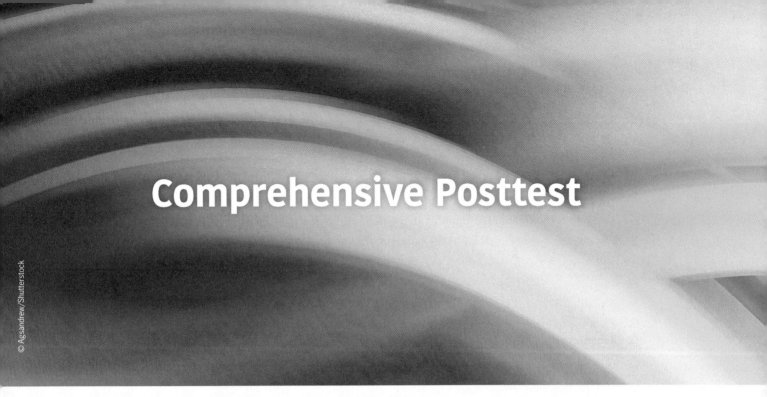

Comprehensive Posttest

Posttest Instructions

The questions in this section are formatted after the pattern of the questions on the sleep technician board examination. The content of these questions is based on the text in this book and other current sleep texts. Select the best answer for each question. The correct answers are provided at the end of the test, along with a brief explanation.

Domain 1: Study Performance/Instrumentation

1. Which filter settings are most appropriate for the associated channel types?

	A	B	C	D
EEG	0.1/15	0.3/35	1.0/70	1.0/70
EOG	0.1/15	0.3/35	1.0/70	1.0/70
ECG	0.3/15	0.3/70	0.3/15	1.0/70
EMG	1.0/100	10/70	1.0/35	5.0/35

2. The E2 electrode is placed out and up from the outer canthus of the right eye, and E1 is placed out and down from the outer canthus of the left eye. If the E2 channel on the polysomnograph is channel 4 and E1 is channel 5, what will the waves on these channels do when the patient looks up?
   A. Move toward each other
   B. Both move up
   C. Both move down
   D. Move away from each other

3. What is the purpose of the low-frequency filter?
   A. Eliminating undesired fast frequencies
   B. Eliminating undesired slow frequencies
   C. Adjusting signal amplitude
   D. Calibrating DC amplifiers

4. What should a technician do first to make sure the proper test is being performed?
   A. Contact the physician
   B. Review the chart for the physician's order
   C. Ask the patient for a chief complaint
   D. Perform physiological calibrations

5. The symbol "G1" represents
   A. The exploring electrode
   B. The reference electrode
   C. The patient ground
   D. The output of a differential amplifier to the polysomnograph

6. If G1 receives a signal of −100 μV at the same time G2 receives a signal of −50 μV, what is the output signal?
   A. −50 μV
   B. +50 μV
   C. −150 μV
   D. +150 μV

7. Which of the following is a process performed by a differential amplifier?
   A. Recording the differences in the voltages of two inputs
   B. Recording the differences in the voltages of the active input and ground
   C. Recording the differences in the voltages of an exploring electrode and the patient ground connection
   D. Recording only identical voltages received by its two inputs

8. If G1 and G2 simultaneously receive an input of 50 μV, what is the output signal?
   A. 0
   B. −100 μV
   C. +100 μV
   D. −50 μV

9. The frequency of an EEG signal
   A. Can be determined by counting the number of waveforms recorded during 1 second
   B. Can be determined by counting the number of waveforms recorded during one epoch
   C. Cannot be determined without using a water column manometer
   D. Depends on the paper speed

10. How is the amplitude of a wave determined?
    A. By reading the sensitivity setting on the polysomnography
    B. By comparing the relative height of the sleep waveforms against the patient's awake EEG
    C. By comparing the height of the patient's EEG slow waves to the patient's alpha waves
    D. By comparing the height of the waveform against a calibration signal of known value

11. The purpose of a high-frequency filter is
    A. To attenuate undesirable fast frequencies
    B. To attenuate undesirable slow frequencies
    C. To eliminate undesirable DC voltages from the signal output
    D. B and C are both correct

12. In polysomnography, what is the sensitivity setting?
    A. The offset between the electrical and the mechanical baselines
    B. The ratio of pen response to the settings of the low- and high-frequency filter settings
    C. The ratio of input signal voltage to the amplitude of the pen deflection
    D. The ratio of input signal voltage to the voltage of the calibration signal

13. An appropriate sensitivity setting for an EEG channel is:
    A. 5–7 μV/mm
    B. 10–12 μV/mm
    C. 20 μV/mm
    D. 10–100 μV/mm

14. Amplitude is a measure of
    A. Impedance
    B. Voltage
    C. Current
    D. Resistance

15. Adjusting the sensitivity from 5 µV/mm to 10 µV/mm will
    A. Double the pen deflection
    B. Increase the pen deflection by five times
    C. Reduce the pen deflection by one-half
    D. Reduce the pen deflection by five times

16. The standard paper speed used for a sleep study is
    A. 30 mm/sec
    B. 10 mm/sec
    C. 5 mm/sec
    D. 1 mm/sec

17. Which of the following filter settings would be most appropriate for EEG channels on a sleep study?
    A. LFF = 10 Hz, HFF = 100 Hz
    B. LFF = 1 Hz, HFF = 30 Hz
    C. LFF = 0.3 Hz, HFF = 30 Hz
    D. LFF = 0.1 Hz, HFF = 0.5 Hz

18. Which of the following filter settings are the most appropriate for recording EMG channels?
    A. LFF = 10 Hz, HFF = 100 Hz
    B. LFF = 1 Hz, HFF = 30 Hz
    C. LFF = 0.3 Hz, HFF = 30 Hz
    D. LFF = 0.1 Hz, HFF = 0.5 Hz

19. Which of the following filter settings should be used for recording airflow and respiratory effort?
    A. LFF = 10 Hz, HFF = 100 Hz
    B. LFF = 1 Hz, HFF = 30 Hz
    C. LFF = 0.3 Hz, HFF = 30 Hz
    D. LFF = 0.1 Hz, HFF = 0.5 Hz

20. What is a major difference between AC and DC amplifiers?
    A. DC amplifiers have a greater sensitivity range than AC amplifiers
    B. AC amplifiers have a high-frequency filter, whereas DC amplifiers do not
    C. AC amplifiers have a low-frequency filter, whereas DC amplifiers do not
    D. DC amplifiers have a polarity switch, whereas AC amplifiers do not

21. The quality and accuracy of a sleep recording is mostly determined by
    A. The type of equipment used to collect the data
    B. Proper electrode application
    C. The selective use of filters
    D. The type of software program used to analyze the data

22. The purpose of physiologic calibrations is to
    A. Establish certain scoring references for the sleep study
    B. Verify signal derivations for each channel
    C. Confirm the integrity of the signals
    D. All of the above

23. The recording of eye movements is based on
    A. Muscle activity produced by the right and left outer canthus
    B. Voltages from the frontal EEGs
    C. The electrical potential difference between the cornea and the retina
    D. The electrical potential difference between the right eye and the left eye

24. If the low-frequency filter is increased from 0.3 Hz to 1 Hz in an EEG channel, how will this affect the recording?
    A. The 1-Hz setting will decrease the amplitude of alpha waves
    B. The 1-Hz setting will decrease the frequency of alpha waves

    C. The 1-Hz setting will decrease the amplitude of slow waves
    D. A and C are correct

25. The right and left outer canthus electrodes (E2 and E1) are referenced to M2. According to polarity convention, an eye movement to the right should result in
    A. An upward pen deflection in both eye channels
    B. A downward pen deflection in both eye channels
    C. An upward pen deflection in the E2 channel and a downward pen deflection in the E1 channel
    D. A downward pen deflection in the E2 channel and an upward pen deflection in the E1 channel

26. Amplitude is a measurement of the _____ of a waveform, whereas frequency is a measurement of the _____ of a waveform.
    A. Speed, shape
    B. Shape, speed
    C. Height, shape
    D. Height, speed

27. EEG amplitude is measured in _____, whereas EEG frequency is measured in _____.
    A. Microvolts, Hertz
    B. Volts, Hertz
    C. Millivolts, cycles per second
    D. Microvolts, volts

28. Which of the following equations is true regarding sensitivity?
    A. Sensitivity = pen deflection/voltage
    B. Voltage = sensitivity/pen deflection
    C. Sensitivity = voltage/pen deflection
    D. Pen deflection = sensitivity/voltage

29. The low-frequency filter is most closely associated with
    A. The high-frequency filter
    B. The sensitivity of the amplifier
    C. The time constant
    D. The input signal

30. Which of the following is the recommended impedance level for EEG electrodes?
    A. Less than 20,000 ohms
    B. Less than 5 ohms
    C. Less than 5 kohms
    D. At least 20,000 ohms

31. A sleep study usually includes all but which of the following measurements?
    A. EOG
    B. ERG
    C. Respiratory effort
    D. EMG

32. The measured distance from the nasion to the inion is 36 cm. What is the distance from Cz to Pz?
    A. 1.8 cm
    B. 3.6 cm
    C. 7.2 cm
    D. 18 cm

33. The measured distance from the nasion to the inion is 32 cm. What is the distance from the inion to Oz?
    A. 1.6 cm
    B. 3.2 cm
    C. 6.4 cm
    D. 16 cm

34. The measured distance from Cz to T4 is 14 cm. What is the distance from C4 to T4?
    A. 1.4 cm
    B. 2.8 cm
    C. 3.5 cm
    D. 7.0 cm

35. The measured distance from pre-auricular to pre-auricular is 40 cm. What is the distance from Cz to C3?
  A. 2.0 cm
  B. 4.0 cm
  C. 8.0 cm
  D. 10 cm

36. The circumference of the patient's head is 56 cm. What is the distance from Oz to O1?
  A. 2.8 cm
  B. 5.6 cm
  C. 11.2 cm
  D. 28 cm

37. The circumference of the patient's head is 60 cm. What is the distance from O2 to T4?
  A. 3.0 cm
  B. 6.0 cm
  C. 12.0 cm
  D. 15.0 cm

38. Which EEG electrode site is half the distance from F8 to Fz?
  A. F4
  B. Fp2
  C. F6
  D. F2

39. Which EEG electrode site is half the distance from O1 to T3?
  A. Oz
  B. P3
  C. C3
  D. T5

40. The distance from Fp1 to O1 through C3 is 24 cm. What is the distance from C3 to P3?
  A. 2.4 cm
  B. 4.8 cm
  C. 6.0 cm
  D. 9.6 cm

41. The distance from Fp2 to T4 is 10 cm. What is the distance from Fp2 to F8?
  A. 2.0 cm
  B. 2.5 cm
  C. 5.0 cm
  D. 10 cm

42. Which electrode site is located half the distance between Fp2 and C4?
  A. P4
  B. O2
  C. T4
  D. F4

43. The circumference of the patient's head is 50 cm. What is the distance from T3 to Oz?
  A. 2.5 cm
  B. 5.0 cm
  C. 10 cm
  D. 12.5 cm

44. Which electrode site is half the distance from T3 to T4?
  A. Tz
  B. Cz
  C. T5
  D. P4

45. G1 = 60 μV, G2 = 10 μV. What is the output signal voltage?
  A. 70 μV
  B. 50 μV
  C. −50 μV
  D. −70 μV

46. Which of these is a possible result of referencing electrodes with dissimilar metals to each other?
    A. Galvanized skin response
    B. Fire
    C. Seizure
    D. Electric shock

47. Which of these is a DC channel?
    A. C3–M2
    B. Chin EMG
    C. E1
    D. SpO_2

48. Which of these types of wires is best for recording EEG activity?
    A. Snap lead
    B. Cup electrode
    C. Motion detector
    D. Clip lead

49. Which of these can be a disadvantage to using a gold cup?
    A. Difficult to break
    B. Increased cost
    C. Low impedances
    D. Requires disposable electrodes

50. The rate at which a wave repeats itself or oscillates is called its
    A. Frequency
    B. Amplitude
    C. Sensitivity
    D. Filter

51. A change in sensitivity produces a change in the
    A. Voltage of the incoming signal
    B. Frequency of the wave
    C. Height of the wave
    D. Color of the wave

52. The frequency of a waveform can be altered by adjusting its
    A. Sensitivity setting
    B. Filter
    C. Color
    D. Paper speed

53. Which of these LFF settings is preferred for an EEG channel?
    A. 0.5 Hz
    B. 3.0 Hz
    C. 10 Hz
    D. 35 Hz

54. Which of these settings is preferred for the HFF in an EMG channel?
    A. 5 Hz
    B. 10 Hz
    C. 30 Hz
    D. 70 Hz

55. Which of these HFF settings is preferred in the airflow channel?
    A. 0.5 Hz
    B. 1.0 Hz
    C. 5.0 Hz
    D. Off

56. Which of these HFF settings is preferred in an EEG channel?
    A. 5 Hz
    B. 10 Hz
    C. 35 Hz
    D. Off

57. In which of these channels is the shape of the waves most important?
    A. SpO_2
    B. EEG
    C. EMG
    D. Body position

58. Which of these is the best sensitivity setting for an EEG channel?
    A. 7 μV/mm
    B. 7 μV/cm
    C. 10 μV/mm
    D. 10 μV/cm

59. Which of these montages typically includes a full or expanded EEG hookup?
    A. Baseline
    B. CPAP
    C. Seizure
    D. MSLT

60. Which of these montages includes the use of a thermal and pressure channel to measure airflow?
    A. Baseline
    B. Seizure
    C. MSLT
    D. CPAP

61. What percentage of the circumference of the head is T5 from T3?
    A. 5%
    B. 10%
    C. 20%
    D. 25%

62. Where should the chin EMG electrodes be placed?
    A. Jaw and above chin
    B. Above and below chin
    C. Mentalis and jaw
    D. Tibialis and mentalis

63. Which of these electrode sites is not typically used in a baseline montage?
    A. Leg EMG
    B. E2
    C. Arm EMG
    D. Thoracic belt

64. The exploring electrode detects a voltage of −20 μV. The output voltage is 50 μV. What voltage did the reference electrode detect at this time?
    A. −30 μV
    B. 30 μV
    C. −70 μV
    D. 70 μV

65. Which muscle are the leg EMG electrodes placed on?
    A. Posterior tibialis
    B. Anterior tibialis
    C. Submentalis
    D. Mentalis

66. G1 and G2 both equal −25 μV. What is the output voltage?
    A. −25 μV
    B. −50 μV
    C. 0 μV
    D. 50 μV

67. Which of these electrodes is located 20% of the horizontal measurement of the head (pre-auricular point to pre-auricular point) to the left of Cz?
    A. T3
    B. C3
    C. C4
    D. P3

68. The E2 electrode is placed out and up from the outer corner of the right eye, and the E1 electrode is placed out and down from the outer corner of the left eye. If the montage has the E2 channel as channel 5 and the E1 channel as channel 6, what will the waves on these channels do when the patient looks up?
    A. Move toward each other
    B. Move away from each other
    C. Both move up
    D. Both move down

69. G1 = −80 µV and the output voltage is 20 µV. What is the voltage at G2?
    A. −100 µV
    B. −60 µV
    C. 60 µV
    D. 100 µV

70. Which electrode site is half the distance from Fp2 to T4?
    A. T6
    B. F8
    C. F4
    D. F6

71. What percentage of the vertical measurement of the head (nasion to inion) is Pz from the inion?
    A. 5%
    B. 20%
    C. 30%
    D. 50%

72. The distance from pre-auricular point to pre-auricular point is 36 cm. What is the distance from the left pre-auricular point to T3?
    A. 1.8 cm
    B. 3.6 cm
    C. 7.2 cm
    D. 18 cm

73. The measurement from T6 to Pz is 8 cm. What is the distance from P4 to Pz?
    A. 2 cm
    B. 4 cm
    C. 6 cm
    D. 8 cm

74. The measurement from F7 to F3 is 6 cm. What is the distance from F3 to Fz?
    A. 1.5 cm
    B. 2.0 cm
    C. 3.0 cm
    D. 6.0 cm

75. What electrode site is located half the distance from O2 to C4?
    A. T6
    B. P4
    C. T4
    D. P6

76. Which electrode site is 10% above the inion?
    A. Fpz
    B. T3
    C. Oz
    D. T4

77. A stress loop can be most helpful when applying which electrodes?
    A. Chin EMGs
    B. Leg EMGs
    C. EEGs
    D. ECGs

78. An EEG channel presents a high-amplitude, low-frequency artifact. Which of these is the most likely cause?
    A. EMG artifact
    B. ECG artifact
    C. Sweat artifact
    D. 60-Hz artifact

79. When using a sensitivity setting of 5 uV/mm, a 75-uV signal will result in a pen deflection of:
    A. 5 mm
    B. 7 cm
    C. 10 cm
    D. 15 mm

80. During physiologic calibrations, you notice a 60-Hz artifact in the leg EMGs. What is the best method of correcting this?
    A. Decrease the HFF to 35 Hz for this channel.
    B. Apply the line filter.
    C. Change the LFF setting for this channel.
    D. Reapply or replace the recording electrodes for this channel.

81. Which of the following actions should the technologist *not* take in response to a low amplitude in the airflow channel?
    A. Check for paradoxical breathing
    B. Increase the gain setting to improve signal quality
    C. Check or replace the airflow sensor
    D. Recalibrate the amplifier

82. Electrical interference can best be prevented if which of the following actions is taken?
    A. The 60-Hz filter is applied.
    B. The high-frequency filter is set at 15 Hz
    C. The impedances of input electrodes are similar
    D. Two ground leads are used

83. The polysomnograph has a leakage current of 200 μA. What should the technician do about this?
    A. Plug the equipment into an ungrounded plug to avoid a ground loop
    B. Do not use the equipment until the leakage current is lowered
    C. Continue to record because this leakage current is within acceptable limits
    D. Use an extra grounding electrode on the patients

84. During the night, the technician notices a gradual decline of the SpO_2 by 8%. Which of the following would help determine the cause of this event?
    I. Airflow and respiratory effort before the decrease in SaO_2
    II. Quality of the signal from the oximeter
    III. Placement of the oxygen sensor
    IV. Pigment of the patient's skin

    A. I and IV only
    B. I, II, and III only
    C. I, III, and IV only
    D. II, III, and IV only

85. Which of these sensors generates its own voltages and may be plugged directly into the head box?
    I. Thermocouple
    II. Thermistor
    III. Piezoelectric crystal band
    IV. Inductive plethysmograph

A. I and III only
B. I and IV only
C. II and III only
D. II and IV only

86. Tracing the signal pathway from the patient to the output of the polysomnograph can be beneficial for
    A. Troubleshooting equipment problems
    B. Gaining better understanding of the equipment
    C. Verifying correct signal derivations
    D. All of the above

87. Wires attached to the patient may be dangerous if
    A. The polysomnograph is not grounded
    B. Excessive electrical leakage is present
    C. The wires come in contact with an electrical outlet or other source of electrical current
    D. All of the above

88. A ground loop may occur when
    A. An exploring electrode is referenced to a ground electrode
    B. The patient is attached to more than one diagnostic device, each with its own patient ground connection
    C. Two or more electrodes are referenced to the same electrode
    D. All of the above

89. Which one or more of the following statements is true regarding notch filters?
    A. They are routinely used in all channels to help eliminate unwanted power line frequency interference
    B. They should not be used routinely in EEG recordings because they may camouflage a bad signal or unstable electrical environment
    C. They should only be used when absolutely necessary—for example, if minor 60-Hz interference occurs in one of the leg EMG channels
    D. B and C are correct

90. Which of the following is not true of muscle artifact?
    A. It is often seen when the patient is anxious or tense
    B. It will likely resolve once the patient falls asleep
    C. It can obscure relevant waveforms making scoring difficult.
    D. It is best corrected by using the notch filter

91. If a 60-Hz artifact is present during physiologic calibrations, the technologist should
    A. Change the signal derivation to a backup electrode and then initiate the study
    B. Wait until the patient falls asleep to see if the problem goes away
    C. Find the source of the problem and correct it before beginning the study
    D. Use a 60-Hz notch filter to eliminate the artifact

92. Slow-frequency artifact appearing in an EEG channel
    A. May be identified by a lack of correlation to EEG or EOG channels
    B. Can impair the accuracy of the recording
    C. May appear similar to EEG slow waves
    D. All of the above

93. Which of the following factors is most likely to cause a 60-Hz artifact?
    A. High and unequal electrode impedances
    B. Incorrect low- and high-frequency filter settings
    C. Incorrect placement of the reference electrodes
    D. Direct pressure against one of the electrodes

94. Which one or more of the following factors is most likely to cause electrode popping?
    A. Electrodes not firmly attached to the face or scalp
    B. Poor patient ground connection
    C. Direct pressure against an electrode
    D. A and C are correct

95. Which of the following conditions is most likely to cause slow wave artifact in the EEG or EOG channels?
    A. Muscle tension
    B. Sweat

C. Incorrect placement of the reference electrodes
D. A and C are correct

96. The optimal method of correcting undesirable artifacts while the patient is asleep is by
   A. Changing the input signal derivations
   B. Temporarily reducing the amplifier sensitivity of the channels affected by the artifact
   C. Applying 60-Hz notch filters to the channels affected by the artifact
   D. Changing the low- and high-frequency filters

97. During a recording, an identical slow wave artifact appears in three EEG channels sharing a common reference. The appropriate response is to
   A. Eliminate the artifact by double referencing the input signal derivation
   B. Eliminate the artifact by raising the low-frequency filters to 1 Hz
   C. Eliminate the artifact by re-referencing the input signal derivation to a backup reference electrode
   D. Either A or C is appropriate

98. If a high-frequency artifact appears in a single EEG channel that shares a reference electrode with other channels, the appropriate response is to
   A. Eliminate the artifact by re-referencing the input signal derivation to a backup reference electrode
   B. Eliminate the artifact by double referencing the input signal derivation
   C. Eliminate the artifact by changing the input signal derivation to a backup exploring electrode
   D. Eliminate the artifact by reducing the high-frequency filter to 15 Hz

99. If a mixed-frequency artifact appears in a channel because of a faulty electrode and no backup derivation is available, the appropriate response is to
   A. Try different low- and high-frequency filter setting combinations until the artifact is minimized
   B. Apply the 60-Hz filter
   C. Weigh the importance of the missing channel against the interruption to the patient's sleep study, then either enter the patient's room and fix the electrode or wait until an appropriate time to do so
   D. Reduce the sensitivity of the channel to minimize the artifact

100. A strong ECG artifact in an EMG channel:
   A. May be caused by poor electrode placement
   B. May be caused by high electrode impedances
   C. Is often unavoidable because EMG derivations are bipolar
   D. A and B are correct

101. If a low-frequency artifact appears in all the EEG and EOG channels, the appropriate response is to
   A. Double-reference all the channels
   B. Raise the low-frequency filters to 1 Hz
   C. Attempt to cool the patient by using a fan or air conditioner; then, if necessary, temporarily raise the low-frequency filters to 1 Hz
   D. Reduce the high-frequency filters to 15 Hz

102. Double referencing may be beneficial for
   A. Reducing ECG artifact in the EEG or eye channels
   B. Reducing sweat or respiration artifact in the EEG or eye channels
   C. Reducing popping artifact in the EEG or eye channels
   D. All of the above

103. If the thermistor becomes removed during a study, causing a flat line in the airflow channel, the best solution is to
   A. Try re-referencing the airflow channel to one of the respiratory effort channels
   B. Continue increasing the amplifier sensitivity until a signal response is seen
   C. Turn off the channel
   D. Enter the patient's room quietly and readjust the thermistor

104. When an artifact is present, changing the high- and low-frequency filters
   A. Is the best way to maintain an artifact-free recording
   B. Is only effective if the underlying physiological signals are still intact
   C. Should only be used as a last resort when other methods of correcting the artifact are unavailable
   D. B and C are correct

105. The preferred type of amplifier in polysomnography is
   A. Single-ended
   B. Triple-ended
   C. Differential
   D. Multifrequency

106. High and unequal electrode impedances
   A. Are common causes of recording artifact
   B. Inhibit the flow of physiological signals from the patient
   C. Promote the passage of interfering signals to the differential amplifier
   D. All of the above

107. The polarity convention for electrophysiology states that when G1 is more negative than G2, the pen
   A. Will not deflect
   B. Will deflect up
   C. Will deflect down
   D. None of the above

108. How far will the pen deflect if the sensitivity is 10 µV/cm and the input voltage is 75 µV?
   A. 75 mm
   B. 7.5 mm
   C. 10 cm
   D. 75 cm

109. What is the sensitivity setting if the pen deflects 1.5 mm and the input voltage is 75 µV?
   A. 5 µV/mm
   B. 5 µV/mm
   C. 50 µV/mm
   D. 500 µV/mm

110. What is the input voltage if the sensitivity is 5 µV/cm and the pen deflection is 10 cm?
   A. 500 µV
   B. 50 µV
   C. 5 µV
   D. 2 µV

111. Which of the following can cause 60-Hz interference?
   A. A faulty ground
   B. Electrical devices plugged in near the patient
   C. An open circuit
   D. All of the above

112. In most sleep systems, which of these devices is the patient head box directly plugged into?
   A. DC amplifier
   B. Wall outlet
   C. AC amplifier
   D. Polysomnograph

113. Which of these is a direct current (DC) channel?
   A. C3–M2
   B. Chin EMG
   C. E1
   D. SpO$_2$

114. Which of these is not a device that detects respiratory effort?
   A. Piezoelectric crystal band
   B. Cardiopneumograph
   C. Inductive plethysmograph
   D. Capnometer

115. What is the primary difference between thermistors and thermocouples?
   A. Thermocouples generate their own electricity, whereas thermistors do not
   B. Thermistors measure room temperature, whereas thermocouples measure airflow
   C. Thermistors generate their own electricity, whereas thermocouples do not
   D. Thermistors use two dissimilar metals

116. Which of these devices uses a cuff-and-bladder system?
    A. Inductive plethysmograph
    B. Mercury strain gauge
    C. Pneumatic respiratory transducer
    D. Esophageal balloon

117. A pH probe helps diagnose which of the following?
    A. Central sleep apnea
    B. Severe obstructive sleep apnea
    C. Primary snoring
    D. Esophageal reflux

118. Common mode rejection ratio (CMRR) refers to
    A. The ratio of protons to electrons in a neuron
    B. The ability of an amplifier to eliminate unwanted signals
    C. The ability of an electrode to conduct electricity
    D. The ratio of current to resistance

119. Which of these stores and releases energy in an alternating current circuit?
    A. Coulomb
    B. Amplifier
    C. Capacitor
    D. Resistor

120. What is the maximum allowable leakage in diagnostic equipment?
    A. $10\ \mu A$
    B. $100\ \mu A$
    C. $1,000\ \mu A$
    D. $10,000\ \mu A$

121. A frequency response curve is
    A. The slight curve that can be seen due to the pivot point of the pen
    B. The downward, or falling, slope of the calibration wave
    C. A visual representation of the filter and sensitivity settings for a channel
    D. A visual representation of the amplifier's ability to eliminate frequencies outside the filter settings

122. The rise time is the time it takes the pen to reach what percentage of its deflection?
    A. 33%
    B. 37%
    C. 63%
    D. 67%

123. The fall time is the amount of time for the pen to return to _____ of its baseline during amplifier calibrations
    A. 33%
    B. 37%
    C. 63%
    D. 67%

124. Which action is appropriate when noting an electrical impedance of 4 kohms in the M1 electrode during the initial impedance check?
    A. Use a notch filter
    B. Reprep the skin and replace electrode
    C. Re-reference to an alternate derivation
    D. None of these

125. During amplifier calibrations, the polysomnograph displays signals of
    A. $0\ \mu V$ and $100\ \mu V$
    B. $5\ \mu V$ and $-5\ \mu V$
    C. $50\ \mu V$ and $-50\ \mu V$
    D. $100\ \mu V$ and $-100\ \mu V$

126. The fall time constant is also referred to as the
    A. Rise time constant
    B. Balance voltage

C. Signal decay
D. Pen response

127. Which of these factors does not tend to increase impedances?
    A. Increased site preparation
    B. Broken or faulty wires
    C. Dirty electrodes
    D. Poor application

128. Which of these does not tend to increase leakage current?
    A. Shorter power cords
    B. Power strips
    C. Battery backups
    D. Parallel placement of wires

129. Which of these channel types produces a square calibration wave?
    A. EEG
    B. EMG
    C. Respiratory
    D. DC

130. Which of these devices receives and transmits signals from 0 to 1 volt?
    A. Head box
    B. Power box
    C. AC amplifier
    D. DC amplifier

131. Which of these respiratory effort devices uses coiled bands that are stretched during respiration?
    A. Pneumatic respiration transducer
    B. Inductive plethysmograph
    C. Mercury strain gauge
    D. Piezoelectric crystal band

132. A time constant of 1 second is equal to an LFF setting of
    A. 0.16 Hz
    B. 0.53 Hz
    C. 1 Hz
    D. 1.6 Hz

133. Amperes are measured in
    A. Volts/meter
    B. Current/resistance
    C. Coulombs/second
    D. Ohms

134. When electrical signals from external sources interfere with signals derived from the patient, this is referred to as
    A. Resistance
    B. Stray capacitance
    C. Cell potential
    D. Biopotentiality

135. Which of these monitoring devices can be used for long-term circadian rhythm monitoring?
    A. Transcutaneous CO_2
    B. Body position sensor
    C. pH probe
    D. Actigraph

136. At which point of the output waveform is end-tidal CO_2 read on a capnogram?
    A. During the beginning of inspiration
    B. During the beginning of expiration
    C. At the beginning of the expiratory phase
    D. At the end of the expiratory phase

137. What is the danger of using two ground wires on a piece of diagnostic equipment?
    A. Ground loop
    B. Electric shock
    C. Galvanized skin response
    D. Common mode rejection

138. Which of these devices produces its own electricity?
    A. Thermistor
    B. Oximeter
    C. Piezoelectric crystal band
    D. Actigraph

139. What value is provided by oximetry?
    A. SaO_2
    B. SpO_2
    C. PaO_2
    D. None of these

For questions 140–151, please refer to this page of sample calibration waves.

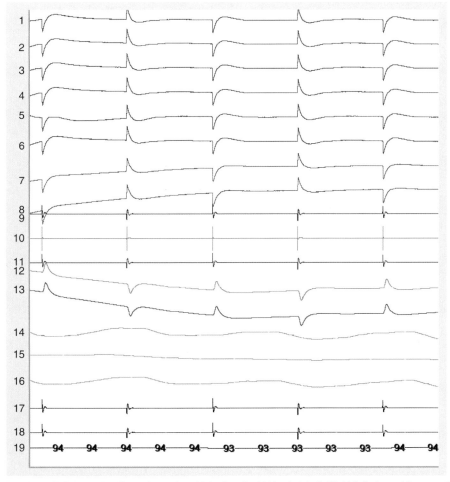

Figure by Lisa M. Endee; produced from a sleep study provided to Stony Brook University School of Health Technology and Management's Polysomnographic Technology Program by Dr. Kala Sury.

140. Which of the following channels is likely to be a leg EMG channel?
    A. 4
    B. 8
    C. 13
    D. 17

141. Which of the following channels is likely to be an airflow channel?
    A. 4
    B. 11
    C. 13
    D. 17

142. Which of the following channels has the highest time constant?
    A. 5
    B. 7
    C. 9
    D. 12

143. Which channel is likely to have a LFF of 0.16 Hz?
    A. 1
    B. 10
    C. 12
    D. 18

144. Which channel is likely to have a LFF of 10 Hz?
    A. 2
    B. 5
    C. 9
    D. 13

145. Which channel is likely to require a sensitivity setting of 20 V/mm?
    A. 3
    B. 6
    C. 9
    D. 12

146. What type of channel is channel 9?
    A. EMG
    B. Respiratory
    C. EEG
    D. EKG

147. Which channel is likely to be the snore channel?
    A. 2
    B. 7
    C. 11
    D. 13

148. What type of channel is channel 2?
    A. EMG
    B. EEG
    C. Respiratory
    D. DC

149. Which of the following channels has the lowest time constant?
    A. 5
    B. 7
    C. 9
    D. 12

150. What type of channel is channel 11?
    A. EMG
    B. Respiratory
    C. EEG
    D. DC

151. What type of channel is channel 8?
    A. EEG
    B. EMG
    C. Respiratory
    D. DC

152. Which of these are common side effects of PAP therapy?
    I.   Heavy snoring
    II. Nasal congestion
    III. Excessive daytime sleepiness
    IV. Dry upper airway

    A. I and II only
    B. I and III only
    C. II and IV only
    D. III and IV only

153. The physician orders a CPAP titration starting at 4 cm H_2O. The CPAP machine has separate controls for EPAP and IPAP. How should the machine controls be set in order to comply with the physician's orders?
    A. IPAP = 4, EPAP = 0
    B. IPAP = 4, EPAP = 4
    C. EPAP = 4, IPAP = 0
    D. EPAP = 8, IPAP = 4

154. What precautions should a technician take when setting up a patient with severe asthma?
    A. Consider the additional parameter of capnography
    B. Avoid the use of respiratory irritants like collodion
    C. Monitor oxygenation and ventilation closely for signs of distress
    D. All of these

155. Which of these items are required to administer oxygen to a patient?
    I.   Flow meter
    II. Water column manometer
    III. Physician's order
    IV. Humidifier

    A. I and II only
    B. I and III only
    C. I, III, and IV only
    D. II, III, and IV only

156. Which of these physiologic calibrations is not performed during an MSLT study?
    A. Clench jaw
    B. Move foot
    C. Eyes closed
    D. Eyes open

157. If the patient does not enter REM sleep during the first four naps of an MSLT, what should the technician do?
    A. Allow the patient to go home
    B. Delay the final nap by one hour
    C. Administer 5 mg of Ambien
    D. Perform the fifth nap as planned

158. What should the technician do if a patient arrives to the sleep lab for a CPAP titration, but the physician's order cannot be located?
    A. Allow the patient to go home
    B. Perform the CPAP titration as directed by the patient
    C. Perform a split night study
    D. Contact the physician

159. Which of these is true regarding a maintenance of wakefulness test?
    A. It is designed to demonstrate the effectiveness of treatment
    B. It is different from the MSLT in that the patient is instructed to remain awake
    C. It is not designed to test the extent of daytime sleepiness
    D. All of the above

160. During which type of study is the patient asked to remain awake for a period of time in a darkened room?
    A. REM behavior disorder study
    B. CPAP titration
    C. MWT
    D. MSLT

161. Which of these studies includes a series of four to five naps?
    A. REM behavior disorder study
    B. CPAP titration
    C. MSLT
    D. MWT

162. What artifact is seen here?

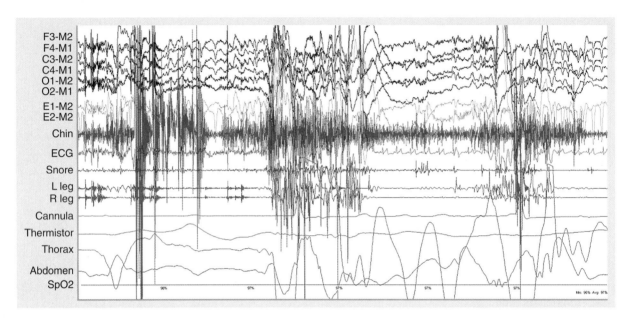

    A. ECG artifact
    B. Movement artifact
    C. Electrode popping
    D. Sweat or slow wave artifact

163. What artifact appears to be causing the high-amplitude, high-frequency activity circled?

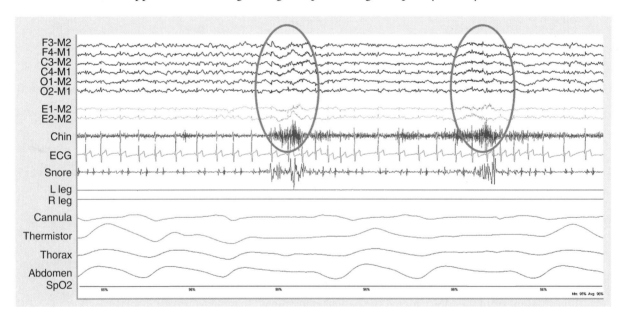

    A. Sweat or slow wave artifact
    B. Movement artifact
    C. 60-Hz artifact or high impedances
    D. Snore artifact

164. What artifact is seen in the snore channel?

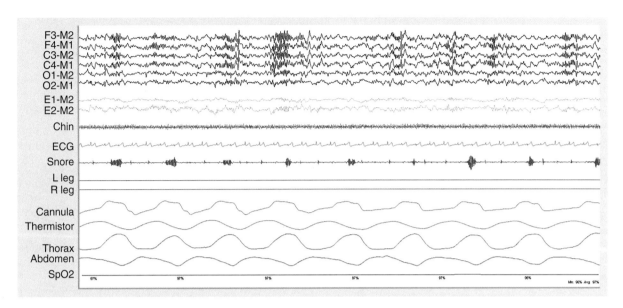

    A. ECG artifact

    B. Movement artifact

    C. High impedances

    D. Sweat or slow wave artifact

165. What artifact is seen in the C3–M2 channel?

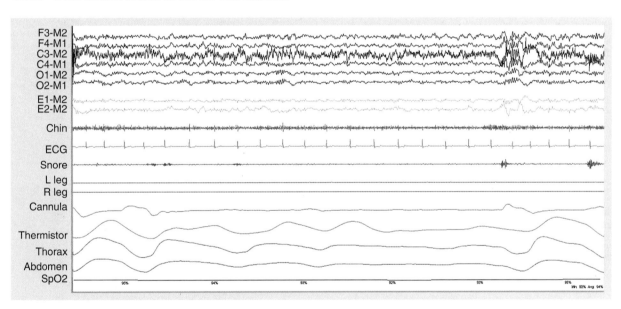

    A. Snore artifact

    B. Movement artifact

    C. ECG artifact

    D. 60-Hz artifact or high impedances

166. What artifact is seen in the snore channel?

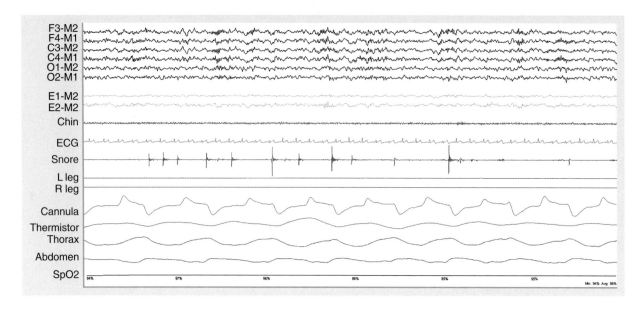

- A. Snore artifact
- B. Electrode popping
- C. Slow wave artifact
- D. This is not an artifact

167. What artifact is seen in the EEG channels?

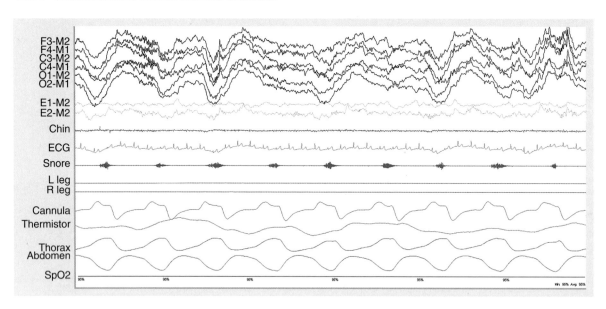

- A. Sweat or slow wave artifact
- B. Snore artifact
- C. Movement artifact
- D. Improper filter settings

168. What artifact is seen in the EEGs, EOGs, and chin EMG?

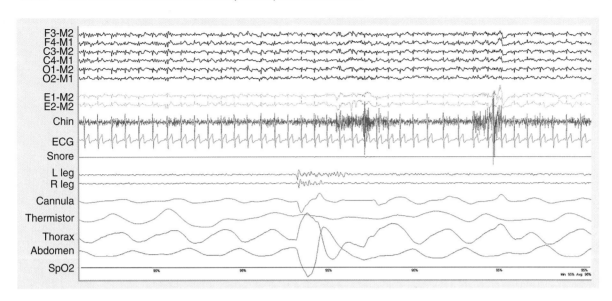

    A. Improper gain settings
    B. Snore artifact
    C. ECG artifact
    D. 60-Hz artifact or high impedances

169. What artifact is seen in the M2 electrode?

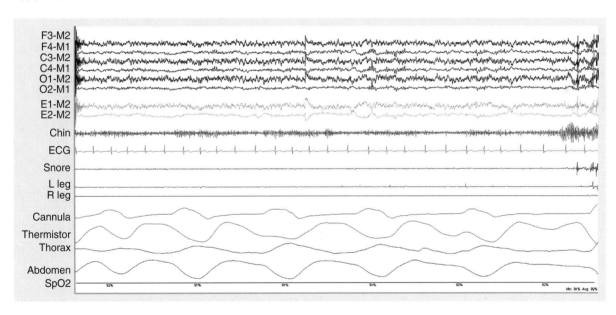

    A. Improper filter settings
    B. ECG artifact
    C. 60-Hz artifact or high impedances
    D. This is not an artifact

170. What artifact is circled in the snore channel?

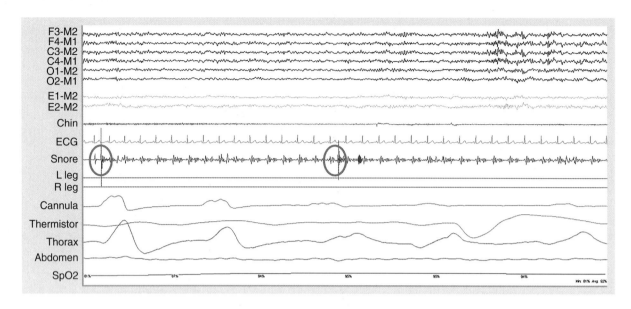

   A. Electrode popping
   B. Snore artifact
   C. Improper gain settings
   D. This is not an artifact

171. What artifact is seen here?

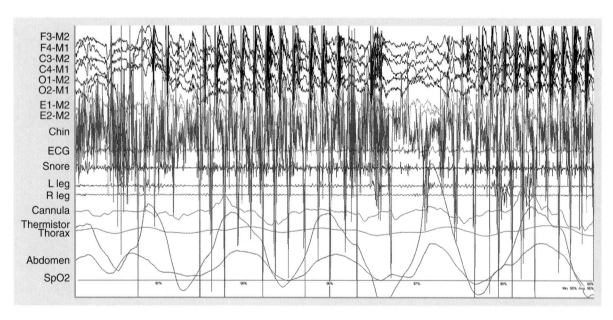

   A. Improper gain settings
   B. Improper filter settings
   C. ECG artifact
   D. 60-Hz artifact

172. What artifact is seen in the EEGs and ECG channel?

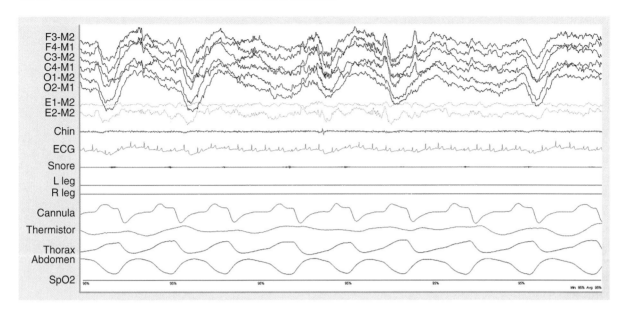

- **A.** Movement artifact
- **B.** Sweat or slow wave artifact
- **C.** Improper gain settings
- **D.** Improper filter settings

173. What artifact is seen here?

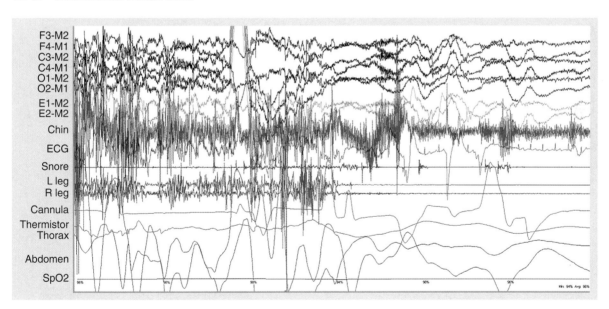

- **A.** Movement artifact
- **B.** ECG artifact
- **C.** Sweat artifact
- **D.** This is not an artifact

174.   What artifact is seen in the chin EMG channel?

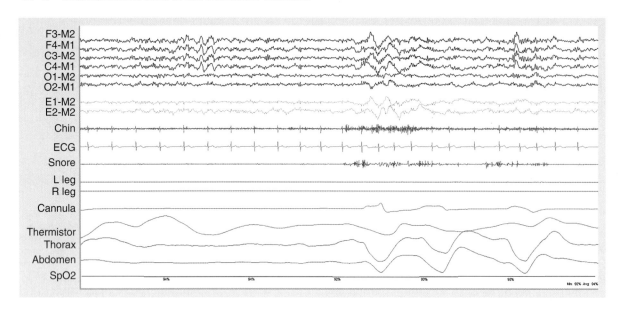

   A.   Snore artifact
   B.   ECG artifact
   C.   Movement artifact
   D.   This is not an artifact

175.   What artifact is seen here?

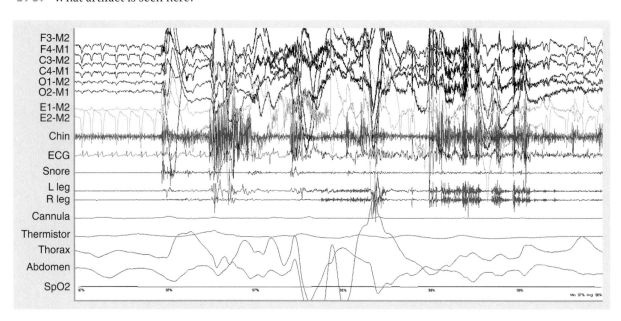

   A.   Snore artifact
   B.   ECG artifact
   C.   Movement artifact
   D.   This is not an artifact

176. What artifact is seen inside the circle?

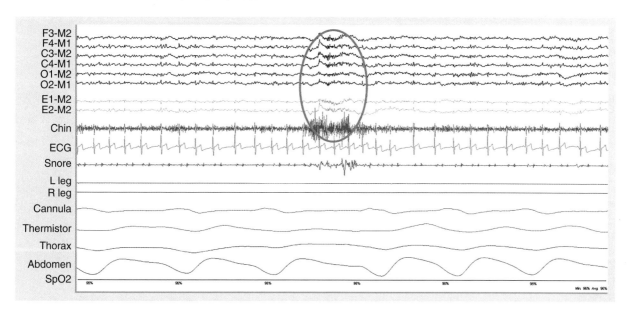

    A. Movement artifact
    B. ECG artifact
    C. Snore artifact
    D. This is not an artifact

177. What artifact is seen here?

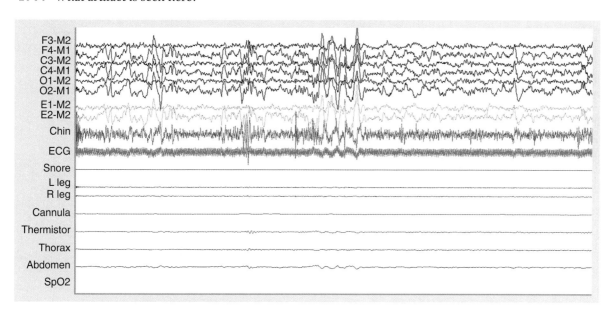

    A. Movement artifact
    B. Improper filter settings
    C. Improper gain settings
    D. 60-Hz artifact

178. What artifact is seen in the chin EMG channel?

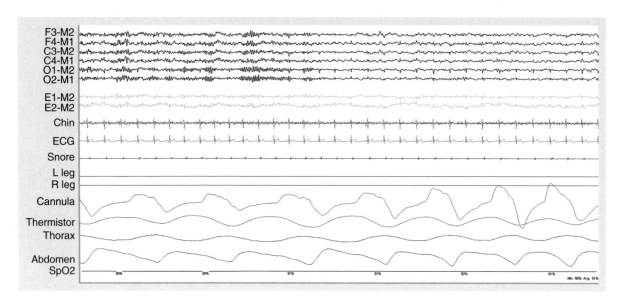

A. ECG artifact
B. Snore artifact
C. Movement artifact
D. This is not an artifact

179. What artifact is circled?

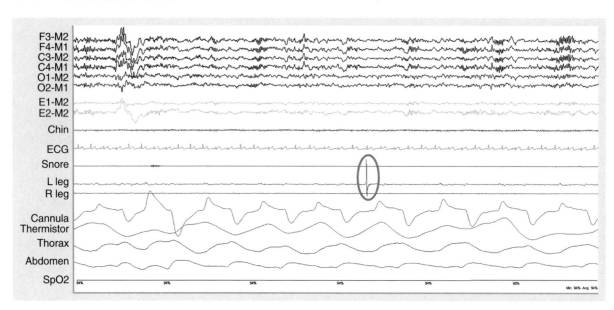

A. ECG artifact
B. Electrode popping
C. Snore artifact
D. This is not an artifact

180. What artifact is seen in the C4–M1 channel?

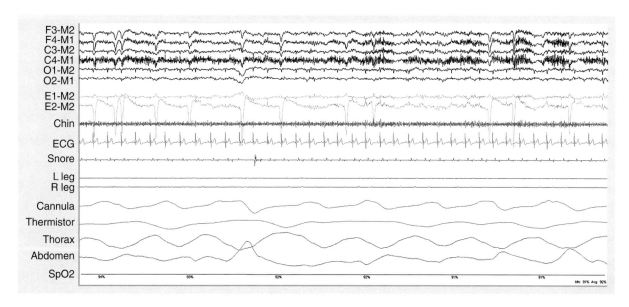

    A. Movement artifact
    B. Electrode popping
    C. High impedances or 60-Hz artifact
    D. ECG artifact

181. What artifact is seen here?

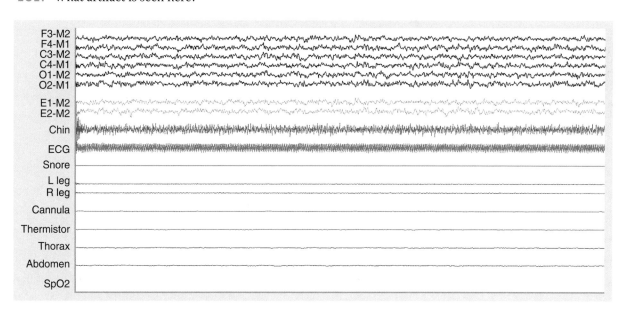

    A. 60-Hz artifact
    B. Improper gain settings
    C. Improper filter settings
    D. This is not an artifact

182. What artifact is seen in the chin EMG channel?

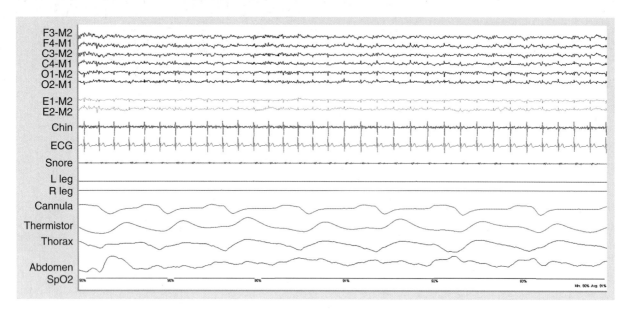

    A. ECG artifact
    B. Electrode popping
    C. Snore artifact
    D. Improper filter settings

183. What artifact is seen in the chin EMG?

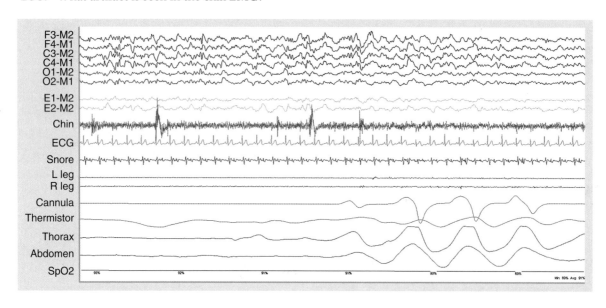

    A. ECG artifact
    B. Snore artifact
    C. Improper filter settings
    D. High impedances or 60-Hz artifact

184. In the image above, what artifact is seen in the snore channel?
    A. ECG artifact
    B. Snore artifact
    C. Improper filter settings
    D. High impedances or 60-Hz artifact

185. What artifact is seen in the chin EMG?

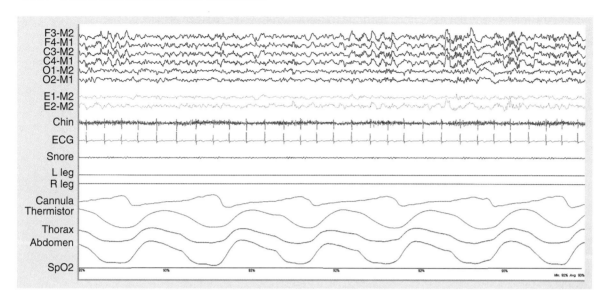

    A. ECG artifact
    B. Snore artifact
    C. Improper filter settings
    D. High impedances or 60-Hz artifact

186. What artifact is circled in the chin EMG channel?

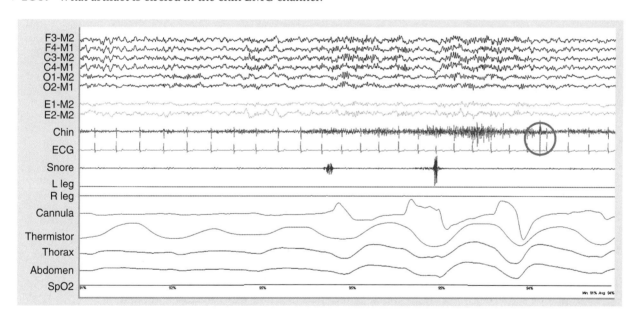

    A. ECG artifact
    B. Snore artifact
    C. Electrode popping
    D. High impedances or 60-Hz artifact

Domain 2: Scoring and Data Processing

187. Which of the following is not associated with the transition from wake to stage N1 sleep?
    A. An increase in alpha activity
    B. Slow-rolling eye movements
    C. Occasional epileptiform activity
    D. A low-voltage, mixed-frequency EEG pattern

188. Which of these characteristics is not a feature of relaxed wakefulness with the eyes open?
    A. Relatively low-voltage, mixed-frequency EEG
    B. Vertex sharp waves
    C. Elevated chin EMG
    D. Rapid eye movements and eye blinks

189. Which of these characteristics is not a feature of relaxed wakefulness with the eyes closed?
    A. Sawtooth waves
    B. Elevated chin EMG
    C. Alpha rhythm
    D. Slow-rolling eye movements

190. What is the frequency of alpha waves?
    A. <2 Hz
    B. 4–7 Hz
    C. 8–13 Hz
    D. >13 Hz

191. What is the frequency of theta waves?
    A. <2 Hz
    B. 4–7 Hz
    C. 8–13 Hz
    D. >13 Hz

192. Which of these are characteristics of stage N1 sleep?
    A. Relatively low-voltage, mixed-frequency EEG; slow-rolling eye movements; and a normally active chin EMG
    B. Relatively low-voltage, mixed-frequency EEG; slow-rolling eye movements; and sleep spindles
    C. Alpha activity in the EEG, slow-rolling eye movements, and a normally active chin EMG
    D. Relatively low-voltage, mixed-frequency EEG; slow-rolling eye movements; and absence of muscle activity in the chin EMG

193. Which of these conditions is not likely to contribute to episodes of hypoventilation or hypoxemia or both?
    A. Partial or complete upper-airway obstruction
    B. Chronic obstructive pulmonary disease
    C. Obesity
    D. Diabetes

194. Which of these statements is true regarding hypoventilation during sleep?
    A. It is identified by measuring a reduction in amplitude in the airflow channel tracings
    B. It can be accurately detected by transcutaneous CO_2 monitoring
    C. It may be suspected when the breathing pattern becomes noticeably shallow and rapid
    D. It can be accurately detected by oximetry

195. Frequent EEG arousals during sleep
    A. May lead to excessive daytime sleepiness
    B. May occur with or without discernible sleep stage changes or body movement
    C. May be an indication of sleep-disordered breathing
    D. All of the above

196. An irregular pattern seen in the airflow channel may be an indication of
    A. Artifact caused by body movement
    B. Wakefulness
    C. Sleep-disordered breathing
    D. All of the above

197. Which of these characteristics is not normally seen at sleep onset?
   A. Slow-rolling eye movements
   B. Decreased chin EMG amplitude
   C. Increase in EEG frequency
   D. Decrease in EEG frequency

198. In most sleepers, what happens to the chin EMG at sleep onset?
   A. It increases in frequency.
   B. It decreases in frequency.
   C. It increases in amplitude.
   D. It decreases in amplitude.

199. What is the oxygen desaturation criteria to score a hypopnea
   A. 1%
   B. 3%
   C. 4%
   D. 10%

200. Which of these events can be caused by titrating CPAP too quickly?
   A. Hypopnea
   B. Obstructive apnea
   C. Central apnea
   D. Mixed apnea

201. What is a primary difference between an apnea and a hypopnea?
   A. An apnea lasts longer than a hypopnea
   B. A hypopnea lasts longer than an apnea
   C. An apnea is a full cessation of airflow (at least a 90% decrease), whereas a hypopnea is a decrease in airflow
   D. A hypopnea is a full cessation of airflow (at least a 90% decrease), whereas an apnea is a decrease in airflow

202. What is the required duration of an apnea?
   A. 5 seconds
   B. 10 seconds
   C. 20 seconds
   D. There is no duration requirement for an apnea

203. What is the term used for opposite effort patterns in the chest and abdomen (the abdomen contracting while the thorax is expanding and vice versa)?
   A. Paradoxical breathing
   B. Cheyne–Stokes breathing
   C. Central apnea syndrome
   D. Hypoventilation syndrome

204. What respiratory event is characterized by a slow waxing and waning pattern seen in the airflow and effort belts?
   A. Mixed apneas
   B. Paradoxical breathing
   C. Upper-airway resistance
   D. Cheyne–Stokes breathing

205. What respiratory event is characterized by a cessation in respiratory effort at the same time as a cessation in airflow?
   A. Hypopnea
   B. Obstructive apnea
   C. Central apnea
   D. Mixed apnea

206. Which of these is not characteristic of REM sleep?
   A. Stabilization of blood pressure
   B. Increased consumption of oxygen by the brain
   C. Decreased muscle tone
   D. Heart rhythm irregularities

207. The sleep latencies for MSLT naps are as follows: 6 min, 7 min, 10 min, 1 min, 6 min. What is the mean sleep latency?
    A. 4 min
    B. 6 min
    C. 10 min
    D. 12 min

208. Using the sleep latencies from the previous question, what is the mode sleep latency?
    A. 5 min
    B. 6 min
    C. 7 min
    D. 10 min

209. The sleep latencies for MSLT naps are as follows: 8 min, 7 min, 11 min, 14 min, 1 min. What is the median sleep latency?
    A. 8 min
    B. 7 min
    C. 2 min
    D. 10 min

210. Lights out for an MSLT nap occurred at 08:00. Sleep onset occurred at 08:10. At what time should lights on occur?
    A. 08:20
    B. 08:25
    C. 08:30
    D. When the patient awakens on his or her own

211. REM sleep is dominant during which portion of the night?
    A. First third
    B. Second third
    C. Final third
    D. First half

212. Which of the following is not part of the narcolepsy tetrad?
    A. Excessive daytime sleepiness
    B. Nocturnal myoclonus
    C. Cataplexy
    D. Sleep paralysis

213. The sleep stage formerly called *active sleep* in pediatric patients is similar to what adult stage of sleep?
    A. Stage R
    B. Stage N1
    C. Stage N2
    D. Stage N3

214. The sleep stage formerly called *quiet sleep* in pediatric patients is similar to what adult stage of sleep?
    A. Stage R
    B. Stage N1
    C. Stage N2
    D. Stage N3

215. In what age group are high-amplitude, low-frequency EEG waves most often seen?
    A. Infants
    B. Adolescents
    C. Middle-aged adults
    D. Older adults

216. How many limb movements are required in a series of periodic limb movements?
    A. 2
    B. 4
    C. 6
    D. There is no minimum requirement.
    E. Coffee in the morning

217. What is the primary difference between PLMD and RLS?
     A. PLMD includes separate leg movements during sleep, whereas RLS consists of continuous leg movements during sleep
     B. PLMD is the former name for RLS
     C. PLMD occurs during REM sleep only
     D. RLS can occur during wakefulness

218. Which of the following is not required to include a leg movement in a PLM sequence?
     A. EEG arousals
     B. Amplitude
     C. Interval
     D. Duration

219. Which of these events occur during wake?
     A. Low-voltage, mixed-frequency EEG pattern and rapid eye movements
     B. Eye blinks and increased muscle tone
     C. Beta frequency EEG patterns and slow-rolling eye movements
     D. Slow-rolling eye movements and increased muscle tone

220. Which of these best defines a K-complex?
     A. A minimum of 0.5 seconds in duration
     B. A minimum of 0.5 seconds in duration with a 75-μV amplitude
     C. Biphasic with a minimum 0.5-second duration and 75-μV amplitude
     D. Biphasic with a minimum 0.5-second duration

221. Which of these best defines an EEG arousal during NREM sleep?
     A. An increase in EEG frequency for at least 3 seconds
     B. A shift in EEG frequency for at least 3 seconds
     C. An EEG burst of 8 to 10 Hz for at least 5 seconds
     D. An increase in chin EMG tone for at least 5 seconds

222. Which of these best describes the end of a period of REM?
     A. The absence of rapid eye movements for at least 3 minutes
     B. A sustained increase in chin EMG amplitude with slow-rolling eye movements
     C. 8- to 10-Hz activity in the EEG channels
     D. The disappearance of sawtooth waves in the EEGs

223. Which of the following best describes an epoch of stage N3 sleep?
     A. At least 50% of the epoch contains waves of *five* cycles per second or slower that have amplitudes greater than 75 μV peak to peak
     B. At least 50% of the epoch contains waves of five cycles per second that are greater than 75 μV peak to peak
     C. At least 20% of the epoch contains waves of two cycles per second or slower that have amplitudes greater than 75 μV peak to peak
     D. At least 20% of the epoch contains waves of two cycles per second or slower that have amplitudes greater than 50 μV peak to peak

224. The scoring technologist notices sudden bursts of high-amplitude, high-frequency activity in all channels. These bursts occur six times during the study at 1-hour intervals. These are most likely
     A. Generalized seizures
     B. Impedance checks
     C. Bruxism
     D. Movement arousals

225. EEG waves with frequencies of 4 to 7.5 Hz are
     I. The most common background sleep frequency
     II. Barbiturate related
     III. Seen in stage REM sleep
     IV. Indicative of night terrors

     A. I and III only
     B. I and IV only
     C. II and III only
     D. II and IV only

226. Alpha rhythm during wake with the eyes closed is best viewed from which area of the brain?
    A. Temporal
    B. Central
    C. Occipital
    D. Frontal

227. Stage N1 is characterized by
    A. A relatively low-voltage, mixed-frequency EEG with a prominence of activity in the 2–7 cps range
    B. A relatively low-voltage, mixed-frequency EEG with distinctive sawtooth waves
    C. A relatively low-voltage, mixed-frequency EEG with a prominence of activity in the 8–13 cps range
    D. The presence of sleep spindles or K-complexes (or both) and the absence of high-amplitude, slow EEG activity

228. What stage of sleep was previously called *transitional sleep* or *drowsy sleep*?
    A. Stage N1
    B. Stage N2
    C. Stage N3
    D. REM

229. Low-frequency, high-amplitude waves are most prevalent during which stage?
    A. Stage N1
    B. Stage N2
    C. Stage N3
    D. REM

230. About how long is a typical period of stage N1?
    A. 0–1 minutes
    B. 1–7 minutes
    C. 20 minutes
    D. 30 minutes

231. What is the amplitude requirement for an EEG slow wave?
    A. 25 µV
    B. 50 µV
    C. 75 µV
    D. There is no amplitude requirement for an EEG slow wave

232. What is the amplitude requirement for a K-complex?
    A. 10 Hz
    B. 25 Hz
    C. 75 Hz
    D. There is no amplitude requirement for a K-complex

233. What characteristics of EEG waves are taken into account when determining sleep stages?
    I. Amplitude
    II. Frequency
    III. Dampening
    IV. Shape

    A. I and II only
    B. I, II, and IV only
    C. III and IV only
    D. All of these

234. Low-voltage, mixed-frequency EEG waves are the prominent pattern in which stages?
    I. Wake
    II. Stage N1
    III. Stage N2
    IV. REM

    A. I and II only
    B. II and IV only
    C. I, II, and IV only
    D. All of these

235. Which of the following can be used as an epoch score?
    A. Movement time
    B. Movement arousal
    C. Major body movement
    D. Movement epoch

236. When scoring sleep stages, how many seconds should each page display?
    A. 10
    B. 30
    C. 60
    D. 120

237. An epoch containing rapid eye movements, high tonic EMG, and alpha waves should be scored as
    A. Wake
    B. Stage N1
    C. Stage N3
    D. REM

238. Which of these can influence the amplitude of an EEG wave?
    I.   Electrical impedance
    II.   Inter-electrode distance
    III. Cerebral activity
    IV.   Electrode placement

    A. I only
    B. I, II, and IV only
    C. II, III, and IV only
    D. All of these

239. When the exploring electrode and reference electrode are extremely close to each other, the amplitude of the resulting wave is _____. When they are far apart from each other, the amplitude of the resulting wave is _____.
    A. Low, high
    B. Average, high
    C. High, low
    D. Average, low

240. What stages can alpha waves appear in?
    A. Wake or REM only
    B. Wake only
    C. Wake or stage N1 only
    D. Any stage

241. If 30% of an epoch consists of EEG slow waves, but K-complexes and sleep spindles are also in the same epoch, what should it be scored as?
    A. Stage N2
    B. Stage N3
    C. Major body movement
    D. Wake

242. What frequency are EEG slow waves?
    A. 0.5–2
    B. <0.5
    C. <2
    D. >0.5

243. Which of these best describes beta spindles?
    A. High-amplitude bursts of EEG activity greater than 13 Hz
    B. Low-amplitude bursts of EEG activity in the range of 8–13 Hz
    C. High-amplitude bursts of EEG activity in the range of 8–13 Hz
    D. Low-amplitude bursts of EEG activity greater than 13 Hz

244. A patient was in stage N2, but an EEG arousal occurred without a following sleep spindle or a K-complex. If the next epoch continues with this pattern, it should be scored as
    A. Stage N1
    B. Stage N2
    C. Wake
    D. REM

245. What is the minimum duration requirement for sleep spindles?
    A. 0.5 seconds
    B. 2 seconds
    C. 3 seconds
    D. There is no duration requirement for sleep spindles

246. When are V waves most commonly seen?
    A. At the end of wakefulness
    B. At the end of stage N1
    C. At sleep onset (beginning of stage N1)
    D. During REM

247. Sleep onset is defined as
    A. The first epoch of any stage of sleep
    B. The first three continuous epochs of sleep
    C. The first three continuous epochs of stage N1 or the first epoch of any other stage of sleep
    D. The point at which alpha waves disappear

248. The average adult spends approximately what percentage of total sleep time in stage N2?
    A. 5%
    B. 10%
    C. 25%
    D. 50%

249. Approximately what percentage of the total sleep time is spent in REM?
    A. 5%
    B. 10%
    C. 25%
    D. 50%

250. EEG arousals cannot be scored
    A. Within 3 seconds of each other
    B. Within 10 seconds of each other
    C. Within 30 seconds of each other
    D. Within the same 30-second epoch of each other

251. A patient is in stage N2 when the chin EMG increases dramatically in amplitude for 5 seconds AND then returns to its original amplitude. No changes are seen in the EEGs during the time period. How should this 5-second period be scored?
    A. It should not be scored
    B. It should be scored as an EEG arousal
    C. It should be scored as a snore
    D. It should be scored as movement

252. A 3-second-long period of alpha intrusion during sleep
    A. Is considered an EEG arousal
    B. Is not considered an EEG arousal unless it is preceded by at least 10 seconds of uninterrupted sleep
    C. Is not considered an arousal unless the entire preceding epoch is alpha free
    D. Is not considered an arousal

253. Ectopic beats that originate below the Bundle of His and occur earlier than expected are
    A. Premature ventricular contractions
    B. Premature atrial contractions
    C. Nodal escape beats
    D. Junctional escape beats

254. On the sleep report, the total recording time is 480 minutes, and the sleep latency is 3 minutes. The patient is asleep at lights on. The total amount of time the patient is awake after sleep onset and before the final awakening is 21 minutes. What is the total sleep time?
    A. 418 minutes
    B. 456 minutes
    C. 462 minutes
    D. Not enough information

255. During a sleep study, the respiratory effort channels suddenly flatten. The airflow channel during this time consists of oscillations of extremely low amplitude with a frequency of approximately 65 Hz. The respiratory rate just before this event was 16 breaths per minute. Which of the following is the most likely conclusion?
    A. The patient is hyperventilating
    B. The airflow device needs to be repositioned
    C. The flow channel's HFF is too high
    D. The patient is having central apneas

256. A computer-generated sleep study report indicates a sleep latency of 15 minutes. The scoring technologist's review indicates a sleep latency of 6.0 minutes. Which of the following is most likely the cause of this discrepancy?
    A. Inaccuracy in the total epoch count
    B. Inaccurate computer clock time
    C. Failure to mark lights on
    D. Failure to mark lights out

257. A patient's ECG tracing shows an irregular R–R rhythm with no visible alterations to the P, QRS, and T waves. Which arrhythmia is this?
    A. Premature atrial contractions
    B. Sinus arrhythmia
    C. Second-degree AV block type II
    D. Third-degree AV block

258. A rapid, bizarre, wide QRS complex with no P wave is referred to as a
    A. Sinus tachycardia
    B. Ventricular tachycardia
    C. Premature ventricular contraction
    D. Normal sinus rhythm

259. Atrial beats that arise earlier than expected, with a normal QRS complex are
    A. Premature atrial contractions
    B. Premature ventricular contractions
    C. Normal sinus rhythm
    D. Atrial flutter

For Questions 260–289, identify the cardiac rhythm that is described.

260. There is a P wave for every QRS complex. The rate is 70 beats per minute and the QRS complex is within normal limits.

261. The P wave is seen as rapid flutter waves. The ventricular rate is regular or irregular and slower. The QRS complex is within normal limits.

262. The baseline wave is irregular, and P waves are absent. Ventricular response (QRS) is irregular, slow, or rapid.

263. There is no relationship between the P waves and the QRS complexes. The QRS rate is slower than the P rate.

264. The P wave precedes each QRS complex, but the PR interval is 0.2 seconds.

265. The P wave is sawtoothed. The atrial rate is rapid (250–350 beats per minute). The ventricular rhythm is usually regular. The ventricular rate is 40–90 bpm but may be higher. The QRS complex is within normal limits.

266. Diseased tissues of the AV node conduct each impulse earlier in the refractory period. Eventually, an impulse is absent. The next impulse is conducted normally.

267. There is a total absence of ventricular activity, although some activity may be present in the atria. There is a flat line on the ECG.

268. There is no P wave. The QRS complex occurs earlier than expected, is wide (0.12 sec or greater), and has a bizarre-looking configuration and an increased amplitude.

269. There is a sustained rhythm of three or more PVCs in a row.

270. The P wave is normal in size. The atrial rate is greater than 100 bpm. The ventricular rate is greater than 90 bpm. The QRS complex is within normal limits.

271. The P wave is not discernible. The atrial rate and rhythm cannot be determined. The ventricular rhythm is chaotic, with no pattern or regularity. The ventricular rate cannot be determined. The duration of the QRS complex is not discernible.

272. There are intermittent blocks of sinus impulses in the AV node. Dropped beats occur without warning.

273. The P wave may or may not be present. There is no conduction of the atrial impulse to the ventricles. QRS complexes are absent.

274. The P wave is normal in size. The ventricular rate is less than 40 bpm. The QRS complex is within normal limits.

275. Ectopic beats originating low in the ventricles occur earlier than expected.

276. The atria and ventricles depolarize independently from each other.

277. The atrial rhythm is characterized by disorganized atrial activity without discernible P waves.

278. The P wave is usually absent but may be obscured by the QRS complex. The atrial rate cannot be determined. The ventricular rate is 100 to 250 bpm. The QRS complex is wide and bizarre looking, usually with increased amplitude.

279. There is a suddenly dropped QRS complex without prior PR lengthening.

280.   Electrical impulses flow normally from the SA node through the atria but are delayed at the AV node. The P wave is normal in size. The PR interval is prolonged (greater than 0.20 seconds) but is constant in duration. The QRS complex is within normal limits.

281.   The P–P intervals are constant. The PR interval progressively lengthens with each cycle until a P wave appears without a QRS complex. The QRS complex is within normal limits.

282.   The sinus rhythm is greater than 100 bpm.

283.   There are premature and abnormally shaped P waves. The PR interval is typically within normal limits but may be short or slightly prolonged. The QRS complex is usually within normal limits and normal configuration.

284.   There is a rapid, disorganized depolarization of the ventricles. The ECG tracing consists of a wavy baseline. Large waves indicate coarse fibrillation, and small waves indicate fine fibrillation.

285.   There is a progressive lengthening of the PR interval with intermittently dropped beats.

286.   The sinus rhythm is less than 40 bpm.

287.   There is a complete block of all supraventricular impulses from reaching the ventricles. The atrial rate is usually faster than normal.

288.   Two PVCs in a row.

289.   Three or more PVCs in a row.

For the following test questions, please refer to the sample epochs on the next several pages.
290.   What stage is this?

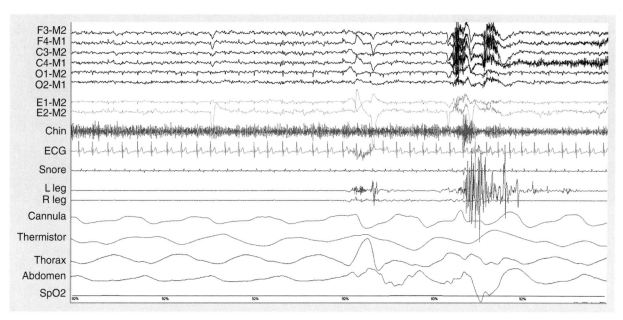

291. What stage is this?

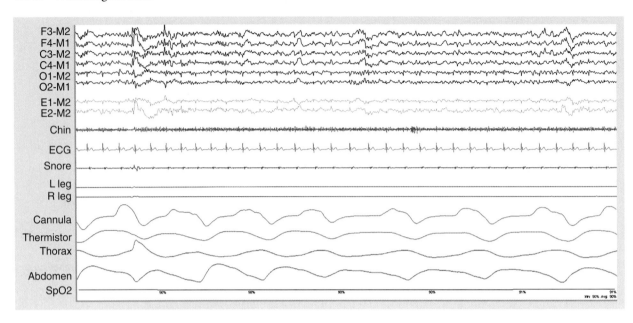

292. What stage is this?

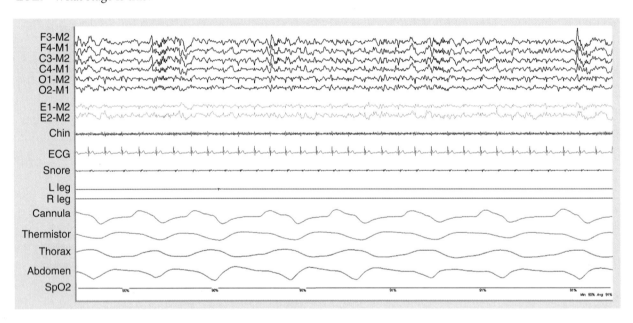

293. What stage is this?

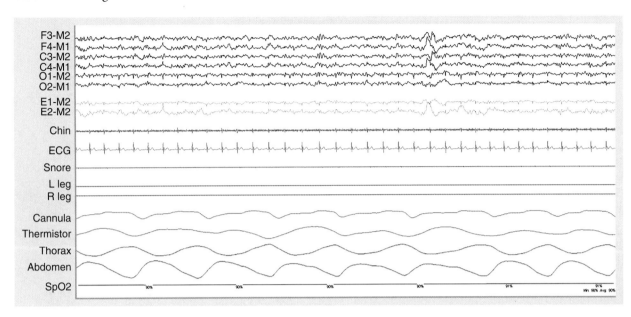

294. What stage is this?

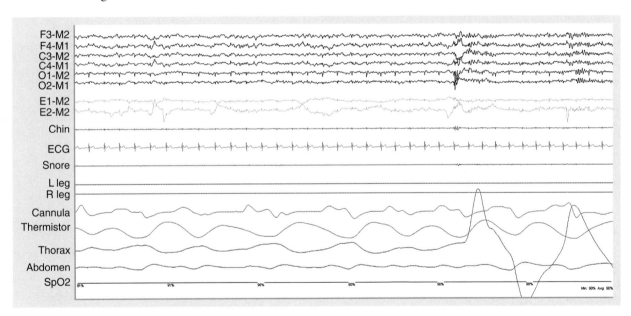

295. What stage is this?

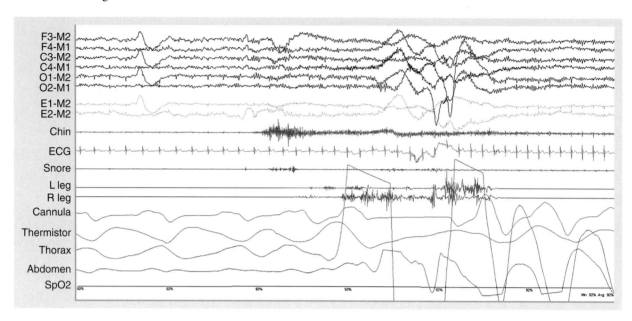

296. What stage is this?

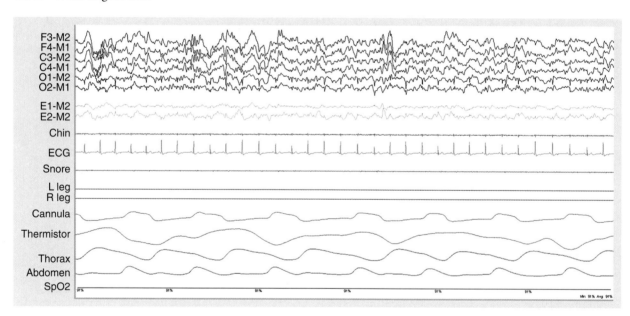

297. What stage is this?

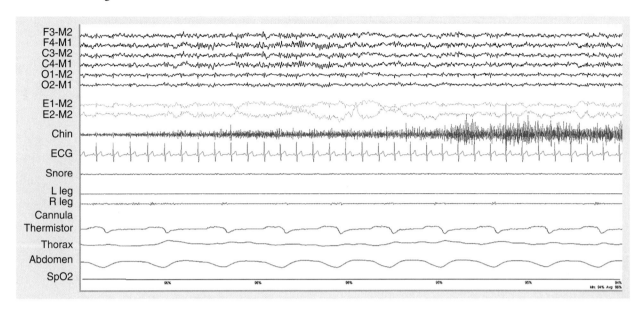

298. What stage is this?

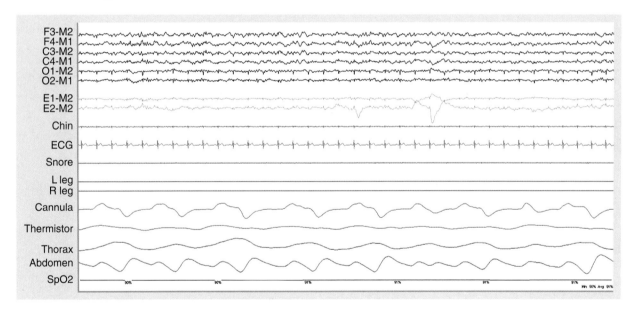

299. What stage is this?

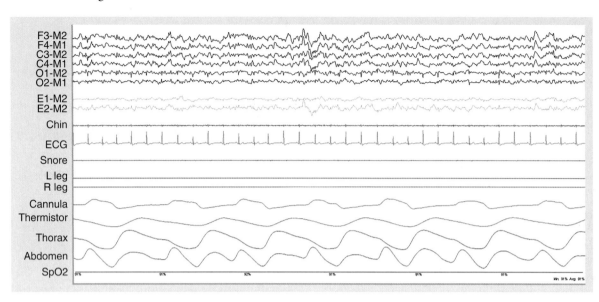

300. What stage is this?

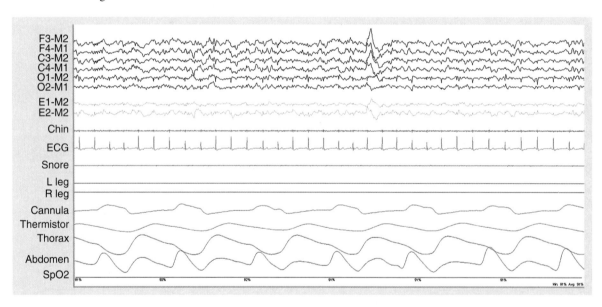

301. What stage is this?

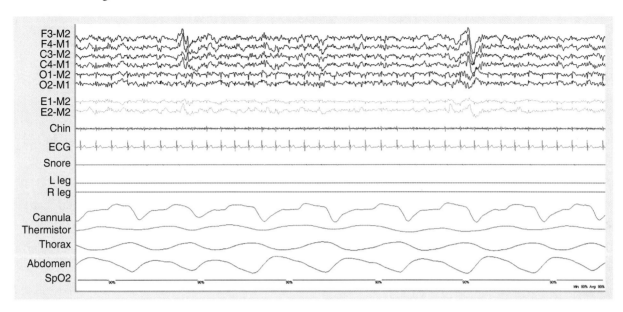

302. What stage is this?

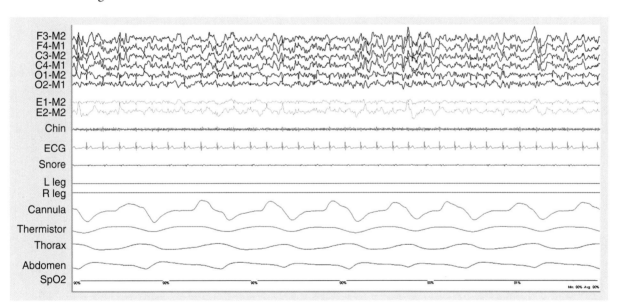

303. What stage is this?

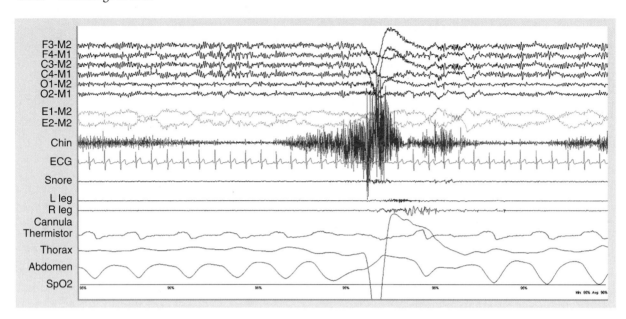

304. What stage is this?

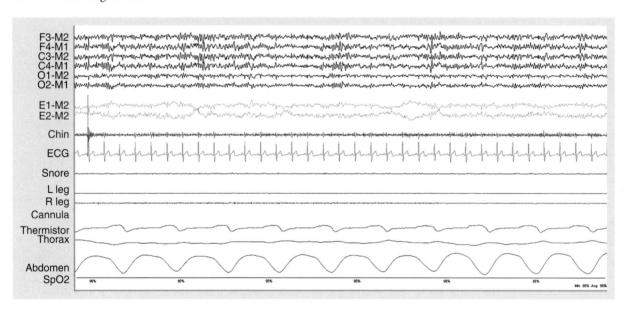

305. What stage is this?

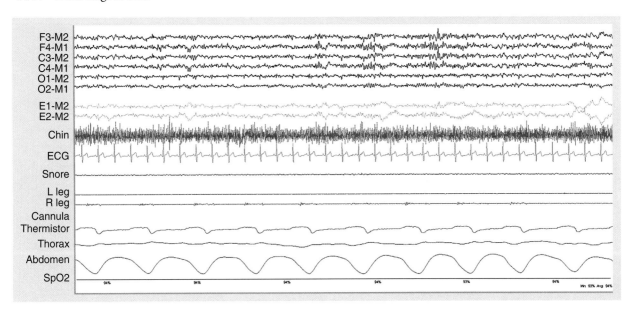

306. What stage is this?

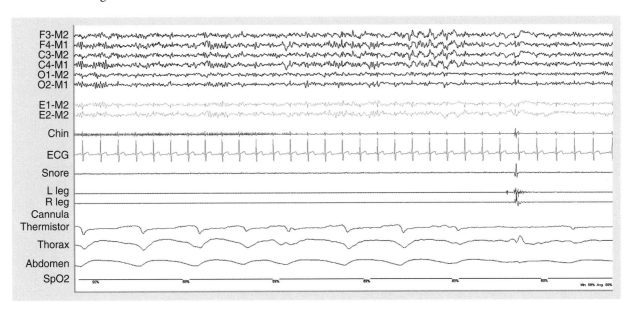

307. What stage is this?

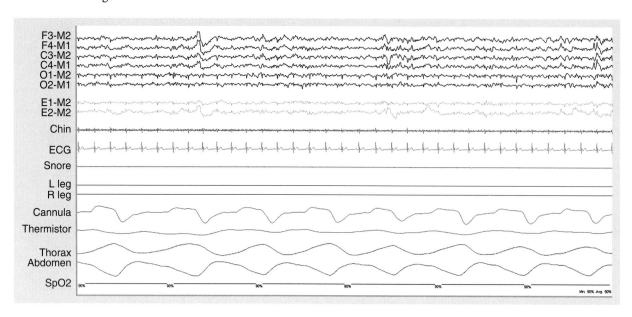

308. What stage is this?

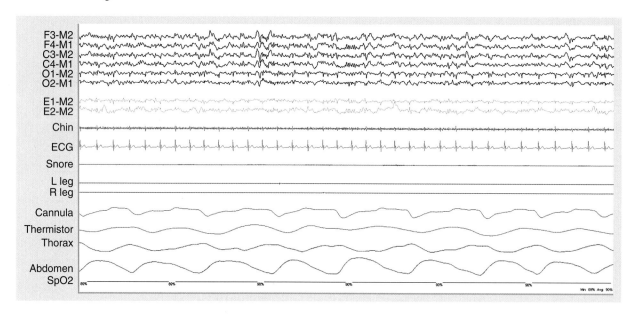

309. What stage is this?

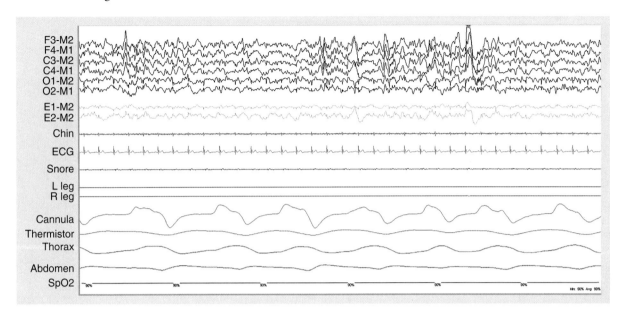

310. What stage is this?

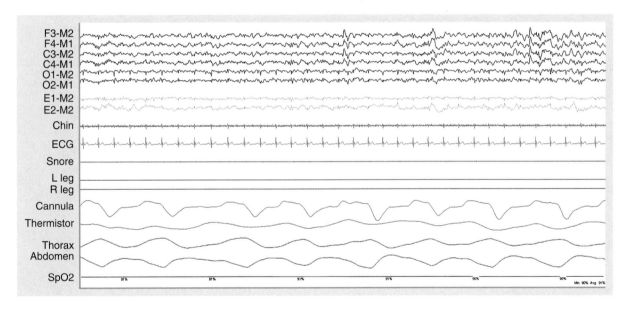

311. What stage is this?

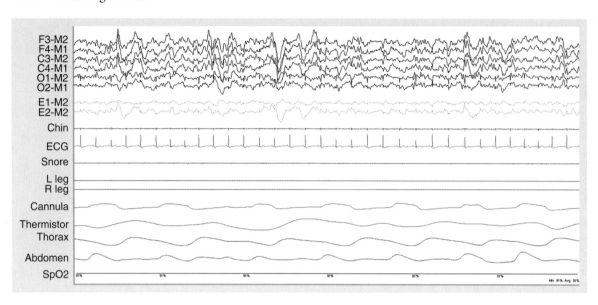

312. What stage is this?

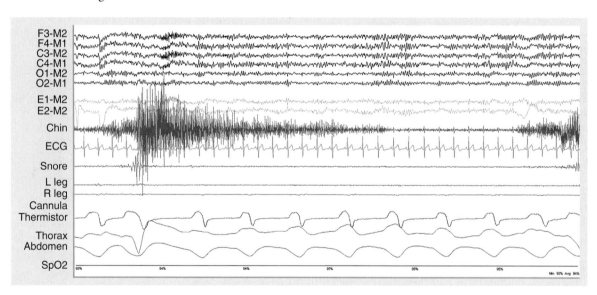

313. What stage is this?

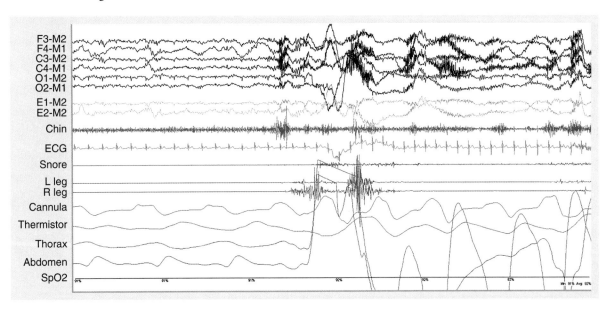

314. What stage is this?

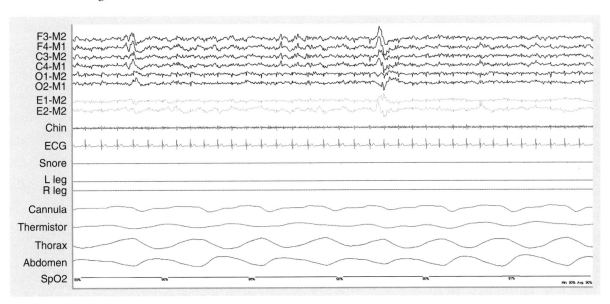

315.   What stage is this?

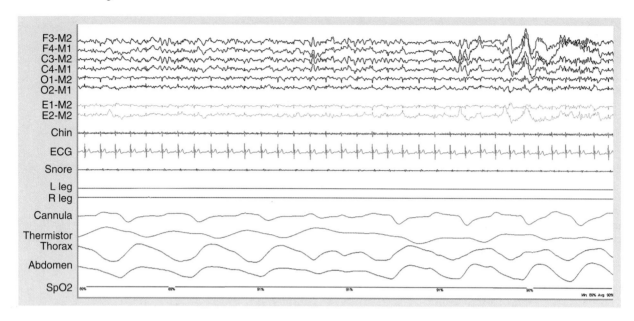

316.   What stage is this?

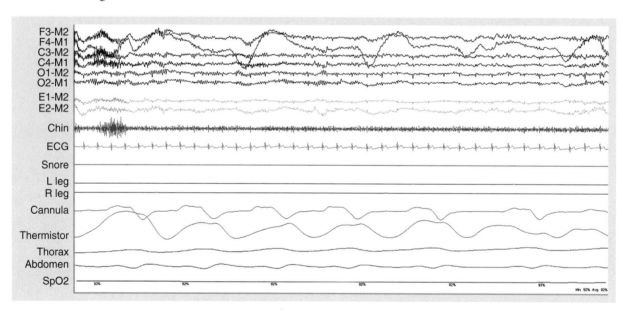

317. What stage is this?

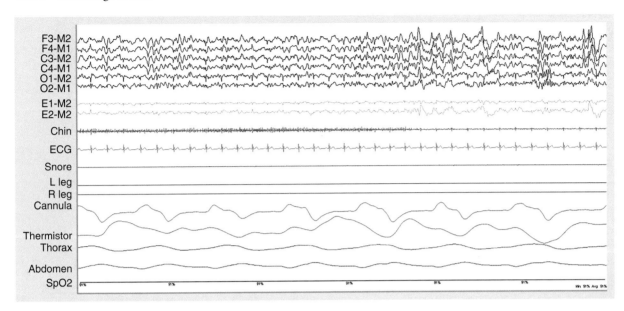

318. What stage is this?

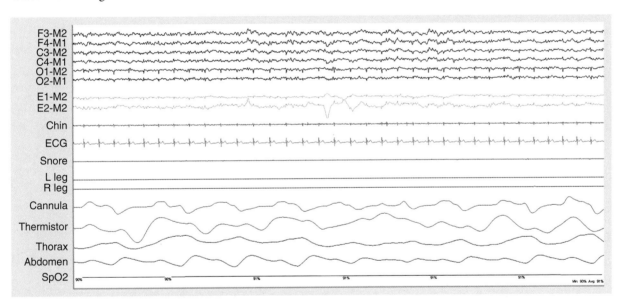

319. What stage is this?

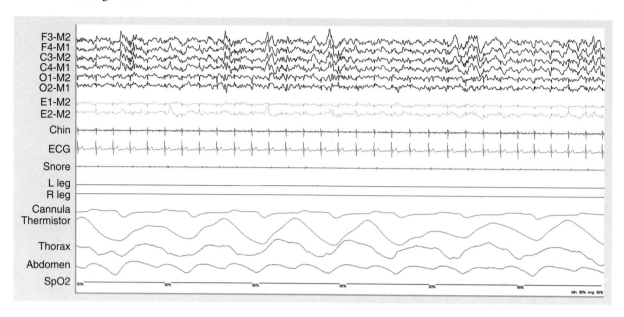

320. What stage is this?

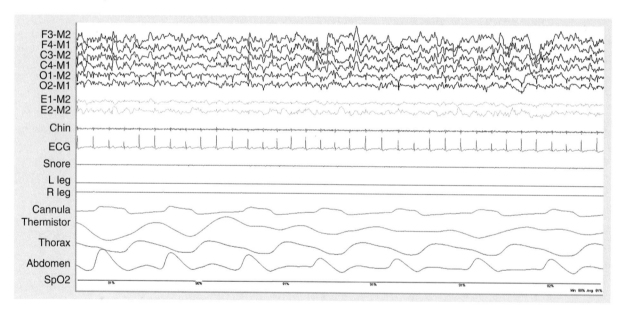

321. What stage is this?

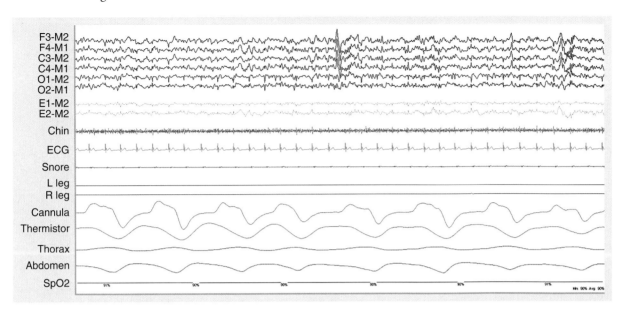

322. What stage is this?

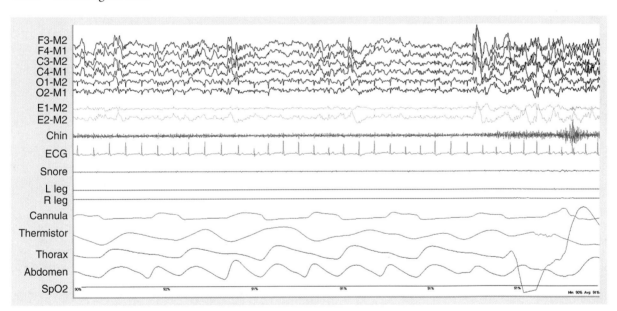

323. What stage is this?

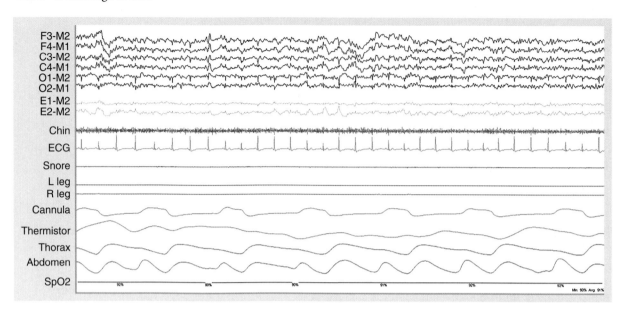

324. What stage is this?

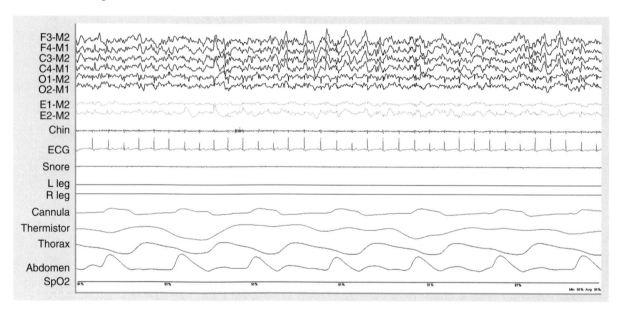

325. What stage is this?

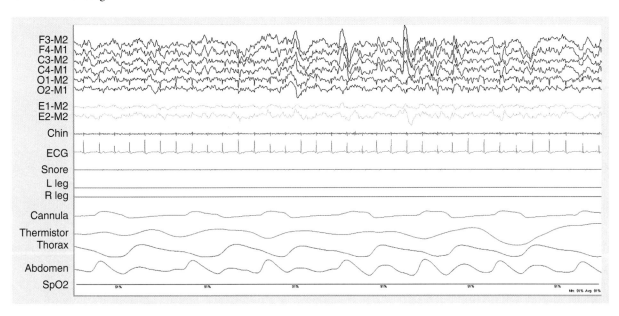

326. What stage is this?

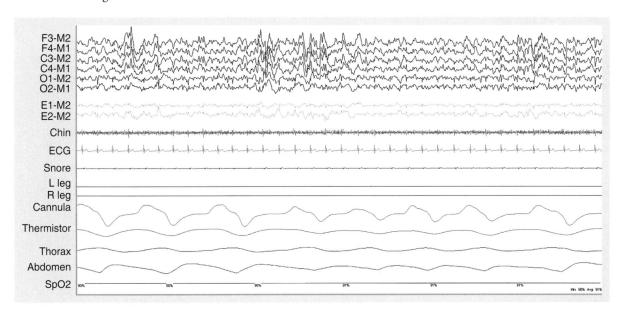

327. What stage is this?

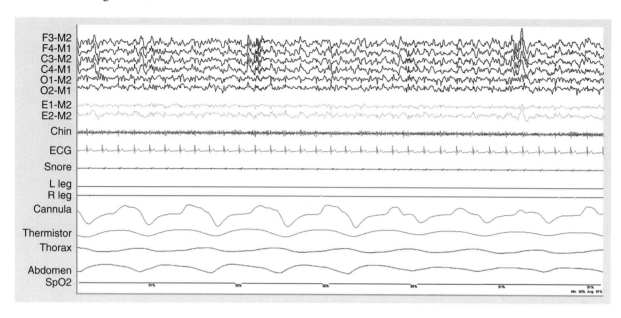

328. What stage is this?

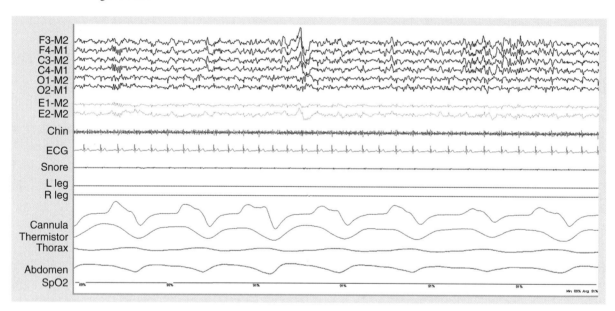

329. What stage is this?

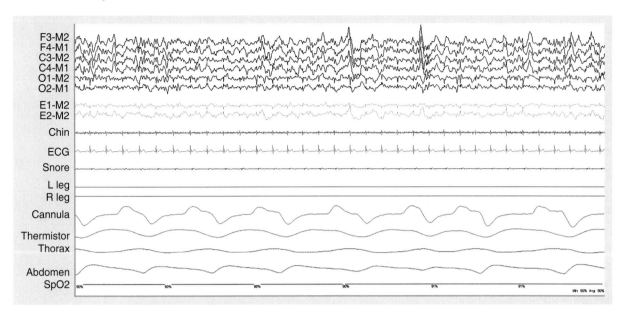

330. What stage is this?

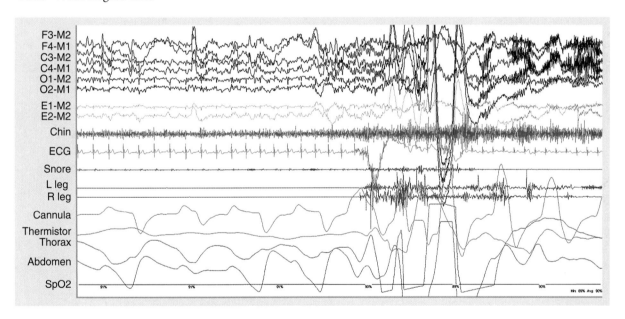

331. What stage is this?

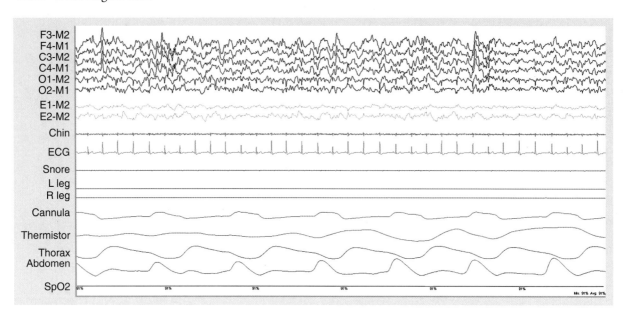

332. What stage is this?

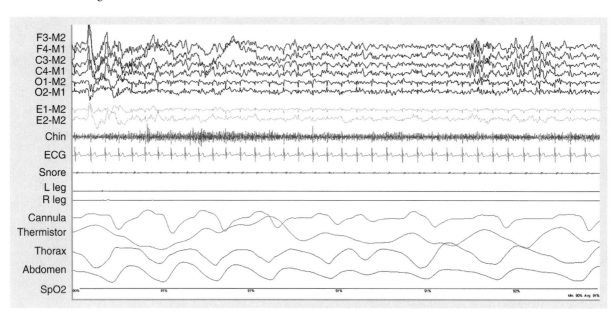

333. What stage is this?

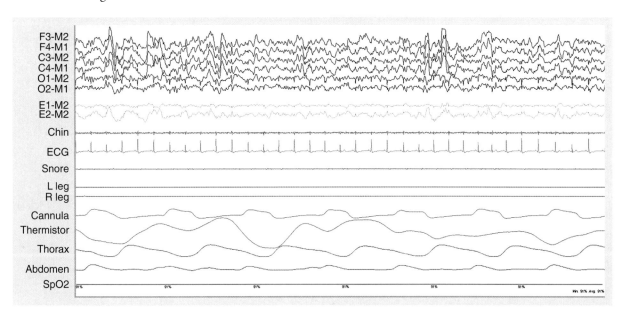

334. What stage is this?

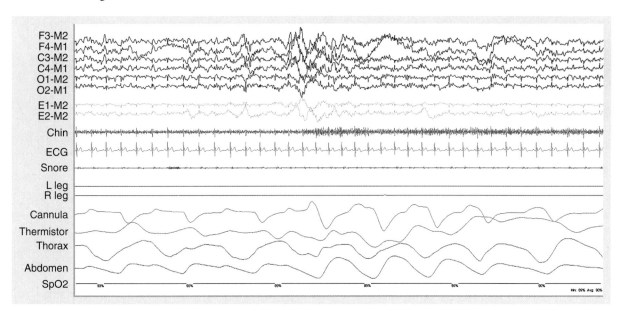

335. What stage is this?

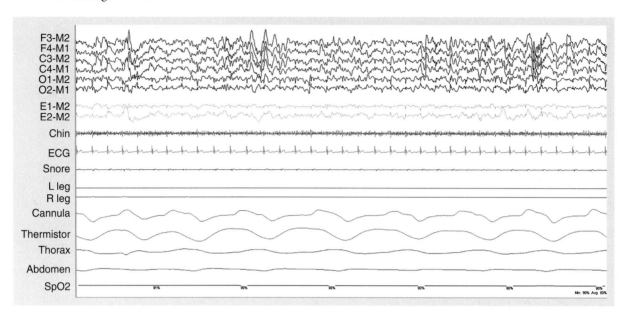

336. What stage is this?

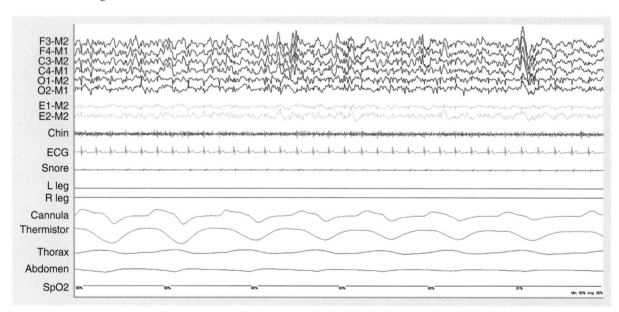

337. What stage is this?

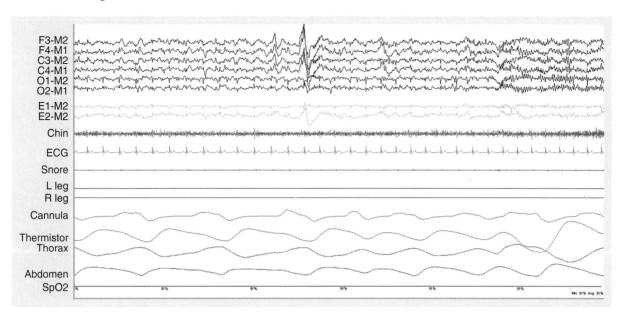

338. What stage is this?

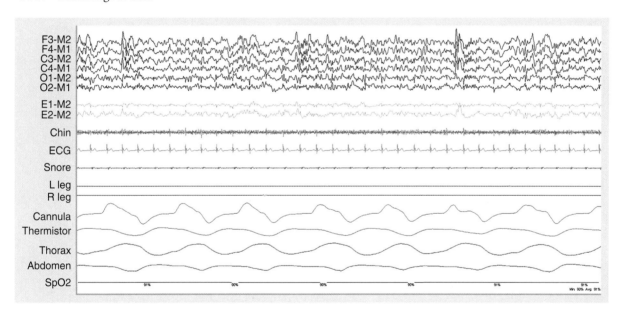

339. What stage is this?

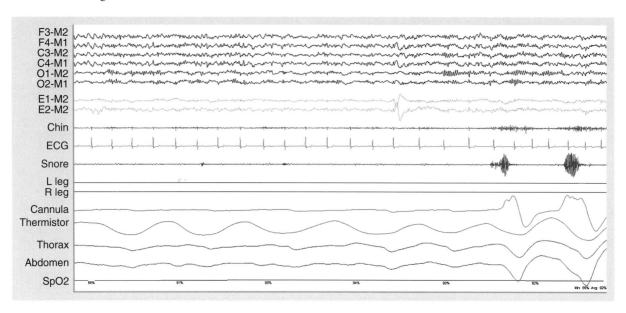

340. What stage is this?

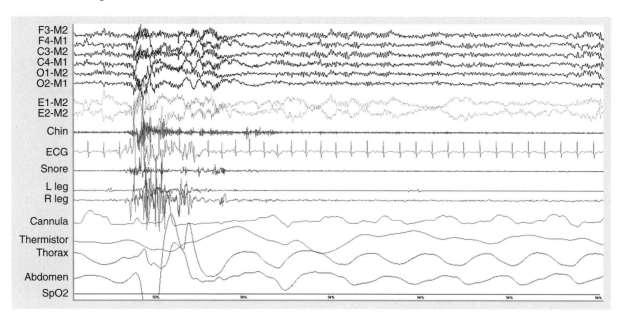

341. What stage is this?

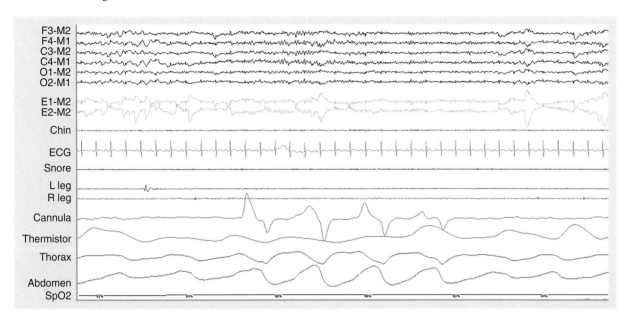

342. What stage is this?

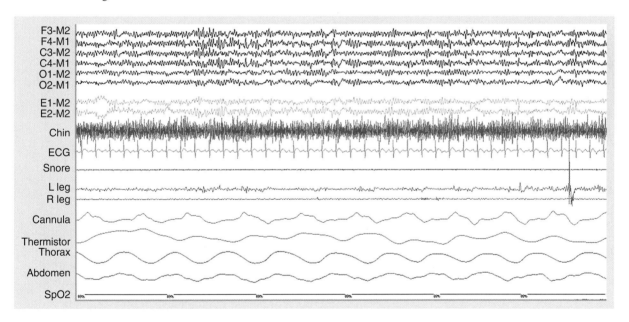

343. What stage is this?

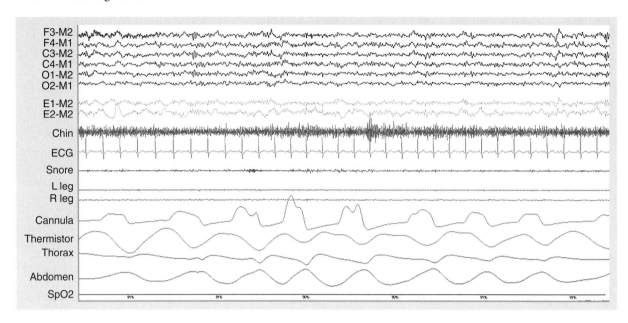

344. What stage is this?

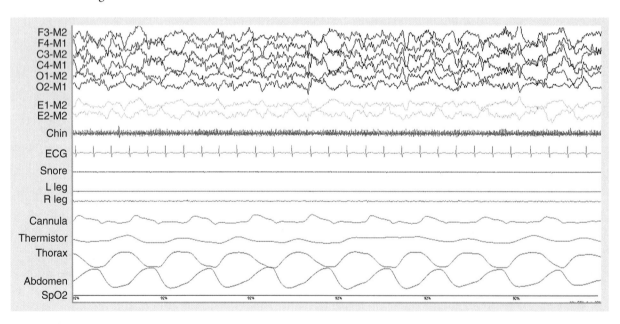

345. What stage is this?

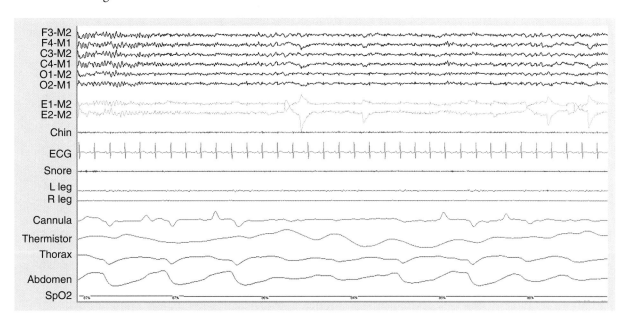

346. What stage is this?

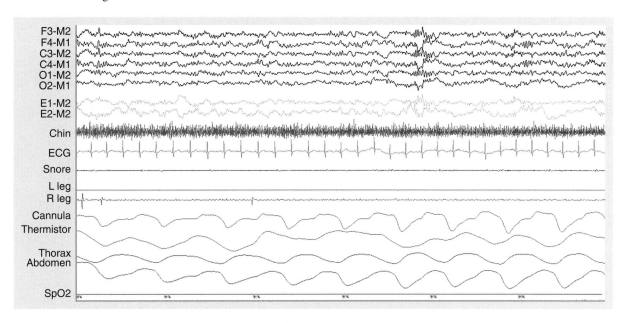

347. What stage is this?

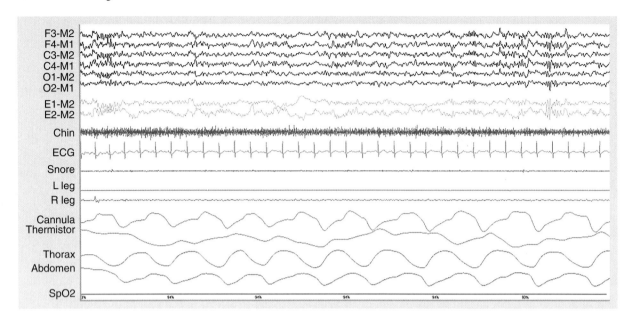

348. What stage is this?

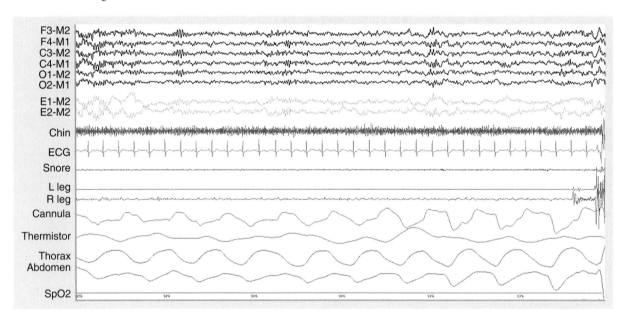

349. What stage is this?

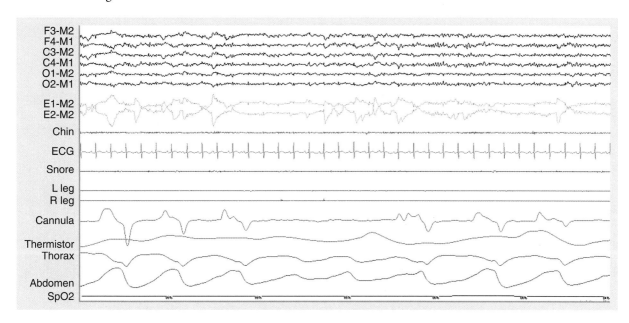

350. What stage is this?

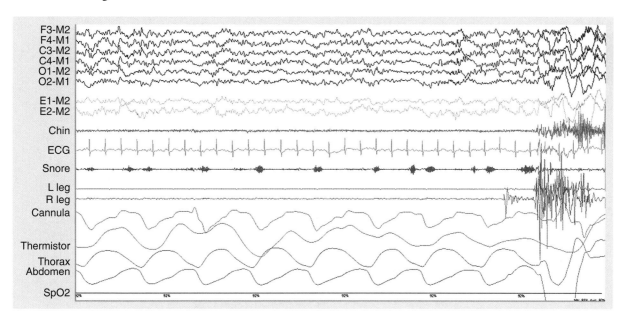

351. What stage is this?

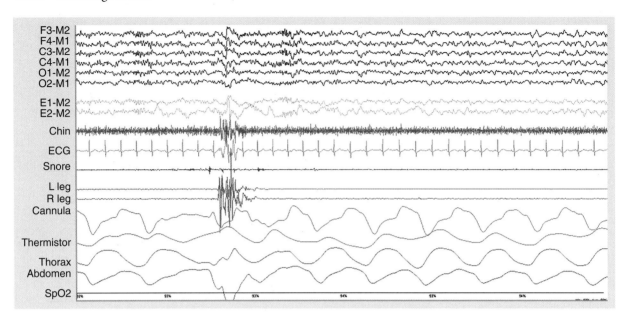

352. What stage is this?

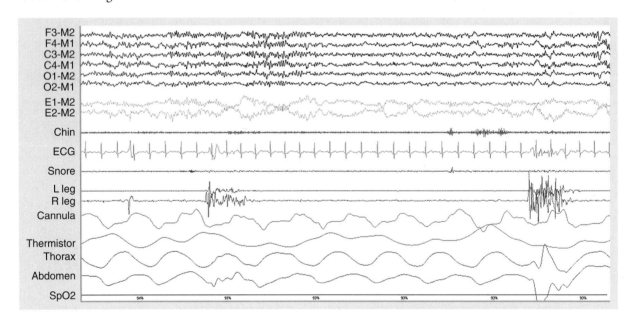

353. What stage is this?

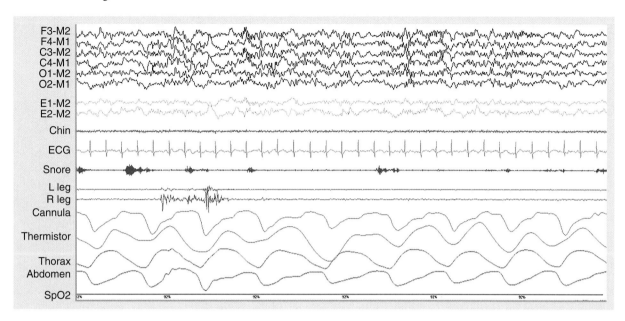

354. What stage is this?

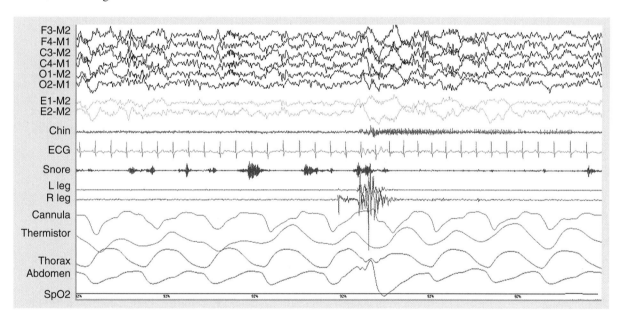

355. What stage is this?

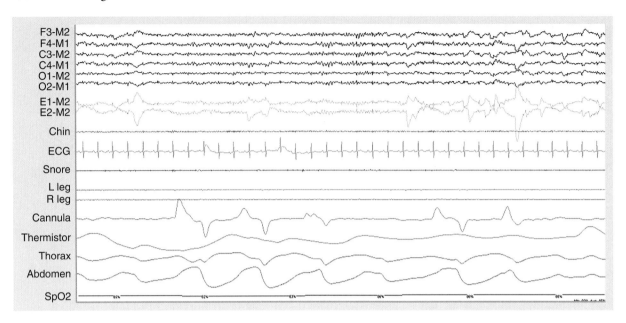

356. What stage is this?

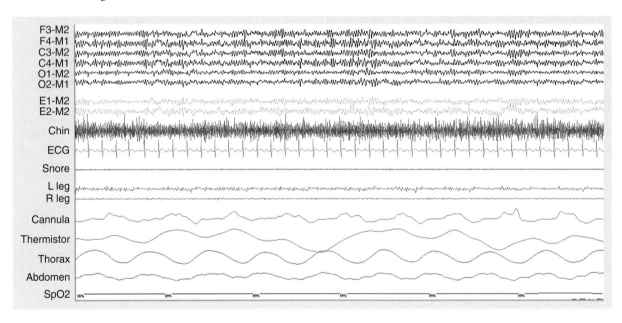

357. What stage is this?

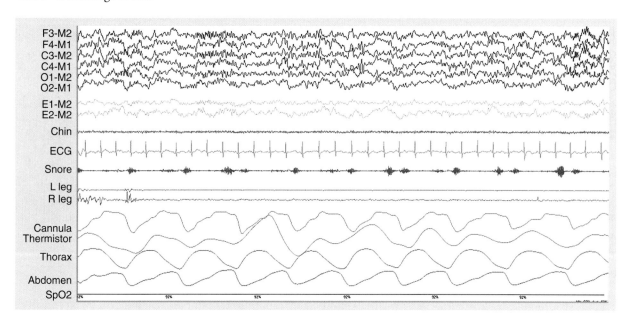

358. What stage is this?

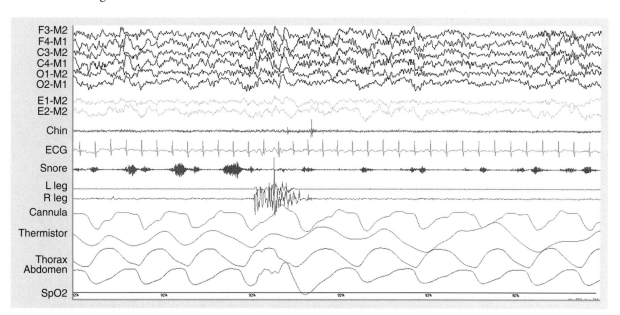

359. What stage is this?

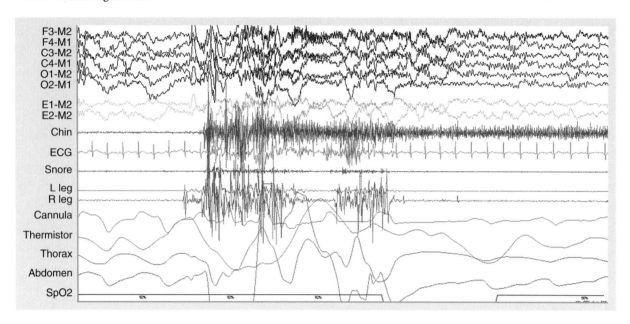

360. What stage is this?

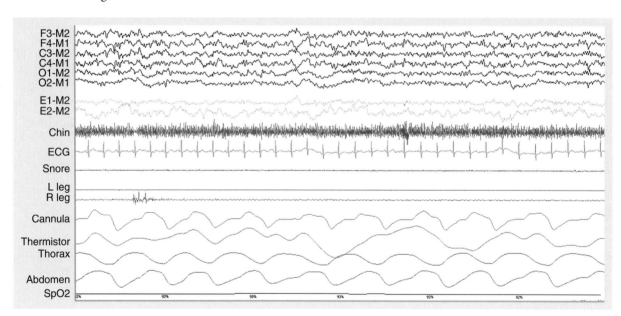

361. What stage is this?

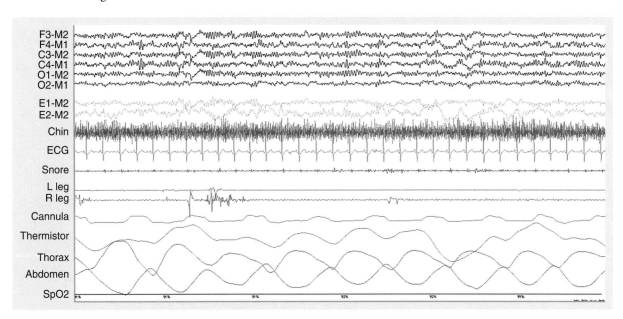

362. What stage is this?

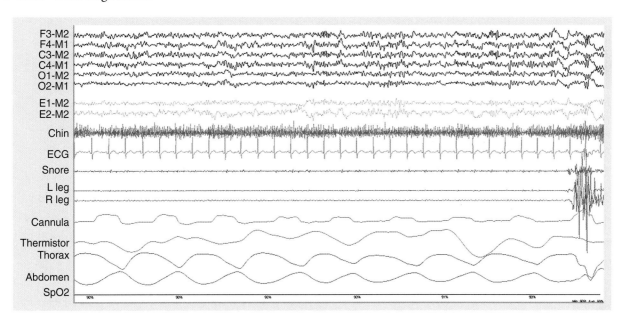

363. What stage is this?

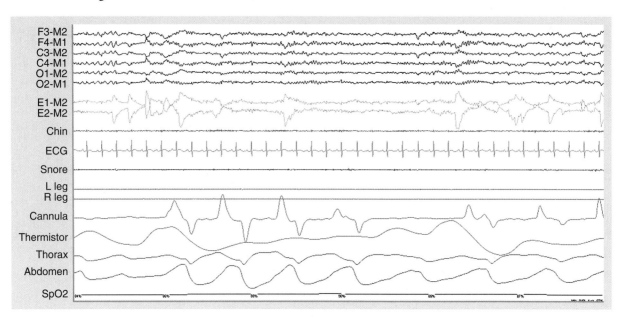

364. What stage is this?

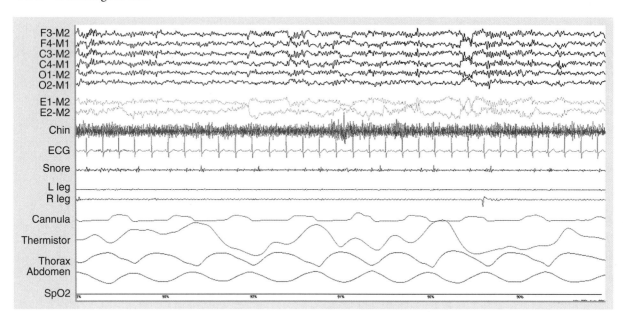

365. What stage is this?

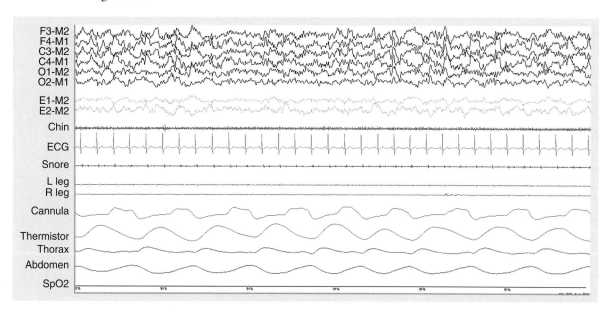

366. What stage is this?

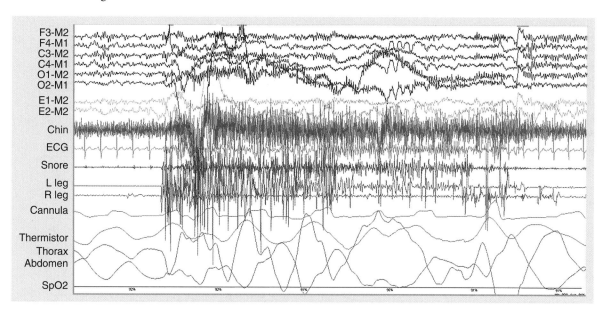

367. What stage is this?

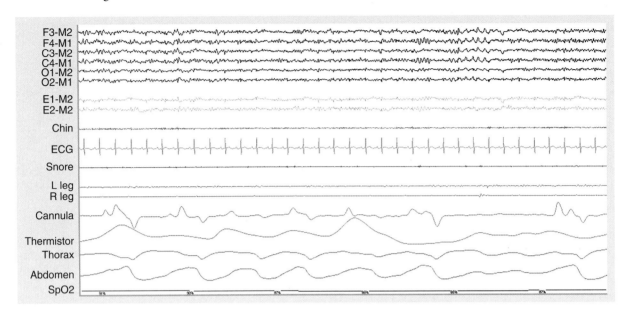

368. What stage is this?

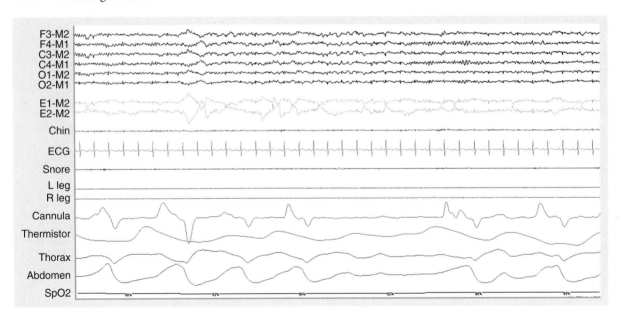

369. What stage is this?

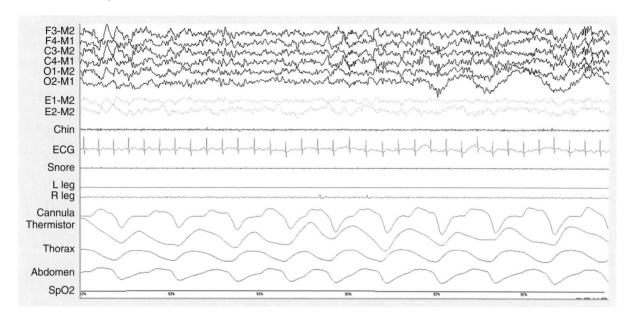

370. What stage is this?

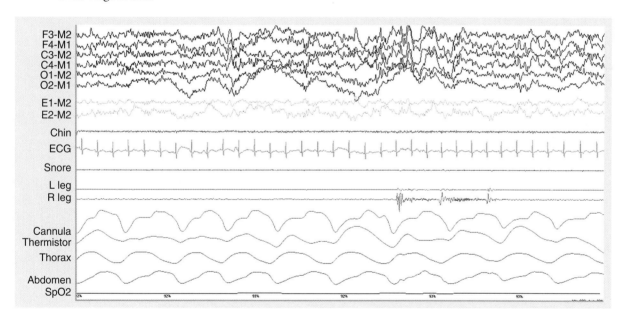

371. What stage is this?

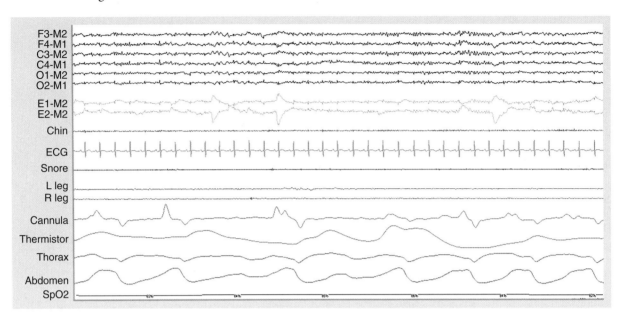

372. What stage is this?

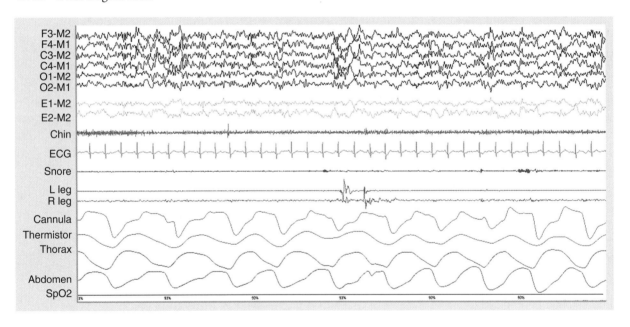

373. What stage is this?

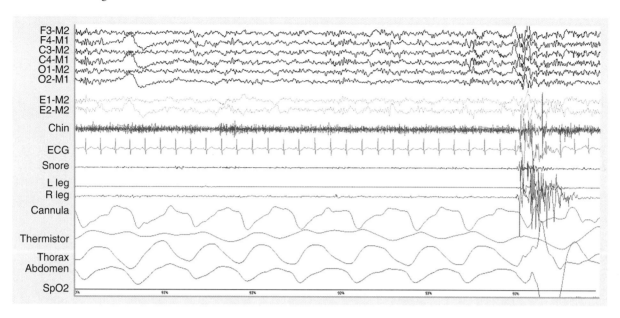

374. What stage is this?

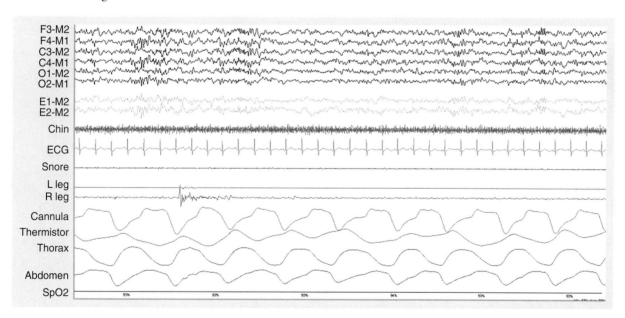

375. What stage is this?

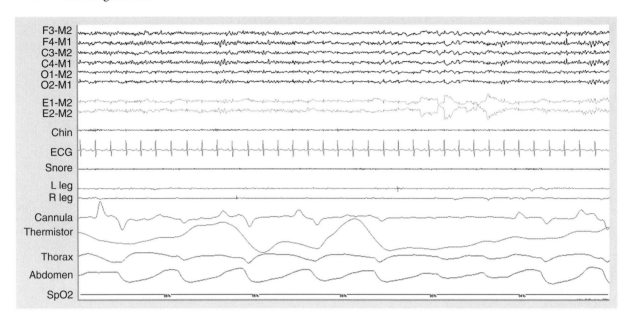

376. What stage is this?

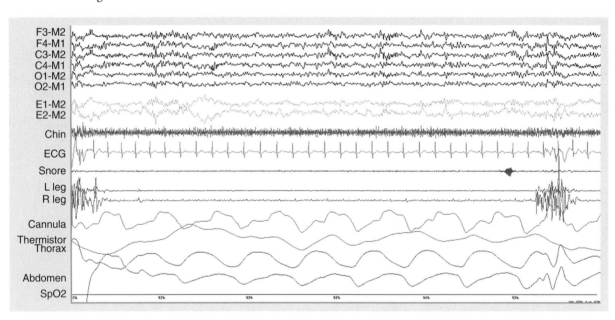

377. What stage is this?

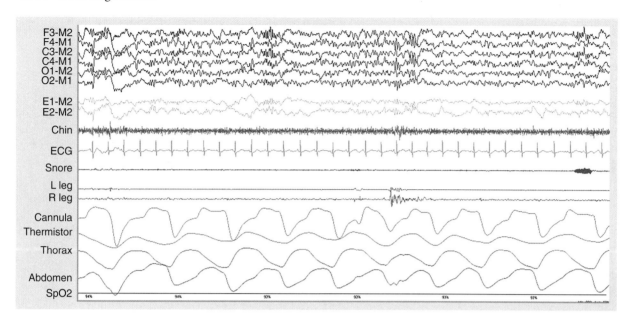

378. What stage is this?

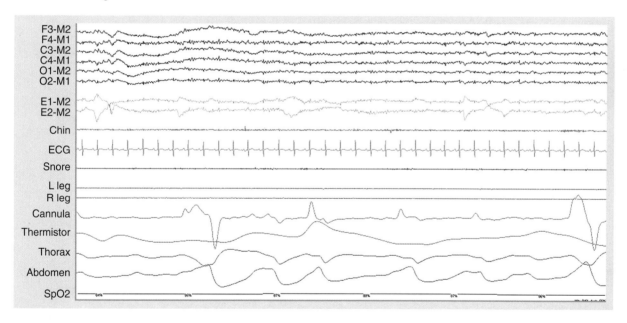

379. What stage is this?

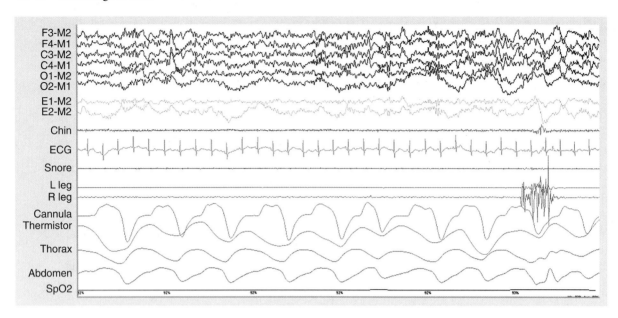

380. What stage is this?

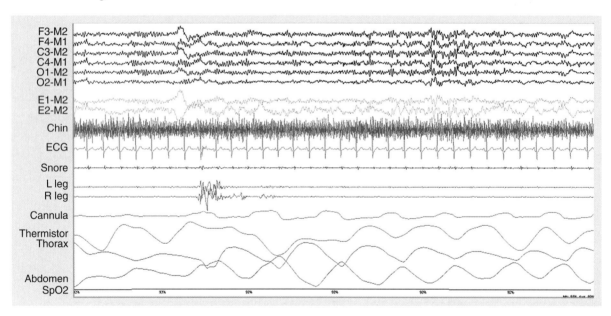

381. What stage is this?

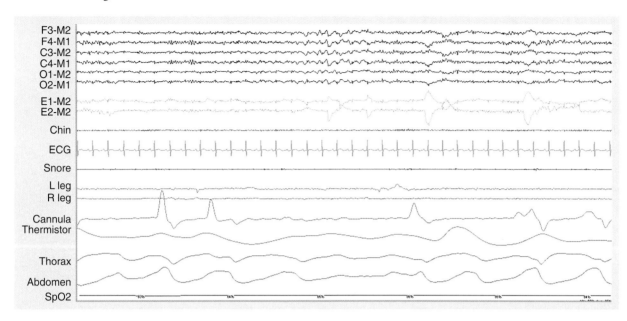

382. What stage is this?

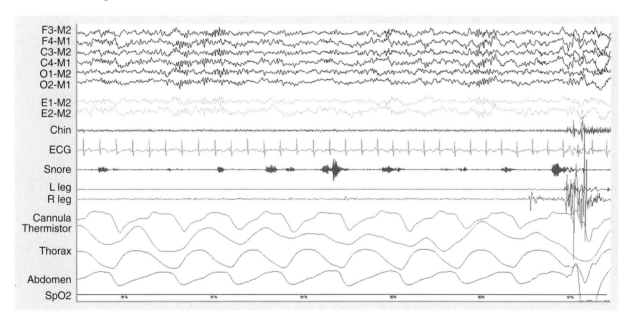

383. What stage is this?

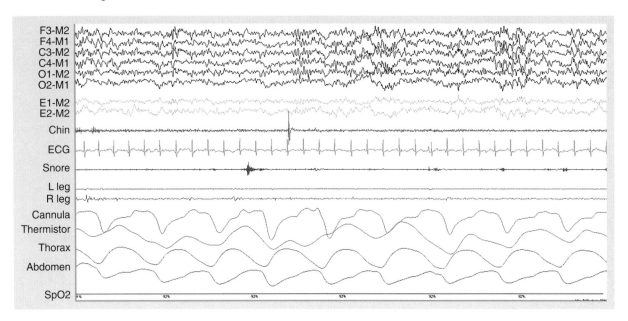

384. What stage is this?

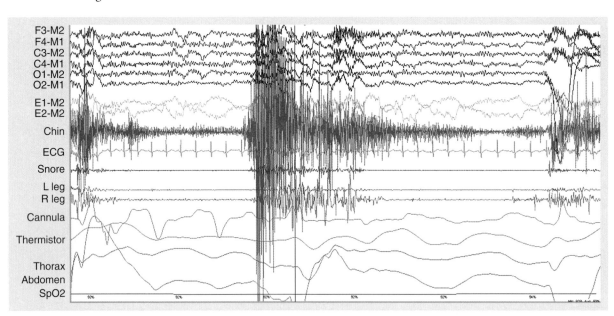

385. What stage is this?

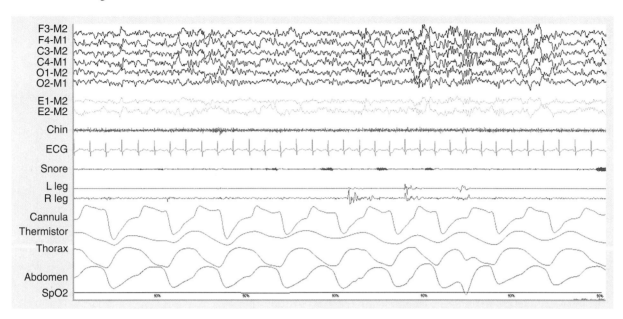

386. What stage is this?

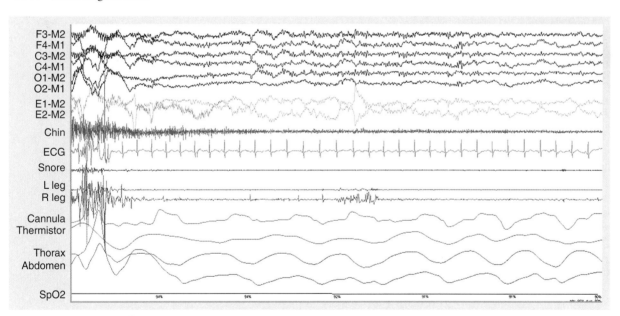

387. What stage is this?

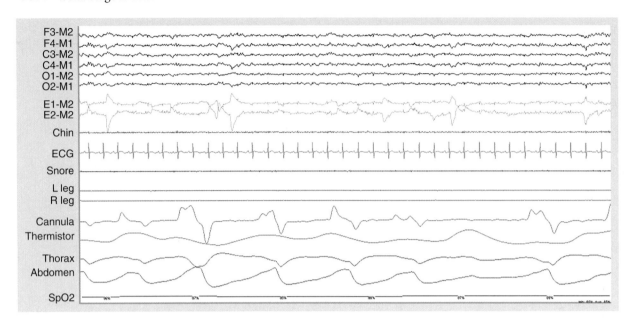

388. What stage is this?

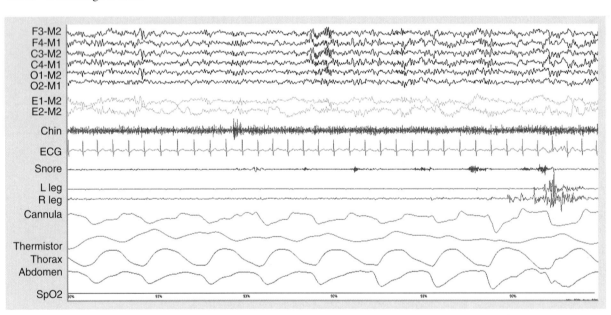

389. What stage is this?

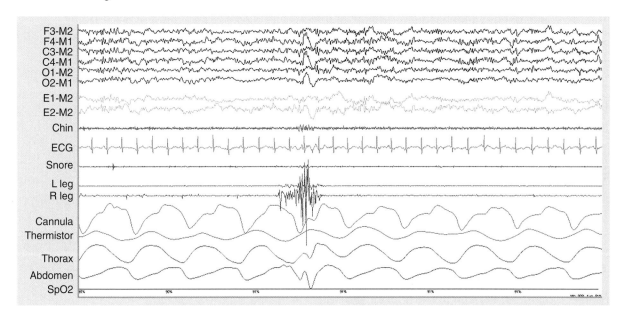

390. What event is seen in the first circle?

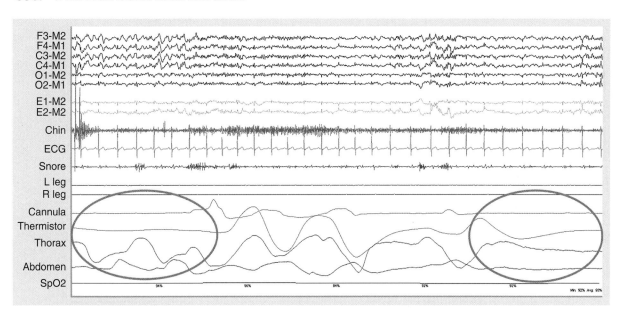

    A. Obstructive apnea
    B. Hypopnea
    C. Central apnea
    D. Mixed apnea

391. What event is seen in the second circle?
    A. Obstructive apnea
    B. Hypopnea
    C. Central apnea
    D. Mixed apnea

392. What event is likely causing the interruptions seen in the EEGs, EOGs, chin EMG, and snore channel?

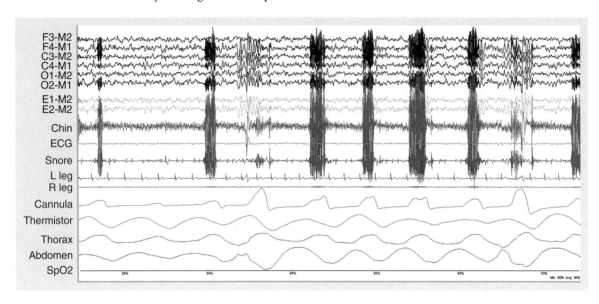

    A. Bruxism
    B. Snores
    C. Respiratory disturbances
    D. Leg movements

393. What event is circled?

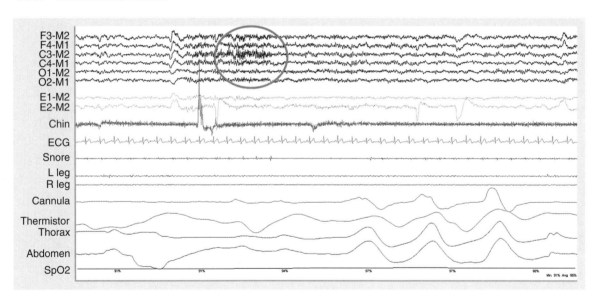

    A. Beta spindles
    B. Nocturnal seizure
    C. EEG arousal
    D. Alpha intrusion

394. What event is circled in red?

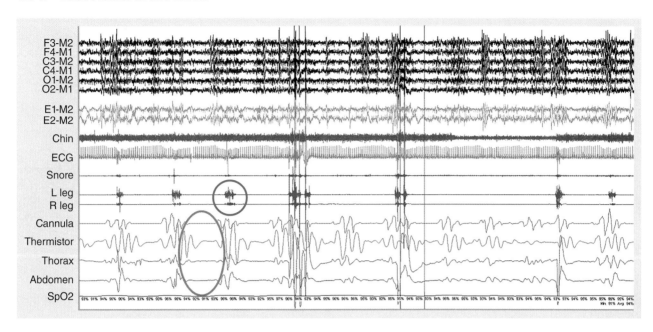

A. Central apnea

B. Mixed apnea

C. Obstructive apnea

D. This is not a scorable event

395. What event is circled in blue?

A. Periodic limb movement

B. Isolated limb movement

C. Sleep start

D. This is not a scorable event

396. What event is circled?

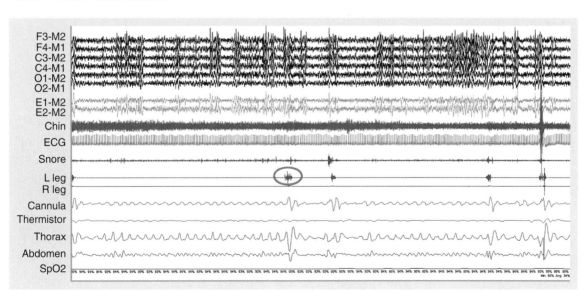

A. Limb movement

B. Snore

C. Sleep start

D. This is not a scorable event

397. What event is circled in blue?

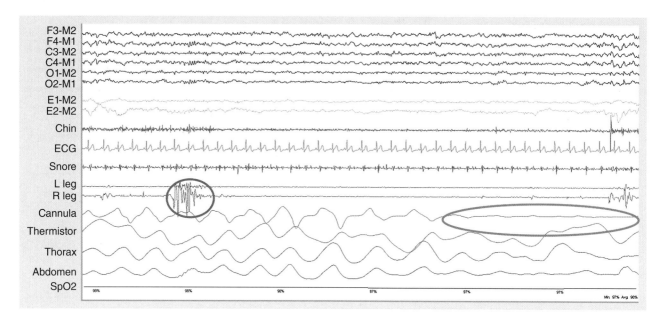

- **A.** Snore
- **B.** Sleep start
- **C.** EEG arousal
- **D.** Limb movement

398. What event is circled in red?
- **A.** Central apnea
- **B.** Mixed apnea
- **C.** Hypopnea
- **D.** Obstructive apnea

399. What event is circled?

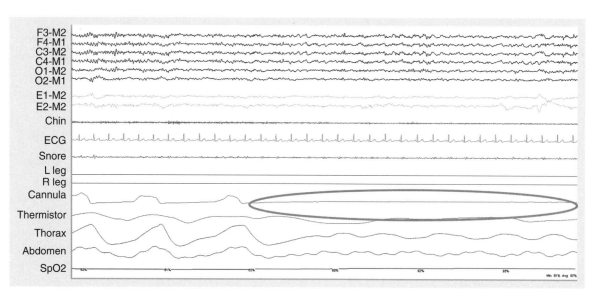

- **A.** Central apnea
- **B.** Mixed apnea
- **C.** Hypopnea
- **D.** Obstructive apnea

400. Immediately following this epoch is a 4% oxygen desaturation. What event is circled?

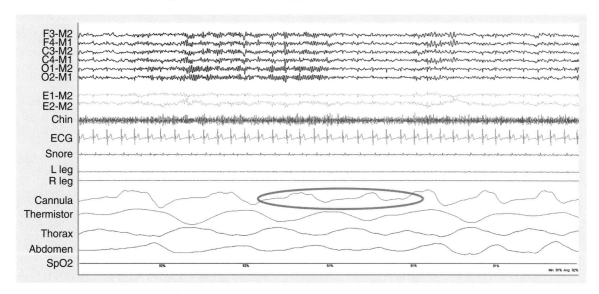

A. This is not a scorable event
B. Upper-airway resistance
C. Hypopnea
D. Obstructive apnea

401. What other event is seen in this epoch?
A. EEG arousal
B. Snore
C. Limb movement
D. Cheyne–Stokes breathing

402. This is a 300-second page. What event is circled?

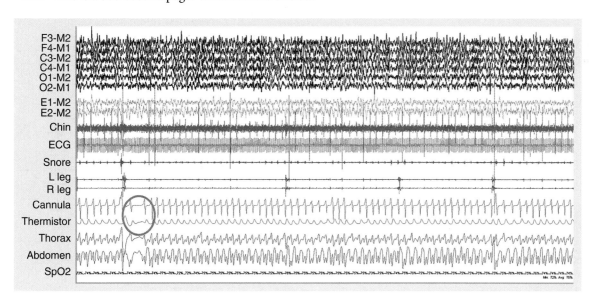

A. Central apnea
B. Mixed apnea
C. Hypopnea
D. Obstructive apnea

403. What classification of leg movements is seen in the previous image?
- **A.** Periodic limb movements
- **B.** Hypnic myoclonus
- **C.** Isolated limb movements
- **D.** These are not scorable events

404. What event is seen in this epoch?

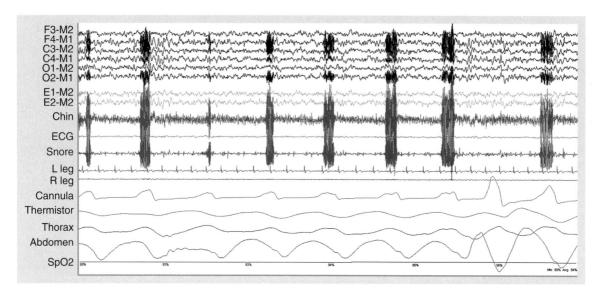

- **A.** Snoring
- **B.** Bruxism
- **C.** Periodic limb movements
- **D.** EEG arousals

405. What event is circled in red?

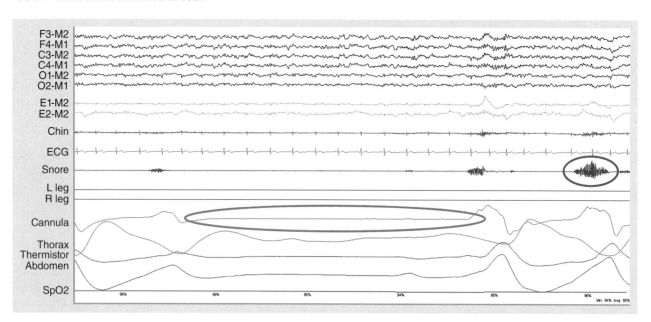

- **A.** Central apnea
- **B.** Mixed apnea
- **C.** Hypopnea
- **D.** Obstructive apnea

406. What event is circled in blue?
- A. Leg movement
- B. Snore
- C. Bruxism
- D. This is not a scorable event

407. What event is circled in this 60-second epoch?

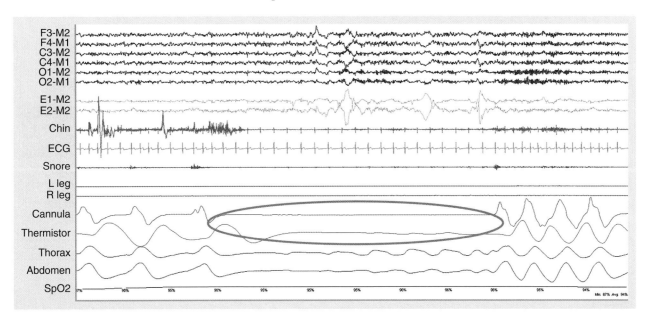

- A. Central apnea
- B. Mixed apnea
- C. Hypopnea
- D. Obstructive apnea

408. What event is associated with this event?
- A. EEG arousal
- B. Limb movement
- C. Bruxism
- D. Sleep start

409. What event is circled in red?

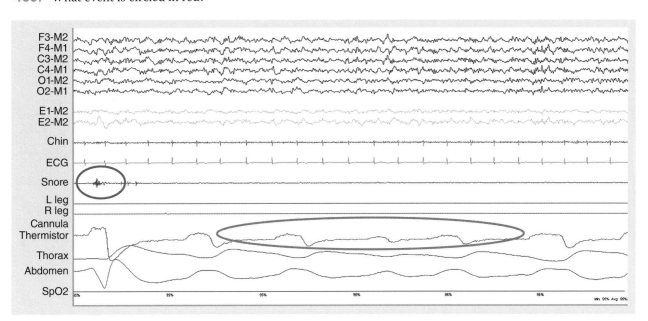

    A. Central apnea
    B. Mixed apnea
    C. Hypopnea
    D. Obstructive apnea

410. What event is circled in blue?
    A. Snore
    B. Bruxism
    C. Leg movement
    D. This is not a scorable event

411. What event is circled in red?

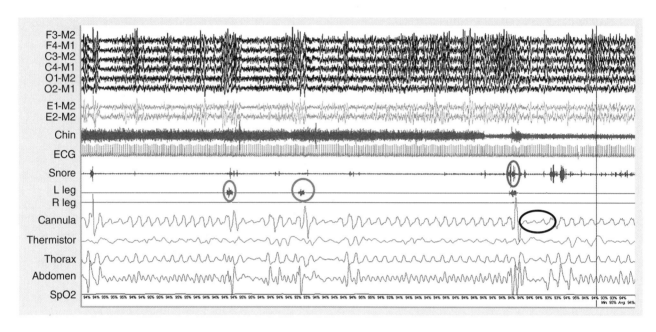

    A. Limb movements
    B. Snores
    C. EEG arousals
    D. These are not scorable events

412. What event is circled in blue?
    A. Limb movement
    B. Snore
    C. Bruxism
    D. This is not a scorable event

413. What event is circled in black?
    A. Central apnea
    B. Mixed apnea
    C. Hypopnea
    D. Obstructive apnea

414. What event is circled?

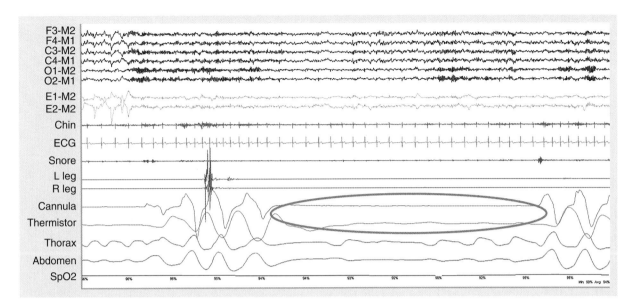

    A. Central apnea
    B. Mixed apnea
    C. Hypopnea
    D. Obstructive apnea

Domain 3: Perform Therapeutic Treatment

415. The patient's baseline SpO_2 is below the wake limits on the lab's protocol. The medical director orders supplemental O_2 at 2 L/min. During the night, the patient's TCO_2 levels increase by 12 mm Hg, and the respiratory rate decreases to six breaths per minute. What should the technician do?
    A. Decrease the O_2 flow rate and contact the physician
    B. Recalibrate the transcutaneous CO_2 monitor
    C. This outcome is desirable and the technician should continue monitoring
    D. Add bi-level PAP with a backup rate

416. The physician's orders are to begin the study with oxygen at 12 L/min. What should the technician do?
    A. Start the study at 2 L/min, because this is probably what was intended
    B. Call the physician to verify the order for 12 L/min
    C. Perform the study without supplemental oxygen
    D. Start the study at 12 L/min as the order stated

417. What is the standard device used to verify CPAP pressure?
    A. CPAP pressure channel on the PSG
    B. Dial manometer
    C. Water column manometer
    D. Digital manometer

418. Which of these is not required for in-home CPAP use?
    A. An interface device
    B. A humidifier
    C. A CPAP machine
    D. A physician's order

419. How can the use of CPAP decrease blood pressure?
    A. The change in ventilatory pattern leads to hypoxemia
    B. The positive airway pressure reduces the variability of cardiac output
    C. The CPAP creates a patent airway
    D. The change in ventilatory pattern leads to an increase in CO_2 retention

420. Which of the following is a common complaint immediately following a PAP titration?
    A. Nasal dryness and sneezing
    B. Severe headaches and blurred vision
    C. Severe heartburn and indigestion
    D. Memory impairment

421. Sudden apneas in a patient successfully treated with CPAP during REM and NREM sleep in the first half of the night might be explained by which of the following?
    A. The patient moves to his or her right or left side.
    B. The temperature in the room has increased.
    C. The patient enters into N3 sleep.
    D. The patient moves to a supine position

422. Which of the following statements is true regarding patients with central sleep apnea?
    A. They always respond well to CPAP
    B. They never respond well to CPAP
    C. They may respond well to CPAP
    D. None of the above

423. If a patient has OSA and the obstruction is at the nasal passages, which of these would be the most appropriate treatment?
    A. CPAP
    B. Surgery
    C. Tracheotomy
    D. Oxygen therapy

424. The optimal CPAP pressure is best determined in which stage of sleep and in which body position?
    A. N3, supine
    B. N3, prone
    C. REM, supine
    D. REM, side

425. Which of these is true regarding CPAP?
    A. It should be tried only if a uvulopalatopharyngoplasty (UPPP) has failed
    B. It is the medical therapy of choice for sleep apnea
    C. It maintains upper-airway patency by virtue of receptors stimulated by the associated increase in lung volume
    D. It is rarely tolerated

426. During which sleep state is respiration controlled the same as during wake in normal sleepers?
    A. REM
    B. NREM
    C. Both of the above
    D. None of the above

427. When performing a CPAP titration, what is the desired RDI?
    A. <5
    B. <10
    C. >15
    D. >20

428. Which of these is a treatment for central sleep apnea?
    A. Bi-level PAP
    B. Tricyclic antidepressants
    C. Stimulants
    D. CPAP

429. Patients with a hypoxic drive
    A. Breathe based on the level of carbon dioxide in their blood
    B. Typically live 5–10 years longer than those with a hypercapneic drive
    C. Do not respond well to CPAP
    D. Respond well to supplemental oxygen

430. On a PAP machine, the amount of air the patient is breathing is called the
   A. Leak
   B. Tidal volume
   C. Pressure
   D. Estimated patient flow

Domain 4: Therapy Adherence and Management

431. Which of the following is not a predisposing factor for OSA?
   A. Getting older
   B. Thick neck
   C. Being male
   D. Epileptiform activity

432. OSA can lead to which of the following cardiovascular problems?
   A. Complete heart block
   B. Myocardial infarction
   C. Pulmonary hypertension
   D. All of the above

433. Which of these is true regarding Cheyne–Stokes breathing?
   A. Cyclic SpO_2 decreases
   B. Respiration improves during REM sleep
   C. Waxing and waning pattern in airflow and respiratory effort channels
   D. All of the above

Answer the following questions (434–446) about arterial blood gases.

434. Which of these values is considered normal for the pH level?
   A. 6.9–7.1
   B. 7.0–7.35
   C. 7.35–7.45
   D. 7.45–7.75

435. Which of these values is considered normal for the PCO_2?
   A. 10–20
   B. 20–30
   C. 30–40
   D. 40–50

436. Which of these values is considered normal for the HCO_3?
   A. 10–20
   B. 15–25
   C. 17–27
   D. 32–42

437. What is the pH a measurement of?
   A. The amount of oxygen in the blood
   B. The thickness of the blood
   C. The amount of hemoglobin in the blood
   D. The level of acidity of the blood

438. Heavy smokers have which of the following?
   A. A decreased HCO_3
   B. An increased HCO_3
   C. A normal HCO_3
   D. An HCO_3 of 0

439. The PCO_2 is a measurement of what?
   A. The type of carbon dioxide in the blood
   B. The acidity of the carbon dioxide in the blood
   C. The amount of carbon dioxide in the blood
   D. The amount of hemoglobin in the blood

440. Which of these base excess (BE) levels is considered normal?
     A. −2.5 to 0
     B. 0 to 2.5
     C. −2.5 to +2.5
     D. −5.0 to +5.0

441. What is the range for normal adult hemoglobin (HB) levels?
     A. 6–11 g/dL
     B. 12–17 g/dL
     C. 18–23 g/dL
     D. None of these

442. What might an HB level of 8 indicate?
     A. HIV
     B. Anemia
     C. Hardening of the arteries
     D. A normal hemoglobin level

443. What is the PO_2 a measurement of?
     A. Oxygen
     B. Carbon dioxide
     C. Carbon monoxide
     D. Acidity

444. Which of these PaO_2 levels is considered normal?
     A. 25–50
     B. 50–75
     C. 75–100
     D. None of these

445. Which of these SaO_2 levels is considered normal?
     A. >75
     B. >80
     C. >88
     D. >92

446. What does the SaO_2 measure?
     A. The percentage of hemoglobin that is saturated with oxygen
     B. The percentage of the tissue that is saturated with blood
     C. The actual amount of oxygen in the blood
     D. None of the above

447. What would a low PO_2 be likely to contribute to?
     A. An increased PCO_2
     B. A decreased SaO_2
     C. An increased pH
     D. An increased HB

448. Increased acidity in the blood produces which of the following?
     A. A decreased pH
     B. An increased pH
     C. A decreased SaO_2
     D. An increased SaO_2

449. Which of the following is within normal ranges?
     A. BE of 3.5
     B. PCO_2 of 25
     C. PO_2 of 59
     D. pH of 7.0

450. What is the main difference between SpO_2 and SaO_2?
     A. How they are detected
     B. There are no differences.
     C. Blood saturation versus hemoglobin saturation
     D. Saturation of oxygen versus actual measurement of oxygen

451. Which of these is not a common characteristic in patients with OSA?
    A. Obesity
    B. Snoring
    C. Large, thick neck
    D. Low body mass index (BMI)

452. Which of the following statements is not true regarding the sleep of normal healthy young adults?
    A. NREM sleep and REM sleep oscillate in a cycle of approximately 90 minutes
    B. REM sleep predominates in the final third of the night
    C. REM sleep usually comprises 20–25% of the night
    D. Stage N2 sleep generally comprises approximately 25% of the night

453. Which of the following should sleep technicians be aware of?
    A. Some patients may be at a higher risk for cardiac arrhythmias during sleep than during wake
    B. Patients with medical conditions such as COPD or neuromuscular disorders may have significantly more severe symptoms during sleep
    C. Electrodes attached to a patient's body may pose a hazard to the patient
    D. All of the above

454. Which of these is considered to be the circadian rhythm oscillator?
    A. Hippocampus
    B. Suprachiasmatic nucleus
    C. Reticular activating system
    D. Cerebellum

455. How many minutes is the length of the average human sleep cycle?
    A. 15
    B. 60
    C. 90
    D. 120

456. Research using MSLTs has shown that physiological sleepiness in normal human adults is
    A. Constant throughout the day with little variation
    B. Greatest in the morning
    C. Greatest in the evening
    D. Greatest in the afternoon

457. Which of these statements is true regarding blood pressure in REM sleep?
    A. It increases during REM sleep
    B. It decreases slightly during REM sleep
    C. It remains the same during REM sleep
    D. It falls dramatically during REM sleep

458. Why is REM sleep often referred to as paradoxical sleep?
    A. Those deprived of REM sleep are no different from normal
    B. The body is paralyzed, although the EEG resembles a waking pattern
    C. EEG patterns are unrelated to dream content
    D. Infants have a higher percentage of REM than adults

459. Which of these practices encourages good sleep?
    A. Go to bed hungry
    B. Drink heavily before going to bed
    C. Go to bed at a regular time whether sleepy or not
    D. Get out of bed at a regular time

460. Which of these is true regarding narcoleptics?
    A. Sedatives do not make them sleepy
    B. They are only occasionally sleepy
    C. They are sleepy nearly all of the time
    D. They are nearly all males

461. In which age group are nocturnal sleep and daytime alertness usually at optimal levels?
    A. Children
    B. Adolescents
    C. Young adults
    D. Older adults

462. Which of these is characterized by a feeling of falling or floating at sleep onset stopped by a sudden jerk and EEG arousal or awakening?
    A. Cataplexy
    B. Epilepsy
    C. Sleep start
    D. Hypnagogic hallucination

463. The most important source of information for diagnosing a sleep schedule disturbance is
    A. An MSLT report
    B. An overnight PSG report
    C. History obtained from the bed partner
    D. A sleep diary

464. Which of these is not a change in sleep that occurs with increasing age?
    A. Decreased N3 sleep
    B. Change in the distribution of REM sleep throughout the night
    C. Decreased REM latency
    D. More frequent reports of dreams

465. When all other factors are equal, alertness on awakening is
    A. Increased if awakened from N3 sleep
    B. Increased if awakened from REM sleep
    C. Independent of the stage from which awakened
    D. Decreased if awakened from stage N2

466. Which of the following is true regarding sleep in old age?
    A. N3 sleep remains constant until about ages 60–65
    B. A typical sleep efficiency for the average 65 year old is <50%
    C. REM occupies about 25% of total sleep time from ages 20 through 70
    D. The average sleep latency is 30 minutes

467. Which of the following statements is true regarding adolescent sleep?
    A. Adolescents need less sleep than children
    B. The need for sleep increases with age
    C. The first REM period in adolescents may be exceptionally short
    D. Adolescents' proportion of N3 is the same as for adults

468. Which of the following statements is true regarding children's sleep?
    A. They have a long sleep latency
    B. They have poorly developed N3 sleep
    C. They have 95% sleep efficiency
    D. They have many spontaneous arousals

469. Which of these often leads to sleep-onset REM periods in normal sleepers?
    A. Withdrawal from benzodiazepines
    B. Recovery from a marathon race
    C. Afternoon naps
    D. REM deprivation

470. Which of these medical conditions can lead to insomnia during infancy?
    A. Food allergies
    B. Gastroesophageal reflux
    C. Otitis media
    D. All of the above

471. A loud noise will most likely awaken an adolescent during which stage of sleep?
    A. N3
    B. REM sleep
    C. N2
    D. It makes no difference

472. Which of these structures is responsible for sending signals from the body to the cortex?
    A. Thalamus
    B. Raphe nuclei
    C. Suprachiasmatic nuclei
    D. Midbrain

473. Bruxism is
    A. More common in the elderly than in infants
    B. Periodic kicking of the legs during sleep
    C. Characterized by clenching or grinding teeth during sleep
    D. Refusal to comply with CPAP

474. Which structure of the brain blocks signals from the thalamus to the cortex?
    A. Medulla oblongata
    B. Spinal cord
    C. Reticular activating neurons
    D. Hypothalamus

475. Which of these EEG waveforms is seen as a result of signals from the thalamus being blocked?
    A. Alpha waves
    B. K-complexes
    C. Sleep spindles
    D. Slow waves

476. What might be seen in a patient with lesions in the suprachiasmatic nucleus?
    A. Inability to sleep
    B. Altered circadian rhythm
    C. Inability to wake
    D. Lack of REM sleep

477. Which of these is responsible for EEG arousals and awakenings?
    A. Reticular activating system
    B. Hypothalamus
    C. Spinal cord
    D. Hippocampus

478. Which structure is strongly affected by light?
    A. Thalamus
    B. Suprachiasmatic nucleus
    C. Hippocampus
    D. Hypothalamus

479. Which neurotransmitter is at its highest levels during wakefulness and REM sleep?
    A. Acetylcholine
    B. Histamine
    C. Noradrenaline
    D. Dopamine

480. Which of these is not a common characteristic of normal REM sleep?
    A. Rapid eye movements
    B. Myoclonia
    C. Increased muscle tone
    D. Sawtoothed EEG waves

481. Which of these neurotransmitters does not activate the cerebral cortex?
    A. Histamine
    B. Glutamate
    C. Noradrenaline
    D. All of these are involved in activating the cerebral cortex

482. Which of these structures of the brain does not play a major role in REM sleep?
    A. Medulla oblongata
    B. Hippocampus
    C. Pons
    D. Raphe nuclei

483. Skeletal muscles during REM sleep are
    A. Paralyzed
    B. Mildly active
    C. Moderately active
    D. Highly active

484. A lack of muscle atonia during REM sleep is
    A. Normal
    B. Impossible
    C. A characteristic of REM behavior disorder
    D. Usually caused by lesions or damage to the thalamus

485. REM sleep comprises approximately what percentage of the sleep period?
    A. 5%
    B. 10%
    C. 25%
    D. 50%

486. The human circadian rhythm oscillates approximately every
    A. Minute
    B. Hour
    C. 90 minutes
    D. Day

487. What does blood pressure do during sleep?
    A. Decreases
    B. Varies greatly
    C. Increases
    D. Remains the same as during wake

488. During what stage of sleep does the core body temperature drop?
    A. N1
    B. N2
    C. N3
    D. REM

489. Which of these is often seen after sleep deprivation?
    A. Increased REM latency
    B. Decreased N3 sleep
    C. Stage N2 rebound
    D. N3 and REM rebounds

490. Which of these stages is seen during the majority of the circadian rhythm?
    A. Wake
    B. N2
    C. N3
    D. REM

491. Which of these stages of sleep is considered to be a transitional stage of sleep?
    A. N1
    B. N2
    C. N3
    D. REM

492. Stage N1 comprises approximately what percentage of the sleep period?
    A. 5–10%
    B. 20–25%
    C. 25–50%
    D. >50%

493. During what part of the night is N3 the most prevalent?
    A. The first third
    B. The middle third
    C. The final third
    D. The entire night

494. What is the average sleep efficiency in normal adult humans?
    A. 25%
    B. 50%
    C. 70%
    D. 90%

495. During which portion of the night is REM sleep the most prevalent?
    A. The first third
    B. The middle third
    C. The final third
    D. The entire night

496. Which of the following statements regarding sleep and aging is true?
    A. EEG arousals decrease with age
    B. N2 decreases with age
    C. N3 decreases with age
    D. Sleep efficiency increases with age

497. EEGs in older adults typically have _____ a than EEGs in younger adults.
    A. Higher frequency
    B. Lower frequency
    C. Higher amplitude
    D. Lower amplitude

498. Which mammal sleeps with half of its brain at a time to increase survival?
    A. Lion
    B. Dolphin
    C. Cat
    D. Chimpanzee

499. Which of these suppresses REM?
    A. Caffeine
    B. Cocaine
    C. Alcohol
    D. Aspirin

500. Which of these helps increase the depth of sleep in narcoleptics?
    A. Warm milk before retiring
    B. Watching television in bed
    C. Increased exercise
    D. Coffee in the morning

Posttest Answers and Explanations

1. B

   An EEG LFF of 0.1 may increase the perception of stage N3 because of slow wave or sweat artifact. The LFF of 1.0 for the EMG in C is too low and may allow slow waves to be recorded, and the HFF of 35 in the EMG in D is too low and may attenuate the EMG amplitude.

2. A

   Eye movement toward an electrode results in a positive (downward) pen deflection because the cornea of the eye is positive with respect to the retina.

3. B

   The LFF is designed to eliminate unwanted slow frequencies. DC amplifiers do not have low-frequency filters.

4. B

   Medical testing and treatments always require a physician's order. The sleep technician should review the patient chart before any type of testing is performed in the sleep lab.

5. A

   G1 is the exploring electrode, or the first signal input. G2 is the second input, or the reference electrode.

6. A

   Output voltages are determined by subtracting G2 from G1: $-100 - (-50) = -50$.

7. A

   Differential amplifiers measure the difference between two signals.

8. A

   Signal output is determined by subtracting G2 from G1.

9. A

   Frequency is measured in cycles per second or Hertz (Hz). The easiest method of determining the frequency is to count the number of cycles in 1 second.

10. D

    Calibrations are performed for many purposes, one of which is to produce a wave to use as a measuring standard.

11. A

    High-frequency filters are used to eliminate undesired fast frequencies.

12. C

    Sensitivity equals input signal voltage divided by pen deflection.

13. A

According to the AAST technical guidelines, the sensitivity setting for an EEG channel should be set between 5 μV/mm and 7 μV/mm.

14. B

The amplitude of a wave is a measure of the voltage of the signal.

15. C

Increasing the sensitivity decreases the pen deflection, whereas decreasing the sensitivity increases the pen deflection.

16. B

The paper speed used in polysomnography is 10 mm/sec, which produces a 30-second epoch.

17. C

The settings in C present the most appropriate filter settings, but the settings in B would also be acceptable.

18. A

These settings should be used when recording EMGs. The HFF can be set to at least 70 Hz, and the LFF should be set at or close to 10 Hz.

19. D

Of the options given, the settings in D are the most appropriate settings for respiratory channels. However, ordinarily the HFF would be set slightly higher than this.

20. B

DC amplifiers do not use high-frequency filters because the changes in voltages are extremely slow.

21. B

The main factor determining the quality of the signals in a sleep study is the quality of the electrode application.

22. D

Physiologic calibrations are performed for all of these reasons.

23. C

The cornea is positive with respect to the retina. Therefore, if the patient looks toward the electrode, the signal produced will be positive, causing a downward pen deflection.

24. C

Increasing the LFF will have no effect on alpha waves or other fast waves but will attenuate slower EEG waves.

25. D

The positive charge given to the E2 electrode will give a positive or downward deflection in the E2 channel and a negative or upward deflection in the E1 channel.

26. D

Amplitude is a measurement of the height of a wave, and frequency is a measurement of the speed of a wave.

27. A

Amplitude can be measured in volts, microvolts, or millivolts, but EEG amplitude is measured in microvolts. EEG frequency is measured in Hertz, which is a measurement of cycles per second.

28. C

Sensitivity is measured in μV/mm, which is a measurement of voltage divided by pen deflection.

29. C

The time constant is closely associated with the low-frequency filter.

30. C

The electrode impedances should be less than 5,000 (5 K) ohms. The lower the impedances, the cleaner the resulting signal will be.

31. B

A sleep study does not typically include ERG, which is a recording of electrical activity in the retina.

32. C

Cz to Pz is 20% of the total distance from the nasion to the inion. Twenty percent of 36 cm is 7.2 cm.

33. B
The distance from the inion to Oz is 10% of the distance from the inion to the nasion. Ten percent of 32 cm is 3.2 cm.

34. D
C4 is the midpoint between Cz and T4. Half of 14 cm is 7.0 cm.

35. C
The distance from Cz to C3 is 20% of the distance from ear to ear. Twenty percent of 40 cm is 8.0 cm.

36. A
The distance from Oz to O1 is 5% of the total circumference of the head. Five percent of 56 cm is 2.8 cm.

37. C
The distance from O2 to T4 is 20% of the total circumference of the head. Twenty percent of 60 cm is 12.0 cm.

38. A
F4 is half the distance from F8 to Fz.

39. D
T5 is half the distance from O1 to T3.

40. C
The distance from C3 to P3 represents 25% of this measurement. Twenty-five percent of 24 cm is 6 cm.

41. C
F8 is located half the distance from T4 to Fp2. Half of 10 cm is 5 cm.

42. D
F4 is half the distance from C4 to Fp2.

43. D
T3 to Oz is 25% of the total circumference of the head. Twenty-five percent of 50 cm is 12.5 cm.

44. B
Cz is located half the distance from T4 to T3.

45. B
Output voltage is determined by subtracting G2 from G1: $60 - 10 = 50$.

46. A
Galvanized skin response is a possible side effect of referencing dissimilar metals to each other.

47. D
The oximeter is a DC device that estimates the SpO_2.

48. B
Cup electrodes generally provide the lowest impedances and are built and shaped for scalp placement.

49. B
Gold cups can be more expensive than other types of wires, although they usually provide lower impedances.

50. A
Frequency refers to how fast a wave oscillates or repeats and is measured in cycles per second or Hertz (Hz).

51. C
The sensitivity setting adjusts the height of the wave.

52. B
Frequency filters work by filtering frequencies above and below given points. Therefore, adjusting frequency filters can directly affect the frequency of a wave.

53. A
The recommended LFF setting for EEG channels in a sleep study is 0.3 Hz. For this question, the closest frequency, and therefore best choice, is 0.5 Hz.

54. D
Of the options provided, 70 Hz is the best HFF setting for EMG channels.

55. C
Of these options, 5.0 Hz is the best HFF setting for the airflow channel.

56. C
The recommended setting for the HFF in EEG channels is 35 Hz.

57. B
The shape of EEG waves is reviewed closely when determining sleep stages.

58. A
The recommended sensitivity setting for EEG channels is 5–7 µV/mm.

59. C
Seizure montages often include a full or expanded EEG hookup to rule out the possibility of seizure activity.

60. A
Baseline PSG studies include the collection of airflow from both a thermal sensor and a nasal–oral pressure transducer.

61. B
The distance from T5 to T3 is 10% of the circumference of the head.

62. B
The chin EMG electrodes should be placed above and below the chin, one above and two below.

63. C
Arm EMGs are recorded during a REM behavior-disorder study.

64. C
The reference voltage is equal to the voltage detected by the exploring electrode minus the output voltage: $-20 - 50 = -70$.

65. B
The leg EMG electrodes should be placed on the anterior tibialis, which runs along the outside of the shin bone.

66. C
When the input signals are identical, they cancel each other out, and the output voltage is 0 µV.

67. B
This describes the site for C3.

68. A
Looking up will cause a positive signal to enter the E2 electrode and a negative charge to enter the E1 electrode. Thus, according to polarity convention, the resulting wave in the E2 channel will go down, and the resulting wave in the E1 channel will go up. With E2 placed above E1 on the montage, these two waves will move toward each other.

69. A
$-80 - (-100)$ is the same calculation as $-80 + 100$, which equals 20.

70. B
F8 is located halfway between Fp2 and T4.

71. C
Oz is 10% of this distance from the inion, and Pz is 20% from Oz, making the total distance 30% of the vertical measurement of the head.

72. B
The distance from the left pre-auricular point to T3 is 10% of the total distance from ear to ear. Ten percent of 36 cm is 3.6 cm.

73. B
P4 is half the distance from T6 to Pz. Half of 8 cm is 4 cm.

74. D
F7 and Fz are the same distance from F3.

75. B
P4 is located half the distance from O2 to C4.

76. C
Oz is located 10% of the vertical measurement of the head above the inion.

77. B
Stress loops are helpful in the application of leg EMGs because they can decrease the likelihood of these leads being pulled off.

78. C
ECG artifact has a high amplitude but not a low frequency. EMG and 60-Hz artifacts have a high frequency. Sweat artifact has a high amplitude and a low frequency.

79. D
Sensitivity = voltage/amplitude; changing the formula around gives amplitude = voltage/sensitivity. So amplitude = 75 μV/5μV/mm or 15 mm.

80. D
A line or notch filter should only be used when electrical interference affects the recording. Changing the HFF will not affect what is recorded. The LFF will not have an effect on a high-frequency artifact. The best solution is to replace the electrode.

81. D
Low signal amplitude does not indicate a malfunction in the amplifier.

82. C
The principles of common mode rejection cause electrical interference to be eliminated when impedances are similar between electrodes.

83. B
Instrument chassis leakage current should be below 100 μA for safety in usage.

84. B
A poor quality signal should be distinguished from real changes in ventilation.

85. A
Thermocouples and piezoelectric belts generate their own voltages. Thermistors and inductive plethysmographs require external electrical sources.

86. D
All of these are reasons for following the signal pathway.

87. D
All of these situations pose potential dangers to patient safety.

88. B
Ground loops can occur when there is more than one ground, causing a variance in the pathways of least resistance.

89. D
A notch or line filter is useful when artifacts from outside electrical sources are present, but it should not be used to make a channel look cleaner.

90. D
The notch filter is appropriate for 60-Hz artifact not muscle activity.

91. C
A 60-Hz filter should not be used to correct artifact unless necessary.

92. D
All of these statements are true about slow-frequency artifacts.

93. A
Electrode impedances are the leading cause of 60-Hz artifact.

94. D
Electrodes not firmly attached, as well as direct pressure against electrodes, can cause electrode popping.

95. B
Sweat artifact manifests itself as a slow wave in the EEG and EOG channels.

96. A
If re-referencing is possible, this is the preferred method of correcting artifacts.

97. C
Re-referencing is the most appropriate method of eliminating this artifact. Double referencing will not eliminate the artifact because it uses both references.

98. C
Changing the reference source will not affect this signal because the source of the artifact is the exploring electrode. The best way to correct this artifact is to change the exploring electrode.

99. C

The electrode will need to be replaced.

100. D

Both of these can cause ECG artifacts in EMG channels.

101. C

This artifact is most likely caused by sweat. The best method of correcting this is by cooling the patient.

102. A

ECG artifact in the EEG channels may be reduced or eliminated by double referencing if both reference electrodes detect the pulse.

103. D

Re-adjusting the thermistor is the appropriate method to correct this problem.

104. D

Changing the filter settings is only effective if the signals are intact.

105. C

Differential amplifiers are used in polysomnography because they use reference electrodes.

106. D

All of these statements are true regarding high and unequal impedances.

107. B

The polarity convention states that negative signals will produce an upward pen deflection, whereas positive signals will produce a downward pen deflection.

108. A

Sensitivity equals voltage divided by pen deflection; 75 μV divided by 10 $\mu V/cm$ is 7.5 cm, which equals 75 mm.

109. B

The quantity 75 μV divided by 1.5 mm equals 50 $\mu V/mm$.

110. B

The quantity 5 $\mu V/cm$ multiplied by 10 cm is 50 μV.

111. D

All of these can cause 60-Hz interference.

112. C

In most sleep systems, the patient head box is plugged directly into the AC amplifier.

113. D

The SpO_2 is detected by an oximeter, which is a DC device.

114. D

A capnometer detects CO_2 levels.

115. A

Thermocouples use dissimilar metals to generate electricity and measure changes in temperature. Thermistors use a single metal that detects changes in temperature; they require an electrical source.

116. C

Respiratory transducers use an air-filled bladder inside a respiratory belt. As the air inside the bladder gets pushed to the transducer from expansion of the abdomen and thorax, a waveform is created on the polysomnograph.

117. D

Esophageal reflux is the presence of acids from the stomach in the esophagus. A pH probe detects the acidity of the esophagus.

118. B

The common mode rejection ratio refers to the amplifier's ability to eliminate unwanted signals. The higher the ratio, the more capable the amplifier.

119. C

Capacitors store energy and then release it.

120. B

The maximum allowable leakage for diagnostic equipment is 100 μA (microamps).

121. D

A frequency-response curve is a graphical display of the amplifier's ability to eliminate unwanted frequencies outside the filter settings.

122. C

The rise time constant is the amount of time it takes for a calibration wave to reach 63% of the pen's deflection.

123. B

The fall time constant is the amount of time for a calibration wave to return to 37% of the pen's deflection.

124. D

An impedance value of 4 kilo ohms is appropriate, so no action is necessary.

125. C

Most amplifiers use standard alternating signals of 50 µV and −50 µV during calibrations.

126. C

Another name for the fall time constant is *signal decay*.

127. A

Preparing the skin more usually decreases impedances, although too much scrubbing on the skin can be abrasive and harmful to the patient.

128. A

Short power cords often decrease leakage current. Power strips and battery backups add more connections, which can increase leakage current. Placing power cords alongside each other can also increase leakage current.

129. D

Calibration waves in DC channels are square because they do not have frequency filters.

130. D

Direct current amplifiers receive signals from DC devices and use those signals to output a signal from 0 to 1 volts.

131. B

Inductive plethysmography uses coiled bands inside an elastic belt that produce a waveform on the polysomnograph as they are stretched.

132. A

The time constant $= 1/(2\pi LFF)$; $1/(2 \times 3.14 \times 1) = 1/(6.28) = 0.16$

133. C

Amperes are measured in coulombs/second, which is a frequency reading.

134. B

Stray capacitance refers to electrical signals interfering with physiologic potentials derived from the patient.

135. D

An actigraph provides long-term data (up to several days) regarding movement activity. This information can give useful information regarding a patient's circadian rhythm.

136. D

$ETCO_2$ is read at the end of the expiratory phase or plateau.

137. B

Double grounding any type of equipment can be extremely hazardous and will likely lead to electric shock.

138. C

When the crystals inside a piezoelectric crystal band are stretched, they produce their own electric potentials.

139. B

SaO_2 and PaO_2 are values attained via blood labs. SpO_2 is the saturation of oxygen via pulse oximetry.

140. D

Leg channels are EMG channels that have LFF settings that are set at approximately 10 Hz. Because a high LFF setting will result in a shorter time constant, the calibration signal will return to baseline fairly quickly. Comparing the channel options, channels 4, 8, and 13 all have long time posttants but channel 17 does not.

141. C

Airflow channels have the lowest LFF settings of all of the channels. Because a low LFF setting will result in a longer time constant, the airflow channel will be indicated by the calibration signal with the most gradual return to baseline.

142. D

The highest time constant will be indicated by the calibration signal with the most gradual return to baseline.

143. C

An LFF of 0.16 indicates a high time constant. The highest time constant will be indicated by the calibration signal with the most gradual return to baseline.

144. C

An LFF of 10 indicates a low or short time constant. The low time constant will be indicated by the calibration signal with the fastest return to baseline.

145. C

EEG channels sensitivity settings are recommended at 5–7 μV/mm. EMG channels may require higher sensitivity settings to visualize muscle activity.

146. A

Channel 9 is an EMG channel.

147. C

Channels 2, 7, and 13 all have high time constants. A snore channel would need to have a lower time constant (or higher LFF setting).

148. B

Channel 2 is an EEG channel because of the filter settings. Calibration waves for EEG channels return to baseline gradually. Note that the top eight channels all have identical calibrations waves indicating identical LFF settings. These represent the EEG and EOG channels.

149. C

The lowest time constant will be seen in the channel with the calibration signal that returns to baseline most quickly.

150. A

EMG channels have higher LFF settings and shorter time constants.

151. A

This channel is an EEG channel because of the filter settings. Calibration waves for EEG channels return to baseline gradually. Note that the top eight channels all have identical calibrations waves indicating identical LFF settings. These represent the EEG and EOG channels.

152. C

Nasal congestion and a dry upper airway are common side effects of PAP therapy, but it decreases snoring and daytime sleepiness.

153. B

CPAP occurs when IPAP and EPAP have identical settings.

154. D

Capnography can provide additional information on ventilatory status. Vapors from collodion may lead to an asthma attack in some patients.

155. B

Oxygen always requires a physician's order. A water column manometer measures CPAP pressure. Humidification may increase comfort but is not required.

156. B

Leg leads are not used during an MSLT study.

157. A

If the first four naps do not produce REM sleep, a fifth nap is not necessary unless the lab protocol states otherwise.

158. D

A sleep study should never be performed without a physician's order.

159. D

All of these are true regarding MWTs.

160. C

An MWT is a maintenance of wakefulness test in which a patient attempts to remain awake in a relaxing environment.

161. C

A multiple sleep latency test consists of 45 naps during the daytime.

162. B

Movement artifact

163. D

Snore artifact

164. A

ECG artifact

165. D

High impedances or 60-Hz artifact

166. B

Electrode popping

167. A

Sweat or slow wave artifact

168. C

ECG artifact

169. C

High impedances or 60-Hz artifact

170. A

Electrode popping

171. A

The activity in the chin EMG channel is intruding and obscuring other channels. Muscle artifact can also be seen in the EEG channels.

172. B

Sweat or slow wave artifact

173. A

Movement artifact

174. B

ECG artifact

175. C

Movement artifact

176. C

Snore artifact

177. D

A 60-Hz artifact (head box is disconnected)

178. A

ECG artifact

179. B

Electrode popping

180. C

High impedances or 60-Hz artifact. Muscle artifact can also been seen in the F4 and C3 channels.

181. A

60-Hz artifact (head box is disconnected)

182. A

ECG artifact

183. D

High impedances or 60-Hz artifact

184. A

ECG artifact

185. A

ECG artifact

186. C

187. A

Alpha activity decreases with sleep onset.

188. B

Vertex sharp waves are seen in the latter end of stage N1 sleep.

189. A

Sawtooth waves are characteristic of REM sleep.

190. C

Alpha waves are 8–13 Hz.

191. B

Theta waves range from 4 to 7 Hz.

192. A

These are the characteristics of stage N1 sleep.

193. D

All the other conditions mentioned are likely to contribute to hypoventilation or hypoxemia.

194. A

Hypoventilation during sleep is a slight reduction in the airflow amplitude for an extended period of time.

195. D

All of these may be true regarding frequent EEG arousals during sleep.

196. D

All of these factors can contribute to irregular patterns in the airflow channel.

197. C

All of these are characteristics associated with sleep onset except for an increase in EEG frequency.

198. D

The chin EMG slightly decreases in amplitude at sleep onset.

199. B

The required desaturation for a hypopnea is 3% when the decrease in airflow is at least 30% in the absence of an EEG arousal.

200. C

Central apneas can be caused by increasing the CPAP too quickly.

201. C

An apnea is a full cessation of airflow, whereas a hypopnea is a decrease in airflow.

202. B

A full cessation of airflow must be at least 10 seconds long to classify as an apnea.

203. A

This pattern describes paradoxical breathing.

204. D

This respiratory pattern describes Cheyne–Stokes breathing.

205. C

This pattern describes a central apnea.

206. A

Blood pressure increases during REM sleep.

207. B

The sum of the latencies is 30 minutes. Thirty minutes divided by five naps is a mean, or an average, of 6 minutes/nap.

208. B

The mode is the number that occurs most frequently.

209. A
The median is the number that is in the middle of the other numbers when they are placed in numerical order.

210. B
The nap should end 15 minutes after sleep onset.

211. C
REM is seen most frequently during the final third of the night.

212. B
Nocturnal myoclonus is an old name for periodic limb movement disorder and is not part of the narcolepsy tetrad.

213. A
Pediatric active sleep is similar in EEG patterns and other physiological parameters to REM sleep in adults.

214. D
Pediatric quiet sleep is similar in EEG patterns and other physiological parameters to stage N3 in adults.

215. A
EEG slow waves are most prevalent in younger subjects.

216. B
A series of at least four limb movements is required to classify as periodic limb movement.

217. D
Restless legs syndrome can occur during wakefulness, whereas periodic limb movement disorder occurs only during sleep.

218. A
Duration, amplitude, and interval requirements exist for scoring periodic limb movements, but they do not require an associated EEG arousal.

219. B
Eye blinks and increased muscle tone are characteristics of wakefulness.

220. D
A K-complex is at least 0.5 seconds long but has no minimum amplitude requirement.

221. B
An EEG arousal is a shift in EEG frequency for at least 3 seconds.

222. B
The amplitude of EMG signals is higher during NREM sleep than during REM.

223. C
This is the definition of stage N3 sleep.

224. B
Impedance checks are sometimes performed during the night at periodic intervals, and should always be documented by the night technician.

225. A
Barbiturate-related EEGs are at least 13 Hz and are called *beta spindles*. Night terrors occur in stage N3, which has slower frequencies.

226. C
Alpha waves are most easily seen in the occipital channels.

227. A
This is the definition for stage N1 sleep.

228. A
These are all terms formerly given to stage N1 sleep.

229. C
These most accurately describe slow waves, which are seen in N3.

230. B
Periods of stage N1 are usually quite brief because this is merely a transition from being awake to sleep.

231. C
A slow wave must be at least 0.5 seconds long and 75 µV in amplitude.

232. D

There is no amplitude requirement for a K-complex, but there is a duration requirement of 0.5 seconds.

233. B

The frequency, amplitude, and shape of EEG waves are taken into account when determining sleep stages. Pen dampening is the curvature of the peak of a calibration wave on an analogue polysomnograph.

234. B

Although other characteristic waves are seen in N1 and REM, most EEG waves during these stages are low voltage, mixed frequency.

235. C

A major body movement is an option for an epoch score. Movement time was used under the rules set forth by Allan Rechtschaffen and Anthony Kales but is not used currently.

236. B

Sleep studies are typically displayed at 30 seconds/page, whereas EEG studies use a paper speed of 10 seconds/page. When scoring respiratory events, a slower paper speed of 120 or even 300 seconds may be more appropriate.

237. A

Rapid eye movements are often seen during wakefulness because the patient may be watching television, reading, or blinking.

238. D

Increased electrical impedances and interelectrode distances increase wave amplitude. If electrodes are placed in the proper location, EEG waves are viewed at their highest amplitude.

239. A

When electrodes are close to each other, they are transmitting similar signals. Therefore, the amplifier will differentiate mostly equal voltages, and the result will be a low-amplitude wave.

240. D

When alpha waves appear during sleep, this is called *alpha intrusion*. This can occur in any stage of sleep.

241. B

Epochs of N3 sleep often contain sleep spindles and K-complexes as well as slow waves.

242. A

EEG slow waves are 0.5–2 Hz.

243. A

Beta spindles are high-amplitude bursts of EEG activity with a frequency of at least 13 Hz.

244. A

If an arousal occurs during N2, the following sleep stage is scored as N1 until a sleep spindle or K-complex occurs.

245. A

Sleep spindles must be at least 0.5 seconds in duration. There is no amplitude requirement for sleep spindles.

246. B

V waves (formerly called *vertex sharp waves*) are seen mainly during the transition from stage N1 to stage N2.

247. A

This is the definition of sleep onset given by the American Academy of Sleep Medicine. Answer C is the definition of sleep onset under the rules developed by Allan Rechtschaffen and Anthony Kales.

248. D

Stage N2 is the most prominent stage of sleep.

249. C

Approximately 25% of the TST is spent in REM for normal adult sleepers.

250. B

EEG arousals must be preceded by at least 10 seconds of uninterrupted sleep.

251. A

A snore can only be scored in the snore channel, and an EEG arousal can only be scored by activity in the EEG channels. Movement is not scored as an event.

252. B
An EEG arousal is at least 3 seconds in duration and must be preceded by at least 10 seconds of uninterrupted sleep.

253. A
This characterizes a premature ventricular contraction, or PVC. PVCs are often seen in patients with obstructive sleep apnea.

254. B
Total sleep time is the total recording time minus the time spent awake between the beginning of the study and the end of the study.

255. D
The flattened signals in the respiratory effort channels indicate a central event.

256. D
Failure to mark lights out on a digital system can cause a variety of problems in the statistical readings on the sleep report.

257. B
This describes sinus arrhythmia.

258. C
This describes a PVC.

259. A
This describes a PAC.

260. Normal sinus rhythm
261. Atrial flutter
262. Atrial fibrillation
263. Third-degree AV block
264. First-degree AV block
265. Atrial flutter
266. Second-degree AV block Mobitz 1
267. Asystole
268. Premature ventricular contraction
269. Ventricular tachycardia
270. Sinus tachycardia
271. Ventricular fibrillation
272. Second-degree AV block Mobitz 2
273. Asystole
274. Sinus bradycardia
275. Premature ventricular contraction
276. Third-degree AV block
277. Atrial fibrillation
278. Ventricular tachycardia
279. Second-degree AV block Mobitz 2
280. First-degree AV block
281. Second-degree AV block Mobitz 1
282. Sinus tachycardia
283. Premature atrial contraction
284. Ventricular fibrillation
285. Second-degree AV block Mobitz 1
286. Sinus bradycardia
287. Third-degree AV block
288. Couplet
289. Ventricular tachycardia
290. W
291. N2
292. N2
293. N2

294. R
295. W
296. N3
297. N1
298. R
299. N2
300. N2
301. N2
302. N3
303. W
304. W
305. N1
306. R
307. N2
308. N2
309. N3
310. N2
311. N3
312. W
313. W
314. N2
315. N2
316. W
317. N2
318. R
319. N3
320. N3
321. N2
322. N2
323. N1
324. N3
325. N3
326. N3
327. N2
328. N2
329. N3
330. W
331. N3
332. N2
333. N3
334. N2
335. N3
336. N3
337. N2
338. N2
339. R
340. W
341. R
342. W
343. N1
344. N3
345. R
346. N1
347. N1
348. N1
349. R
350. N2

351. N2
352. N1
353. N2
354. N3
355. R
356. W
357. N2
358. N2
359. W
360. N2
361. W
362. N1
363. R
364. N1
365. N3
366. W
367. R
368. R
369. N2
370. N3
371. R
372. N2
373. N1
374. N2
375. R
376. N1
377. N2
378. R
379. N3
380. W
381. R
382. N2
383. N2
384. W
385. N2
386. W
387. R
388. N2
389. N1
390. A
     Obstructive apnea
391. C
     Central apnea
392. A
     Bruxism
393. C
     EEG arousal
394. A
     Central apnea
395. D
     This is not a scorable leg movement because it occurs just after a respiratory event.
396. A
     Limb movement
397. D
     Limb movement

398. C
Hypopnea

399. D
Obstructive apnea

400. C
Hypopnea

401. A
EEG arousal (alpha intrusion)

402. A
Central apnea

403. A
Periodic limb movements

404. B
Bruxism

405. A
Central apnea

406. B
Snore

407. D
Obstructive apnea

408. A
EEG arousal

409. C
Hypopnea

410. A
Snore

411. A
Limb movements

412. B
Snore

413. C
Hypopnea

414. D
Obstructive apnea

415. A
The physician should be informed of the patient's increasing CO_2 levels. It is likely the result of oxygen-induced hypoventilation. Reducing the oxygen flow may restore the patient's respiratory drive.

416. B
The oxygen flow rate of 12 L/min is abnormally high, so the order should be verified.

417. C
PAP machines are calibrated to water column manometers because this is the true measure of cm H_2O.

418. B
Humidification may increase comfort and tolerance but is not required.

419. D
The positive airway pressure lowers blood pressure by decreasing the variance in cardiac output.

420. A
Following the first night on CPAP, patients often complain of dryness.

421. D
Obstructions in the upper airway are usually more frequent and severe when the patient is in the supine position.

422. C
Some patients with central sleep apnea respond well to CPAP whereas others do not.

423. B
Surgery of the nasal passages would be the most appropriate treatment.

424. C
Obstructions are usually most severe during REM and in the supine position. Therefore, these are the most appropriate conditions under which to determine the optimal CPAP level.

425. B
When tolerated by the patient, CPAP is the preferred treatment option for OSA.

426. B
Breathing during REM is generally not the same as it is during wake.

427. A
The RDI is the respiratory disturbance index and refers to the average number of respiratory events, including RERAs, per hour. Most physicians and labs use an RDI of less than 5 as the goal of a CPAP titration.

428. A
Bi-level PAP is a treatment for central apneas.

429. C
Patients with a hypoxic drive breathe based on the level of oxygen in the blood rather than CO_2 levels. Therefore, they typically do not respond well to CPAP.

430. B
The tidal volume is the actual amount of air the patient is breathing.

431. D
Epileptiform activity does not affect the likelihood of OSA.

432. D
OSA can lead to all of these.

433. D
All of these can be seen in patients with Cheyne–Stokes breathing.

434. C
435. B
436. C
437. D
438. B
439. C
440. C
441. B
442. B
443. A
444. C
445. D
446. A
447. B
448. A
449. C
450. A
451. B
All of these are common features of OSA except for a low BMI. The body mass index is a calculation based on height and weight. As weight increases, BMI increases.

452. D
Stage N2 makes up approximately 50% of normal adult sleep.

453. D
All of these can be true about patients in the sleep lab.

454. B
The suprachiasmatic nucleus is the pacemaker of the circadian rhythm.

455. C

The average sleep cycle in adult humans is approximately 90 minutes.

456. D

These studies have shown the highest level of daytime sleepiness to be in the afternoon.

457. A

Blood pressure is not stable during REM.

458. B

REM is referred to as *paradoxical* because EEG patterns during REM are similar to those seen in wake with the eyes open, but the body is paralyzed.

459. D

This is one of many sleep hygiene techniques.

460. C

Most narcoleptics tend to be sleepy nearly all of the time.

461. A

Children are usually able to get the highest quality sleep of any age group.

462. C

These are characteristics of sleep starts.

463. D

Viewing a record of a patient's sleep schedule is the most useful tool in diagnosing a sleep schedule disturbance.

464. D

With age comes decreases in N3 sleep, changes in REM sleep, and decreases in REM latency and sleep latency.

465. B

Patients awakened from N3 sleep are usually sleepy and groggy, whereas patients awakened from REM sleep are more alert.

466. C

N3 sleep begins decreasing dramatically during middle adulthood. Sleep efficiency remains fairly constant at around 90–95% for normal adults of all ages, and sleep latency decreases slightly with age.

467. C

Adolescents tend to have extremely short REM periods at the beginning of the night, probably because of the large amounts of N3 sleep that occur during this time.

468. C

Children tend to have short sleep latencies and high sleep efficiencies.

469. C

Following REM sleep deprivation, normal sleepers often have sleep-onset REM periods.

470. D

All of these can lead to insomnia during infancy.

471. D

Loud noises can awaken a person from any stage of sleep. Awakenings from softer noises may vary according to the sleep stage.

472. A

The thalamus is the primary structure for relaying information from the body to the cortex.

473. C

Bruxism is characterized by grinding teeth and clenching the jaw during sleep.

474. C

When the neurons in the reticular activating system deactivate, the electrical signals from the thalamus to the cortex are blocked, resulting in a loss of consciousness.

475. C

Sleep spindles are seen when the signals from the thalamus to the cortex are blocked.

476. B

The suprachiasmatic nucleus is the circadian rhythm's pacemaker.

477. A

The RAS activates the brain from unconsciousness and altered consciousness.

478. B

The suprachiasmatic nucleus is strongly affected by light.

479. A

Acetylcholine is at its highest levels during REM and wake.

480. C

Normal REM sleep is associated with a decrease in muscle tone.

481. D

All of these neurotransmitters activate the cerebral cortex.

482. D

The raphe nuclei are primarily involved in NREM sleep.

483. A

Skeletal muscles are paralyzed during REM sleep.

484. C

Patients with REM behavior disorder have continued muscle tone in REM sleep.

485. C

Approximately 25% of the total sleep time is spent in REM sleep.

486. C

The length of the average circadian rhythm in humans is 90 minutes.

487. A

Blood pressure decreases slightly during sleep.

488. D

The body does not maintain its core temperature during REM.

489. D

Following sleep deprivation, long N3 and REM rebounds are commonly seen.

490. A

Approximately two-thirds of the 24-hour cycle is spent awake.

491. A

Stage N1 sleep is considered to be a transition between wakefulness and sleep.

492. A

Approximately 5–10% of the night is spent in stage N1 sleep. This percentage tends to increase with EEG arousals and awakenings.

493. A

Periods of N3 are longest during the first third of the night.

494. D

Normal sleepers are asleep for at least 90% of the time they are in bed.

495. C

REM periods are longest during the final third of the night.

496. C

N3 decreases dramatically with age and in some cases is absent in older adults.

497. D

EEG amplitude tends to decrease with age.

498. B

A dolphin sleeps with only half a brain at a time to defend itself from predators.

499. C

Alcohol increases N3 and decreases REM.

500. C

Exercising at least 4–6 hours before bedtime can increase the depth of sleep and is often recommended for narcoleptics.

Appendix A: Patient Hookup

This section contains step-by-step information regarding patient-hookup procedures. Although electrode-application processes may vary among technicians, proper placement on the head and body remains key to performing a quality sleep study.

International 10/20 System

The following EEG electrode sites are used in a standard overnight sleep study:

- F3
- F4
- C3
- C4
- O1
- O2
- M1
- M2
- Cz, Fz, or Fpz (often used as ground and main reference)

Step 1: Locate the Four Landmarks

- The nasion is the bridge of the nose.
- The inion is the most prominent point of the occipital bone.
- The pre-auricular points are just in front of the notches in the middle of each ear.

Step 2: Measure and Mark Between the Nasion and Inion

Measure the distance between the nasion and inion across the top of the head. Calculate 10% of the total distance and mark this distance above the nasion and the inion. Mark the halfway point (50%) of the total distance, providing the first mark for Cz. Mark 20% down from the halfway point toward the front of the head, giving the first mark for Fz.

Step 3: Measure and Mark Between the Pre-Auricular Points

Measure the distance between pre-auricular points ensuring the tape crosses the first mark for Cz. Mark 10% of the total distance up on each side. Mark the 50% point. This point reveals the exact location of Cz. Mark 20% down from the halfway point on the left and right sides, giving the first marks for C3 and C4.

Step 4: Measure and Mark Circumference

Measure the circumference of the head through all of the 10% marks, starting and ending above the nasion. Mark 50% in the front and back of the head (Fpz and Oz). Mark 5% of the total circumference on each side of Fpz and Oz, giving the locations Fp1 and Fp2 in the front and O1 and O2 in the back. Mark an additional 10% to the left and right of Fp1 and Fp2 for locations F7 and F8.

Step 5: Measure and Mark the Sides

Measure from Fp1 to O1 over the top of the head. Mark 50%, giving the exact location for C3. Mark 25% toward the front, giving the first mark for F3. Do the same on the right side, from Fp2 to O2, giving the exact location for C4 and the first mark for F4.

Step 6: Measure and Mark F7 to F8

Measure from F7 to F8 through the first marks for F3, Fz, and F4. Mark the 50% point, giving the exact location for Fz. Mark 25% on the left and right, giving the exact location for F3 and F4.

Step 7: Apply the Electrodes

For a standard sleep study, electrodes are placed at the locations measured for F3, F4, C3, C4, O1, O2. In addition, M1 and M2 reference electrodes are placed high on the mastoid behind each ear. A ground electrode is also placed, usually on Fpz, Cz, or Fz. Depending on the recording system, a reference to the ground may also be used.

Face Electrodes

The following electrodes or sensors are placed on the face:

- E1 (left eye)
- E2 (right eye)
- Airflow
- Chin EMG

The placement details described in this section refer to the adult patient.

E1 (Left Eye)

E1 is found by locating the left outer canthus, or the point at which the upper and lower eyelids meet. Measure 1 cm directly below and 1 cm laterally to the left outer canthus to locate the E1 site. Prepare the site and apply the electrode. Cup electrodes are preferred; use a small piece of tape to hold the electrode in place.

E2 (Right Eye)

E2 is found by locating the right outer canthus, or the point at which the upper and lower eyelids meet. Measure 1 cm directly above and 1 cm laterally to the right outer canthus to locate the E2 site. Prepare the site and apply the electrode. Cup electrodes are preferred; use a small piece of tape to hold the electrode in place.

Airflow Sensors

An oronasal thermal airflow sensor and a nasal pressure transducer are placed just below the nares, with the mouth piece directly in front of the mouth. The wire or tubing is usually directed over the ears to hold the sensor in place. A small piece of tape may be applied to the wire or tubing on each side of the face to prevent the sensor from slipping over the nose.

Chin EMG

Three electrodes are placed for the chin EMG: two for recording and one for a backup. The first electrode is placed centrally 1 cm above the inferior edge of the mandible, or the lower point of the chin. This electrode is used as a primary source of EMG recording, while either of the other two electrodes can be used as the other source.

Two electrodes are placed below the mandible to serve as the second active electrode for the chin EMG channel. These electrodes are placed 2 cm below the inferior edge of the mandible and 2 cm to the left and right. Either electrode may be used; the other is used as a backup in case either of the other two fails.

Body Electrodes

The following electrodes or sensors are placed on the body:

- Snore microphone or sensor
- EKG
- Thoracic belt
- Abdominal belt
- Body position sensor
- L leg EMG
- R leg EMG
- Oximeter

Snore Microphone or Sensor

The snore sensor is placed and secured with tape in the middle of the throat, where vibrations from a cough or snore are felt the strongest. A snore microphone, which records noises from snoring rather than vibrations in the upper airway, can be placed on the face or on the clothing.

EKG Leads

Two EKG leads are used in polysomnography. The exploring electrode is placed low on the left rib cage, vertically aligned with the left hip. The reference electrode is placed high on the right chest and horizontally aligned with the right shoulder. Using this method, the QRS complex is upright. Often, a backup electrode is placed on the middle of the left clavicle.

Respiratory Effort Belts

Two respiratory effort belts are placed on the patient: one around the thorax directly above the nipple line and one around the abdomen at the level of the umbilical. The sensor is placed in the center of the front side of the patient. The belt is pulled to fit snugly around the patient without restricting movement from respirations.

Body Position Sensor

The body position sensor is placed on the front of the thoracic belt. Most body position sensors indicate the direction it should be placed by an arrow or a small stick figure.

Leg EMG Electrodes

Two leg EMG electrodes are placed on each leg, longitudinally and symmetrically in the middle of the anterior tibialis muscle. They are placed approximately 2–3 cm apart from each other and aligned vertically. Because large leg movements may be frequent in many patients, special care should be taken to ensure these leads are applied securely against the skin. Tape and stress loops are often used to help prevent removal of leg EMG electrodes during sleep.

Oximeter Finger Sensor

The oximeter finger sensor is placed on the fingertip of any of the three middle fingers on either hand. When using a flexible sensor like the one shown here, the red light on one end should be aligned through the fingertip with the sensing device. The oximeter estimates the blood oxygen saturation by measuring the brightness of the light after it passes through the blood in the fingertip. Alternative placements include the toes and earlobes.

EEG Measurement Guide

	5%	10%	20%	25%	50%	
10 cm				2.5 cm	5.0 cm	
12 cm				3.0 cm	6.0 cm	
14 cm				3.5 cm	7.0 cm	F7 to F8
16 cm				4.0 cm	8.0 cm	
18 cm				4.5 cm	9.0 cm	
20 cm				5.0 cm	10.0 cm	
22 cm				5.5 cm	11.0 cm	
24 cm				6.0 cm	12.0 cm	Fp to O
26 cm				6.5 cm	13.0 cm	
28 cm		2.8 cm	5.6 cm	7.0 cm	14.0 cm	
30 cm		3.0 cm	6.0 cm	7.5 cm	15.0 cm	
32 cm		3.2 cm	6.4 cm	8.0 cm	16.0 cm	
34 cm		3.4 cm	6.8 cm	8.5 cm	17.0 cm	
36 cm		3.6 cm	7.2 cm	9.0 cm	18.0 cm	
38 cm		3.8 cm	7.6 cm	9.5 cm	19.0 cm	Nasion to Inion
40 cm		4.0 cm	8.0 cm	10.0 cm	20.0 cm	
42 cm		4.2 cm	8.4 cm	10.5 cm	21.0 cm	
44 cm		4.4 cm	8.8 cm	11.0 cm	22.0 cm	
46 cm		4.6 cm	9.2 cm	11.5 cm	23.0 cm	
48 cm		4.8 cm	9.6 cm	12.0 cm	24.0 cm	
50 cm	2.5 cm	5.0 cm	10.0 cm	12.5 cm	25.0 cm	
52 cm	2.6 cm	5.2 cm	10.4 cm	13.0 cm	26.0 cm	
54 cm	2.7 cm	5.4 cm	10.8 cm	13.5 cm	27.0 cm	
56 cm	2.8 cm	5.6 cm	11.2 cm	14.0 cm	28.0 cm	Circumference
58 cm	2.9 cm	5.8 cm	11.6 cm	14.5 cm	29.0 cm	
60 cm	3.0 cm	6.0 cm	12.0 cm	15.0 cm	30.0 cm	
62 cm	3.1 cm	6.2 cm	12.4 cm	15.5 cm	31.0 cm	
64 cm	3.2 cm	6.4 cm	12.8 cm	16.0 cm	32.0 cm	
66 cm	3.3 cm	6.6 cm	13.2 cm	16.5 cm	33.0 cm	

Left side labels: Ear to Ear (spanning rows 28 cm through 40 cm)

Appendix B: Artifacts

This section contains information to assist the technician in identifying and correcting signal artifacts and sleep diagnostic equipment malfunctions that may occur during a sleep study. The connection diagram shown is for a variety of digital sleep systems; however, not all systems are configured the same. Lab protocol should always be followed when correcting equipment malfunctions and signal artifacts. For more detailed information regarding artifacts and troubleshooting, please refer to *Essentials of Polysomnography*, third edition.

EKG Artifact

EKG artifact is characterized by the EKG waveform appearing in other channels. When it is present in one electrode, it is usually corrected by moving or replacing the affected electrode. Alternately, if the patient is asleep, a backup channel can be used. When EKG artifact appears in multiple channels, the source is likely the reference electrode. In this case, correction includes moving or replacing the reference electrode, using an alternate reference electrode (re-referencing) or double referencing (using common mode rejection to cancel out the artifact).

Movement Artifact

Movement artifact consists of high-amplitude, high-frequency electrical signals entering several channels at once. It is corrected by waiting until the patient stops moving.

Slow-Wave Artifact

Slow-wave artifacts can be attributed to sweat, respiratory movements, or sway. Slow artifact is characterized by low-frequency, often high-amplitude waves appearing in EEG, EKG, or other channels. Sweat artifact is corrected by cooling the patient, while respiratory artifact is corrected by adjusting the patient's head on the pillow or re-referencing to the opposite mastoid.

Snore Artifact

Snore artifact is characterized by periodic bursts of high-frequency activity associated with snores that occurs in a channel other than the snore channel. It can be corrected by moving any affected electrode.

Sixty-Hz Interference

Sixty-Hz interference exists when high-frequency signals from external electrical sources enter a channel. This is usually the result of poor electrode application and thus, corrected best by replacing the electrode.

Muscle Artifact

Muscle artifact appears as high frequency activity in a channel that is not designed to collect muscle activity. It is commonly seen in the EEG and EOG channels when a patient is anxious or clenches the jaw or grinds his or her teeth. Muscle artifact tends to gradually disappear as the patient relaxes and enters sleep.

Electrode Popping

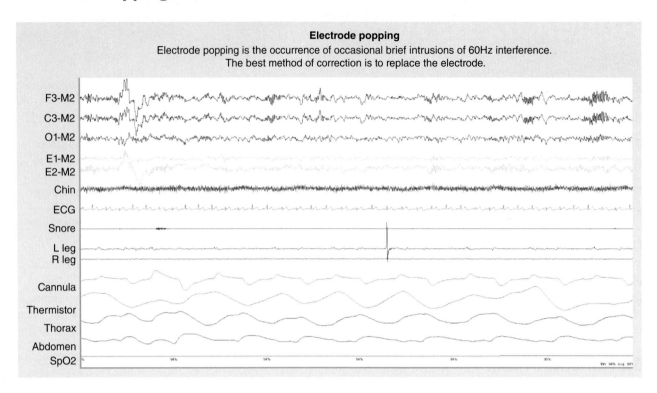

Electrode popping

Electrode popping is the occurrence of occasional brief intrusions of 60Hz interference.
The best method of correction is to replace the electrode.

Pen Blocking

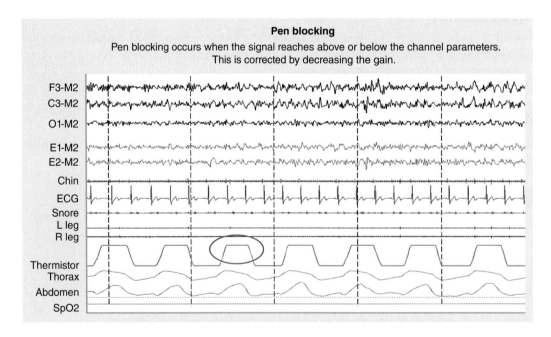

Pen blocking

Pen blocking occurs when the signal reaches above or below the channel parameters.
This is corrected by decreasing the gain.

Improper Gain Setting

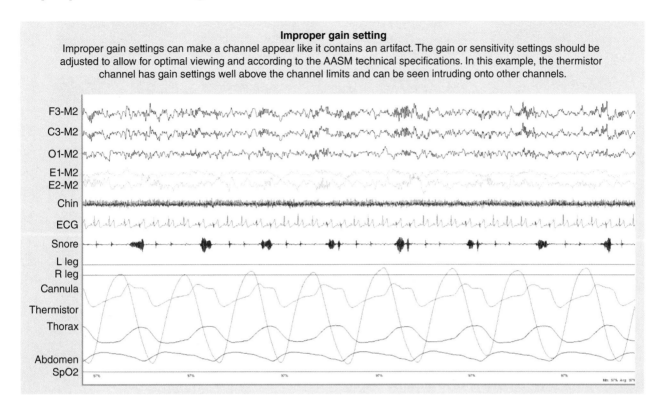

Improper gain setting

Improper gain settings can make a channel appear like it contains an artifact. The gain or sensitivity settings should be adjusted to allow for optimal viewing and according to the AASM technical specifications. In this example, the thermistor channel has gain settings well above the channel limits and can be seen intruding onto other channels.

Improper Filter Setting

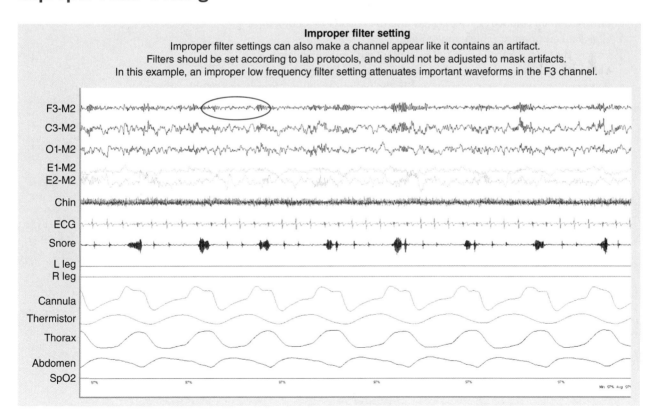

Improper filter setting

Improper filter settings can also make a channel appear like it contains an artifact.
Filters should be set according to lab protocols, and should not be adjusted to mask artifacts.
In this example, an improper low frequency filter setting attenuates important waveforms in the F3 channel.

Correcting Artifacts

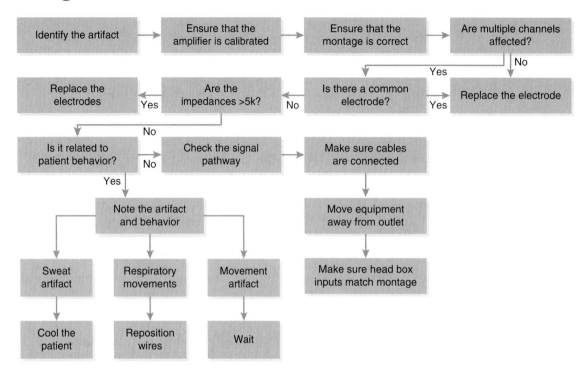

Items to Check When an Unknown Artifact is Present:

- ❑ Perform electrode impedances to ensure they are within acceptable ranges.
- ❑ Perform amplifier calibrations to ensure the amplifier is communicating properly with the polysomnography.
- ❑ Check for patient movement or activity that may be contributing to the artifact.
- ❑ Ensure that the montage settings and channel properties are correct.
- ❑ Ensure that all lead wires are plugged into the correct head box inputs.
- ❑ Check all equipment cable connections.
- ❑ Ensure that the electrodes are not in contact with metal jewelry.
- ❑ Ensure that the power to all pieces of equipment is turned on.
- ❑ Power off any unnecessary equipment in the patient room or close to the signal pathway.
- ❑ Ensure that the paper speed is correct (30 sec/pg or 10mm/sec).

Appendix C: Scoring

This section is designed as a quick reference to help the technician and scoring technologist identify sleep stages and sleep-related events. When identifying sleep stages, the stage of the previous epoch should be taken into account. For more detailed information regarding sleep-stage and event scoring, please refer to *Essentials of Polysomnography*, third edition.

Stage W (Wake)

Stage W (Wake)

Identifying characteristics:
- EEG's show mixed but often high frequency pattern when eyes are open
- Occipital EEG's show alpha rhythm (see below) in 8–13Hz range when eyes are closed
- Eye blinks may occur
- Large body movements are common
- Chin EMG amplitude is high

Alpha Waves

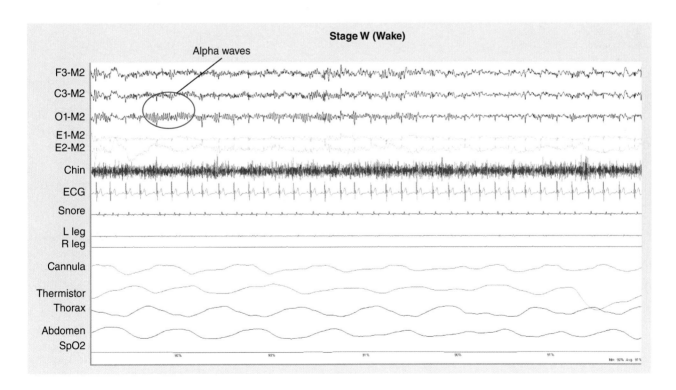

Stage W (Wake)

Alpha waves

F3-M2
C3-M2
O1-M2
E1-M2
E2-M2
Chin
ECG
Snore
L leg
R leg
Cannula
Thermistor
Thorax
Abdomen
SpO2

Stage N1

Stage N1

Identifying characteristics:

- EEG's show a low voltage, mixed frequency pattern in the theta range (see below) of 4–7Hz
- Vertex sharp waves (V waves) are commonly seen in the central EEG's
- EOG's often show slow eye movements (SEM's)
- Chin EMG amplitude is slightly decreased from wake

Theta waves

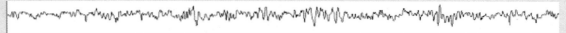

Theta Waves

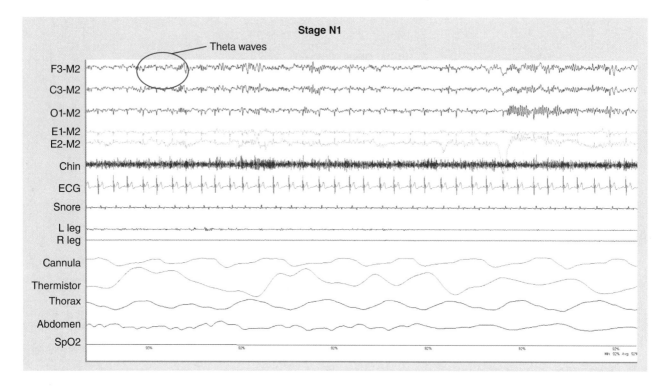

Stage N2

Stage N2

Identifying characteristics:

- EEG's show sleep spindles, bursts of 11–16Hz activity lasting at least 0.5 seconds, most prominent in the central electrodes
- EEG's show K complexes, sharp, negative waves followed by slower positive components lasting at least 0.5 seconds, seen most prominently in the frontal electrode channels
- Background EEG rhythm is usually within theta ranges
- Not usually associated with significant eye movements

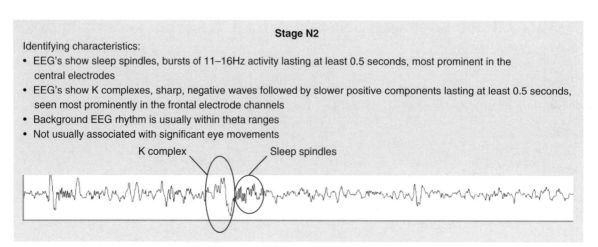

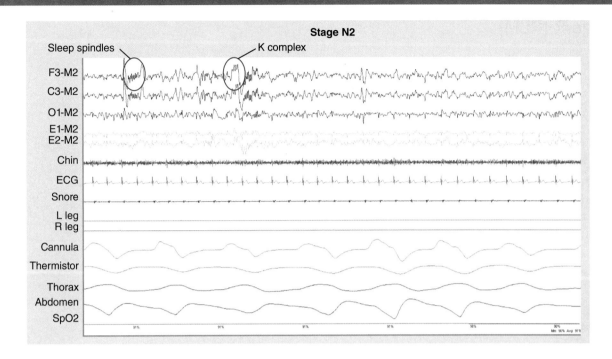

Stage N2

Stage N3

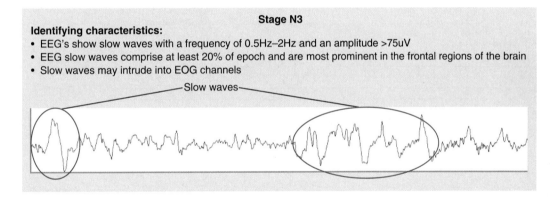

Stage N3

Identifying characteristics:

- EEG's show slow waves with a frequency of 0.5Hz–2Hz and an amplitude >75uV
- EEG slow waves comprise at least 20% of epoch and are most prominent in the frontal regions of the brain
- Slow waves may intrude into EOG channels

Slow waves

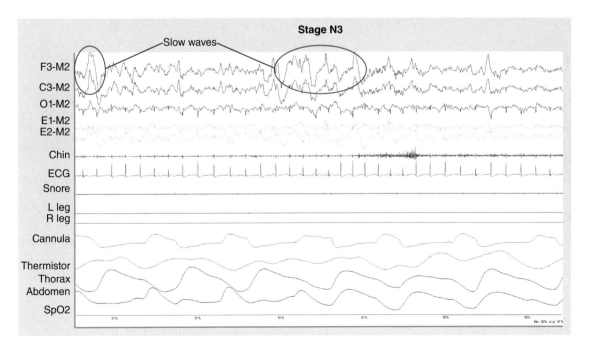

Stage N3

Stage R (REM)

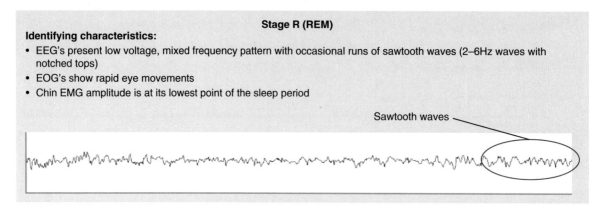

Stage R (REM)

Identifying characteristics:
- EEG's present low voltage, mixed frequency pattern with occasional runs of sawtooth waves (2–6Hz waves with notched tops)
- EOG's show rapid eye movements
- Chin EMG amplitude is at its lowest point of the sleep period

Sawtooth waves

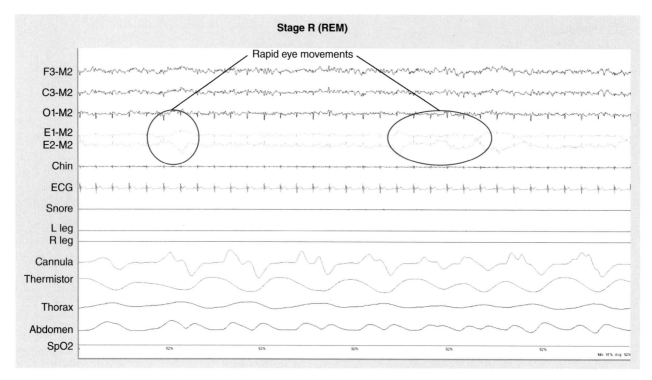

Stage R (REM)

Rapid eye movements

Sleep Events

EEG Arousals

Identifying Characteristics

- An abrupt shift in EEG frequency (including alpha, theta, and frequencies greater than 16 Hz) that lasts at least 3 seconds.
- Must be preceded by at least 10 seconds of sleep.
- An EEG arousal in REM sleep requires an increase in chin EMG amplitude for at least 1 second.

Significance

- An EEG arousal represents a disruption to normal sleep. Although common, they may be a sign of a more serious underlying sleep disturbance.
- EEG arousals often occur in association with other sleep-related events, such as apneas, snores, or leg movements.
- Frequent EEG arousals often lead to excessive daytime sleepiness (EDS).

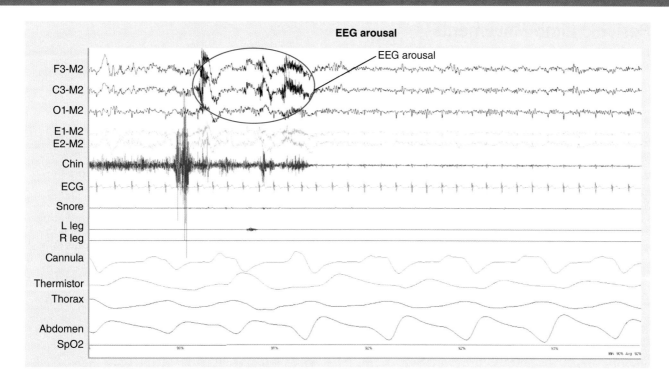

Beta Spindles

Identifying Characteristics

- Bursts of high-frequency (>14 Hz), high-amplitude EEG waves.
- Can occur in any stage of sleep and should not be confused with sleep spindles.

Significance

- Beta spindles are sometimes called *drug spindles* and may be the result of the use of benzodiazepines or barbiturates.
- Beta spindles are often the result of chronic pain.
- Beta spindles may be seen in patients with Parkinson's disease or fibromyalgia.

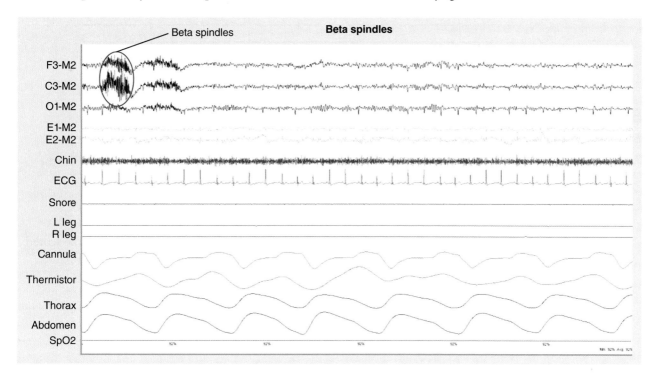

Periodic Limb Movements

Identifying Characteristics

- A limb movement is at least 8μV in amplitude above the resting EMG level and is between 0.5 and 10 seconds in duration.
- A PLM series consists of at least four limb movements.
- PLMs must be at least 5 seconds and no greater than 90 seconds apart from each other.
- Movements from different legs occurring within 5 seconds of each other are counted as a single limb movement.
- Limb movements occurring within 0.5 seconds preceding or following a respiratory event are not scored.

Significance

- Frequent episodes of PLMs can indicate periodic limb movement disorder.
- Limb movements can disturb the sleep of both the patient and the bed partner by causing EEG arousals or awakenings.

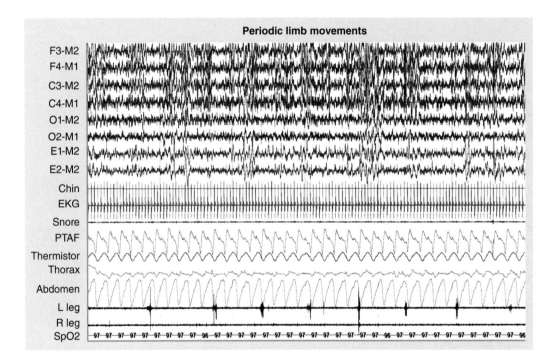

Bruxism

Identifying Characteristics

- Episodes of bruxism consist of brief (phasic) or sustained (tonic) elevations in chin EMG at least double the amplitude of the background chin EMG level.
- Brief elevations of chin EMG are scored as bruxism if they are 0.25–2 seconds in duration and if at least three episodes occur in sequence.
- Sustained elevations of chin EMG must last at least 2 seconds to be scored.
- A period of at least 3 seconds of stable background chin EMG must occur before a new episode can be scored.
- Heavy tooth grinding may cause muscle artifact in the snore channel, EEGs, and EOGs.

Significance

- Bruxism can cause damage to the teeth by grinding down the enamel.
- Bruxism can awaken the patient or the bed partner, causing EEG arousals or awakenings.

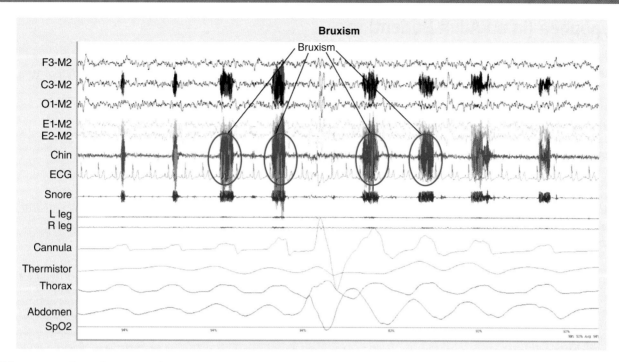

Obstructive Apnea (in an Adult Patient)

Identifying Characteristics

- Complete (>90% decrease in amplitude) cessation of airflow in oronasal thermal sensor.
- Must last at least 10 seconds.
- Continuation of respiratory effort throughout the event (may be slightly increased or decreased).
  - Paradoxical breathing (respiratory effort asynchrony) often noted.

Significance

- Obstructive apneas are often associated with oxygen desaturations, EEG arousals, or awakenings.
- Frequent obstructive apneas may indicate the presence of obstructive sleep apnea syndrome.
- Apneas can lead to EDS, hypertension, memory loss, and various cardiovascular and metabolic disorders.
- Apneas tend to interrupt the sleep cycle, often decreasing the amount of REM sleep achieved.
- Obstructive apneas are also often associated with snoring and hypopneas.

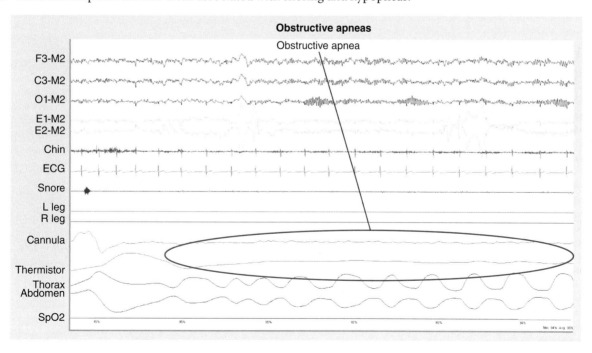

Hypopnea (in an Adult Patient)

Identifying Characteristics

- Decrease (≥30%) in amplitude in nasal pressure signal excursion (PAP device flow [titration]) with a continuation of respiratory effort.
- Must be associated with an oxygen desaturation of at least 3% or an EEG arousal.
- Event must be at least 10 seconds in duration

Significance

- Hypopneas are associated with oxygen desaturations, EEG arousals, or awakenings.
- Frequent hypopneas may indicate the presence of obstructive sleep apnea syndrome.
- Hypopneas can lead to EDS, hypertension, memory loss, and various cardiovascular and metabolic disorders.
- Hypopneas tend to interrupt the sleep cycle, often decreasing the amount of REM sleep achieved.
- Hypopneas are also often associated with snoring and obstructive apneas.

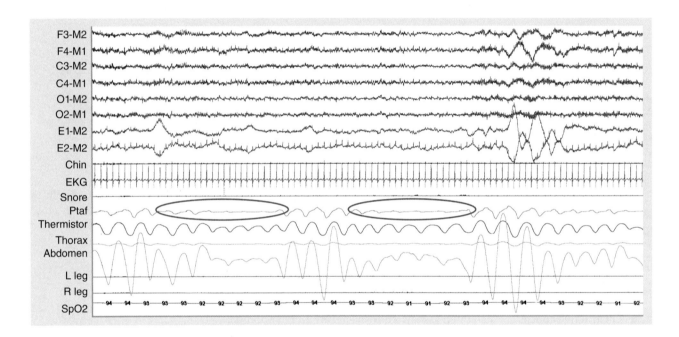

Central Apnea (in an Adult Patient)

Identifying Characteristics

- Complete (>90% decrease in amplitude) cessation of airflow in oronasal thermal sensor.
- Must last at least 10 seconds.
- Complete cessation of respiratory effort throughout the event.

Significance

- Central apneas are occasionally associated with oxygen desaturations, EEG arousals, or awakenings.
- Frequent central apneas may indicate the presence of central sleep apnea syndrome.
- Apneas can lead to EDS, hypertension, memory loss, and various cardiovascular and metabolic disorders.
- Apneas tend to interrupt the sleep cycle, often decreasing the amount of REM sleep achieved.
- Central apneas are often the result of low CO_2 levels in the blood and may be caused by high PAP levels.

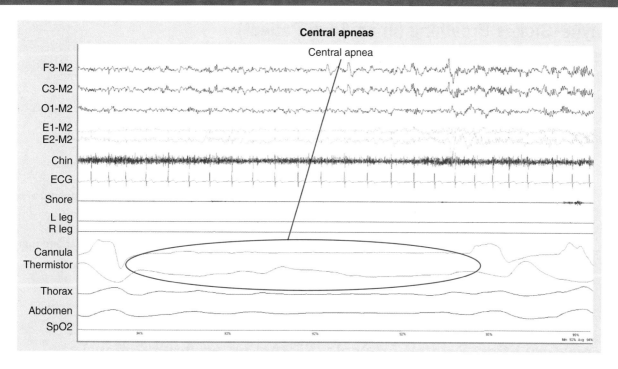

Central apneas

Mixed Apnea (in an Adult Patient)

Identifying Characteristics

- Complete (>90% decrease in amplitude) cessation of airflow in oronasal thermal sensor.
- Must last at least 10 seconds.
- Complete cessation of respiratory effort during the first portion of the event with a return of respiratory effort before the end of the event.

Significance

- Mixed apneas are usually associated with oxygen desaturations, EEG arousals, or awakenings.
- Frequent mixed apneas may indicate the presence of obstructive sleep apnea syndrome or central sleep apnea syndrome.
- Apneas can lead to EDS, hypertension, memory loss, and various cardiovascular and metabolic disorders.
- Apneas tend to interrupt the sleep cycle, often decreasing the amount of REM sleep achieved.

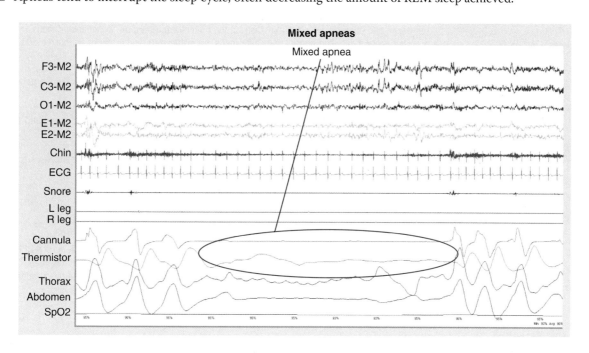

Mixed apneas

Cheyne–Stokes Breathing (in an Adult Patient)

Identifying Characteristics

- At least three consecutive central apneas or central hypopneas separated by a crescendo–decrescendo breathing pattern with a cycle length of ≥40 seconds.
- There must be at least five central apneas or central hypopneas per hour of sleep in more than 2 hours of recording.

Significance

- Cheyne–Stokes breathing cannot typically be detected on a 30-second epoch. The paper speed must be increased to accurately view this breathing pattern.
- Cheyne–Stokes breathing is typically seen in patients with congestive heart failure, stroke, or traumatic brain injury and may be observed in those on opioid medications.
- Oxygen desaturations are often associated with this breathing pattern.
- Cheyne–Stokes breathing can lead to EDS, hypertension, memory loss, and various cardiovascular and metabolic disorders.
- Cheyne–Stokes breathing tends to interrupt the sleep cycle, often decreasing the amount of REM sleep achieved.
- Cheyne–Stokes breathing can also occur during wake.

Respiratory Effort Related Arousals (RERAs) (in an Adult Patient)

Identifying Characteristics

- An EEG arousal that is associated with a sequence of breaths lasting at least 10 seconds that exhibit decreased airflow of <30 % or are associated with increasing respiratory effort or snoring.

Significance

- RERAs are often associated with oxygen desaturations or awakenings or both.
- RERAs can lead to EDS, hypertension, memory loss, and various cardiovascular and metabolic disorders.
- RERAs tend to interrupt the sleep cycle, often decreasing the amount of REM sleep achieved.
- RERAs are most commonly seen in patients with obstructive respiratory events such as apneas, hypopneas, and snoring.

Sleep Study Times, Formulas, and Calculations

Lights Out	The beginning of the study, or the time at which the patient first attempts to fall asleep. Lights, television, and other devices that may distract the patient are turned off. Impedance checks, amplifier calibrations, and physiologic calibrations are completed, and artifacts are corrected before lights out.
Lights On	The end of the study, or the point in time when the technician enters the room to wake the patient. Posttest calibrations are performed after lights on.
Total Recording Time (TRT)	The total time in minutes from lights out to lights on. This is calculated by using lights out and lights on times, or by adding total sleep time + total wake time.
Total Sleep Time (TST)	The total time spent asleep. This can be calculated by adding the time spent in each sleep stage or by subtracting the total wake time from the total recording time.
Sleep Efficiency (SE)	The percentage of total recording time the patient was asleep. SE = TST/TRT.
Total Wake Time (TWT)	The total amount of time spent awake during the study. TWT = TRT – TST.
% Stage R	The percentage of total sleep time spent in stage R, or REM sleep. Percent stage R = total REM time/TST. For normal sleepers, the % stage R should be approximately 25%. Percentages for other stages of sleep are calculated the same, but norms may vary according to age and other factors.

Sleep Onset	The time at which sleep first occurs after lights out. This is defined as the first epoch of sleep, regardless of the stage. It is usually marked by the first epoch of stage N1.
Sleep Latency	The amount of time in minutes from lights out to sleep onset. This calculation is especially important in MSLT reports. In an MSLT, the mean, median, and mode sleep latencies are often calculated.
Mean Sleep Latency	The average sleep latency for all MSLT naps. It is calculated by adding the sleep latencies from the naps and dividing by the number of naps. If the sleep latencies for five naps were 2, 3, 4, 8, and 8 minutes, the mean sleep latency is 5 minutes.
Median Sleep Latency	When viewing the sleep latencies from the naps in an MSLT in increasing numerical order, the median sleep latency is the middle number. For example, if the sleep latencies from the naps in an MSLT were 2, 3, 4, 8, and 8 minutes, the median sleep latency is 4 minutes.
Mode Sleep Latency	When viewing the sleep latencies from MSLT naps, the mode sleep latency is the number that occurs the most number of times. For example, if the sleep latencies for five MSLT naps were 2, 3, 4, 8, and 8 minutes, the mode sleep latency is 8 because it occurs more frequently than the other numbers.
Stage R Latency	The amount of time in minutes from sleep onset to stage R onset.
Stage R Onset	The first epoch of stage R.
Apnea Hypopnea Index (AHI)	The total number of apneas and hypopneas per hour of sleep. AHI = (apneas + hypopneas)/TST.
Respiratory Disturbance Index (RDI)	The total number of apneas, hypopneas, and RERAs per hour of sleep. RDI = (apneas + hypopneas + RERAs)/TST in hours.
Periodic Limb Movement Index (PLM Index)	The total number of limb movements that are part of a PLM sequence per hour of sleep (see chapter 2 for PLM qualifications). PLM Index = total number of PLMs/TST in hours
Arousal Index (AI)	The total number of EEG arousals per hour of sleep. AI = EEG arousals/TST in hours.
Wake After Sleep Onset (WASO)	Total time in minutes awake after the first epoch of sleep. WASO = TRT − TST − sleep latency.

Norms and Averages

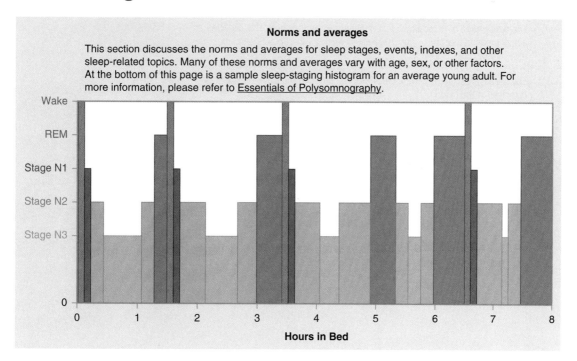

Norms and averages

This section discusses the norms and averages for sleep stages, events, indexes, and other sleep-related topics. Many of these norms and averages vary with age, sex, or other factors. At the bottom of this page is a sample sleep-staging histogram for an average young adult. For more information, please refer to Essentials of Polysomnography.

Sleep Efficiency	Sleep efficiencies of 90–100% are considered normal for healthy young adults. Decreased sleep efficiencies may indicate a sleep disturbance caused by apneas, limb movements, or other sleep-related events. Napping can also decrease sleep efficiency. Sleep efficiency tends to decrease with age. Older adults often have 70–80% sleep efficiency, whereas infants often enjoy 95–100% sleep efficiency.
Sleep Latency	A sleep latency of 10–20 minutes is considered normal. A decreased sleep latency may indicate EDS, while an increased sleep latency may indicate insomnia.
Stage R Latency	A REM latency of 90-120 minutes is typically considered normal. A decreased REM latency may indicate EDS or narcolepsy, while an increased REM latency may be indicative of insomnia or sleeping too much.
% Stage N1	The average percentage of the TST spent in stage N1 is 5–10%, regardless of age. Increases in stage N1 may indicate a disruption to sleep caused by respiratory events, limb movements, or other sleep-related events.
% Stage N2	The average percentage of the TST spent in stage N2 is approximately 45–50%. This tends to increase with age as the percentage of N3 decreases.
% Stage N3	The average percentage of the TST spent in stage N3 is 20–25% for normal, healthy young adults. This is much greater in infants and children and gradually decreases with age. Stage N3 may be completely absent in some patients by age 60.
% Stage R	The average percentage of the TST spent in REM sleep, regardless of age, is 20–25%. Decreases in REM may indicate a disruption to sleep caused by respiratory events, limb movements, or other sleep-related events. Increases in REM may indicate rebound sleep from treatment such as PAP.
Respiratory Disturbance Index (RDI)	An RDI >five events per hour may indicate obstructive sleep apnea syndrome. Severity levels vary from lab to lab and may include other factors in addition to the RDI.
Periodic Limb Movement Index (PLM Index)	A PLM index >15 in adults or >5 in children is considered abnormal and may be indicative of PLMD if other requirements are met.

Arterial Blood Gas Values

Gas	Description	Normal Levels
SaO_2	The percentage of hemoglobin that is saturated with oxygen. This provides an actual measurement of oxygen saturation, whereas the SpO_2 is an estimated measure by pulse oximetry.	95–100%
PCO_2	The partial pressure of carbon dioxide or the amount of carbon dioxide gas dissolved in the blood.	35–45 mm Hg
pO_2	The partial pressure of oxygen or the measurement of oxygen levels in the blood (this refers to the amount of oxygen rather than the percentage of saturation).	80–100 mm Hg
pH	The acidity level of the blood. A decreased pH is usually the result of a high CO_2, which leads to more acidity in the blood.	7.35–7.45
BE	Base excess. The amount of acid required to return the blood to normal pH levels.	–2.0 to 2.0 mEq/L
HB	The actual amount of hemoglobin in the blood. A low level may indicate anemia.	12–16 g/dL
HCO_3	Bicarbonate level regulated by the kidneys. An important factor in determining and regulating the pH of the blood. Smokers often have a high HCO_3.	22–26 mEq/L

Appendix D: EKG Rhythms

This section is designed as a quick reference to help the technician and scoring technologist identify EKG rhythms and arrhythmias. The samples in this section were derived using a two-lead EKG, which is the setup most commonly used in polysomnography. For more information regarding normal and abnormal EKG rhythms, please refer to *Essentials of Polysomnography,* third edition.

Reading EKGs

Reading EKG's

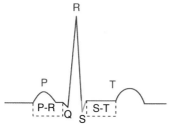

The EKG waveform consists of four basic waves: The P Wave, the QRS Complex, the T Wave, and the U Wave. In many cases, the U wave is not visible or easily discernible. Time axis distances between these waveforms are carefully reviewed. These intervals include the PR Interval, the ST segment, and the QT interval. The length of the QRS complex is also reviewed as an important time interval in the EKG.

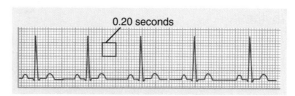

Normal EKG ranges:

PR Interval	0.12–0.20 sec
QRS Complex	0.04–0.10 sec
QT Interval	0.36–0.44 sec

A rate of 60–100 beats per minute (bpm) is normal for adults. The rate can be calculated by counting the QRS complexes in a minute, or in 10 seconds and multiplying by 6. Each large box on EKG paper is 0.20 seconds. Therefore, the EKG can be calculated by dividing the number of large boxes between R waves into 300.

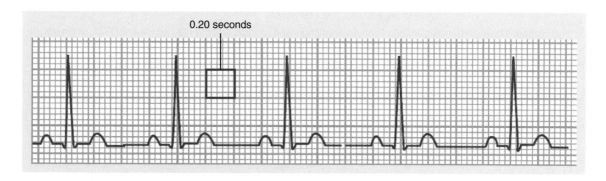

Sinus Rhythms
Normal Sinus Rhythm

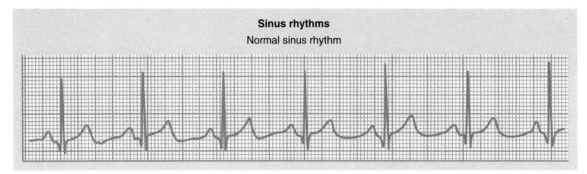

Rate:	60–100 bpm
Rhythm:	Regular
QRS:	< 0.10 sec
P waves:	Uniform and upright in appearance
PR interval:	0.12–0.20 sec

Description: The rhythm is regular, the P waves are upright and uniform, and the PR interval and QRS complexes are within normal ranges.

Sinus Arrhythmia

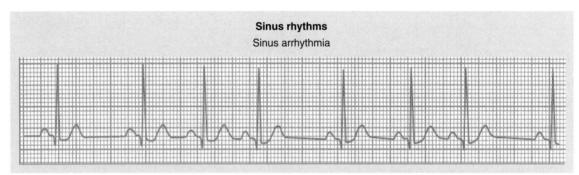

Rate:	Usually 60–100 bpm, but may vary
Rhythm:	Irregular
QRS:	< 0.10 sec
P waves:	Uniform and upright in appearance
PR interval:	0.12–0.20 sec

Description: The rhythm is irregular, the P waves are upright and uniform, and the PR interval and QRS complexes are within normal ranges. This is similar to a normal sinus rhythm, but the rate is variable.

Sinus Bradycardia

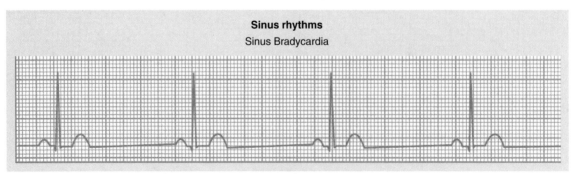

Rate:	< 60 bpm
Rhythm:	Regular
QRS:	< 0.10 sec
P waves:	Uniform and upright in appearance
PR interval:	0.12–0.20 sec

Description: The rhythm is regular, the P waves are upright and uniform, and the PR interval and QRS complexes are within normal ranges. This is similar to a normal sinus rhythm, but the rate is slower than normal.

Sinus Tachycardia

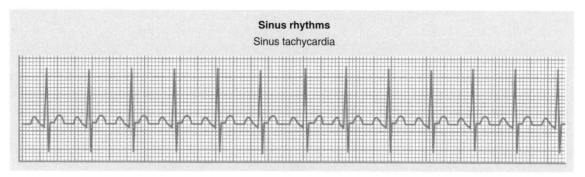

Sinus rhythms
Sinus tachycardia

Rate:	> 100 bpm
Rhythm:	Regular
QRS:	< 0.10 sec
P waves:	Uniform and upright in appearance
PR interval:	0.12–0.20 sec

Description: The rhythm is regular, the P waves are upright and uniform, and the PR interval and QRS complexes are within normal ranges. This is similar to a normal sinus rhythm, but the rate is faster than normal.

Atrial Rhythms

Premature Atrial Complex (PAC)

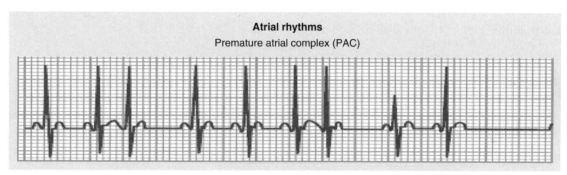

Atrial rhythms
Premature atrial complex (PAC)

Rate:	Usually normal, but depends on the underlying rhythm
Rhythm:	Irregular due to PAC's
QRS:	Usually < 0.10 sec, but may be prolonged
P waves:	P wave of early beat differs from sinus P waves
PR interval:	Varies from 0.12–0.20 sec

Description: A PAC is an abnormal beat that originates in the atria and occurs prior to the next expected beat. The rhythm is irregular due to the beat occurring early. PACs are often not a concern in patient without heart disease as they can result from caffeine use.

Atrial Flutter

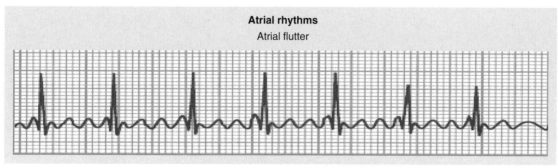

Atrial rhythms
Atrial flutter

Rate:	Atrial rate 250–350 bpm. Ventricular rate is variable.
Rhythm:	Atrial rhythm regular. Ventricular rhythm is usually regular.
QRS:	Usually < 0.10 sec, but may be widened
P waves:	Sawtoothed "flutter" waves
PR interval:	Not measurable

Description: This rhythm is characterized by fast flutter waves for P waves. The tracing shows normal QRS complexes with a faster atrial rate. This is a more dangerous EKG rhythm, and rarely occurs in the absence of heart disease.

Atrial Fibrillation

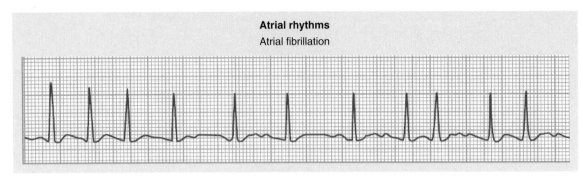

Atrial rhythms
Atrial fibrillation

Rate:	Atrial rate usually > 400 bpm
Rhythm:	Atrial and ventricular rates are very irregular
QRS:	Usually < 0.10 sec
P waves:	No identifiable P waves
PR interval:	None

Description: This rhythm is characterized by unorganized activity in the atria. In this case, the atria are quivering rather than contracting. Atrial fibrillation is usually the result of heart disease. Signs and symptoms of decreased cardiac output may also be present.

Junctional Rhythms

Premature Junctional Contractions (PJCs)

Rate:	Underlying rate; may be slow
Rhythm:	Irregular due to PJC
QRS complex:	Normal < 0.10 seconds
P waves:	Present before, during, or after QRS; may be inverted
PR interval:	Absent or short

Description: A PJC is an abnormal beat that occurs prior to the next expected p wave. It is identified by an inverted or abnormal p wave and a short PR interval. PJCs are often seen in patients with underlying heart disease.

Supraventricular Tachycardia (SVT)

Rate:	150–250
Rhythm:	Regular
QRS complex:	Normal < 0.10 seconds
P waves:	Mixed with T wave
PR interval:	Normal but difficult to measure

Description: SVT is an abnormally fast heart rhythm that typically starts and ends abruptly. Its fast rate makes often makes the visualization of p waves difficult. The rhythm may be related to stress and exertion or occur because of an abnormal electrical conduction pathway or underlying illness like heart, lung, or thyroid disease.

Ventricular Rhythms

Premature Ventricular Contraction

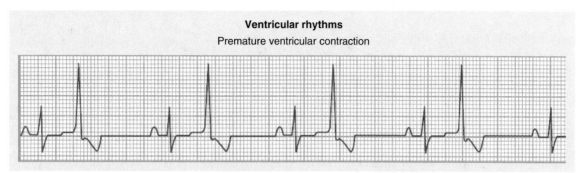

Ventricular rhythms
Premature ventricular contraction

Rate:	Atrial and ventricular rates depend on the underlying rhythm
Rhythm:	Irregular due to the PVC
QRS:	Wide and bizarre. T wave may be opposite direction of QRS.
P waves:	There is no P wave associated with the PVC
PR interval:	None with the PVC

Description: PVC's are some of the most commonly-occurring ectopic beats seen during a sleep study, as they are often associated with OSA and its associated hypoxia. PVC's are characterized by wide, bizarre QRS complexes that begin earlier than the next expected beat.

PVCs occurring in groups or patterns are classified as follows:

Unifocal PVCs:	Originate from the same location and therefore look the same as each other
Multifocal PVCs:	Different origins and therefore different from each other
Bigeminy:	A PVC in every other beat
Trigeminy:	A PVC in every third beat
Couplet:	Two PVCs in a row
Ventricular tachycardia:	Three or more PVCs in a row

PVCs are not usually considered dangerous unless they occur frequently or consecutively. Isolated PVCs may occur in otherwise healthy individuals.

Ventricular Tachycardia

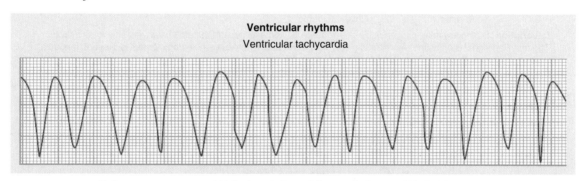

Ventricular rhythms
Ventricular tachycardia

Rate:	Atrial rate not discernible, ventricular rate 100–250 bpm
Rhythm:	Atrial rhythm not discernible, ventricular rhythm is regular
QRS:	> 0.12 sec
P waves:	May be present or absent. If present, they have no relationship with the QRS complex
PR interval:	Not discernible

Description: V-Tach is characterized by 3 or more PVC's in a row. This is considered dangerous, and requires intervention. CPR may be required.

Ventricular Fibrillation

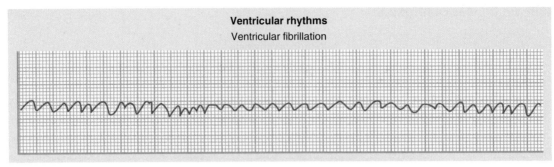

Ventricular rhythms
Ventricular fibrillation

Rate:	Cannot be determined
Rhythm:	Rapid and chaotic
QRS:	Not discernible
P waves:	Not discernible
PR interval:	Not discernible

Description: V-Fib is a very severe and dangerous rhythm in which the heart is quivering rather than contracting. There are no discernible waveforms during V-Fib. Immediate action should be taken, including activating the emergency response team and performing CPR and defibrillation.

Ventricular Standstill (Asystole)

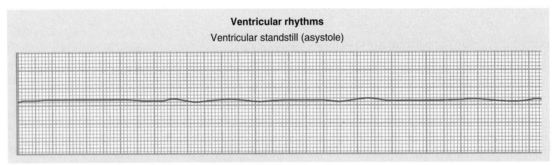

Ventricular rhythms
Ventricular standstill (asystole)

Rate:	Cannot be determined
Rhythm:	Atrial rate may be discernible. Ventricular rate indiscernible.
QRS:	None
P waves:	Usually not discernible
PR interval:	Not measurable

Description: During asystole, the ventricules have absolutely no activity, and the atria have very little to no activity. The resulting signal is a flat line. Asystole is a very severe EKG arrhythmia, as no cardiac output is present. Immediate action must be taken when this rhythm is seen, including activating the emergency response team and performing CPR. Asystole is characterized by a cardiac pause of at least 3 seconds.

AV Blocksa

First-Degree AV Block

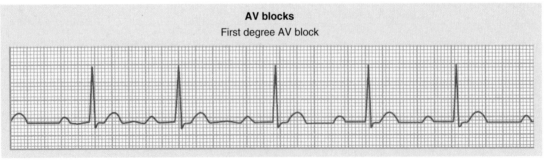

AV blocks
First degree AV block

Rate:	Normal
Rhythm:	Normal
QRS:	< 0.10 sec
P waves:	Normal in size and configuration
PR interval:	Prolonged (> 0.20 sec), but constant

Description: An AV block is a block between the atria and the ventricles, and is characterized on the EKG as a disassociation between the P wave and the QRS complex that follows it. In first degree AV block, the rate and rhythm are normal but the PR interval is prolonged. Intervention is not usually necessary.

Second-Degree AV Block Type 1 (Wenckebach, Mobitz 1)

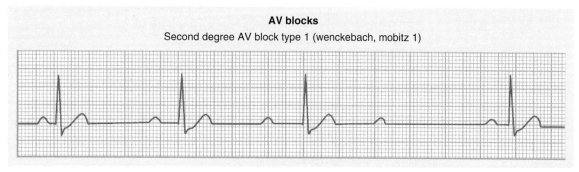

AV blocks
Second degree AV block type 1 (wenckebach, mobitz 1)

Rate:	Atrial rate > ventricular rate, but both are in normal ranges
Rhythm:	Atrial rhythm is regular, ventricular rhythm is irregular
QRS:	< 0.10 sec, but is dropped periodically
P waves:	Normal in size and configuration
PR interval:	Lengthens in each cycle until a P wave occurs without a QRS

Description: A second degree AV block is characterized by a QRS complex the is missed or skipped periodically. Second degree AV blocks are classified as either Type 1 or Type 2. Type 1 occurs when the PR interval gradually increases until this QRS complex is missed. This is usually asymptomatic, but can be a sign of hypotension.

Second-Degree AV Block Type 2 (Non-Wenckebach, Mobitz 2)

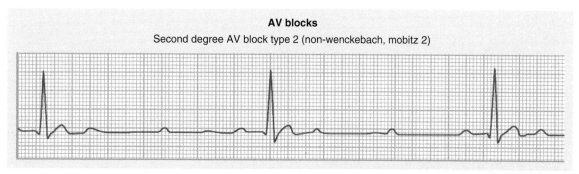

AV blocks
Second degree AV block type 2 (non-wenckebach, mobitz 2)

Rate:	Atrial rate > ventricular rate, but both are in normal ranges
Rhythm:	Atrial rhythm is regular, ventricular rhythm is irregular
QRS:	< 0.10 sec, but is dropped periodically
P waves:	Normal in size and configuration
PR interval:	May be normal or prolonged, but is constant for each QRS

Description: Second degree AV block, type 2 occurs when the QRS complex is suddenly skipped, without warning. If this rhythm is noted, the patient should be carefully assessed for symptoms and worsening status.

Third-Degree (Complete) AV Block

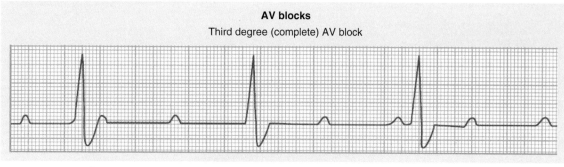

AV blocks
Third degree (complete) AV block

Rate:	Atrial rate > ventricular rate
Rhythm:	Atrial and ventricular rhythms are regular
QRS:	May be narrow or wide, depending on the escape pacemaker
P waves:	Normal in size and configuration
PR interval:	None since there is no relationship between the P waves and the QRS complexes

Description: Third degree, or complete AV block is a complete lack of association between the atria and the ventricles. As a result, the P waves and QRS complexes perform independently. This results in a decreased cardiac output and may lead to asystole. Immediate intervention is required including activating the emergency response team.

Appendix E: Procedures and Protocol

This section is designed as a quick reference to help the technician or technologist perform common tasks in the sleep lab in an organized, systematic manner. It is also provides sample protocols for titrations, technician notes, and MSLT studies. The protocols provided in this section are for use as a learning tool only. Lab protocols should always be followed.

Order of Operations for a Sleep Study

Before Patient Arrival

- ❏ Review the patient chart for physician's order, medical history, and symptoms.
- ❏ Prepare the patient tray with all items necessary for the hookup procedure.
- ❏ Prepare the patient room by ensuring cleanliness and order.
- ❏ Connect the diagnostic equipment and follow the signal pathway.
- ❏ Select an appropriate montage for the type of study being performed.
- ❏ Perform pretest amplifier calibrations to ensure equipment connectivity.

After Patient Arrival

- ❏ Provide and explain patient questionnaires and have the patient complete them.
- ❏ Perform patient hookup and provide patient education.
- ❏ Perform pretest physiological calibrations according to lab protocol.

During the Study

- ❏ Keep thorough and accurate technician notes and documentation.
- ❏ Maintain patient safety and the integrity of the recording.
- ❏ If a PAP study, initiate and titrate PAP therapy safely and according to lab protocols.
- ❏ Finish the study and perform posttest physiologic and amplifier calibrations.

After the Study

- ❏ Discharge the patient.

Items for the Patient Tray

- ❏ EEG paste
- ❏ Tape
- ❏ CPAP masks
- ❏ EEG marker or pen
- ❏ Cotton swabs
- ❏ Alcohol prep pads
- ❏ Precut gauze pads
- ❏ Measuring tape
- ❏ Gloves
- ❏ Prepping gels and pastes
- ❏ Hair clips
- ❏ Clipboard with questionnaires and handouts
- ❏ Electrodes, sensors, and lead wires

Physiologic Calibrations

- ❑ Close eyes: Patient lies still in the supine position and relaxes with eyes closed for 30 seconds. Technician looks for alpha waves in occipital EEGs.
- ❑ Open eyes: Patient lies in the supine position and relaxes with eyes open for 30 seconds (blinking is allowed). Alpha waves should disappear.
- ❑ Look left and right: Patient looks left and right only with the eyes while keeping the head still. This mimics the eye movements seen during REM.
- ❑ Look up and down: Patient looks up and down only with the eyes, keeping the head still. This mimics eye movements seen during stage N1.
- ❑ Blink: The technologist instructs the patient to blink five times while keeping the head still. This provides a reference for revealing blinks later in the study.
- ❑ Grind teeth: The technologist instructs the patient to grind his or her teeth or mimic chewing for at least 5 seconds. This provides a reference for increased in chin EMG activity.
- ❑ Snore: The technologist instructs the patient to simulate a snore or hum for at least 5 seconds. This helps set a standard for snore levels during the night.
- ❑ Breathe normally: The technologist instructs the patient to breathe normally to ensure that airflow and effort signals are optimal and synchronized.
- ❑ Hold breath: Patient takes a deep breath and holds it for 5–10 seconds, mimicking a central apnea.
- ❑ Breathe through nose: The technologist instructs the patient to breathe only through his or her nose for approximately 10 seconds. This ensures that nasal breathing is captured.
- ❑ Breathe through mouth: The technologist instructs the patient to breathe only through his or her mouth for approximately 10 seconds. This ensures that oral breathing is captured.
- ❑ Respiratory effort: Patient moves the chest and abdomen in and out while holding the breath, mimicking an obstructive apnea
- ❑ Move feet: Patient lightly moves the left foot or wiggles the toes on the left foot, followed by the right. This mimics the leg movements seen during wake and sleep.

Technician Notes

The following items should be included in the technician's notes, in addition to other items indicated by the lab protocol:

- ❑ Patient name, first and last
- ❑ Patient date of birth
- ❑ Patient height and weight
- ❑ Referring physician
- ❑ Interpreting physician
- ❑ Technician/Technologist name and credentials
- ❑ Patient medications
- ❑ Brief medical history
- ❑ Type of study being performed
- ❑ Date of the sleep study
- ❑ Lights out and lights on times
- ❑ Amplifier calibration times
- ❑ Physiologic calibration times
- ❑ Any time the technician enters the patient room
- ❑ Nocturia (patient using the restroom)
- ❑ Technical difficulties, including artifacts and equipment problems
- ❑ How artifacts and equipment problems were corrected
- ❑ Any time the test is stopped
- ❑ Patient complaints
- ❑ PAP level changes
- ❑ Mask type and size
- ❑ Oxygen flow level
- ❑ Snoring levels
- ❑ Leg movements, respiratory events, and other events
- ❑ Unusual events or personal observations

Sample Diagnostic PSG Montage

Channel	LFF (Hz)	HFF (Hz)	Sensitivity (µV/mm)	Sampling Rate (Hz)	Impedance (kOhm)
F4–M1	0.3	35	7	500	<5
C4–M1	0.3	35	7	500	<5
O2–M1	0.3	35	7	500	<5
E1–M2	0.3	35	7	500	<5
E2–M2	0.3	35	7	500	<5
Chin	10	100	2	500	<10
EKG	0.3	70	20	500	<10
L leg	10	100	7	500	<10
R leg	10	100	7	500	<10
Snore	10	100	7	500	
Oronasal thermal airflow	0.1	15	7	100	
Nasal pressure transducer	DC or <0.03	100	7	100	
Thorax	0.1	15	7	100	
Abdomen	0.1	15	7	100	
SpO$_2$	N/A	N/A	N/A	25	
Heart rate	N/A	N/A	N/A	25	
Position	N/A	N/A	N/A	1	

Sample PAP Montage

Channel	LFF (Hz)	HFF (Hz)	Sensitivity (µV/mm)	Sampling Rate (Hz)	Impedance (kOhm)
F4–M1	0.3	35	7	500	<5
C4–M1	0.3	35	7	500	<5
O2–M1	0.3	35	7	500	<5
E1–M2	0.3	35	7	500	<5
E2–M2	0.3	35	7	500	<5
Chin	10	100	2	500	<10
EKG	0.3	70	20	500	<10
L leg	10	100	7	500	<10
R leg	10	100	7	500	<10
Snore	10	100	7	500	
CPAP flow	0.1	15	7	100	
Thorax	0.1	15	7	100	

Channel	LFF (Hz)	HFF (Hz)	Sensitivity (µV/mm)	Sampling Rate (Hz)	Impedance (kOhm)
Abdomen	0.1	15	7	100	
SpO$_2$	N/A	N/A	N/A	25	
Heart rate	N/A	N/A	N/A	25	
Position	N/A	N/A	N/A	1	
Pressure	N/A	N/A	N/A	1	

Sample REM Behavior Disorder Montage

Channel	LFF (Hz)	HFF (Hz)	Sensitivity (µV/mm)	Sampling Rate (Hz)	Impedance (kOhm)
F4–M1	0.3	35	7	500	<5
C4–M1	0.3	35	7	500	<5
O2–M1	0.3	35	7	500	<5
E1–M2	0.3	35	7	500	<5
E2–M2	0.3	35	7	500	<5
Chin	10	100	2	500	<10
EKG	0.3	70	20	500	<10
L leg–R leg	10	100	7	500	<10
L arm–R arm	10	100	7	500	<10
Snore	10	100	7	500	
Oronasal thermal airflow	0.1	15	7	100	
Nasal pressure transducer	DC or <0.03	100	7	100	
Thorax	0.1	15	7	100	
Abdomen	0.1	15	7	100	
SpO$_2$	N/A	N/A	N/A	25	
Heart rate	N/A	N/A	N/A	25	
Position	N/A	N/A	N/A	1	

Sample Seizure Disorder Montage

Channel	LFF (Hz)	HFF (Hz)	Sensitivity (µV/mm)	Sampling Rate (Hz)	Impedance (kOhm)
Fp1–T3	0.3	35	7	500	<5
T3–01	0.3	35	7	500	<5
Fp2–F4	0.3	35	7	500	<5
F4–02	0.3	35	7	500	<5

Channel	LFF (Hz)	HFF (Hz)	Sensitivity (µV/mm)	Sampling Rate (Hz)	Impedance (kOhm)
Fp1–F3	0.3	35	7	500	<5
F3–C3	0.3	35	7	500	<5
Fp2–F4	0.3	35	7	500	<5
F4–C4	0.3	35	7	500	<5
Fpz–Fz	0.3	35	7	500	<5
Fz–Cz	0.3	35	7	500	<5
Cz–Oz	0.3	35	7	500	<5
E1–M2	0.3	35	7	500	<5
E2–M2	0.3	35	7	500	<5
Chin	10	100	2	500	<10
EKG	0.3	70	20	500	<10
L leg–R leg	10	100	7	500	<10
L arm–R arm	10	100	7	500	<10
Snore	10	100	7	500	
Oronasal thermal airflow	0.1	15	7	100	
Nasal pressure transducer	DC or <0.03	100	7	100	
Thorax	0.1	15	7	100	
Abdomen	0.1	15	7	100	
SpO$_2$	N/A	N/A	N/A	25	
Heart rate	N/A	N/A	N/A	25	
Position	N/A	N/A	N/A	1	

Sample MSLT Montage

Channel	LFF (Hz)	HFF (Hz)	Sensitivity (µV/mm)	Sampling Rate (Hz)	Impedance (kOhm)
F4–M1	0.3	35	7	500	<5
C4–M1	0.3	35	7	500	<5
O2–M1	0.3	35	7	500	<5
E1–M2	0.3	35	7	500	<5
E2–M2	0.3	35	7	500	<5
Chin	10	100	2	500	<10
EKG	0.3	70	20	500	<10

Sample CPAP Protocol

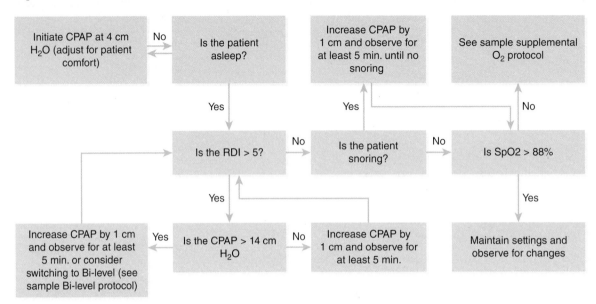

Sample Bi-Level PAP Protocol

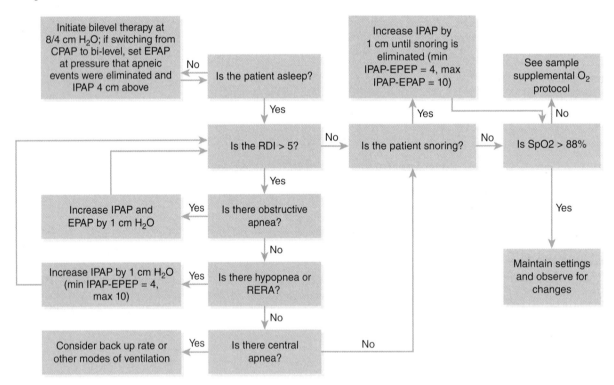

Sample Split Night Protocol

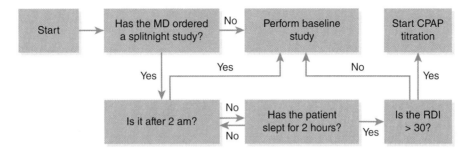

Sample Supplemental O₂ Protocol

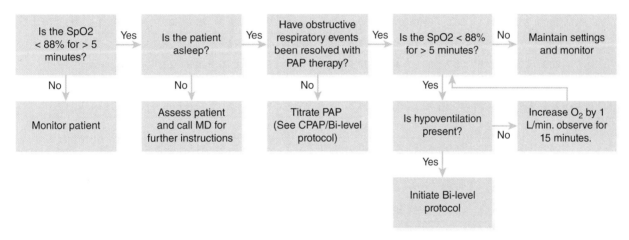

MSLT Procedures

- ❏ Begin the first nap 1½ to 3 hours after lights on from the overnight PSG.
- ❏ Perform amplifier and physiologic calibrations at the beginning and end of each nap.
- ❏ End the nap after 20 minutes if the patient has not had at least one epoch of any stage of sleep.
- ❏ If the patient achieves any stage of sleep for an epoch during the first 20 minutes, end the nap 15 minutes after sleep onset (first epoch of any stage of sleep).
- ❏ Each nap begins 2 hours after the previous nap began.
- ❏ The patient should remain awake and as alert as possible between naps. The technician should ensure that the patient does not lie down or fall asleep.
- ❏ The patient should not be allowed to consume any caffeine or alcohol between naps.
- ❏ The patient should eat a healthy breakfast and lunch. The patient should take prescribed medications as normally scheduled unless directed otherwise.
- ❏ The technician should document lights out and lights on times, sleep-onset times, sleep latencies, REM onsets, REM latencies, and all activities between naps.

Body Mass Index (BMI) Table

Body mass index (BMI) table
BMI = Weight (lbs) × 703/Height (Inches)^2
Inches

Pounds	60	61	62	63	64	65	66	67	68	69	70	71	72	73	74
120	23.5	22.7	22.0	21.3	20.6	20.0	19.4	18.8	18.3	17.8	17.3	16.8	16.3	15.9	15.4
130	25.4	24.6	23.8	23.1	22.4	21.7	21.0	20.4	19.8	19.2	18.7	18.2	17.7	17.2	16.7
140	27.4	26.5	25.7	24.9	24.1	23.3	22.6	22.0	21.3	20.7	20.1	19.6	19.0	18.5	18.0
150	29.4	28.4	27.5	26.6	25.8	25.0	24.3	23.5	22.9	22.2	21.6	21.0	20.4	19.8	19.3
160	31.3	30.3	29.3	28.4	27.5	26.7	25.9	25.1	24.4	23.7	23.0	22.4	21.7	21.2	20.6
170	33.3	32.2	31.2	30.2	29.2	28.3	27.5	26.7	25.9	25.2	24.4	23.8	23.1	22.5	21.9
180	35.2	34.1	33.0	32.0	31.0	30.0	29.1	28.3	27.4	26.6	25.9	25.2	24.5	23.8	23.2
190	37.2	36.0	34.8	33.7	32.7	31.7	30.7	29.8	28.9	28.1	27.3	26.6	25.8	25.1	24.4
200	39.1	37.9	36.7	35.5	34.4	33.4	32.3	31.4	30.5	29.6	28.8	28.0	27.2	26.4	25.7
210	41.1	39.8	38.5	37.3	36.1	35.0	34.0	33.0	32.0	31.1	30.2	29.4	28.5	27.8	27.0
220	43.1	41.7	40.3	39.1	37.8	36.7	35.6	34.5	33.5	32.6	31.6	30.7	29.9	29.1	28.3
230	45.0	43.5	42.2	40.8	39.6	38.4	37.2	36.1	35.0	34.0	33.1	32.1	31.3	30.4	29.6
240	47.0	45.4	44.0	42.6	41.3	40.0	38.8	37.7	36.6	35.5	34.5	33.5	32.6	31.7	30.9
250	48.9	47.3	45.8	44.4	43.0	41.7	40.4	39.2	38.1	37.0	35.9	34.9	34.0	33.1	32.2
260	50.9	49.2	47.7	46.2	44.7	43.4	42.1	40.8	39.6	38.5	37.4	36.3	35.3	34.4	33.5
270	52.8	51.1	49.5	47.9	46.4	45.0	43.7	42.4	41.1	40.0	38.8	37.7	36.7	35.7	34.7
280	54.8	53.0	51.3	49.7	48.2	46.7	45.3	43.9	42.7	41.4	40.3	39.1	38.1	37.0	36.0
290	56.8	54.9	53.2	51.5	49.9	48.4	46.9	45.5	44.2	42.9	41.7	40.5	39.4	38.3	37.3
300	58.7	56.8	55.0	53.3	51.6	50.0	48.5	47.1	45.7	44.4	43.1	41.9	40.8	39.7	38.6
310	60.7	58.7	56.8	55.0	53.3	51.7	50.1	48.7	47.2	45.9	44.6	43.3	42.1	41.0	39.9
320	62.6	60.6	58.7	56.8	55.0	53.4	51.8	50.2	48.8	47.4	46.0	44.7	43.5	42.3	41.2

- Underweight < 18.5
- Normal 18.5–24.9
- Overweight 25–29.9
- Obese 30–40
- Morbidly obese > 40

Body Mass Index Table (Metric)

Body mass index table (Metric)
BMI = Weight (kg)/Height (Meters)^2
Meters

	1.50	1.53	1.57	1.60	1.63	1.67	1.70	1.73	1.77	1.80	1.83	1.87	1.90	1.93	1.96
50	22.2	21.4	20.3	19.5	18.8	17.9	17.3	16.7	16.0	15.4	14.9	14.3	13.9	13.4	13.0
55	24.4	23.5	22.3	21.5	20.7	19.7	19.0	18.4	17.6	17.0	16.4	15.7	15.2	14.8	14.3
60	26.7	25.6	24.3	23.4	22.6	21.5	20.8	20.0	19.2	18.5	17.9	17.2	16.6	16.1	15.6
65	28.9	27.8	26.4	25.4	24.5	23.3	22.5	21.7	20.7	20.1	19.4	18.6	18.0	17.5	16.9
70	31.1	29.9	28.4	27.3	26.3	25.1	24.2	23.4	22.3	21.6	20.9	20.0	19.4	18.8	18.2
75	33.3	32.0	30.4	29.3	28.2	26.9	26.0	25.1	23.9	23.1	22.4	21.4	20.8	20.1	19.5
80	35.6	34.2	32.5	31.3	30.1	28.7	27.7	26.7	25.5	24.7	23.9	22.9	22.2	21.5	20.8
85	37.8	36.3	34.5	33.2	32.0	30.5	29.4	28.4	27.1	26.2	25.4	24.3	23.5	22.8	22.1
90	40.0	38.4	36.7	35.2	33.9	32.3	31.1	30.1	28.7	27.8	26.9	25.7	24.9	24.2	23.4
95	42.2	40.6	38.5	37.1	35.8	34.1	32.9	31.7	30.3	29.3	28.4	27.2	26.3	25.5	24.7
100	44.4	42.7	40.6	39.1	37.6	35.9	34.6	33.4	31.9	30.9	29.9	28.6	27.7	26.8	26.0
105	46.7	44.9	42.6	41.0	39.5	37.6	36.3	35.1	33.5	32.4	31.4	30.0	29.1	28.2	27.3
110	48.9	47.0	44.6	43.0	41.4	39.4	38.1	36.8	35.1	34.0	32.8	31.5	30.5	29.5	28.6
115	51.1	49.1	46.7	44.9	43.3	41.2	39.8	38.4	36.7	35.5	34.3	32.9	31.9	30.9	29.9
120	53.3	51.3	48.7	46.9	45.2	43.0	41.5	40.1	38.3	37.0	35.8	34.3	33.2	32.2	31.2
125	55.6	53.4	50.7	48.8	47.0	44.8	43.3	41.8	39.9	38.6	37.3	35.7	34.6	33.6	32.5
130	57.8	55.5	52.7	50.8	48.9	46.6	45.0	43.4	41.5	40.1	38.8	37.2	36.0	34.9	33.8
135	60.0	57.7	54.8	52.7	50.8	48.4	46.7	45.1	43.1	41.7	40.3	38.6	37.4	36.2	35.1
140	62.2	59.8	56.8	54.7	52.7	50.2	48.4	46.8	44.7	43.2	41.8	40.0	38.8	37.6	36.4
145	64.4	61.9	58.8	56.6	54.6	52.0	50.2	48.4	46.3	44.8	43.3	41.5	40.2	38.9	37.7
150	66.7	64.1	60.9	58.6	56.5	53.8	51.9	50.1	47.9	46.3	44.8	42.9	41.6	40.3	39.0

Kg (left axis label)

- ☐ Underweight < 18.5
- ☐ Normal 18.5–24.9
- ☐ Overweight 25–29.9
- ☐ Obese 30–40
- ☐ Morbidly obese > 40

Appendix F: Drugs and Medications

This appendix lists commonly used drugs that are known to affect sleep in specific ways. The list includes each drug's name, its brand name, its drug type, any indications it has, and its known effects on sleep. This list does not necessarily include every drug that may affect sleep, nor does it include every side effect for the drugs listed.

A

Acebutolol (Sectral) Beta blocker. For angina and arrhythmias. Associated with insomnia. Increases REM.

Accupril (Quinapril) ACE inhibitor. For hypertension, congestive heart failure. Increases fatigue.

Adderall *See* Amphetamine.

Adipex *See* Phentermine.

Alcohol Suppresses REM and N3 sleep. Increases N2, apnea and sleep fragmentation in the latter half of the sleep period.

Aldactone *See* Spironolactone.

Aldomet *See* Methyldopa.

Alprazolam (Xanax) Hypnotic. Decreases REM, N1, N3, leg movements, sleep latency. Increases N2 and spindle activity, apneas.

Allopurinol (Zyloprim) Acid reducer.

Amantadine (Symmetrel) Antiviral. For Parkinson's and influenza A. Drowsiness and hallucinations.

Ambien *See* Zolpidem.

Amitriptyline Tricyclic antidepressant. Increases TST, sleep efficiency, and N2 and N3 sleep. Suppresses REM. Associated with drowsiness, sleepwalking, PLMD.

Amphetamine (Adderall) Stimulant. For ADHD. Decreases sleep efficiency, TST, and REM. Increases WASO, sleep latency, N1 sleep, and R latency.

Anafranil *See* Clomipramine.

Apresoline *See* Hydralazine.

Aspirin Suppresses N3, increases N2.

Atenolol (Tenormin) Beta blocker. For HTN and arrhythmias. Suppresses REM. Associated with insomnia.

B

Bromfed *See* Brompheniramine.

Brompheniramine (Bromfed) Antihistamine. For allergies. Associated with drowsiness. Suppresses REM.

Bupropion (Wellbutrin) Antidepressant. Increases insomnia.

Buspirone Antianxiety. Increases insomnia.

C

Caffeine Suppresses N3. Stimulant. Associated with insomnia.

Carbamazapine (Tegretol) Anticonvulsant. For epilepsy. Associated with drowsiness. Suppresses REM.

Catapres *See* Clonidine.

Chlorpromazine (Thorazine) Tranquilizer. Increases REM.

Cimetidine (Tagamet) Acid reducer. For ulcers. Increases N3.

Clomipramine (Anafranil) Tricyclic antidepressant. Increases TST, sleep efficiency, and N2 and N3 sleep. Suppresses REM. Associated with drowsiness, sleepwalking, PLMD.

Clonazepam (Klonopin) Anticonvulsant. For seizures and panic disorders. Decreases REM, N2, leg movements. Increases N3.

Clonidine (Catapres) For hypertension. Suppresses REM. Increases N2, N3, EDS, insomnia, nightmares, sleepwalking, sedation.

Cocaine Stimulating effects. Prolongs sleep latency. Reduces TST. Associated with cardiac arrhythmias, bruxism, and sleep disruption.

Corgard *See* Nadolol.

Cylert *See* Pemoline.

Cyproheptadine (Periactin) Antihistamine. Associated with drowsiness. Suppresses REM. Increases N3.

D

Dalmane *See* Flurazepam.

Depakene *See* Valproic acid.

Desipramine (Norpramin) Tricyclic antidepressant. Increases TST, sleep efficiency, and N2 and N3 sleep. Suppresses REM. Associated with drowsiness, sleepwalking, PLMD.

Diazepam (Valium) For anxiety, panic disorders. Increases TST and sleep efficiency. Suppresses REM and N3 sleep. Increases N2, spindle activity, apnea, and restless legs.

Diethylpropion (Tenuate) Simulant, appetite suppressant. For obesity. Increases insomnia.

Dilantin *See* Phenytoin.

Dolophine *See* Methadone.

Donnatal *See* Scopolamine.

Doxepin (Sinequan) Tricyclic antidepressant. Increases TST, sleep efficiency, and N2 and N3 sleep. Suppresses REM. Associated with drowsiness, sleepwalking, PLMD.

E

Eldepryl *See* Selegiline.

Ephedrine (Rynatuss) Bronchodilator. For asthma, COPD. Simulating effects. Associated with insomnia.

Ethosuximide (Zarontin) Anticonvulsant. For seizures. Suppresses N3, REM. Increases N1, leg movements, insomnia.

Eulexin *See* Flutamide.

F

Fenofibrate (Tricor) Lipid regulator. Increases insomnia, nightmares.

Fluoxetine (Prozac) Antidepressant. Increases WASO, N1, arousals. Decreases REM sleep significantly. Associated with insomnia, slow eye movements in NREM and PLMD.

Flurazepam (Dalmane) Sedative used for insomnia. Increases TST and sleep efficiency. Suppresses REM and N3 sleep. Increases N2, spindle activity, apnea, and restless legs.

Flutamide (Eulexin) Antiandrogenic, anticancer. Increases insomnia, nightmares, drowsiness, somnolence, fatigue.

G

Guanfacine (Tenex) For hypertension. Suppresses REM.

H

Halcion *See* Triazolam.

Halotussin *See* Pseudoephedrine.

Heroin Opioid. Increases N1, central apnea. Decreases REM, N3, TST, sleep efficiency.

Hydralazine (Apresoline) For hypertension. Increases sleep disturbances.

K

Klonopin *See* Clonazepam.

L

Levodopa (Sinemet) Dopamine precursor. For Parkinson's. Decreases N3, REM. Increases N2, leg movements,

insomnia, nightmares, sleep disturbances, hallucinations, vocalizations.

Lithium (Lithobid) Antimanic. For depression, mania. Decreases REM, REM latency, N1. Increases N3, insomnia, sleepwalking.

Lithobid *See* Lithium.

Lovastatin (Mevacor) For high cholesterol. Increases insomnia.

Ludiomil *See* Maprotiline.

M

Maprotiline (Ludiomil) Cyclic antidepressant. Suppresses REM.

Matulane *See* Procarbazine.

Methadone (Dolophine) Narcotic analgesic. Decreases REM, leg movements. Increases N1, apneas.

Methyldopa (Aldomet) For hypertension. Decreases N3, REM. Increases insomnia, nightmares, drowsiness, sedation, sleep disturbances.

Methylphenadate (Ritalin) Stimulant. For ADHD. Decreases sleep efficiency, TST, and REM. Increases WASO, sleep latency, N1 sleep, and R latency.

Metoclopramide (Reglan) For heartburn, ulcers. Suppresses REM. Increases drowsiness.

Metoprolol (Toprol) Beta blocker. For hypertension, angina, arrhythmias. Suppresses REM. Increases sleep disturbances.

Mevacor *See* Lovastatin.

Midazolam Sedative. Decreases N3, REM, N1, leg movements, sleep latency. Increases N2, apneas.

Minipress *See* Prazosin.

Morphine Opioid analgesic. Increases N1, central apnea. Decreases REM, N3, TST, sleep efficiency.

N

Nadolol (Corgard) Beta blocker. For hypertension, angina, arrhythmias. Suppresses REM.

Nardil *See* Phenelzine.

Norpramin *See* Desipramine.

Nortriptyline (Pamelor) Tricyclic antidepressant. Increases TST, sleep efficiency, N2 and N3 sleep. Suppresses REM. Associated with drowsiness, sleepwalking, PLMD.

P

Pamelor *See* Nortriptyline.

Pemoline (Cylert) Stimulant. For ADHD, narcolepsy. Decreases sleep efficiency, TST, and REM. Increases WASO, sleep latency, N1 sleep, and R latency.

Periactin *See* Cyproheptadine.

Perphenazine (Trilafon) Tranquilizer. Sedation.

Phenelzine (Nardil) MAO inhibitor. For depression, bulimia. Suppresses REM.

Phenergan *See* Promethazine.

Phenobarbital Sedative, anticonvulsant. Decreases N3, REM, leg movements. Increases N2.

Phentermine (Adipex) Amphetamine. For obesity. Increases insomnia.

Phenytoin (Dilantin) Anticonvulsant. For epilepsy. Decreases REM, sleep latency. Increases N3.

Pindolol (Visken) Beta blocker. For hypertension, angina. Suppresses REM. Increases nightmares, drowsiness, fatigue.

Prazosin (Minipress) For hypertension. Increases drowsiness, sedation.

Procarbazine (Matulane) For Hodgkin's disease. Increases insomnia, nightmares, drowsiness, fatigue.

Promethazine (Phenergan) Sedative. Increases drowsiness, sedation.

Prozac *See* Fluoxetine.

Pseudoephedrine (Halotussin) Decongestant. Increases sleep disturbances.

Q

Quinapril *See* Accupril.

R

Reglan *See* Metoclopramide.

Restoril *See* Temazepam.

Ritalin *See* Methylphenadate.

Rynatuss *See* Ephedrine.

S

Salmeterol (Serevent) Bronchodilator. For asthma, COPD. Improves quality of sleep.

Scopolamine (Donnatal) Antispasmodic, sedative. Decreases REM. Increases REM latency, N2, leg movements, sedation.

Sectral *See* Acebutolol.

Selegiline (Eldepryl) MAO inhibitor. For Parkinson's. Decreases N3, REM, sleep latency. Increases N2, insomnia.

Serevent *See* Salmeterol.

Simvastatin (Zocor) Cholesterol reducer. Increases insomnia.

Sinemet *See* Levodopa.

Sinequan *See* Doxepin.

Sonata *See* Zaleplon.

Spironolactone (Aldactone) Diuretic. May increase sleep fragmentation as a result of increased need to void.

Stelazine *See* Trifluoperazine.

Suvorexant (Belsomra) Orexin receptor antagonist. Used for sleep onset and maintenance insomnia. Decreases sleep and REM latency. Increases sleep efficiency and R time.

Symmetrel *See* Amantadine.

T

Tagamet *See* Cimetidine.

Tegretol *See* Carbamazapine.

Temazepam (Restoril) Hypnotic. Increases TST and sleep efficiency. Suppresses REM and N3 sleep. Increases N2, spindle activity, apnea, and restless legs.

Tenex *See* Guanfacine.

Tenormin *See* Atenolol.

Tenuate *See* Diethylpropion.

Theophylline (Uniphyl) Bronchodilator. For asthma, COPD. Decreases N2. Increases N1, stimulating effects, insomnia, sleep disturbances.

Thioridazine Tranquilizer. Increases N3, sleepwalking.

Thorazine *See* Chlorpromazine.

Toprol *See* Metoprolol.

Triazolam (Halcion) Hypnotic used for insomnia. Increases TST and sleep efficiency. Suppresses REM and N3 sleep. Increases N2, spindle activity, apnea and restless legs.

Tricor *See* Fenofibrate.

Trifluoperazine (Stelazine) Tranquilizer. Increases sleep disturbances.

Trilafon *See* Perphenazine.

U

Uniphyl *See* Theophylline.

V

Valium *See* Diazepam.

Valproic acid (Depakene) Anticonvulsant. For seizures. Decreases REM. Increases N3.

Visken *See* Pindolol.

W

Wellbutrin *See* Bupropion.

X

Xanax *See* Alprazolam.

Z

Zaleplon (Sonata) Hypnotic used for insomnia. Increases TST, SE and N2 sleep. Mild suppressant effects on N3 and REM.

Zarontin *See* Ethosuximide.

Zocor *See* Simvastatin.

Zolpidem (Ambien) Hypnotic used for insomnia. Decreases leg movements. Increases TST, SE, and N2 sleep. Mild suppressant effects on N3 and REM. Increased risk of falls in elderly patients.

Zyloprim *See* Allopurinol.

Glossary

A

AAST *See* American Association of Sleep Technologists.

ABG *See* Arterial blood gas.

Acclimatization Techniques used to familiarize patients with PAP therapy.

Accredited Sleep Technologist Education Program (A-STEP) A program developed by the American Academy of Sleep Medicine to standardize sleep technology education.

ACE inhibitor Angiotensin-converting enzyme inhibitor. Heart medications that widen or dilate blood vessels to treat high blood pressure and heart failure.

Acetylcholine A chemical in the brain responsible for activating the cortex.

Actigraph A device used to measure movement, usually over long periods of time.

Adaptive support ventilation (ASV) A mode of PAP therapy that adapts ventilation on a breath-by-breath basis to prevent apnea and maintain consistent minute ventilation.

Adenoidectomy The surgical removal of the adenoids for reasons which include impaired breathing through the nose, chronic infections, or recurrent earaches.

Adenotonsillectomy An operation to remove both the adenoids and tonsils.

Advanced sleep–wake phase syndrome (ASPS) A circadian rhythm disorder in which the sleep–wake cycle is advanced (early) with respect to clock time.

AHI *See* Apnea–hypopnea index.

ALMA *See* Alternating leg muscle activation.

Alpha intrusion The presence of EEG alpha waves during sleep.

Alpha wave An EEG waveform seen during relaxed wakefulness while the eyes are closed. The frequency of alpha waves is 8–13 Hz.

Alternating leg muscle activation (ALMA) A sleep disorder characterized by repetitive movements in alternating legs.

Alveolar hypoventilation A disorder characterized by periods of shallow breathing or decreased airflow associated with oxygen desaturations and EEG arousals.

Ambulatory sleep study Refers to a portable sleep study that can be performed in a patient's home, living facility, or within the floors of the hospital.

American Association of Sleep Technologists (AAST) A society designed to provide education and training for sleep technologists.

American Society of Electroneurodiagnostic Technologists (ASET) An organized group or society dedicated to the education and training of END and EEG technologists.

Amplifier calibrations A test to determine the validity of signals from the amplifier to the polysomnograph.

Amplitude The voltage of an electrical signal.

Analogue polysomnography Recording bioelectric potentials using a pen-and-paper system.

Anterior tibialis The muscle on the outer side of the shinbone.

Antiarrhythmic A group of medications that are used to suppress abnormal rhythms of the heart,

Antiepileptic drug (AED) A diverse group of pharmacological agents used in the treatment of epileptic seizures. Also called anticonvulsants.

Antihistamines Medications that treat allergic rhinitis and other allergies.

Antihypertensive A class of medications that are used to lower systemic blood pressure.

Anti-inflammatories Used to describe a class of medications that reduce inflammation or swelling.

Apnea–hypopnea index (AHI) The average number of hypopneas and apneas per hour of sleep.

Apneic events A respiratory event characterized by cessation of airflow

Arousal A shift in EEG frequency for at least 3 seconds. This represents a brief awakening or an interruption to sleep.

Arousal index The total number of EEG arousals per hour of sleep time.

Arterial blood gas (ABG) A test of blood taken from the arteries that shows levels of certain gases in the blood.

Artifact An undesired signal intruding into a channel on a sleep study.

ASET *See* American Society of Electroneurodiagnostic Technologists.

ASPS *See* Advanced sleep–wake phase syndrome.

Association of Sleep Disorders Centers (ASDC) The original organization of sleep specialists that was established in 1975. In 1999, the name of this organization was changed to the American Academy of Sleep Medicine.

A-STEP *See* Accredited Sleep Technologist Education Program.

Asystole *See* Ventricular standstill.

Ataxic breathing An abnormal pattern of breathing characterized by irregular pauses and periods of apnea.

Atria The two upper chambers of the heart that receive the blood and force it into the ventricles.

Atrial fibrillation Unorganized activity in the atria that results in an atrial rate greater than 400 beats per minute.

Atrial flutter An EKG rhythm characterized by fast flutter waves for P waves. The atrial rate is 250–350 beats per minute.

Atrioventricular (AV) node The point of the heart that is responsible for the conduction of the electrical impulses from the atria to the ventricles.

Auto adjusting continuous positive airway pressure device A PAP machine that monitors changes in respirations and adjusts the pressure automatically as needed.

Automatic behavior A behavior that is performed without conscious knowledge and that does not appear to be under conscious control.

Automatic scoring A sleep diagnostic software feature that assigns sleep stages and detects significant events on the sleep recording.

AV block An EKG event in which a block has occurred between the atria and the ventricles.

AV bundle A part of the heart that carries electrical impulses down the septum to the ventricles.

AV node *See* Atrioventricular node.

Average volume assured pressure support (AVAPS) A form of non-invasive positive pressure ventilation that adjust the pressure support to maintain a target average ventilation over several breaths.

AWAKE Acronym for "Alert, Well, And Keeping Energetic." A group designed to support those with sleep apnea.

B

Barbiturate A drug that acts as a central nervous system depressant and can produce a range of effects from mild sedation to death.

Bariatric surgery A surgical procedure to help with weight loss by altering the digestive track.

Baseline montage A montage for a baseline or diagnostic sleep study.

Bedwetting *See* Nocturnal enuresis.

Behavioral insomnia of childhood A sleep disorder common in children and characterized by difficulty initiating or maintaining sleep. The disorder is often the result of poor sleep habits and can lead to sleep deprivation and daytime detriments.

Benign sleep myoclonus of infancy (BSMI) A sleep disorder characterized by limb movements during sleep in infants.

Benzodiazepine A class of medications that act on gamma-aminobutyric acid-A (GABA-A) receptors in the central nervous system and are used for a variety of medical conditions.

Berlin Questionnaire A series of questions designed to demonstrate the likelihood of a patient having sleep apnea.

Beta blocker A class of medications that prevent the stimulation of the adrenergic receptors responsible for increased cardiac action. They are used to control heart rhythm, treat angina, and reduce high blood pressure.

Beta spindles High-frequency, usually high-amplitude EEG waveforms with a frequency greater than 13 Hz. Beta spindles are usually associated with drug use or anxiety.

Beta waves An EEG activity with a frequency range between 12.5 and 30 Hz that is associated with normal waking consciousness.

Bigeminy An EKG rhythm in which every other beat is a PVC.

Bi-level PAP Bi-level pressure device used to treat sleep apnea, including EPAP for exhalation and a higher IPAP for inhalation.

Biocalibrations A series of simple tasks performed by the patient that ensure tracing reliability on the sleep study. These are also known as *physiologic calibrations*.

Biofeedback A mind-body technique that involves using visual or auditory feedback to gain control over bodily functions. It is used in the treatment of sleep disorders to help control misperceptions related to sleep.

Bipolar channel Refers to a data channel derived from output from two active electrodes

Bipolar montage A channel setup based on recordings from two exploring electrodes.

BMI *See* Body mass index.

Board of Registered Polysomnographic Technologists (BRPT) A board that registers sleep technologists by use of a comprehensive examination.

Body mass index (BMI) A calculation of height and weight.

Body position sensor A monitoring device usually placed on the middle of the thoracic belt to detect the patient's body position.

Body rocking *See* Rhythmic movement disorder.

Bright light therapy (BLT) A therapeutic modality for the treatment of circadian rhythm disorders, among other medical issues, that includes the use of timed exposure to daylight or specific wavelengths of light.

Bruxism A sleep disorder characterized by jaw clenching or teeth grinding during sleep. Bruxism is common in adolescents and, in many cases, tends to decrease with age.

BSMI *See* Benign sleep myoclonus of infancy.

Bundle branches Three branches from the Bundle of His in the heart that run along the interventricular septum.

C

Calcium channel blocker A group of medications that disrupt the movement of calcium through calcium channels. Used as antihypertensive agents.

Calibration A process of testing and adjusting diagnostic equipment in response to varying voltages of a known value. This process ensures reliability in recorded signals.

Canthus Corners of either the eye, where upper and lower eyelids meet. The outer canthus is used as a landmark for placing EOG electrodes.

Capnogram A direct monitor of the inhaled and exhaled concentration or partial pressure of carbon dioxide.

Capnograph A recording of carbon dioxide levels over a period of time.

Capnography The monitoring of the concentration or partial pressure of carbon dioxide in the respiratory gases.

Cataplexy A common symptom of narcolepsy characterized by a brief loss of muscle tone with resulting weakness, often in the knees or legs. This is usually triggered by a strong emotion such as anger or laughter.

Catathrenia *See* Sleep-related groaning.

Central apnea A complete cessation of airflow and respiratory effort for at least 10 seconds during sleep.

Central apnea index A parameter describing the number of central apneas per hour of sleep; calculated by dividing the total number central apneas by the total sleep time and multiplying by a factor of 60.

Central sleep apnea (CSA) A disorder characterized by the presence of central apneas.

Cheyne–Stokes breathing A sleep disorder characterized by a series of crescendos and decrescendos or waxing and waning patterns in respiratory rate and tidal volume.

Chin EMG A PSG channel displaying a recording of muscle activity from the chin.

Chronic insomnia disorder A sleep disorder characterized by the inability to initiate or maintain sleep for more than 3 months.

Chronic pain Used to describe a medical syndrome lasting at least twelve weeks associated with frequent dull pain.

Chronotherapy A treatment for circadian rhythm disorders that adjusts sleeping and awakening times in an attempt to reset the biological clock.

Circadian rhythm The cycle of fluctuations in biological and behavioral functions seen in mammals and other living things. The suprachiasmatic nucleus is the pacemaker for the circadian rhythm and is strongly affected by light.

Circadian rhythm sleep disorders A class of sleep disorders characterized by disruptions to the normal circadian rhythm.

Cleaning log A document that is used to track the maintenance and cleaning of materials and supplies.

Cognitive Behavioral Therapy (CBT) A psycho-social therapeutic intervention that focuses on changing unhelpful cognitive distortions and behaviors and developing personal coping strategies.

Cognitive control The process by which goals or plans influence behavior.

Common mode rejection The ability of a differential amplifier to eliminate a common-mode voltage from the output.

Common mode rejection ratio A rating of the ability of a differential amplifier to eliminate identical inputs.

Compensatory pause A long pause after an abnormal beat

Complex sleep apnea A sleep disorder characterized by the presence of obstructive, central, and sometimes mixed respiratory events during sleep. It can include the emergence of central apnea while undergoing treatment of obstructive sleep apnea with positive airway pressure therapy.

Confusional arousal An event characterized by awakening with disorientation and decreased mentation.

Congenital central alveolar hypoventilation Syndrome (CCHS) A rare lifelong and life-threatening disorder characterized by shallow breathing and resulting in a shortage of oxygen and a buildup of carbon dioxide in the blood.

Congestive heart failure (CHF) A chronic condition in which the heart doesn't pump blood as well as it should.

Conjugate eye movements Refers to movement of both eyes in the same direction

Consent form A documentation of a patient's permission/agreement to a specific test or procedure.

Continuing education unit (CEU) A unit of credit equal to 10 hours of participation in an accredited program designed for professionals with certificates or licenses to practice various professions.

Continuous positive airway pressure (CPAP) A device for treating obstructive sleep apnea and other sleep-related breathing disorders.

Control III A hospital-grade disinfectant used against a broad spectrum of bacteria, viruses, and fungi.

Couplet An EKG rhythm characterized by two PVCs in a row.

CPAP *See* Continuous positive airway pressure.

CPAP montage A montage for a CPAP titration.

CSA *See* Central sleep apnea.

Cup electrode The term used to describe a sensor that includes a gold or silver cup that holds electrode conductive paste.

Current The rate of flow of electric charge past a point or region.

Cycles per second Number of times a wave repeats itself or oscillates in 1 second. Measured in Hertz (Hz).

D

Delayed sleep–wake phase syndrome A circadian rhythm disorder in which the sleep–wake cycle is delayed (late) with respect to clock time.

Delta sleep The former name for stage N3. Under the rules developed by Allan Rechtschaffen and Anthony Kales, delta sleep was the combination of what are now known as stages 3 and 4.

Deoxyhemoglobin The form of hemoglobin without oxygen, the predominant protein in red blood cells.

Desensitization Techniques used to assist patients having difficulty acclimating to PAP therapy.

Diagnostic (baseline) polysomnograph report A document that summarizes all of the objective data recorded during a diagnostic sleep study.

Differential amplifier An amplifier used in polysomnography that works by comparing the difference between two incoming voltages and outputting a signal based on the difference.

Digital polysomnography Recording bioelectric signals during sleep on a computerized polysomnograph.

Disaster plan Includes having a comprehensive emergency management protocols including mitigation, preparedness, response, and recovery.

Diuretic Any substance that promotes diuresis, the increased production of urine.

DME *See* Durable medical equipment.

Dominant posterior rhythm A normal EEG rhythm seen in infants and children while awake, relaxed with the eyes closed.

Dopamine A hormone and neurotransmitter that plays a role regulating sleep, mood, and pain, among other things.

Double referencing Using cables to connect two reference leads to each other in order to decrease or eliminate artifact.

Durable medical equipment (DME) Includes medical equipment such as wheelchairs, walkers, and PAP machines that are prescribed by a physician.

Duration of action The length of time that a particular drug is effective.

E

E1 The electrode site for recording activity of the left eye.

E2 The electrode site for recording activity of the right eye.

ECG *See* Electrocardiogram.

ECG arrhythmia An abnormal heart rate or rhythm.

ECG artifact The appearance of the ECG electrical activity in a channel other than the ECG channel.

Ectopy A term used to describe an irregular heart beat or rhythm.

EDS *See* Excessive daytime sleepiness.

EEG *See* Electroencephalogram.

EEG arousal *See* Arousal.

EKG *See* Elektrocardiogram.

EKG arrhythmia The absence of a rhythm in the EKG channel.

Electrical baseline The vertical position of a pen when the power to the amplifier is turned on.

Electrical noise *See* Sixty-Hertz interference.

Electrocardiogram (ECG) Recording of electrical activity of the heart. Also spelled *Elektrocardiogram*.

Electrode popping An artifact characterized by occasional brief bursts of 60-Hz activity.

Electroencephalogram (EEG) The recording of electrical potentials from the brain.

Electromyogram (EMG) The recording of electrical potentials generated by a muscle.

Electroocculogram (EOG) The recording of eye movements and activity in a sleep study.

Elektrokardiogram (EKG) Alternate spelling for Electrocardiogram (ECG).

EMG *See* Electromyogram.

End tidal CO$_2$ A reading of carbon dioxide levels in the blood as measured by expired air.

Environmental sleep disorder A secondary sleep disorder caused by a sleep disorder present in a bed partner, poor sleep hygiene, or other factors.

EOG *See* Electroocculogram.

EPAP *See* Expiratory positive airway pressure.

Epilepsy A disorder in which nerve cell activity in the brain is disturbed, causing seizures.

Epileptiform discharge EEG activity indicating a seizure.

Epoch In polysomnography, a page of the sleep study recording. The standard paper speed in polysomnography is 10 mm/sec, which produces a 30-second epoch.

Epworth Sleepiness Scale (ESS) An index of sleepiness during the day as perceived by patients, derived from the answers to eight questions.

Esophageal balloon A device inserted into the esophagus to measure small changes in airway resistance.

Esophageal pressure The amount of pressure produced by the esophagus. This is measured by inserting a small balloon into the esophagus, and helps detect upper-airway resistance.

Excessive daytime sleepiness / Excessive daytime somnolence (EDS) Difficulty maintaining wakefulness or feelings or drowsiness of tiredness during the waking hours.

Excessive fragmentary myoclonus A sleep disorder characterized by frequent small twitches of fingers, toes, or muscles of the mouth during wake or sleep.

Expiratory positive airway pressure (EPAP) Positive airway pressure during the exhalation or expiratory phase of respiration. EPAP and IPAP are identical during CPAP and dissimilar during bi-level PAP.

Exploding head syndrome A sleep disorder characterized by an imagined loud noise or sense of explosion in the head while falling asleep or awakening.

F

Fall time The amount of time for a calibration wave to fall from the peak to 37% of the peak.

Fibrillation Unorganized activity, usually referring to the heart.

Fibromyalgia A disorder characterized by widespread musculoskeletal pain accompanied by fatigue, sleep, memory and mood issues.

First night effect Negative effects of the first night in a sleep lab, often resulting in increased sleep latency and decreased sleep efficiency.

First-degree AV block An EKG rhythm characterized by a prolonged PR interval.

Fisher & Paykel A medical supply company that specializes in products that improve respiratory and sleep functions.

Free-running circadian rhythm A circadian rhythm sleep disorder in which an individual's biological clock fails to synchronize to a 24-hour day and instead sleep time gradually delays by minutes to hours every day. Also known as Non-24-hour Sleep Wake Disorder.

Frequency Measured in cycles per second (cps) or Hertz (Hz), the number of times a wave oscillates in 1 second.

Frequency response curve A graphical depiction of an amplifier's ability to filter unwanted signals at varying frequencies.

Full face mask A CPAP mask that covers both the nose and the mouth.

G

G1 *See* Grid 1.

G2 *See* Grid 2.

Gain control Sensitivity control of the amplifier.

Gastric reflux A digestive disease in which stomach acid or bile enters the esophagus and creates a burning pain in the lower chest area.

Genioglossus advancement A surgical procedure where the tongue muscle that is attached to the lower jaw is pulled forward, making the tongue firmer and less collapsible during sleep.

Graveyard shift Used to describe working during the overnight hours.

Grid 1 / Gate 1 (G1) Refers to the first input terminal on a differential amplifier or the exploring electrode.

Grid 2 / Gate 2 (G2) This refers to the second input terminal on a differential amplifier, or the reference electrode.

Ground In polysomnography, a common reference for all electrodes to use as a measurement tool for voltage differences.

Ground loop When two grounds are used, a signal can loop through both grounds and cause interference.

Group therapy A form of psychotherapy in which one or more therapists treat a small group of patients with similar disorders together as a group. This type of therapy utilizes personal interaction with people who have shared experiences to help each individual process, cope, and grow.

H

Half-life The time it takes for the concentration of a drug in the body to be reduced by 50%.

Head banging *See* Rhythmic movement disorder.

Health Insurance Portability and Accountability Act of 1996 (HIPAA) A congressional regulation enacted to improve efficiency in healthcare, eliminate waste, combat fraud, and ensure that individual health information is protected, kept private and confidential.

Heart rate Measured in beats per minute (bpm), the speed at which the heart beats.

Hertz (Hz) A measure of frequency referring to the number of cycles per second (cps).

HFF *See* High-frequency filter.

High impedances Increased resistance to the flow of electricity, resulting in poor signal tracings.

High-altitude periodic breathing A disorder characterized by periodic breathing patterns at altitudes above 12,000 feet.

High-frequency filter (HFF) A tool or device on a polysomnograph that sets a limitation to the high-frequency signals that are allowed to pass through the amplifier.

Histamine A compound released by cells in response to injury and in allergic and inflammatory reactions

Histogram A display of sleep stages achieved throughout the sleep period.

Home sleep test (HST) An ambulatory sleep study that is performed in the patient's home. Subtypes can include the collection of between four and seven variables.

HST report A document that summarizes all of the objective data recorded during a home sleep study.

Hybrid mask A type of CPAP mask that combines an oral mask with a nasal pillow.

Hyoid suspension A surgical procedure in which the hyoid bone and its muscle attachments to the tongue and airway are pulled forward with the aim of increasing airway size.

Hypercapnea Excess levels of carbon dioxide (CO_2) in the blood.

Hypercapneic respiratory drive When the drive to breathe is based on carbon dioxide levels in the blood.

Hyperoxemia An increase in arterial oxygen partial pressure to a level greater than 120 mmHg.

Hypersomnia Excess lengths of levels of sleep or daytime sleepiness. Often used as a synonym for EDS.

Hypersomnolence A condition where a person experiences significant episodes of sleepiness, even after having 7 hours or more of quality sleep.

Hypertension A disease characterized by high blood pressure.

Hypnagogic Referring to the transition from wakefulness to sleep.

Hypnagogic foot tremor (HFT) A sleep disorder characterized by rhythmic leg or foot movements at sleep onset.

Hypnagogic hallucination A vivid, often frightening, dreamlike experience that occurs during the transition from wake to sleep. This common symptom of narcolepsy can occur separately from narcolepsy in cases of sleep deprivation.

Hypnic jerk *See* Sleep start.

Hypnogram *See* Histogram.

Hypnopompic Refers to the transition from sleep to wakefulness.

Hypnotics Medications designed to induce sleep.

Hypocapnea Having too little carbon dioxide in the blood.

Hypoglossal nerve stimulation A novel therapuetic option for the treatment of obstructive sleep apnea that involves an implantable device which stimulates the upper airway during sleep to prevent airway collapse.

Hypopnea A decrease in airflow for at least 10 seconds caused by a partial obstruction in the upper airway.

Hypopneic events A respiratory event characterized by reduction in airflow by 30%

Hypoxemia The state of having habitually low oxygen levels in the blood.

Hypoxic respiratory drive When the drive to breathe is based off of oxygen levels rather than carbon dioxide levels.

I

Idiopathic central alveolar hypoventilation A rare, life-long condition characterized by impaired ventilatory response to hypercapnia (elevated carbon dioxide levels) and hypoxemia (reduced oxygen levels)

Idiopathic hypersomnia A sleep disorder of unknown cause in which a person is excessively sleepy during the day and has great difficulty being awakened from sleep.

Idiopathic insomnia Lifelong insomnia that appears to have no discernible cause.

Impedance Resistance to the flow of electricity. In polysomnography, EEG electrode impedances should be kept below 5,000 Ohms.

Impedance check A procedure that is performed prior to lights off and after lights on to measure electrode impedances.

Infection control Refers to the prevention of healthcare associated infections through handwashing and the use of various barrier devices

Inion An anatomical landmark on the back of the head where the occipital bone protrudes from the skull. This landmark is used in the international 10/20 system of electrode placement to locate electrode sites.

Insomnia A class of sleep disorders characterized by the inability to initiate or maintain sleep or the perception of the inability to sleep.

Inspiratory positive airway pressure (IPAP) Positive airway pressure during the inhalation or inspiratory phase of respiration. EPAP and IPAP are identical during CPAP and dissimilar during bi-level PAP.

Insufficient sleep syndrome A sleep disorder characterized by consistent lack of sufficient sleep

International 10/20 electrode placement system A standard system of EEG electrode placement that uses specified anatomical landmarks and measurement percentages to locate EEG sites.

International Agency for Research on Cancer An intergovernmental agency forming part of the World Health Organization whose role is to conduct and coordinate research into the causes of cancer.

International Classification of Sleep Disorders (ICSD) A manual developed to establish and maintain standards for the evaluation, diagnosis, and treatment of sleep disorders.

Internodal pathways The electrical impulse pathways followed by the heart follow, from the SA node to the AV node.

Interscorer reliability An assessment system used to improve and verify consistency among scoring technologists in scoring of sleep studies

Irregular sleep–wake rhythm A circadian rhythm disorder characterized by irregular bedtimes or awakening times.

Isomorphism Acting out dreams.

J

Jet lag disorder A sleep disorder characterized by a disturbance to sleep induced by travel to a new time zone.

Jumper cables Wires that connect two leads to each other before the signal enters the head box.

Junctional escape rhythm A cardiac rhythm with a rate of 40-60 beats per minute that originates from the atrioventricular junction and occurs when the rate of depolarization of the sinoatrial node falls below the rate of the atrioventricular node.

K

K-complex A distinct EEG waveform characterized by a sharp negative deflection followed by a slower positive component. K-complexes often occur immediately before sleep spindles and are indicative of stage N2, although they can also occur in stage N3.

Klein-Levin syndrome A disorder that has recurrent hypersomnia as one of its symptoms.

L

Laser-assisted uvuloplasty (LAUP) A procedure performed under local anesthesia in which a laser is used to vaporize the tissue of the uvula and a portion of the palate as a way to treat snoring and mild sleep apnea.

Late-onset central hypoventilation with hypothalamic dysfunction A rare disorder that often presents after 1.5 years of age in otherwise healthy children. It is characterized by dramatic weight gain, hypoventilation, and poor respiratory control. The majority of those affected will require ventilator support either during sleep only or 24-hours per day.

Leg movement An event recorded during a sleep study that may indicate a disturbance to sleep.

Light therapy Also called phototherapy. Consists of timed exposure to daylight or specific wavelengths of light to help treat circadian rhythm disorders among other medical disorders.

Limb movement index A parameter describing the number of limb movement per hour of sleep; calculated by dividing the total number of limb movements by the total sleep time and multiplying by a factor of 60.

Limit-setting disorder A sleep disorder characterized by the inadequate enforcement of consistent bedtimes by a caretaker.

Line filter *See* Notch filter.

Low-amplitude, mixed-frequency (LAMF) activity Used to describe EEG activity between 4 and 7 cycles per second that is observed during many sleep stages.

Low-frequency filter A tool or device on a polysomnograph that sets a limitation to the low-frequency signals that are allowed to pass through the amplifier.

M

Machine calibrations A procedure that is performed prior to lights off and after lights on to verify the integrity of the recording and all channel property settings.

Maintenance of wakefulness test (MWT) A sleep study in which the patient is given several opportunities to remain awake while in a relaxed, darkened environment.

Mallampati classification A rating of the degree of obstruction in the upper airway. Used in anesthesia to predict a difficult intubation and in sleep consultations to predict obstructive sleep apnea.

Material safety data sheet (MSDS) Information provided by the manufacturer of a potentially hazardous product that discloses proper uses and potential dangers.

Maxillomandibular advancement (MMA) A form of facial skeletal surgery that advances the jaws to expand the airway.

Mechanical baseline The vertical placement of a pen when the power to the amplifier is turned off.

Melatonin A hormone secreted by the pineal gland that affects wakefulness.

MI *See* Myocardial infarction.

Microarousal A brief EEG arousal or a partial awakening from sleep.

Micrognathia Small jaw or mandible.

Microsleep A brief period of sleep of which the individual may not be aware. Episodes of microsleep are often associated with excessive daytime sleepiness.

Mixed apnea A full cessation of airflow for at least 10 seconds that begins central (no associated respiratory effort) and ends obstructive (respiratory effort).

Monoamine oxidase inhibitors (MAOI) Members of a drug class that work by inhibiting the activity of monoamine oxidase enzymes; they are powerful anti-depressants, as well as effective therapeutic agents for panic disorder and social phobia.

Montage The defined arrangement of channels and signal derivations on a polysomnogram.

Morphology Refers to the shape of a waveform.

Motion detector A sensor that detects movement.

Movement arousal An EEG arousal during which the patient moves.

Movement artifact An unwanted signal caused by movements from the patient.

Multiple sleep latency test (MSLT) A daytime sleep study consisting of four to five short naps of approximately 20 minutes each at 2-hour intervals. Sleep latency is measured for each nap, and REM periods during these naps are considered abnormal. The MSLT is commonly used to assist in the diagnosis of narcolepsy.

Multiple sleep latency test (MSLT) montage The collection of data channels needed to perform an MSLT test; includes EEG, chin EMG, EOG, and EKG channels.

Muscle artifact The appearance of high frequency muscle activity in a channel not meant to collect muscle activity.

Muscle atonia OK as is.

MWT *See* Maintenance of wakefulness test.

Myocardial infarction (MI) A heart attack.

Myoclonus A term referring to extremely brief muscle contractions or twitches.

N

Narcolepsy A central hypersomnia characterized by excessive sleepiness that is usually associated with REM phenomena such as hypnogogic hallucinations and sleep paralysis. Categorized as type I (with cataplexy) or type II (without cataplexy).

Narcolepsy Tetrad The term used for the four clinical features common to narcolepsy; excessive daytime sleepiness, sleep paralysis, cataplexy, and hypnagogic hallucinations.

Narcolepsy type I Narcolpesy associated with cataplexy.

Narcolepsy type II Narcolpesy not associated with cataplexy.

Nasal CPAP mask A CPAP mask that covers only the nose.

Nasal pillow A type of CPAP mask with prongs that rest on the end of the nares.

Nasion An anatomical landmark on the top or bridge of the nose where the forehead and nose meet. This landmark is used in the international 10/20 system of electrode placement to locate electrode sites.

National Sleep Foundation (NSF) A non-profit organization, founded in 1990, that promotes public understanding of sleep and sleep disorders.

Night shift Used to describe working during the overnight hours.

Night terror A sleep disorder characterized by a partial arousal from stage N3 sleep in which the individual has strong feelings of terror or fear. On wakening, the person typically does not remember the event. Night terrors are considered normal in young children. Also referred to as *sleep terrors*.

Nightmare A frightening or otherwise unpleasant dream. Nightmares are common in children and in patients with post-traumatic stress disorder (PTSD).

Nocturnal enuresis Also called *sleep enuresis* or *bedwetting*, this sleep disorder is characterized by urination during sleep.

Nocturnal seizure A seizure occurring during sleep.

Nocturnal seizure disorder study montage The collection of data channels needed to perform an seizure montage study; includes all baseline PSG channels with additional EEG channels.

Non–24-hour sleep–wake rhythm disorder A circadian rhythm sleep disorder in which an individual's biological clock fails to synchronize to a 24-hour day and instead sleep time gradually delays by minutes to hours every day. Also known as Free Running Circadian Rhythm Disorder.

Nonbenzodiazepine Used to describe a class of psychoactive drugs that are very benzodiazepine-like in nature.

Non-REM (NREM) sleep A term referring to the stages of sleep except for REM sleep. This includes stages N1, N2, and N3.

Nonsteroidal anti-inflammatory drugs (NSAIDs) Members of a drug class that reduces pain, decreases fever, prevents blood clots, and in higher doses, decreases inflammation.

Noradrenaline A neurotransmitter and hormone released during sympathetic activation with properties that increase blood pressure. Also known as norepinephrine.

Normal sinus rhythm (NSR) An EKG rhythm characterized by a normal rate and rhythm; all wave intervals are in normal ranges.

Notch filter A specialized frequency filter used for a small range of frequencies from 50 Hz to 60 Hz. A notch filter helps eliminate AC line frequency interference. This is also known as a *60-Hz filter* or *line filter*.

O

Obesity–hypoventilation syndrome A condition characterized by obesity, hypoxemia, and hypercapnia resulting from daytime and nighttime hypoventilation and often sleep-disordered breathing.

Obstructive apnea A full cessation of airflow for at least 10 seconds during sleep that is associated with a continuation of respiratory effort.

Obstructive apnea index (OAI) A parameter describing the number of obstructive apneas per hour of sleep; calculated by dividing the total number obstructive apneas by the total sleep time and multiplying by a factor of 60.

Obstructive sleep apnea (OSA) A common sleep disorder characterized by the presence of frequent obstructive apneas and hypopneas.

Occupational Safety and Health Administration (OSHA) A US Department of Labor agency with the responsibility of ensuring safety at work and a healthful work environment.

Onset of action The duration of time it takes for a drug to take effect upon administration.

Opioids A class of substances that act on opioid receptors to reduce pain.

Oral appliances Used to describe various devices that are made to fit in the mouth and act to pull the lower jaw forward and create a more patent airway.

Oral mask A CPAP mask that covers only the mouth.

Orexin receptor antagonist A medication used as a sleep aid that inhibits the effect of orexin, a wake promoting chemical in the brain, and thus, promotes sleep.

OSA *See* Obstructive sleep apnea.

Otolaryngologist Physicians trained in the medical and surgical management and treatment of patients with diseases and disorders of the ear, nose, throat, and related structures of the head and neck.

Outer canthus The point at the outside of either eye in which the eyelids meet.

Over-the-counter (OTC) sleep aid The term used to refer to a sleep aid available without a prescription.

Oximeter A device used to estimate blood oxygen saturation levels.

Oxygen desaturation A temporary decrease in blood oxygen level.

Oxygen saturation A measure of oxygen carried by the hemoglobin in the blood.

Oxyhemoglobin Formed by the combination of hemoglobin with oxygen, present in oxygenated blood.

P

P wave A portion of the electrocardiogram that represents atrial depolarization and results contraction of the atria.

PAC *See* Premature atrial complex.

Paper speed In analogue polysomnography, the speed at which the paper is fed into the polysomnograph.

Paradoxical breathing Used to describe out-of-phase chest and abdominal effort that often occurs during airway obstruction.

Paradoxical insomnia A state in which the patient believes he or she slept much less than the amount actually achieved.

Paradoxical intention The identification of a poor practice, habit, or thought and steps taken to eliminate it.

Parasomnia A class of sleep disorders characterized by specific activities occurring during sleep, such as eating and enuresis.

Parkinson's disease A progressive disorder of the central nervous system that affects movement, often including tremors.

Patient chart Hardcopy or electronic record containing a patient's healthcare, demographic and insurance information.

Patient confidentiality Requires health care providers to keep a patient's personal health information private unless consent to release the information is provided by the patient.

Patient tray Refers to the collection of supplies needed to perform a specific procedure.

Pediatric sleep medicine A field of study specializing in the diagnosis and treatment of sleep disorders in infants and children up to 18 years old.

Pen blocking An artifact caused by a high gain setting that causes the signal to reach beyond the upper- or lower-channel parameters. The tracing blocks until the signal again enters the channel boundaries.

Periodic breathing Episodes of repetitive apneas.

Periodic hypersomnolence Episodes of severe sleepiness that occur at intervals over time. This symptom is a hallmark feature of recurrent hypersomnia or Kleine-Levin symdrome.

Periodic limb movement disorder (PLMD) A sleep disorder characterized by repetitive limb movements during sleep. This is also known as periodic limb movements in sleep (PLMS) and nocturnal myoclonus.

Periodic limb movements in sleep (PLMS) *See* Periodic limb movement disorder.

pH probe A device to monitor acidity levels in the esophagus.

Phasic EMG activity Brief leg movements of low amplitude that do not appear to be associated with any other event.

Phasic REM Portions of stage R during which eye movements occur.

Phototherapy A therapeutic modality for the treatment of circadian rhythm disorders, among other medical issues, that includes the use of timed exposure to daylight or specific wavelengths of light.

Physician order Provides directions to the healthcare team regarding medications, procedures, treatments, therapy, diagnostic tests, laboratory tests, etc.

Physiologic calibrations A series of simple tasks performed by the patient that ensure tracing reliability on the sleep study. These are also known as *biologic calibrations*.

Pickwickian syndrome The former name for obesity hypoventilation syndrome, a disorder characterized by obesity with somnolence, chronic hypoventilation, hypoxia, and secondary polycythemia.

Pittsburgh Sleep Quality Index (PSQI) A series of questions in which the patient provides a subjective assessment of their own sleep quality.

Pleural pressure The pressure surrounding the lung, within the pleural space.

PLM index A calculation representing the average number of periodic limb movements per hour of sleep time.

PLMS *See* Periodic limb movement disorder.

Pneumotachography The quantitative and continuous measure of airflow volume and flow rates.

Polarity The positive or negative orientation of an electrical signal.

Polysomnogram (PSG) A recording of various physiologic parameters relating to sleep, such as EEGs, EOGs, EMGs, and respiratory parameters. Commonly referred to as a *sleep study*.

Polyvinylidene fluoride (PVDF) airflow sensors An available option for monitoring airflow during sleep testing as they are responsive to both air temperature and pressure

Positional therapy A behavioral strategy to treat obstructive sleep apnea that involves preventing a patient from sleeping on their back.

Positive airway pressure (PAP) therapy A therapeutic modality for the treatement of sleep related breathing disorders that includes the use of air pressure to overcome airway obstruction and assist in ventilation.

Positive airway pressure (PAP) titration A sleep study in which postive airway pressure therapy is initiatied and titrated to optimize breathing.

Posttest questionnaire A brief survey used after the completion of a sleep study to gain information about a patient's perception of their sleep during the study.

Posttraumatic stress disorder (PTSD) A mental health condition triggered by a terrifying event.

PR interval The time from the onset of the P wave to the start of the QRS complex; reflects conduction through the AV node. The normal PR interval is between 0.12-0.20s.

Preauricular point An anatomical landmark used as a measuring point in the international 10/20 electrode placement system. The preauricular point is located in front of the small notch at the midpoint of the ear.

Premature atrial complex (PAC) An EKG rhythm characterized by the P wave appearing earlier than expected.

Premature junctional contractions (PJCs) Premature cardiac electrical impulses originating from the atrioventricular node of the heart.

Premature ventricular contraction (PVC) An EKG rhythm characterized by a wide, bizarre QRS complex.

Pressure transducer A monitoring device that uses pressure from expired air to detect airflow.

Pretest questionnaire A brief survey used prior to a sleep study to gain relevant information regarding a patient's recent activity, medications, sleep habits.

Primary central sleep apnea An idiopathic sleep disorder characterized by repetitive absence of breathing effort and airflow.

Primary sleep apnea of infancy A life-threatening disorder in which infants have apneas or hypopneas lasting at least 20 seconds.

Primary snoring A sleep disorder characterized by snoring.

Propriospinal myoclonus at sleep onset (PSM) A sleep disorder characterized by body movements at sleep onset.

PSG *See* Polysomnogram.

PSM *See* Propriospinal myoclonus at sleep onset.

Psychophysiological insomnia Insomnia lasting at least a month that is caused by psychophysiological responses to the bedtime routine.

Purkinje fibers Specialized myocardial fibers that conduct electrical impulses that enable the heart to contract.

PVC *See* Premature ventricular contraction.

Q

QRS complex A portion of the electrocardiogram that represents ventricular depolarization and results contraction of the ventricles.

QT interval The time from the start of the Q wave to the end of the T wave; represents the time for ventricular depolarization and repolarization. Normal range is 0.36 to 0.44 second.

Quality assurance Any systematic process used to determine if a product or service meets quality standards.

R

Rapid eye movement (REM) Sleep stage R. REM is characterized by low-voltage, mixed-frequency EEGs, the presence of sawtooth EEG waves, muscle atonia, and rapid eye movements. REM is the sleep stage in which most dreaming occurs.

Rapid eye movement (REM) behavior disorder study Montage The collection of data channels needed to perform an RBD study; includes all baseline PSG channels with additional arm and leg EMG channels.

Rapid maxillary expansion (RME) A procedure performed most commonly in children in which a butterfly brace is placed on the roof of the mouth and is gradually expanded to enlarge the maxillary dental arch and the palate.

RAS *See* Reticular activating system.

RBD *See* REM behavior disorder.

RDI *See* Respiratory disturbance index.

Rebound sleep Sleep after periods of deprivation, which usually consists of decreased sleep latency, increased stage R, and increased N3.

Recurrent hypersomnia A rare sleep disorder characterized by recurrent episodes of severe sleepiness associated with confusion, derealization, apathy, compulsive eating, and hypersexuality. Also known as Kleine-Levin syndrome.

Recurrent isolated sleep paralysis A sleep disorder characterized by the inability to talk or move at sleep onset or upon awakening.

Referential montage A montage that uses common electrodes as references for the exploring electrodes.

Registered Polysomnographic Technologist (RPSGT) An internationally recognized credential, provided by the BRPT, representing the highest certification for health care professionals who clinically assess patients with sleep disorders.

Registered Sleep Technologist (RST) An objectively designed pathway, provided by the ABSM, for trained sleep technologists to demonstrate their knowledge and aptitude in sleep technology.

REM *See* Rapid eye movement.

REM behavior disorder (RBD) A disorder characterized by a lack of normal muscle atonia during REM sleep in which the patient may act out dreams.

REM behavior-disorder study *See* RBD montage.

REM extremity movement A brief limb movement during REM sleep.

REM latency The length of time between sleep onset and REM onset. Normal REM latency is 90–120 minutes. This may be reduced in cases of sleep deprivation.

REM onset The beginning of REM, which is defined as the first 30-second epoch of REM sleep.

REM-related parasomnias Sleep disorders that involve unwanted events or experiences that occur while you are falling asleep, sleeping or waking up from REM sleep.

RERA *See* Respiratory effort–related arousal.

Re-referencing Referencing to another electrode in order to eliminate an artifact.

Resistance *See* Impedance.

Resmed A medical supply company that specializes in products that improve respiratory and sleep functions.

Respiratory artifact The appearance of slow frequency artifact that correlates to the respiratory rate.

Respiratory cycle Refers to one breath and Includes inspiration and expiration

Respiratory disturbance index (RDI) The number of apneas, hypopneas, and RERAs per hour of total sleep time.

Respiratory effort–related arousal (RERA) An EEG arousal caused by a decrease in airflow that does not qualify as an apnea or hypopnea.

Respiratory inductive plethysmography (RIP) A method of evaluating pulmonary ventilation by measuring the movement of the chest and abdominal wall.

Respironics A medical supply company that specializes in products that improve respiratory and sleep functions.

Restless legs syndrome (RLS) A common sleep disorder characterized by creeping or crawling sensations in the legs that usually occur when the patient is awake and not moving.

Restlessness Difficulty staying still or remaining asleep.

Reticular activating system (RAS) A system in the brain causing wakefulness and alertness.

Retrognathia Recessed jaw or mandible.

Rhythm A repeated pattern; may be regular or irregular.

Rhythmic masticatory muscle activity Repetive bursts of jaw muscle activity. This type of activity can be seen in the chin EMG channel on a sleep study. This term is frequently used to describe bruxism.

Rise time The amount of time for a calibration signal to rise from baseline to 63% of the peak.

RLS *See* Restless legs syndrome.

RR interval The time elapsed between two successive R waves of the QRS signal on the electrocardiogram.

S

SA *See* Sinoatrial node.

Sampling rate The designated number of bits recorded per second in a channel.

School of Sleep Medicine Founded to provide high quality continuing education on the nature and treatment of sleep disorders.

Second-degree AV block type I An EKG rhythm in which the PR interval gradually increases until a QRS complex is dropped.

Second-degree AV block type II An EKG rhythm in which a QRS complex is occasionally dropped or skipped without warning.

Sedatives A class of drugs designed to calm and reduce anxiety or excitement.

Seizure activity Abnormal and excessive electrical activity in the brain.

Selective serotonin reuptake inhibitor (SSRI) Members of a drug class that work by blocking the reabsorption of serotonin into neurons, hence increasing levels in the brain. They are primarly used to treat anxiety and depression.

Self-control techniques A form of therapy that seeks to promote behavior change by motivating self-discipline to replace poor habits with healthier ones.

Sensitivity The ratio of signal input to the resulting wave. Sensitivity is usually measured in μV/mm.

Shift work disorder A sleep disorder characterized by working house outside of conventional daytime hours or rotating shifts.

Short-term insomnia disorder A sleep disorder characterized by the inability to initiate or maintain sleep for less than 3 months.

Sinoatrial (SA) node The point of the heart at which the electrical impulse begins. The SA node is the pacemaker of the heart.

Sinus arrhythmia An EKG rhythm in which all parameters are normal except the rhythm varies from beat to beat.

Sinus bradycardia An EKG rhythm in which all parameters are normal except the rate is less than 40 beats per minute.

Sinus tachycardia An EKG rhythm in which all parameters are normal except the rate is more than 90 beats per minute.

Sixty-Hertz filter A unique filter pointed specifically at electrical activity in the 59-Hz to 61-Hz range to eliminate or attenuate 60-Hz activity.

Sixty-Hertz interference High-frequency activity in the 59-Hz to 61-Hz range derived from outside electrical activity.

Sleep A physiologic state characterized by decreased consciousness, metabolism, and movement.

Sleep architecture The pattern of REM and NREM stages of sleep achieved throughout the night.

Sleep debt The amount of sleep an individual did not receive over a period of time but should have. Sleep debt increases with sleep deprivation and can lead to excessive daytime sleepiness.

Sleep deprivation A lack of sufficient sleep.

Sleep diary A log that records sleep and wake times and alertness levels.

Sleep Disorders Testing and Therapeutic Intervention credential A credential used to designate a registered respiratory therapist who has objectively demonstrated the knowledge, skill, and experience of sleep disorders testing and therapeutic intervention.

Sleep efficiency A calculation of total sleep time divided by the total time spent in bed. Normal sleep efficiency is greater than 90%. Decreased sleep efficiency may indicate a sleep disturbance such as insomnia.

Sleep enuresis Also called *nocturnal enuresis* or *bedwetting*, this sleep disorder is characterized by urinating during sleep.

Sleep history questionnaire A comprehensive survey often used prior to, or in conjunction with, the initial sleep consultation to gain a better understanding of the patient's sleep complaints and symptoms.

Sleep hygiene Practices that aid in falling asleep or staying asleep. Sleep hygiene techniques include practices such as going to bed and awakening at consistent times from day to day, using the bed only for sleeping, and avoiding heavy exercise just before retiring.

Sleep latency The length of time from lights out to sleep onset. Sleep latency may be decreased as a result of sleep deprivation, or it may be increased as a result of too much sleep or the presence of insomnia.

Sleep log A diary of an individual's time in bed, estimated total sleep time, lights out time, lights on time, and daily activities. Sleep logs can help clinicians determine circadian rhythm disorders and causes of insomnia.

Sleep onset The first epoch of sleep in a polysomnogram.

Sleep paralysis An event characterized by awakening and not being able to move for a period of time.

Sleep restriction The practice of limiting the amount of time spent in bed in an effort to treat insomnia.

Sleep spindles A burst of 11 Hz to 16 Hz (usually 12–14 Hz) EEG activity lasting at least 0.5 seconds. Sleep spindles are most commonly seen in stage N2 sleep.

Sleep start Also called a *hypnic jerk*, this event is characterized by a sudden jerk or movement at sleep onset, resulting in wakefulness and often alarm.

Sleep state misperception *See* Paradoxical insomnia.

Sleep study report A document that summarizes all of the objective data recorded during a sleep study.

Sleep talking A sleep disorder characterized by talking during sleep. Formerly called *somniloquy*.

Sleep terror A sleep disorder occurring during stage N3 in which the patient jumps out of bed with a loud scream and exhibits dangerous or threatening behaviors.

Sleep-maintenance insomnia Refers to difficulty staying asleep.

Sleep-onset insomnia Refers to difficulty falling asleep.

Sleep-onset REM period (SOREMP) A REM period occurring at or just after sleep onset. This is considered abnormal and is often associated with narcolepsy and excessive daytime sleepiness.

Sleep-related breathing disorders A class of sleep disorders characterized by abnormal breathing during sleep.

Sleep-related bruxism A sleep disorder characterized by either repetitive grinding of the teeth or sustained clenching of the jaw

Sleep-related eating disorder A sleep disorder characterized by eating large amounts of high-calorie foods during sleep.

Sleep-related groaning A sleep disorder characterized by groaning during sleep.

Sleep-related hallucinations The perception of visual, tactile, or auditory experiences during sleep onset or offset

Sleep-related leg cramps A sleep disorder characterized by leg cramps during sleep.

Sleep-related movement disorders A class of sleep disorders characterized by abnormal movements during sleep.

Sleep-related rhythmic movement disorder A sleep disorder characterized by repetitive movements of large muscle groups immediately before and during sleep. Types include head banging and body rocking.

Sleepwalking A sleep disorder characterized by walking during sleep. Formerly called *somnambulism*.

Slow eye movements (SEMs) Conjugate, reasonably regular, sinusoidal eye movements with an initial deflection usually lasting >500 msec.

Slow wave An EEG wave that is at least 75 μV and is 0.5–2 Hz.

Slow wave artifact An unwanted low-frequency, usually high-amplitude signal often caused by sweat.

Snap electrode The term used to describe a silver/silver choride sensor used with disposable adhesive gel electrodes.

Snore artifact A high-frequency artifact caused by vibrations in the upper airway. This is usually seen in the chin EMG, the EEGs, and EOGs.

Snore microphone A monitoring device that reads sounds and converts them to an electrical signal for the polysomnograph to record.

Snore sensor A monitoring device that reads vibrations from the upper airway and delivers them to the polysomnograph to record.

Snoring A sleep disorder characterized by a noise produced during breathing resulting from a partial obstruction of the upper airway. When the tissues of the upper airway vibrate, usually during inhalation, the resulting noise is called a *snore*. Snoring can be extremely disruptive to any bed partner.

Somnambulism The former name for *sleepwalking*.

Somniloquy The former name for *sleep talking*.

Somnoplasty A procedure that uses radiofrequency ablation to treat habitual snoring, chronic nasal obstruction, and obstructive sleep apnea to shrink the tissues of the uvula and soft palate.

SOREMP *See* Sleep-onset REM period.

Split night report A document that summarizes all of the objective data recorded during a split night sleep study; includes diagnostic and titration data.

Split night study A type of sleep study in which the first half of the night is diagnostic and the second half is therapeutic with a CPAP titration.

SpO$_2$ The amount of oxygen in the blood as read by a pulse oximeter.

ST segment The flat, isoelectric section of the ECG between the end of the S wave and the beginning of the T wave; represents the interval between ventricular depolarization and repolarization.

Stage N1 A sleep stage that makes up approximately 5-10 % of total sleep time and is characterized by theta activity, slow eye movements and moderate to high muscle tone.

Stage N2 A sleep stage that makes up approximately 45-50 % of total sleep time and is characterized by theta activity, K-complexes, sleep spindles, and moderate muscle tone.

Stage N3 A sleep stage that makes up approximately 25 % of total sleep time and is characterized by high amplitude, low frequency delta activity and moderate to low muscle tone. Also called slow wave sleep or deep sleep.

Stage R A sleep stage that makes up approximately 25% of total sleep time and is characterized by rapid eye movements and low muscle tone.

Stage W Scored on a sleep study when the patient is awake.

Standard polysomnogram (PSG) A diagnostic sleep study that includes the collection of brain waves, muscle tone, eye movements, heart rate and rhythm, airflow and breathing parameters to diagnose sleep disorders.

Stanford Sleepiness Scale (SSS) A scale consisting of seven statements describing subjective levels of sleepiness or alertness.

Stimulus control A therapuetic modality that seeks to modify behavior in response to certain stimuli.

Sudden infant death syndrome The unexplained death, usually during sleep, of a seemingly healthy baby less than a year old.

Supplemental oxygen Additional oxygen delivered to a patient, usually via nasal cannula.

Suprachiasmatic nucleus (SCN) Nerve clusters located in the hypothalamus that regulate the body's circadian rhythms

Supraventricular tachycardia (SVT) A faster than normal heart rate beginning above the heart's two lower chambers.

Sway artifact *See* Slow wave artifact.

Sweat artifact A slow wave artifact caused by excessive sweat from the patient.

T

T wave A portion of the electrocardiogram that represents ventricular repolarization and results relaxation of the ventricles.

Technologist notes Used to describe the documentation of sleep study data and observations by the recording technologist.

Thalamus A structure in the brain responsible for relaying certain sensory information from the body to different parts of the brain.

Thermal airflow sensors Detects the difference between the temperature of exhaled and ambient air to estimate airflow and detect apneic events.

Thermistor A sensor that measures changes in temperature resulting from a patient's inhalations and exhalations.

Thermocouple A sensor placed in front of the nose and mouth that detects airflow by sensing temperature changes.

Thermoregulation The ability to adjust body temperature.

Theta waves EEG activity in the 4-Hz to 7-Hz frequency range.

Third-degree (complete) AV block An EKG rhythm in which there appears to be no relationship whatsoever between the P wave and the QRS complex.

Tidal volume The estimated volume of air passed in and out of the lungs in a breath, usually measured in liters.

Time axis The horizontal time line of the polysomnogram. If the time axis of a pen is misaligned, signals occurring at identical times in multiple channels will appear to occur at different times from each other.

Time constant The fall time of a calibration wave to 37% of its amplitude. Time constant is synonymous with the low-frequency filter. The low-frequency filter is used to control slow frequency waves.

Titration A steady increase in CPAP levels or oxygen flow applied during a sleep study to determine the optimal level of treatment.

Titration report A document that summarizes all of the objective data recorded during a positive pressure titration study.

Tonic REM Periods of stage R in which no eye movements occur.

Tonsillectomy The surgical removal of the tonsils. Performed for recurrent throat infections and obstructive sleep apnea.

Total recording time (TRT) The length of time from lights out to lights on.

Total sleep time (TST) The amount of time spent during a sleep period. TST can be calculated by adding the amount of time spent in each sleep stage.

Total wake time (TWT) The total time, in minutes, during a sleep study in which the patient was awake.

Tracheostomy A surgical procedure which consists of making an incision on the anterior aspect of the neck and opening a direct airway through an incision in the trachea.

Transcutaneous CO$_2$ A reading of carbon dioxide levels in the blood as measured by a heated sensor placed on the skin.

Transmembrane potential Electrical activity across the cell surfaces.

Treatment-emergent central sleep apnea A sleep disorder characterized by the emergence of central apnea while undergoing treatment of obstructive sleep apnea with positive airway pressure therapy. Previously refered to as complex sleep apnea.

Tricyclic antidepressant (TCA) Members of a drug class that work by increasing levels of norepinephrine and serotonin and are primarily used to treat anxiety and depression.

Trigeminy EKG rhythm in which every third beat is a premature ventricular contraction.

TRT *See* Total recording time.

TST *See* Total sleep time.

TWT *See* Total wake time.

U

UARS *See* Upper-airway resistance syndrome.

Unequivocal sleep Refers to the observation of three consecutive epochs of stage 1 sleep or one epoch of any other sleep stage

Universal precautions A group of practices such as handwashing that reduce or stop the spread of infection.

Upper-airway resistance syndrome (UARS) The former name for a sleep disorder characterized by resistances to flow in the upper airway that lead to EEG arousals and Excessive daytime sleepiness.

Uvulopalatopharyngoplasty (UPPP) A surgical procedure that involves the removal of the tonsils, the posterior surface of the soft palate, and the uvula.

Uvuloplasty A surgical procedure to remove the uvula, the small bit of flesh dangling in the back of the throat.

V

V fib *See* Ventricular fibrillation.

V tach *See* Ventricular tachycardia.

Ventricles The chambers of the heart that receive blood from the atria and pump it to the arteries.

Ventricular escape rhythm A cardiac rhythm with rate of 20-40 beats per minute that originates in the ventricles and occurs whenever higher-lever pacemakers in AV junction or sinus node fail to control ventricular activation.

Ventricular fibrillation (V fib) A severe EKG arrhythmia in which the heart is quivering rather than beating, resulting in no discernible waveforms.

Ventricular standstill (asystole) An EKG arrhythmia in which there is no ventricular activity whatsoever.

Ventricular tachycardia (V tach) An EKG rhythm characterized by three or more consecutive PVCs.

Vital signs Clinical objective measures including heart rate, temperature, respiratory rate, and blood pressure, that indicate the state of a patient's essential body functions.

Voltage The difference in electric potential between two points.

W

Wake after sleep onset (WASO) The amount of time in minutes a patient spends awake during a sleep study after sleep onset.

WASO *See* Wake after sleep onset.

Abbreviations Commonly Used in Polysomnography

AASM	American Academy of Sleep Medicine
AAST	American Association of Sleep Technologists
AB	automatic behavior
ABG	arterial blood gas
ADD	attention deficit disorder
ADHD	attention deficit hyperactivity disorder
AHI	apnea–hypopnea index

AI	arousal index
APAP	autotitrating PAP
BPM	beats per minute
BRPT	Board of Registered Polysomnographic Technologists
CDC	Centers for Disease Control and Prevention
CFIDS	chronic fatigue immune dysfunction syndrome
CFS	chronic fatigue syndrome
CMN	certificate of medical necessity
CNS	central nervous system
CPAP	continuous positive airway pressure
CPS	cycles per second
DME	durable medical equipment
DSPS	delayed sleep phase syndrome
Dx	diagnosis
ECG	electrocardiogram
EDS	excessive Daytime Sleepiness
EEG	electroencephalogram
EKG	electrocardiogram
EMG	electromyogram
EOG	electrooculogram
ENT	ear, nose, and throat
GABA	gamma-aminobutyric acid
GERD	gastroesophageal reflux disease
HH	hypnogogic hallucinations
HLA	human leukocyte antigen
Hx	medical history
Hz	Hertz
IH	idiopathic hypersomnia
IRM	Institute of Respiratory Medicine
IPAP	inspiratory positive airway pressure
LAUP	laser-assisted uvulopalatoplasty
LMN	letter of medical necessity
LTD	long-term disability
MRI	magnetic resonance imagery
MMOA	mandibular maxillary osteotomy and advancement
MSLT	multiple sleep latency test
MWT	maintenance of wakefulness test
NCSDR	National Commission on Sleep Disorders Research
NN	narcolepsy network
NREM	nonrapid eye movement

OCD	obsessive compulsive disorder
ODI	oxygen desaturation index
OH	obstructive hypopnea
OSA	obstructive sleep apnea
OSAS	obstructive sleep apnea syndrome
PAP	positive airway pressure
PCP	primary care physician
PET	positron emission tomography
PLMD	periodic leg movement disorder
PLMS	periodic limb movements in sleep
PND	paroxsymal nocturnal dyspnea
PSG	polysomnogram
PTSD	posttraumatic stress disorder
RCP	respiratory care practitioner
RDI	respiratory disturbance index
REM	rapid eye movement
RERA	respiratory effort–related arousal
RLS	restless leg syndrome
R/O	rule out
Rx	prescription
SAS	sleep apnea syndrome
SAHS	sleep apnea–hypopnea syndrome
SDB	sleep disordered breathing
SE	sleep efficiency

SL	sleep latency
SO	sleep onset
SOREM	sleep-onset REM
SOREMP	sleep-onset REM Period
SRBD	sleep-related breathing disorder
SSRI	selective serotonin reuptake inhibitor
STD	(1) short-term disability; (2) sexually transmitted disease
SWS	slow wave sleep
Sz	schizophrenia
TIB	time in bed
TMT	total movement time
TREM	total REM time
TST	total sleep time
TSW	total slow wave sleep (stage N3)
TT	total time
TWT	total wake time
Tx	treatment
UARS	upper-airway resistance syndrome
UVPPP	uvulopalatopharyngoplasty
VPAP	variable positive airway pressure
WASO	wake after sleep onset
XPAP	any type of positive airway pressure device
YAWN	Young Americans with Narcolepsy

Index

Note: Page numbers followed by *f*, or *t* indicate material in figures, or tables, respectively.

Section 1: Patient Hookup and Measurements

Question 1

What system of measurements is used to locate EEG sites?

Section 1: Patient Hookup and Measurements

Question 3

What landmark in the back of the head is used to begin measuring EEGs?

Section 1: Patient Hookup and Measurements

Question 2

What landmark in the front of the head is used to begin measuring EEGs?

Section 1: Patient Hookup and Measurements

Question 4

What electrode site is circled?

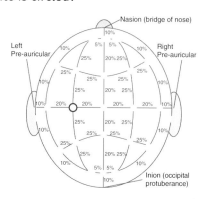

Question 3 Answer:

Inion

Essentials of Polysomnography, Chapter 6

Question 1 Answer:

The international $^{10}/_{20}$ electrode placement system

Essentials of Polysomnography, Chapter 6

Question 4 Answer:

C3

Essentials of Polysomnography, Chapter 6

Question 2 Answer:

Nasion

Essentials of Polysomnography, Chapter 6

Section 1: Patient Hookup and Measurements

Question 5

Which electrode site is circled?

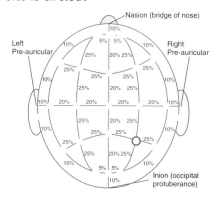

Section 1: Patient Hookup and Measurements

Question 7

Which electrode site is circled?

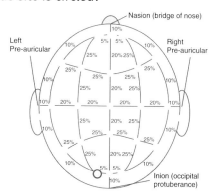

Section 1: Patient Hookup and Measurements

Question 6

Which electrode site is circled?

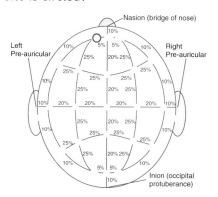

Section 1: Patient Hookup and Measurements

Question 8

Which electrode site is circled?

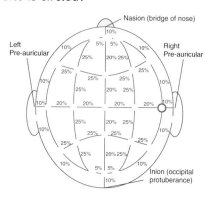

Question 7 Answer:

O1

Essentials of Polysomnography, Chapter 6

Question 5 Answer:

P4

Essentials of Polysomnography, Chapter 6

Question 8 Answer:

T4

Essentials of Polysomnography, Chapter 6

Question 6 Answer:

Fp1

Essentials of Polysomnography, Chapter 6

Section 1: Patient Hookup and Measurements

Question 9

Which electrode site is circled?

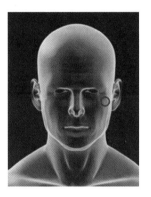

Section 1: Patient Hookup and Measurements

Question 10

Where is E2 located?

Section 1: Patient Hookup and Measurements

Question 11

The distance from the nasion to the inion is 32 cm. What is the distance from Cz to Pz?

Section 1: Patient Hookup and Measurements

Question 12

The distance from the left pre-auricular point to the right pre-auricular point is 36 cm. What is the distance from Cz to T3?

Question 11 Answer:

6.4 cm

Question 9 Answer:

E1

Question 12 Answer:

14.4 cm

Question 10 Answer:

1 cm above and 1 cm lateral to the right outer canthus

Section 1: Patient Hookup and Measurements

Question 13

The distance from Fp1 to O1 (through C3) is 24 cm. What is the distance from Fp1 to F3?

Section 1: Patient Hookup and Measurements

Question 15

Where is the exploring electrode placed on a two-lead EKG for a sleep study?

Section 1: Patient Hookup and Measurements

Question 14

How far above the inferior edge of the mandible is the first chin EMG electrode placed?

Section 1: Patient Hookup and Measurements

Question 16

Where is the reference electrode placed on a two-lead EKG for a sleep study?

Question 15 Answer:

Low on the left rib cage, vertically aligned with the left hip

Question 13 Answer:

6 cm

Question 16 Answer:

High on the right chest, horizontally aligned with the right shoulder

Question 14 Answer:

1 cm

Section 1: Patient Hookup and Measurements

Question 17

Where are the two respiratory effort belts placed?

Section 1: Patient Hookup and Measurements

Question 19

What are some differences between the hookup processes for an adult and those for a pediatric patient?

Section 1: Patient Hookup and Measurements

Question 18

Where are the leg EMG electrodes placed?

Section 1: Patient Hookup and Measurements

Question 20

How is electrical current calculated?

Question 19 Answer:

EOG and EMG electrodes may be adjusted to accommodate smaller facial features in children.

Smaller-sized respiratory effort bands and airflow sensors should be used.

Transcutaneous CO_2 or end-tidal CO_2 monitoring is standard for pediatric baseline studies.

Question 17 Answer:

Around the thorax under the armpits and around the abdomen at the level of the umbilical

Question 20 Answer:

Current (I) equals voltage (V) divided by resistance (R): I = V/R

Question 18 Answer:

Near the middle of the anterior tibialis muscle of each leg, approximately 2–3 cm apart, aligned vertically

Section 2: Diagnostic Equipment

Question 1

What is the difference between an AC signal and a DC signal?

Section 2: Diagnostic Equipment

Question 3

What is the difference between a snore microphone and a snore sensor?

Section 2: Diagnostic Equipment

Question 2

Why are cup electrodes used in electroencephalography?

Section 2: Diagnostic Equipment

Question 4

How does an oximeter estimate the blood oxygen level?

Question 3 Answer:
Snore microphones detect the noise from the snores and can be placed wherever snoring is heard the loudest, close to the nose or mouth or on the throat. Snore sensors record vibrations from the snores and are placed on the throat.

Question 1 Answer:
AC signals can alternate quickly between positive and negative voltages, whereas DC signals change slowly and range from 0 to 1V.

Question 4 Answer:
One end shines a light through the finger while the other end detects the red and infrared light. Hemoglobin-carrying oxygen absorbs mostly infrared light while hemoglobin without oxygen absorbs mostly red light. The pulse oximeter compares the ratio of infrared to red light (oxygenated vs. deoxygenated) and displays a percentage saturation.

Question 2 Answer:
The small, cup-shaped head makes it easy to be placed securely against the scalp and hold conductive paste. They are also made of a highly conductive metal, usually gold or silver–silver chloride.

Section 2: Diagnostic Equipment

Question 5

What is the difference between a thermistor and a thermocouple?

Section 2: Diagnostic Equipment

Question 6

Name four methods of recording respiratory effort.

Section 2: Diagnostic Equipment

Question 7

A 10-μV signal is detected by the exploring electrode (G1) at the same time as a 5-μV signal is detected by the reference electrode (G2). What is the output voltage?

Section 2: Diagnostic Equipment

Question 8

What is the optimal range for impedances in EEG channels?

Question 7 Answer:

5 μV

Question 5 Answer:

Thermocouples detect the rate of temperature change by using two dissimilar metals that are sensitive to temperature change. Thermistors use a Wheatstone bridge circuit to amplify the difference in temperature between expired air and room air.

Question 8 Answer:

< 5,000 ohms (5 kohms)

Question 6 Answer:

(any four of these)
Inductive plethysmography
Piezoelectric crystal belts
Mercury strain gauges
Cardiopneumograph
Pneumatic respiration transducer
Intercostal EMGs
Esophageal balloon
Water-filled catheter
Currently the AASM recommended method is via inductive plethysmography or esophageal manometry

Section 2: Diagnostic Equipment

Question 9

What does a frequency-response curve show?

Section 3: Calibrations and Montages

Question 2

What is the recommended LFF for EEG channels?

Section 3: Calibrations and Montages

Question 1

What is the main difference between a baseline or diagnostic montage and a CPAP montage?

Section 3: Calibrations and Montages

Question 3

What is the recommended sampling rate for EEGs, EOGs, EKGs, and EMGs?

Question 2 Answer:

0.3 Hz

Question 9 Answer:

The amplifier's ability to eliminate unwanted signals through the use of filters.

Question 3 Answer:

500 Hz

Question 1 Answer:

A CPAP montage includes additional channels for CPAP flow, pressure, and leak.

Section 3: Calibrations and Montages

Question 4

What is the recommended HFF setting for EOG channels?

Section 3: Calibrations and Montages

Question 6

What channel types are typically included in an MSLT montage unless otherwise indicated?

Section 3: Calibrations and Montages

Question 5

What is the recommended LFF setting for the SpO_2 channel?

Section 3: Calibrations and Montages

Question 7

What additional channels are typically included when performing a REM behavior disorder study?

Question 6 Answer:

EEG, EOG, Chin EMG, and EKG

Question 4 Answer:

35 Hz

Question 7 Answer:

Arm EMG channels to detect arm movements. Additional EEG channels are also sometimes recommended to rule out seizures.

Question 5 Answer:

The SpO_2 channel is a DC channel. Therefore, no filters are set for this channel.

Section 3: Calibrations and Montages

Question 8

When looking at a calibration wave, what is the rise time?

Section 3: Calibrations and Montages

Question 10

What is the time constant?

Section 3: Calibrations and Montages

Question 9

What filter directly impacts the fall time?

Section 3: Calibrations and Montages

Question 11

Increasing the sensitivity setting from 10 µV/mm to 20 µV/mm will do what to the appearance of the wave?

Question 10 Answer:

The amount of time for a calibration wave to fall from its highest point or peak to 37% of the peak. This is sometimes referred to as the fall time.

Essentials of Polysomnography, Chapter 9

Question 8 Answer:

The amount of time is takes for the wave to travel from its baseline to 63% of its peak. This is usually measured in hundredths of a second.

Essentials of Polysomnography, Chapter 9

Question 11 Answer:

It will cut the height of the wave in half.

Essentials of Polysomnography, Chapter 9

Question 9 Answer:

The low-frequency filter

Essentials of Polysomnography, Chapter 9

Section 3: Calibrations and Montages

Question 12

What waveform characteristic is directly affected by the voltage of the input signal?

Section 4: Artifacts and Troubleshooting

Question 1

Shortly after the patient wakes up, all the signals on the PSG show a high-frequency, high-amplitude artifact obscuring all the tracings. What is the most appropriate course of action?

Section 3: Calibrations and Montages

Question 13

The EEG and EOG channels are difficult to visualize because of a periodic single fast wave approximately every second. What is the likely cause and most appropriate course of action?

Section 4: Artifacts and Troubleshooting

Question 2

During physiologic calibrations, the EEG and EOG channels present a high-amplitude, extremely slow wave artifact. What is the most appropriate course of action?

Question 1 Answer:
Wait for the patient to stop moving because this is most likely movement artifact. After movement has stopped, determine if any leads have detached and reapply if necessary.

Essentials of Polysomnography, Chapter 8

Question 2 Answer:
Take steps to correct sweat artifact, including cooling the patient and replacing the ground lead.

Essentials of Polysomnography, Chapter 8

Question 12 Answer:
Amplitude

Essentials of Polysomnography, Chapter 9

Question 13 Answer:
This likely represents an EKG artifact and can be best corrected by repositioning the M1 and M2 electrodes higher up or to the earlobes.

Essentials of Polysomnography, Chapter 8

Section 4: Artifacts and Troubleshooting

Question 3

During the night, the tech notices that the C3 channel appears slightly darker than the other EEG channels. What should she do first?

Section 4: Artifacts and Troubleshooting

Question 5

When attempting to correct an artifact, the technician notices that the artifact appears in multiple channels. What should he do next?

Section 4: Artifacts and Troubleshooting

Question 4

The airflow channel squares rather than rounds at the peaks. What should the technician do?

Section 4: Artifacts and Troubleshooting

Question 6

What artifact is seen in the chin EMG channel?

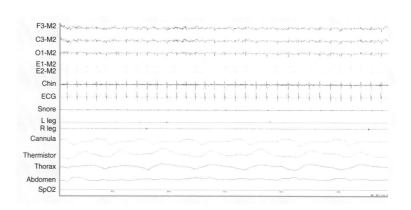

Question 5 Answer:

Check to see if there is a common reference between the affected channels.

Essentials of Polysomnography, Chapter 8

Question 3 Answer:

Run an impedance check. If the impedance in this channel is higher than 5 kohms, the electrode should be reapplied or replaced.

Essentials of Polysomnography, Chapter 8

Question 6 Answer:

EKG artifact

Essentials of Polysomnography, Chapter 8

Question 4 Answer:

Adjust the sensitivity setting to correct the pen blocking artifact.

Essentials of Polysomnography, Chapter 8

Section 4: Artifacts and Troubleshooting

Question 7

What artifact is seen in the EEG channels?

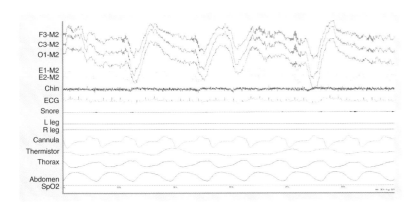

Section 4: Artifacts and Troubleshooting

Question 9

What artifact is circled?

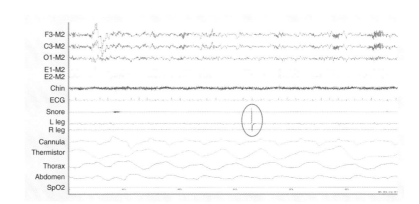

Section 4: Artifacts and Troubleshooting

Question 8

What artifact is seen at the 15-second mark of the epoch?

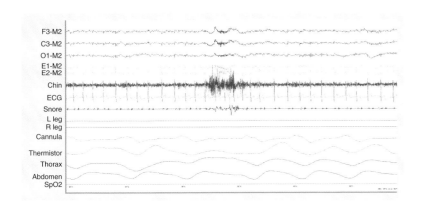

Section 4: Artifacts and Troubleshooting

Question 10

What artifact is shown in the following?

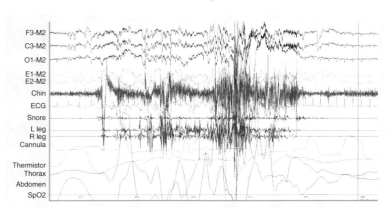

Question 9 Answer:

Electrode popping

Question 7 Answer:

Sweat artifact

Question 10 Answer:

Movement artifact

Question 8 Answer:

Bruxism or teeth grinding

Section 4: Artifacts and Troubleshooting

Question 11

What artifact is shown in the C3 channel?

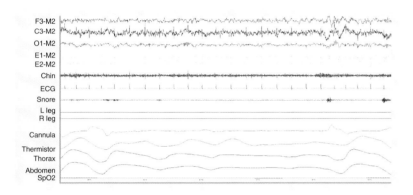

Section 4: Artifacts and Troubleshooting

Question 13

What is wrong with the thermistor channel?

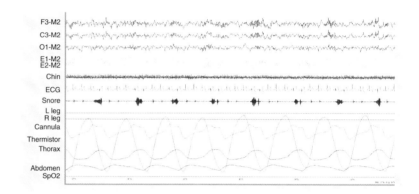

Section 4: Artifacts and Troubleshooting

Question 12

What artifact is shown in the airflow channel?

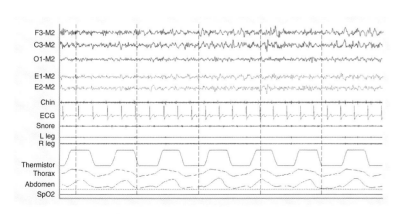

Section 4: Artifacts and Troubleshooting

Question 14

During the night, the patient awakens and kicks off one of the leg EMG leads. What should the technician do?

Question 13 Answer:

The gain or sensitivity setting is too high, causing the signal to intrude into other channels.

Question 11 Answer:

High impedances or 60-Hz artifact

Question 14 Answer:

Enter the patient room and replace the lead.

Question 12 Answer:

Pen blocking

Section 5: Policies and Procedures

Question 1

When reviewing the patient chart, you notice that the physician's orders call for supplemental oxygen at 10 L/min. What should you do?

Section 5: Policies and Procedures

Question 3

During a diagnostic study, the patient has an RDI of 80 after 3 hours of sleep and is desaturating below 70%. What should you do?

Section 5: Policies and Procedures

Question 2

A patient arrives at the lab claiming to be scheduled for a sleep study, but he is not on the schedule. You cannot find a chart for him. What should you do?

Section 5: Policies and Procedures

Question 4

How often should amplifier calibrations be performed?

Question 3 Answer:

Follow the lab protocol. If the lab does not have oxygen or CPAP protocols for this situation, contact the medical director for orders on how to proceed.

Essentials of Polysomnography, Chapter 9

Question 1 Answer:

Contact the physician to verify the accuracy of the order. If the physician is not available, contact the lab manager.

Essentials of Polysomnography, Chapter 9

Question 4 Answer:

Before and after every study, and while troubleshooting equipment problems.

Essentials of Polysomnography, Chapter 9

Question 2 Answer:

Contact the lab manager. Do not perform a study without physician's orders.

Essentials of Polysomnography, Chapter 9

Section 5: Policies and Procedures

Question 5

What should be done during a CPAP titration if obstructive apneas persist?

Section 5: Policies and Procedures

Question 7

What should be used to clean nondisposable sensors?

Section 5: Policies and Procedures

Question 6

What should be done during a CPAP titration if central apneas persist?

Section 5: Policies and Procedures

Question 8

What patient privacy rule did the U.S. Department of Health and Human Services initiate in 1996?

Question 7 Answer:

A disinfectant solution such as control III.

Essentials of Polysomnography, Chapter 3

Question 5 Answer:

Increase CPAP according to lab protocol.

Essentials of Polysomnography, Chapter 9

Question 8 Answer:

The Health Insurance Portability and Accountability Act of 1996 (HIPAA)

Essentials of Polysomnography, Chapter 3

Question 6 Answer:

Decrease CPAP or switch to bi-kevel PAP according to lab protocol.

Essentials of Polysomnography, Chapter 9

Section 5: Policies and Procedures

Question 9

During the night, excessively strong winds build outside, causing the technician to worry for the safety of the patients. What should the technician do?

Section 6: Sleep Stage Scoring

Question 1

What stage is this?

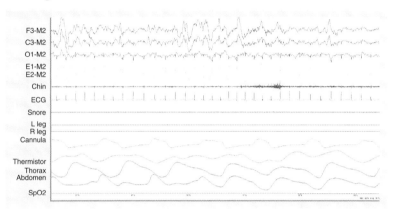

Section 5: Policies and Procedures

Question 10

What type of soap should be used when washing hands?

Section 6: Sleep Stage Scoring

Question 2

What stage is this?

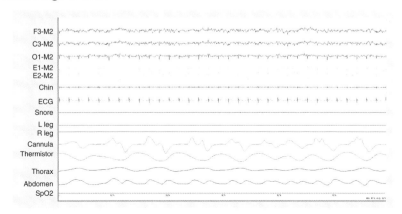

Question 1 Answer:

N3

Essentials of Polysomnography, Chapter 12

Question 2 Answer:

REM

Essentials of Polysomnography, Chapter 12

Question 9 Answer:

Consult the lab's written emergency and disaster plan for tornadoes.

Essentials of Polysomnography, Chapter 3

Question 10 Answer:

Antimicrobial soap

Essentials of Polysomnography, Chapter 3

Section 6: Sleep Stage Scoring

Question 3

What stage is this?

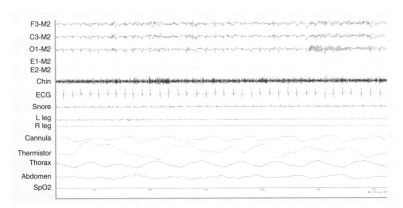

Section 6: Sleep Stage Scoring

Question 5

What stage is this?

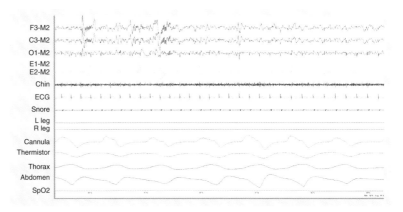

Section 6: Sleep Stage Scoring

Question 4

What stage is this?

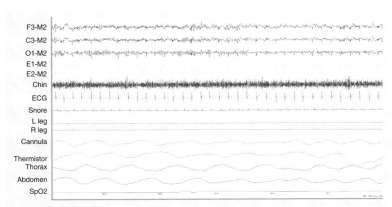

Section 6: Sleep Stage Scoring

Question 6

What is the amplitude requirement for slow waves in N3?

Question 5 Answer:

N2

Question 3 Answer:

N1

Question 6 Answer:

75 µV

Question 4 Answer:

W

Section 6: Sleep Stage Scoring

Question 7

What is the frequency range for slow waves in N3?

Section 6: Sleep Stage Scoring

Question 9

What is the duration requirement for a run of sleep spindles?

Section 6: Sleep Stage Scoring

Question 8

What is the amplitude requirement for a K-complex?

Section 6: Sleep Stage Scoring

Question 10

What is the frequency range for sleep spindles?

Question 9 Answer:

0.5 seconds

Question 7 Answer:

0.5–2 Hz

Question 10 Answer:

11–16 Hz

Question 8 Answer:

There is no amplitude requirement for a K-complex.

Section 6: Sleep Stage Scoring

Question 11

What is the frequency range for alpha waves?

Section 6: Sleep Stage Scoring

Question 13

What is the duration requirement for a K-complex?

Section 6: Sleep Stage Scoring

Question 12

In what channels are alpha waves seen most prominently?

Section 6: Sleep Stage Scoring

Question 14

The EEGs show trains of pointed waves in the 2-Hz to 6-Hz range with a decreased chin EMG. What stage is this?

Question 13 Answer:

0.5 seconds

Essentials of Polysomnography, Chapter 12

Question 11 Answer:

8–13 Hz

Essentials of Polysomnography, Chapter 12

Question 14 Answer:

REM

Essentials of Polysomnography, Chapter 12

Question 12 Answer:

Occipital channels (O1 and O2)

Essentials of Polysomnography, Chapter 12

Section 6: Sleep Stage Scoring

Question 15

The EEGs are a low-voltage, mixed-frequency pattern, and the EOGs show slow eye movements. What stage is this?

Section 6: Sleep Stage Scoring

Question 17

What are the infant sleep stages?

Section 6: Sleep Stage Scoring

Question 16

For what age group are the infant sleep-staging guidelines recommended?

Section 6: Sleep Stage Scoring

Question 18

For what age group are the pediatric sleep-staging guidelines recommended?

Question 17 Answer:

Stage wake (W), stage N (NREM), and stage R (REM)

Question 15 Answer:

N1

Question 18 Answer:

Two months postterm to 18 years

Question 16 Answer:

Infants 0–2 months postterm

Section 6: Sleep Stage Scoring

Question 19

What is the predominant EEG activity seen in pediatric patients in relaxed wakefulness with eyes closed?

Section 7: Event Scoring

Question 2

What events are circled in this 300-second epoch?

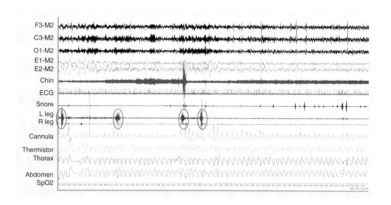

Section 7: Event Scoring

Question 1

What event is circled in this epoch?

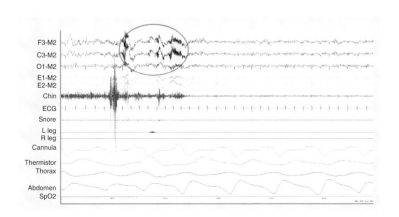

Section 7: Event Scoring

Question 3

What event is circled in this epoch?

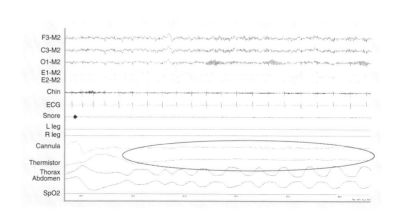

Question 2 Answer:

Periodic limb movements

Essentials of Polysomnography, Chapter 13

Question 19 Answer:

Dominant posterior rhythm (DPR)

Essentials of Polysomnography, Chapter 16

Question 3 Answer:

Obstructive apnea

Essentials of Polysomnography, Chapter 13

Question 1 Answer:

EEG arousal

Essentials of Polysomnography, Chapter 13

Section 7: Event Scoring

Question 4

What event is circled in this epoch?

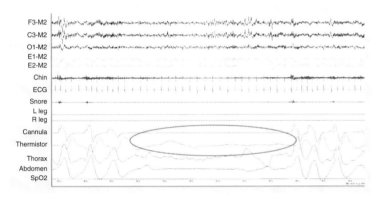

Section 7: Event Scoring

Question 6

What event is circled in this epoch?

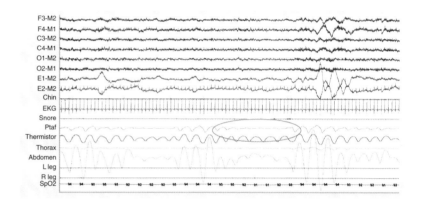

Section 7: Event Scoring

Question 5

What event is circled in this epoch?

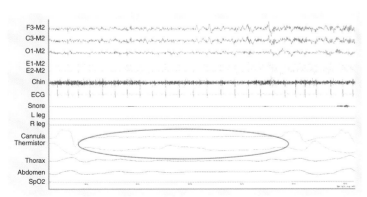

Section 7: Event Scoring

Question 7

What event is circled in this epoch?

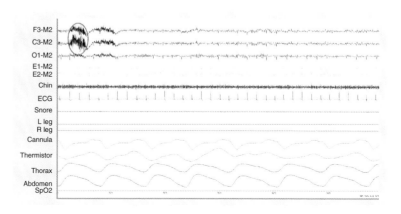

Figure by Lisa M. Endee; produced from a sleep study provided to Stony Brook University School of Health Technology and Management's Polysomnographic Technology Program by Dr. Kala Sury.

Question 6 Answer:

Hypopnea

Question 4 Answer:

Mixed apnea

Question 7 Answer:

Beta spindles

Question 5 Answer:

Central apnea

Section 7: Event Scoring

Question 8

What are the requirements for a series of limb movements to be scored as periodic limb movements?

Section 7: Event Scoring

Question 10

What are the requirements for scoring Cheyne–Stokes breathing?

Section 7: Event Scoring

Question 9

What are the requirements for scoring a hypopnea?

Section 7: Event Scoring

Question 11

How does the pediatric respiratory event duration criteria compare to the adult guidelines?

Question 10 Answer:

There must be at least three consecutive cycles of a waning–waxing pattern in the airflow with a duration of at least 10 seconds each and at least five central apneas or hypopneas per hour of sleep during the night.

Essentials of Polysomnography, Chapter 13

Question 8 Answer:

There must be at least four limb movements, each at least 8 μV above the resting limb movement amplitude and at least 0.5 seconds long, all occurring within 5 to 90 seconds of each other.

Essentials of Polysomnography, Chapter 13

Question 11 Answer:

For OA, MA, and hypopnea, duration must be at least two breaths. For CA, duration is either at least 20 seconds; or at least two breaths associated with either an arousal or an O_2 desaturation of at least 3%; or at least two breaths and associated with a heart rate of less than 50 bpm for 5 seconds.

Essentials of Polysomnography, Chapter 16

Question 9 Answer:

The Ptaf airflow must decrease by 30% to 90% of the original amplitude and be associated with an O_2 desaturation of at least 3% or an EEG arousal.

Essentials of Polysomnography, Chapter 13

Section 8: Electrocardiography

Question 1

What are the normal ranges for the PR interval?

Section 8: Electrocardiography

Question 3

What cardiac activity does the P wave represent?

Section 8: Electrocardiography

Question 2

What are the normal ranges for the QRS complex?

Section 8: Electrocardiography

Question 4

What ECG wave is representative of the ventricular repolarization?

Question 3 Answer:

Contraction of the atria

Essentials of Polysomnography, Chapter 14

Question 1 Answer:

0.12–0.20 seconds

Essentials of Polysomnography, Chapter 14

Question 4 Answer:

T wave

Essentials of Polysomnography, Chapter 14

Question 2 Answer:

0.04–0.10 seconds

Essentials of Polysomnography, Chapter 14

Section 8: Electrocardiography

Question 5

What cardiac activity does the QRS complex represent?

Section 8: Electrocardiography

Question 7

A 10-second ECG strip has 12 QRS complexes. What is the rate?

Section 8: Electrocardiography

Question 6

A 6-second ECG strip has seven QRS complexes. What is the rate?

Section 8: Electrocardiography

Question 8

Describe the types of PVCs, including unifocal, multifocal, bigeminy, trigeminy, couplets, and ventricular tachycardia.

Question 7 Answer:

72 bpm

Essentials of Polysomnography, Chapter 14

Question 5 Answer:

Contraction of the ventricles

Essentials of Polysomnography, Chapter 14

Question 8 Answer:

Unifocal PVCs: Same origins, look the same

Multifocal PVCs: Different origins

Bigeminy: PVC in every other beat

Trigeminy: PVC in every third beat

Couplet: Two PVCs in a row

V tach: Three or more PVCs in a row

Essentials of Polysomnography, Chapter 14

Question 6 Answer:

70 bpm

Essentials of Polysomnography, Chapter 14

Section 8: Electrocardiography

Question 9

Identify the ECG rhythm

Rate: 60–100 bpm

Rhythm: Regular

QRS: <0.10 sec

P waves: Uniform and upright

PR interval: 0.12–0.20 sec

Description: Normal rhythm, rate, and intervals

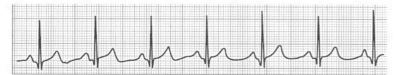

Section 8: Electrocardiography

Question 11

Identify the ECG rhythm.

Rate: <40 bpm

Rhythm: Regular

QRS: <0.10 sec

P waves: Uniform and upright

PR interval: 0.12–0.20 sec

Description: Normal rhythm and intervals. Decreased rate

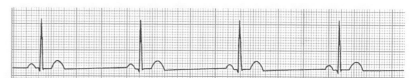

Section 8: Electrocardiography

Question 10

Identify the ECG rhythm

Rate: Usually 60–90 bpm but may vary

Rhythm: Irregular

QRS: <0.10 sec

P waves: Uniform and upright

PR interval: 0.12–0.20 sec

Description: Normal rate and intervals. Irregular rhythm.

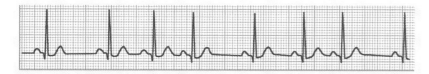

Section 8: Electrocardiography

Question 12

Identify the ECG rhythm.

Rate: >100 bpm

Rhythm: Regular

QRS: <0.10 sec

P waves: Uniform and upright

PR interval: 0.12–0.20 sec

Description: Normal rhythm and intervals. Increased rate.

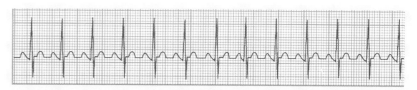

Question 11 Answer:

Sinus bradycardia

Essentials of Polysomnography, Chapter 14

Question 9 Answer:

Normal sinus rhythm (NSR)

Essentials of Polysomnography, Chapter 14

Question 12 Answer:

Sinus tachycardia

Essentials of Polysomnography, Chapter 14

Question 10 Answer:

Sinus arrhythmia

Essentials of Polysomnography, Chapter 14

Section 8: Electrocardiography

Question 13

Identify the ECG rhythm.
Rate: Atrial rate >400
Rhythm: Atrial and ventricular rates are irregular.
QRS: Usually <0.10 sec
P waves: No identifiable P waves
PR interval: None
Description: Unorganized atrial activity.

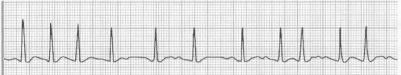

Section 8: Electrocardiography

Question 14

Identify the ECG rhythm.
Rate: Depends on underlying rhythm
Rhythm: Irregular
QRS: >0.12 sec. Wide and bizarre.
P waves: Usually absent
PR interval: None
Description: QRS complexes are wide and begin early.

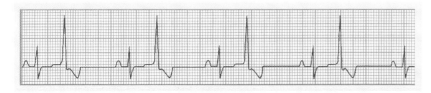

Section 8: Electrocardiography

Question 15

Identify the ECG rhythm.
Rate: Cannot be determined.
Rhythm: Rapid and chaotic
QRS: Not discernible
P waves: Not discernible
PR interval: Not measurable
Description: Heart is quivering rather than contracting.

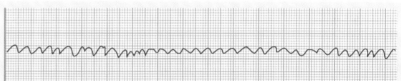

Section 8: Electrocardiography

Question 16

Identify the ECG rhythm.
Rate: Cannot be determined.
Rhythm: Ventricular rate indiscernible
QRS: None
P waves: Not discernible
PR interval: Not measurable
Description: No activity in ventricles.

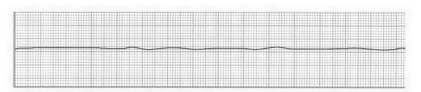

Question 15 Answer:
Ventricular fibrillation (V fib)

Essentials of Polysomnography, Chapter 14

Question 13 Answer:
Atrial fibrillation

Essentials of Polysomnography, Chapter 14

Question 16 Answer:
Ventricular standstill (asystole)

Essentials of Polysomnography, Chapter 14

Question 14 Answer:
Multifocal premature ventricular contractions (PVCs) occurring every other beat (bigeminy)

Essentials of Polysomnography, Chapter 14

Section 8: Electrocardiography

Question 17

Identify the ECG rhythm.
Rate: Normal
Rhythm: Normal
QRS: <0.10 sec
P waves: Normal in size and configuration
PR interval: Prolonged (>0.20 sec) but constant
Description: Normal rate and rhythm. Long PR interval.

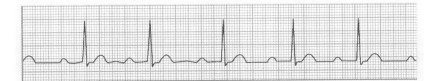

Section 8: Electrocardiography

Question 18

Identify the ECG rhythm.
Rate: Atrial rate > ventricular rate, both in normal ranges
Rhythm: Atrial regular, ventricular irregular
QRS: <0.10 sec but is dropped periodically
P waves: Normal in size and configuration
PR interval: Lengthens with each cycle until QRS drops
Description: Missed QRS after increasing PR intervals.

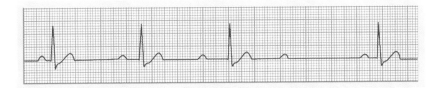

Section 8: Electrocardiography

Question 19

Identify the ECG rhythm.
Rate: Atrial rate > ventricular rate, both in normal ranges
Rhythm: Atrial regular, ventricular irregular
QRS: >0.10 sec but is dropped periodically
P waves: Normal in size and configuration
PR interval: Constant for each QRS
Description: Missed QRS without warning

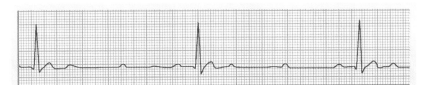

Section 8: Electrocardiography

Question 20

Identify the ECG rhythm.
Rate: Atrial rate > ventricular rate, both in normal ranges
Rhythm: Atrial regular, ventricular regular
QRS: May be narrow or wide
P waves: Normal in size and configuration
PR interval: None
Description: No association between P waves and QRS

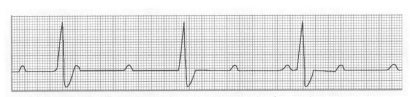

Question 19 Answer:

Second-degree AV block type II (non–Wenckebach, Mobitz II)

Essentials of Polysomnography, Chapter 14

Question 17 Answer:

First-degree AV block

Essentials of Polysomnography, Chapter 14

Question 20 Answer:

Third-degree (complete) AV block

Essentials of Polysomnography, Chapter 14

Question 18 Answer:

Second-degree AV block type I (Wenckebach, Mobitz I)

Essentials of Polysomnography, Chapter 14

Section 9: Reports and Calculations

Question 1

The recording starts at 2232. Physiologic calibrations start 7 minutes later and last for 5 minutes. Three minutes later, the television and lights are turned off and the patient begins trying to sleep. What time does lights out occur?

Section 9: Reports and Calculations

Question 3

Total recording time minus total wake time equals:

Section 9: Reports and Calculations

Question 2

The duration in minutes from lights out to lights on is called:

Section 9: Reports and Calculations

Question 4

How is sleep efficiency calculated?

Question 3 Answer:

Total sleep time (TST)

Essentials of Polysomnography, Chapter 15

Question 1 Answer:

2247

Essentials of Polysomnography, Chapter 15

Question 4 Answer:

SE = TST/TRT

Essentials of Polysomnography, Chapter 15

Question 2 Answer:

Total recording time (TRT)

Essentials of Polysomnography, Chapter 15

Section 9: Reports and Calculations

Question 5

How is the total wake time calculated?

Section 9: Reports and Calculations

Question 7

What is sleep onset?

Section 9: Reports and Calculations

Question 6

How is the % of stage R calculated?

Section 9: Reports and Calculations

Question 8

How is sleep latency calculated?

Question 7 Answer:

The first epoch of sleep regardless of the stage. This is usually the first epoch of stage N1.

Question 5 Answer:

TWT = TRT − TST or TWT = Sleep latency + WASO

Question 8 Answer:

Sleep latency is the time in minutes from lights out to sleep onset.

Question 6 Answer:

% stage R = total REM time/TST

Section 9: Reports and Calculations

Question 9

What is REM onset?

Section 9: Reports and Calculations

Question 11

How is the apnea–hypopnea index (AHI) calculated?

Section 9: Reports and Calculations

Question 10

How is REM latency calculated?

Section 9: Reports and Calculations

Question 12

How is the respiratory disturbance index (RDI) calculated?

Question 11 Answer:

AHI = (apneas + hypopneas)/TST in hours

Essentials of Polysomnography, Chapter 15

Question 9 Answer:

The first epoch of stage R

Essentials of Polysomnography, Chapter 15

Question 12 Answer:

RDI = (apneas + hypopneas + RERAs)/TST in hours

Essentials of Polysomnography, Chapter 15

Question 10 Answer:

REM latency is the time, in minutes, from sleep onset to REM onset.

Essentials of Polysomnography, Chapter 15

Section 9: Reports and Calculations

Question 13

What is WASO and how is it calculated?

Section 9: Reports and Calculations

Question 15

There are 64 limb movements recorded during 287 minutes of sleep. Of these, 41 were part of PLM series. What is the PLM index?

Section 9: Reports and Calculations

Question 14

There are 28 apneas and 45 hypopneas during 328 minutes of sleep. What is the AHI?

Section 10: Sleep Disorders—Insomnias

Question 1

Short-term insomnia

Question 15 Answer:

8.6

Question 13 Answer:

WASO (Wake after sleep onset) = TRT – TST – Sleep latency

Question 1 Answer:

Also known as *acute insomnia*; describes the inability to fall or stay asleep reported for a period of less than 3 months despite adequate opportunity. It is often associated with a specific stressor and if not addressed can lead to chronic insomnia disorder.

Question 14 Answer:

13.4

Section 10: Sleep Disorders—Insomnias

Question 2

Psychophysiological insomnia

Section 10: Sleep Disorders—Insomnias

Question 4

Idiopathic insomnia

Section 10: Sleep Disorders—Insomnias

Question 3

Paradoxical insomnia

Section 10: Sleep Disorders—Insomnias

Question 5

Inadequate sleep hygiene

Question 4 Answer:
Also known as *lifelong insomnia*, this is identified at infancy and persists throughout the life. Appears to be no external cause for this, and no other sleep disorder exists as a contributing factor.

Question 2 Answer:
A type of chronic insomnia caused by a learned response to not fall asleep when planned.

Question 5 Answer:
This disorder consists of practices that encourage poor sleep, such as watching TV in bed, frequently altering bedtimes, not blocking out light and noise during sleep, and drinking alcohol before sleep.

Question 3 Answer:
Also known as *sleep state misperception*, this consists of a complaint of insomnia without any evidence. Use of a sleep diary or sleep log may be appropriate.

Section 10: Sleep Disorders—Insomnias

Question 6

Behavioral insomnia of childhood

Section 10: Sleep Disorders—Sleep-Related Breathing Disorders

Question 2

Cheyne–Stokes breathing pattern

Section 10: Sleep Disorders—Sleep-Related Breathing Disorders

Question 1

Primary central sleep apnea

Section 10: Sleep Disorders—Sleep-Related Breathing Disorders

Question 3

High-altitude periodic breathing

Question 2 Answer:

In this disorder, the airflow shows distinct waning and waxing patterns, usually seen during NREM. Diagnostic criteria includes greater than five central apneas or hypopneas per hour and a crescendo–decrescendo pattern.

Essentials of Polysomnography, Chapter 2

Question 6 Answer:

Also known as *limit-setting disorder*, this condition is characterized by a parent promoting poor sleep hygiene techniques in a child, such as putting toys in the crib or frequently altering feeding times.

Essentials of Polysomnography, Chapter 2

Question 3 Answer:

This disorder is characterized by central apneas and hypopneas occurring during a recent ascent to at least 4,000 meters, or approximately 12,000 feet. The events occur at least five times per hour of sleep.

Essentials of Polysomnography, Chapter 2

Question 1 Answer:

This is characterized by cessations of airflow and concurrent cessations of respiratory effort. It is often seen in the elderly. Diagnostic features include an average of at least five of these events per hour.

Essentials of Polysomnography, Chapter 2

Section 10: Sleep Disorders—Sleep-Related Breathing Disorders

Question 4

Adult obstructive sleep apnea

Section 10: Sleep Disorders—Sleep-Related Breathing Disorders

Question 6

Sleep-related nonobstructive alveolar hypoventilation

Section 10: Sleep Disorders—Sleep-Related Breathing Disorders

Question 5

Pediatric obstructive sleep apnea

Section 10: Sleep Disorders—Sleep-Related Breathing Disorders

Question 7

Congenital central alveolar hypoventilation syndrome

Question 6 Answer:
This disorder is characterized by abnormally elevated arterial PCO_2 (>45 mmHg), or hypercapnia, during sleep.

Question 4 Answer:
This includes repeated apneas and hypopneas with continued respiratory effort. Diagnostic criteria include an RDI > 5 with complaints of EDS, choking, gasping, or snoring, or an RDI > 15 without these complaints.

Question 7 Answer:
This disorder is similar to sleep-related nonobstructive alveolar hypoventilation, but it occurs in infants. Those affected by it experience severe oxygen desaturation and hypercapnia.

Question 5 Answer:
Diagnostic criteria for this disorder include at least one obstructive apnea or hypopnea per hour of sleep.

Section 10: Sleep Disorders—Sleep-Related Breathing Disorders

Question 8

Sleep-related hypoventilation resulting from pulmonary parenchymal or vascular pathology

Section 10: Sleep Disorders—Sleep-Related Breathing Disorders

Question 10

Sleep-related hypoventilation resulting from neuromuscular and chest wall disorders

Section 10: Sleep Disorders—Sleep-Related Breathing Disorders

Question 9

Late-onset central hypoventilation with hypothalamic dysfunction

Section 10: Sleep Disorders—Hypersomnias of Central Origin

Question 1

Narcolepsy type I

Question 10 Answer:

This disorder refers to patients who have difficulty breathing as a result of a chest wall or neuromuscular disorder such as muscular dystrophy or Eaton-Lambert syndrome.

Question 8 Answer:

This disorder is characterized by elevated arterial PCO_2 (>45 mmHg), or hypercapnia, during sleep related to lung diseases such as interstitial pneumonitis or forms of pulmonary hypertension.

Question 1 Answer:

This is characterized by EDS and cataplexy and often includes sleep paralysis and hypnagogic hallucinations. Diagnostic criteria include a mean sleep latency <8 min and two REM onsets during an MSLT.

Question 9 Answer:

This disorder affects young children and is characterized by severe obesity and hypoventilation during the first few years of life. It often requires ventilatory support.

Section 10: Sleep Disorders—Hypersomnias of Central Origin

Question 2

Klein-Levin syndrome

Section 10: Sleep Disorders—Hypersomnias of Central Origin

Question 4

Behaviorally induced insufficient sleep syndrome

Section 10: Sleep Disorders—Hypersomnias of Central Origin

Question 3

Idiopathic hypersomnia with long sleep time

Section 10: Sleep Disorders—Circadian Rhythm Sleep Disorders

Question 1

Delayed sleep–wake phase disorder

Question 4 Answer:
This is more commonly known as *sleep deprivation* or *sleep restriction*, and it is self-induced. These lifestyle choices often result in EDS and longer sleep periods on weekends.

Essentials of Polysomnography, Chapter 2

Question 2 Answer:
This is a rare disorder characterized by repeated episodes of hypersomnia. Patients may sleep 16–18 hours a day during these periods, which may last as long as 4 weeks.

Essentials of Polysomnography, Chapter 2

Question 1 Answer:
This is characterized by a later sleep time than expected. Patients with this disorder are usually adolescents or young adults, and they tend to stay up late at night and wake up late in the morning.

Essentials of Polysomnography, Chapter 2

Question 3 Answer:
This disorder is characterized primarily by sleeping periods lasting more than 10 hours in duration, EDS, and short sleep latency.

Essentials of Polysomnography, Chapter 2

Section 10: Sleep Disorders—Circadian Rhythm Sleep Disorders

Question 2

Advanced sleep–wake phase disorder

Section 10: Sleep Disorders—Circadian Rhythm Sleep Disorders

Question 4

Non–24-hour sleep–wake rhythm disorder

Section 10: Sleep Disorders—Circadian Rhythm Sleep Disorders

Question 3

Irregular sleep–wake rhythm disorder

Section 10: Sleep Disorders—Circadian Rhythm Sleep Disorders

Question 5

Jet lag disorder

Question 4 Answer:

This circadian rhythm is not consistent with the 24-hour clock. The patient's rhythm is often longer than 24 hours and does not seem to be related to the light–dark cycle.

Question 2 Answer:

This is characterized by an earlier sleep time than expected. Patients with this disorder are usually elderly, and they tend to go to bed early at night and wake up early in the morning.

Question 5 Answer:

This occurs when a person travels across two or more time zones, resulting in EDS or insomnia. Other symptoms such as gastrointestinal disturbances or poor performance often occur.

Question 3 Answer:

This disorder is characterized by abnormal sleep and wake times. Although the total sleep time during the 24-hour period may be normal, the sleep periods may come in the form of several naps.

Section 10: Sleep Disorders—Circadian Rhythm Sleep Disorders

Question 6

Shift work disorder

Section 10: Sleep Disorders—Parasomnias

Question 2

Sleepwalking

Section 10: Sleep Disorders—Parasomnias

Question 1

Confusional arousal

Section 10: Sleep Disorders—Parasomnias

Question 3

Sleep terrors

Question 2 Answer:

This is characterized by certain behaviors during slow wave sleep such as sitting up, walking, jumping, and even violent behaviors. Sleepwalking tends to be common in children and adolescents and tends to decline with advanced age.

Question 6 Answer:

Patients with this disorder are assigned to work a shift that causes them to sleep during hours other than the typical nighttime hours. As a result, the patient often experiences EDS and poor performance and judgment.

Question 3 Answer:

These are awakenings from slow wave sleep with feelings of intense fear, a loud scream, and often violent behaviors. After the event, the patient returns to slow wave sleep and has no recollection in the morning.

Question 1 Answer:

This occurs when a person awakens in a confused state, usually when awakening from slow wave sleep. People may not know who they are or what is happening. Speech may be slurred and mentation slow.

Section 10: Sleep Disorders—Parasomnias

Question 4

REM sleep behavior disorder (RBD)

Section 10: Sleep Disorders—Parasomnias

Question 6

Nightmare disorder

Section 10: Sleep Disorders—Parasomnias

Question 5

Recurrent isolated sleep paralysis

Section 10: Sleep Disorders—Parasomnias

Question 7

Other parasomnias

Question 6 Answer:

Common in young children and patients with posttraumatic stress disorder (PTSD), this disorder includes repeated frightening or intense dreams, causing persistent fear after awakening.

Question 4 Answer:

This consists of physical activities during REM sleep. Normal muscle atonia does not occur in REM in these patients. On awakening, the patient is likely to remember the associated dream.

Question 7 Answer:

These are parasomnias that have not as of yet been categorized as either REM related or NREM related.

Question 5 Answer:

This includes episodes of the inability to move during sleep onset (hypnagogic) or awakening (hypnopompic). These periods last a few seconds to several minutes. This disorder occurs in the absence of narcolepsy.

Section 10: Sleep Disorders—Parasomnias

Question 8

Sleep enuresis

Section 10: Sleep Disorders—Parasomnias

Question 10

Exploding head syndrome

Section 10: Sleep Disorders—Parasomnias

Question 9

Parasomnia due to a medication or substance

Section 10: Sleep Disorders—Parasomnias

Question 11

Sleep-related hallucinations

Question 10 Answer:

This is a sleep disorder in which the patient is awakened by an imagined loud noise or sense of explosion in the head while falling asleep or awakening.

Question 8 Answer:

This includes repeated episodes of involuntary urination during sleep. Diagnostic criteria require the patient to be at least 5 years of age and wet the bed at least twice a week. PTSD is often associated.

Question 11 Answer:

These are hallucinations either at sleep onset or upon awakening, often associated with sleep-onset REM periods (SOREMPs), and may be frightening to the patient. These occur in the absence of narcolepsy.

Question 9 Answer:

This diagnosis is used when a parasomnia can be attributed to a drug or medication use or abuse.

Section 10: Sleep Disorders—Parasomnias

Question 12

Sleep talking

Section 10: Sleep Disorders—Sleep-Related Movement Disorders

Question 2

Periodic limb movement disorder (PLMD)

Section 10: Sleep Disorders—Sleep-Related Movement Disorders

Question 1

Restless legs syndrome (RLS)

Section 10: Sleep Disorders—Sleep-Related Movement Disorders

Question 3

Sleep-related leg cramps

Question 2 Answer:

Formerly known as *nocturnal myoclonus*, this affects one-third of adults 60 years of age and older and causes involuntary limb movements during sleep in series of at least four events within 5 to 90 seconds of each other.

Essentials of Polysomnography, Chapter 2

Question 12 Answer:

Sleep talking, also called *somniloquy*, is often considered benign unless it disturbs the sleep significantly. It can occur at any age.

Essentials of Polysomnography, Chapter 2

Question 3 Answer:

This disorder is characterized by intense and sudden muscle cramps in the legs during sleep. These muscle cramps are often painful and result in the patient waking up from sleep, thereby disturbing the sleep period.

Essentials of Polysomnography, Chapter 2

Question 1 Answer:

This is characterized by the irresistible urge to move the body in an effort to stop uncomfortable or odd sensations often described as creeping, crawling feelings in the legs. It often leads to disturbed sleep.

Essentials of Polysomnography, Chapter 2

Section 10: Sleep Disorders—Sleep-Related Movement Disorders

Question 4

Sleep-related bruxism

Section 10: Sleep Disorders—Sleep-Related Movement Disorders

Question 6

Benign sleep myoclonus of infancy

Section 10: Sleep Disorders—Sleep-Related Movement Disorders

Question 5

Sleep-related rhythmic movement disorder (RMD)

Section 10: Sleep Disorders—Sleep-Related Movement Disorders

Question 7

Propriospinal myoclonus at sleep onset (PSM)

Question 6 Answer:

BSMI is a rare disorder that occurs when repetitive leg jerks or movements in sleep have been noted to occur during infancy, typically from birth to 6 months of age.

Question 4 Answer:

This disorder is often discovered by the dentist and is characterized by the repeated grinding of teeth or clenching of the jaw. This is more common in children and teens and is often the result of stress.

Question 7 Answer:

These events are similar to sleep starts but mainly involve body movements in the trunk and neck areas. They typically occur at sleep onset or during brief arousals from sleep.

Question 5 Answer:

Also known as *body rocking* and *head banging*, this is characterized by repetitive body movements during drowsiness or sleep. This is most common in infants and children under 5 years of age.

Section 10: Sleep Disorders—Isolated Symptoms

Question 1

Sleep starts (hypnic jerks)

Section 10: Sleep Disorders—Isolated Symptoms

Question 3

Excessive fragmentary myoclonus

Section 10: Sleep Disorders—Isolated Symptoms

Question 2

Hypnagogic foot tremor (HFT) and alternating leg muscle activation (ALMA)

Section 11: Therapeutic Modalities

Question 1

What is CPAP therapy?

Question 3 Answer:

These events are characterized by frequent small twitches of fingers, toes, or muscles of the mouth during wake or sleep. They are typically benign, occur in NREM sleep, and persist for >20 minutes.

Essentials of Polysomnography, Chapter 2

Question 1 Answer:

These are sudden muscle jerks or movements at sleep onset that are often accompanied by feelings of surprise or fear. They are usually benign, although they can disturb the sleep of the bed partner.

Essentials of Polysomnography, Chapter 2

Question 1 Answer:

CPAP therapy—continuous positive airway pressure—is the most common method of treating obstructive sleep apnea. Positive pressure is delivered to the upper airway to act as a splint to keep the airway clear during sleep.

Essentials of Polysomnography, Chapter 10

Question 2 Answer:

These are rhythmic leg or foot movements at sleep onset. The latter is characterized by movement in one leg followed by movement in the other leg. They are typically benign but can cause brief arousals.

Essentials of Polysomnography, Chapter 2

Section 11: Therapeutic Modalities

Question 2

What is bi-level therapy?

Section 11: Therapeutic Modalities

Question 4

What are the main components needed to initiate PAP therapy?

Section 11: Therapeutic Modalities

Question 3

What are the three main types of interfaces used to deliver PAP therapy?

Section 11: Therapeutic Modalities

Question 5

What are some adverse effects to PAP therapy?

Question 4 Answer:

PAP device, interface, corrugated tubing

Essentials of Polysomnography, Chapter 10

Question 2 Answer:

Bilevel therapy uses pressure applied at two separate levels, a higher pressure during the inspiratory phase (IPAP) and a lower pressure during the expiratory phase (EPAP). Bi-level therapy is used to treat more complex sleep-related breathing disorders, including hypoventilation and Cheyne–Stokes respiration.

Essentials of Polysomnography, Chapter 10

Question 5 Answer:

Nasal dryness, claustrophobia, inability to tolerate pressure, facial soreness, etc.

Essentials of Polysomnography, Chapter 10

Question 3 Answer:

Nasal mask, full face mask, and nasal pillows

Essentials of Polysomnography, Chapter 10

Section 11: Therapeutic Modalities

Question 6

What is included in acclimatization to PAP therapy?

Section 11: Therapeutic Modalities

Question 8

How is bi-level therapy titrated in response to respiratory events during sleep?

Section 11: Therapeutic Modalities

Question 7

When should CPAP therapy be titrated upward?

Section 11: Therapeutic Modalities

Question 9

What defines an optimal PAP titration?

Question 8 Answer:

Upward titration of the IPAP and EPAP by greater than or equal to 1 cm H_2O for apneic events and upward titration of the IPAP pressure by greater than or equal to 1 cm H_2O in response to hypopnea, RERAs, or snoring.

Essentials of Polysomnography, Chapter 10

Question 6 Answer:

Acclimatization includes educating patients about their sleep disorders and the rationale behind the use of PAP therapy to treat it. Central to this is giving a patient the opportunity to handle PAP equipment, make self-adjustments, and ask questions—and providing time for the patient to adjust to the therapy.

Essentials of Polysomnography, Chapter 10

Question 9 Answer:

According to the *AASM Clinical Guidelines for the Manual Titration of PAP Therapy*, an optimal titration is defined as:

- a respiratory disturbance index (RDI) of less than five events for a period of 15 minutes
- SpO_2 >90%
- EEG arousals < 5/hour in supine REM
- snoring eliminated

Essentials of Polysomnography, Chapter 10

Question 7 Answer:

During sleep, if the patient demonstrates two or more obstructive apneas, three or more hypopneas, five or more respiratory effort–related arousals (RERAs), or more than 3 minutes of loud snoring.

Essentials of Polysomnography, Chapter 10

Section 11: Therapeutic Modalities

Question 10

What is chronotherapy?

Section 11: Therapeutic Modalities

Question 12

Name some of the components of Cognitive Behavioral Therapy (CBT).

Section 11: Therapeutic Modalities

Question 11

How is phototherapy used to treat sleep disorders?

Section 11: Therapeutic Modalities

Question 13

How is oral appliance (OA) therapy used to treat OSA?

Question 12 Answer:
CBT strategies can include sleep restriction therapy, stimulus control, paradoxical intention, relaxation, cognitive control, and biofeedback.

Question 10 Answer:
Chronotherapy aims to reset the internal biological clock to the desired time for sleep by systematically and gradually delaying or advancing bedtimes and rise times. It is used to treat various circadian rhythm disorders.

Question 13 Answer:
OA devices are worn during sleep and act to pull the lower jaw forward. By stabilizing the mandible, tongue, and pharyngeal structures in this forward position, the oral appliance can create a more patent airway in patients with mild to moderate OSA who are not tolerant of traditional CPAP therapy.

Question 11 Answer:
Phototherapy, also called *bright light therapy* (BLT), is a treatment that uses purposeful exposure to natural daylight, or specific wavelengths of light using lamps or light boxes to increase alertness and help reset the circadian rhythm.

Section 11: Therapeutic Modalities

Question 14

Which treatment modality includes an implantable pulse generating device that stimulates the tongue during sleep to prevent the collapse of the airway?

Section 11: Therapeutic Modalities

Question 16

What is a uvulopalatopharyngoplasty (UPPP)?

Section 11: Therapeutic Modalities

Question 15

Which treatment modality is the most common major surgical procedure performed on children as the first-line treatment for moderate to severe OSA?

Section 12: Drug Effects on Sleep

Question 1

Alcohol

Question 16 Answer:

A UPPP is an invasive procedure in which the tonsils, uvula, and part of the soft palate are surgically removed to enlarge and stabilize the airway.

Question 14 Answer:

Hypoglossal nerve stimulation

Question 1 Answer:

Suppresses REM, increases stage N3 and apneas. Increases sleep fragmentation.

Question 15 Answer:

Adenotonsillectomy

Section 12: Drug Effects on Sleep

Question 2

Amphetamines

Section 12: Drug Effects on Sleep

Question 4

Benzodiazepines

Section 12: Drug Effects on Sleep

Question 3

Barbiturates

Section 12: Drug Effects on Sleep

Question 5

Caffeine

Question 4 Answer:

Decrease REM and N3, increase latency to REM and N3. Increase fast frequency activity.

Essentials of Polysomnography, Chapter 17

Question 2 Answer:

Reduce sleep efficiency, suppress REM. Delay sleep and REM onset.

Essentials of Polysomnography, Chapter 17

Question 5 Answer:

Suppresses N3. Stimulates.

Essentials of Polysomnography, Chapter 17

Question 3 Answer:

Decrease N3, REM, and leg movements. Increase N2. Significant daytime impairment.

Essentials of Polysomnography, Chapter 17

Section 12: Drug Effects on Sleep

Question 6

Cocaine

Section 12: Drug Effects on Sleep

Question 8

Heroin

Section 12: Drug Effects on Sleep

Question 7

Antidepressants

Section 12: Drug Effects on Sleep

Question 9

Morphine

Question 8 Answer:

Decreases REM, N1, and limb movements. Increases apneas.

Essentials of Polysomnography, Chapter 17

Question 6 Answer:

Stimulating and cardiovascular effects.

Essentials of Polysomnography, Chapter 17

Question 9 Answer:

Decreases REM and leg movements. Increases N1 and apneas.

Essentials of Polysomnography, Chapter 17

Question 7 Answer:

Decrease REM and N3, increase latency to REM and N3.

Essentials of Polysomnography, Chapter 17

Section 12: Drug Effects on Sleep

Question 10

Antiarrhythmic medications

Section 13: Terms and Definitions

Question 2

Actigraph

Section 13: Terms and Definitions

Question 1

Acetylcholine

Section 13: Terms and Definitions

Question 3

Alpha intrusion

Question 2 Answer:

A device used to measure movement, usually over long periods of time

Question 10 Answer:

Nighttime sleep difficulties, insomnia, and nightmares. Decreases stage R sleep.

Question 3 Answer:

The presence of EEG alpha waves (8–13 Hz) during sleep

Question 1 Answer:

A chemical in the brain responsible for activation of the cortex

Section 13: Terms and Definitions

Question 4

Alveolar hypoventilation

Section 13: Terms and Definitions

Question 6

Amplifier calibrations

Section 13: Terms and Definitions

Question 5

Ambulatory sleep study

Section 13: Terms and Definitions

Question 7

Amplitude

Question 6 Answer:

A series of tests to determine the validity of signals from the amplifier to the polysomnograph

Question 4 Answer:

A disorder characterized by hypercapnia, oxygen desaturations and EEG arousals

Question 7 Answer:

The voltage of an electrical signal

Question 5 Answer:

A sleep study using mobile equipment to study the patient in a hospital room or at home

Section 13: Terms and Definitions

Question 8

Anterior tibialis

Section 13: Terms and Definitions

Question 10

Arterial blood gas (ABG)

Section 13: Terms and Definitions

Question 9

Apnea

Section 13: Terms and Definitions

Question 11

Atrioventricular (AV) node

Question 10 Answer:

A test of blood taken from the arteries that shows levels of certain gases in the blood

Question 8 Answer:

The muscle on the outer side of the shinbone where the leg EMG electrodes are placed

Question 11 Answer:

The point of the heart that is responsible for the conduction of the electrical impulses from the atria to the ventricles

Question 9 Answer:

A complete cessation of airflow for at least 10 seconds during sleep, which may be classified as central, obstructive, or mixed

Section 13: Terms and Definitions

Question 12

Attenuation

Section 13: Terms and Definitions

Question 14

AWAKE

Section 13: Terms and Definitions

Question 13

Automatism

Section 13: Terms and Definitions

Question 15

Berlin Questionnaire

Question 14 Answer:

"Alert, Well, And Keeping Energetic," a group designed to support those with sleep apnea

Question 12 Answer:

A marked decrease in the amplitude of a wave

Question 15 Answer:

A series of questions designed to demonstrate the likelihood of a patient having sleep apnea

Question 13 Answer:

Actions performed without intent or awareness

Section 13: Terms and Definitions

Question 16

Bioelectric potentials

Section 13: Terms and Definitions

Question 18

Bipolar montage

Section 13: Terms and Definitions

Question 17

Biofeedback

Section 13: Terms and Definitions

Question 19

Body mass index

Question 18 Answer:

A channel setup based on recordings from two exploring electrodes

Question 16 Answer:

Electrical signals that originate from a living source

Question 19 Answer:

A calculation of height and weight

BMI = weight (lbs) * 703 / height (inches)^2

Question 17 Answer:

A treatment for insomnia in which a patient learns to control biological activity

Section 13: Terms and Definitions

Question 20

Bundle branches

Section 13: Terms and Definitions

Question 22

Canthus

Section 13: Terms and Definitions

Question 21

Calibration

Section 13: Terms and Definitions

Question 23

Capnograph

Question 22 Answer:

Either corner of the eye, where the upper and lower eyelids meet. The outer canthus is used as a landmark for placing EOG electrodes.

Question 20 Answer:

Three branches from the Bundle of His in the heart that run along the interventricular septum

Question 23 Answer:

A recording of carbon dioxide levels over a period of time

Question 21 Answer:

A process of testing and adjusting diagnostic equipment in response to varying voltages of a known value. This process ensures reliability in recorded signals.

Section 13: Terms and Definitions

Question 24

Cardiac arrest

Section 13: Terms and Definitions

Question 26

Cardiovascular

Section 13: Terms and Definitions

Question 25

Cardiopneumograph

Section 13: Terms and Definitions

Question 27

Cataplexy

Question 26 Answer:

Referring to blood vessels and the heart

Question 24 Answer:

A complete cessation of beating in the heart

Question 27 Answer:

A common symptom of narcolepsy characterized by a brief loss of muscle tone with resulting weakness, often in the knees or legs. This is usually triggered by a strong emotion such as anger or laughter.

Question 25 Answer:

A device for measuring respiratory effort that uses two chest electrodes to record changes in impedance by measuring current flow in an AC circuit.

Section 13: Terms and Definitions

Question 28

Catathrenia

Section 13: Terms and Definitions

Question 30

Circadian rhythm

Section 13: Terms and Definitions

Question 29

Chronotherapy

Section 13: Terms and Definitions

Question 31

Clavicle

Question 30 Answer:

The cycle of fluctuations in biological and behavioral functions seen in mammals and other living things. The suprachiasmatic nucleus is the pacemaker for the circadian rhythm and is strongly affected by light.

Question 28 Answer:

Another name for sleep-related groaning

Question 31 Answer:

The collarbone. This is used as a landmark for EKG lead placement.

Question 29 Answer:

A treatment for circadian rhythm disorders that adjusts sleeping and awakening times in an attempt to reset the biological clock.

Section 13: Terms and Definitions

Question 32

Common mode rejection ratio (CMRR)

Section 13: Terms and Definitions

Question 34

Confusional arousal

Section 13: Terms and Definitions

Question 33

Compliance

Section 13: Terms and Definitions

Question 35

DC amplifier

Question 34 Answer:

An event characterized by awakening with disorientation and decreased mentation

Question 32 Answer:

A rating of the ability of a differential amplifier to eliminate identical inputs

Question 35 Answer:

Direct current amplifier. An amplifier that processes slowly changing electrical signals. A DC amplifier does not require the use of frequency filters and does not have negative signals.

Question 33 Answer:

The ability to adhere to or conform with treatment. PAP compliance is tracked closely in patients with OSA.

Section 13: Terms and Definitions

Question 36

Differential amplifier

Section 13: Terms and Definitions

Question 38

Dopamine

Section 13: Terms and Definitions

Question 37

Diurnal

Section 13: Terms and Definitions

Question 39

Double referencing

Question 38 Answer:

A chemical in the brain that is responsible for arousal of the cortex, movement, and responsiveness

Question 36 Answer:

An amplifier used in polysomnography that works by comparing the difference between two incoming voltages and then outputting a signal based on the difference

Question 39 Answer:

Using cables or software settings to link two reference leads to each other to decrease or eliminate artifact

Question 37 Answer:

A term referring to something that occurs during the daytime

Section 13: Terms and Definitions

Question 40

EKG arrhythmia

Section 13: Terms and Definitions

Question 42

Electrical baseline

Section 13: Terms and Definitions

Question 41

EKG dysrhythmia

Section 13: Terms and Definitions

Question 43

Electrical noise

Question 42 Answer:

The vertical position of a pen when the power to the amplifier is turned on

Question 40 Answer:

The absence of a regular rhythm in the EKG channel

Question 43 Answer:

Sixty-Hz artifact. Unwanted signals are received when impedances are high or a poor connection exists.

Question 41 Answer:

An abnormal rhythm in the EKG channel

Section 13: Terms and Definitions

Question 44

Head box

Section 13: Terms and Definitions

Question 46

Electrode popping

Section 13: Terms and Definitions

Question 45

Electrode impedance

Section 13: Terms and Definitions

Question 47

End tidal CO_2

Question 46 Answer:

An artifact characterized by occasional brief bursts of 60 Hz activity

Question 44 Answer:

A box into which the electrodes, sensors, and lead wires are plugged and from which a cable connects the signals to amplifiers, electrode selector switches, and the recording device

Question 47 Answer:

A reading of carbon dioxide levels in the blood as measured by expired air

Question 45 Answer:

Resistance to the flow of electricity from the scalp or body to the sensor or electrode. Impedances below 5 kohms should produce high-quality recordings.

Section 13: Terms and Definitions

Question 48

Environmental sleep disorder

Section 13: Terms and Definitions

Question 50

Epoch

Section 13: Terms and Definitions

Question 49

EPAP

Section 13: Terms and Definitions

Question 51

Epworth Sleepiness Scale (ESS)

Question 50 Answer:
In polysomnography, a page of the sleep study recording. The standard paper speed in polysomnography is 10mm/sec, which produces a 30-second page.

Question 48 Answer:
A secondary sleep disorder caused by a sleep disorder present in a bed partner, poor sleep hygiene, or other factors

Question 51 Answer:
A subjective daytime sleepiness assessment based on 8 different scenarios.

Question 49 Answer:
Expiratory positive airway pressure. Positive airway pressure during the exhalation or expiratory phase of respiration. EPAP and IPAP are identical during CPAP and dissimilar during bi-level PAP.

Section 13: Terms and Definitions

Question 52

Esophageal balloon

Section 13: Terms and Definitions

Question 54

Exploring electrode

Section 13: Terms and Definitions

Question 53

Expiratory phase

Section 13: Terms and Definitions

Question 55

Fibrillation

Question 54 Answer:

An electrode or sensor used to detect electrical activity in a specified area of the head or body

Essentials of Polysomnography, Glossary

Question 52 Answer:

A device inserted into the esophagus to measure small changes in airway resistance

Essentials of Polysomnography, Glossary

Question 55 Answer:

Unorganized activity, usually referring to the heart

Essentials of Polysomnography, Glossary

Question 53 Answer:

The segment of the respiratory cycle in which air is exhaled

Essentials of Polysomnography, Glossary

Section 13: Terms and Definitions

Question 56

Fibromyalgia

Section 13: Terms and Definitions

Question 58

Flattening index

Section 13: Terms and Definitions

Question 57

First night effect

Section 13: Terms and Definitions

Question 59

Frequency response

Question 58 Answer:

A calculation referring to the level of airflow limitation caused by partial obstructions of the upper airway

Question 56 Answer:

A disorder characterized by muscle pain and fatigue

Question 59 Answer:

A graphical depiction of an amplifier's ability to filter unwanted signals at varying frequencies

Question 57 Answer:

Negative effects of the first night in a sleep lab, often resulting in increased sleep latency and decreased sleep efficiency

Section 13: Terms and Definitions

Question 60

G1 curve

Section 13: Terms and Definitions

Question 62

Gamma-aminobutyric acid (GABA)

Section 13: Terms and Definitions

Question 61

G2

Section 13: Terms and Definitions

Question 63

Gain control

Question 62 Answer:
A neurotransmitter involved in relaxation, sleep, decreased emotional reaction and sedation

Essentials of Polysomnography, Glossary

Question 60 Answer:
Grid 1 or gate 1. This refers to the first input terminal on a differential amplifier or the exploring electrode.

Essentials of Polysomnography, Glossary

Question 63 Answer:
An amplifier setting that allows the user to multiply the height of a wave

Essentials of Polysomnography, Glossary

Question 61 Answer:
Grid 2 or gate 2. This refers to the second input terminal on a differential amplifier, or the reference electrode.

Essentials of Polysomnography, Glossary

Section 13: Terms and Definitions

Question 64

Gastroesophageal reflux disease (GERD)

Section 13: Terms and Definitions

Question 66

Ground

Section 13: Terms and Definitions

Question 65

Glutamate

Section 13: Terms and Definitions

Question 67

Ground loop

Question 66 Answer:

In polysomnography, a common reference for all electrodes to use as a measurement tool for voltage differences

Essentials of Polysomnography, Glossary

Question 64 Answer:

A disease characterized by movement of stomach acid upward into the esophagus. These acids often lead to obstructions of the upper airway during sleep.

Essentials of Polysomnography, Glossary

Question 67 Answer:

When two grounds are used, a signal can loop through both grounds causing safety implications and interference.

Essentials of Polysomnography, Glossary

Question 65 Answer:

Excitatory amino acids that project to the cortex, forebrain, and brainstem

Essentials of Polysomnography, Glossary

Section 13: Terms and Definitions

Question 68

Hertz (Hz)

Section 13: Terms and Definitions

Question 70

Histamine

Section 13: Terms and Definitions

Question 69

High-frequency filter (HFF)

Section 13: Terms and Definitions

Question 71

Histogram

Question 70 Answer:

A chemical in the brain responsible for activation of the cortex

Essentials of Polysomnography, Glossary

Question 68 Answer:

A measure of frequency, referring to the number of cycles per second (cps)

Essentials of Polysomnography, Glossary

Question 71 Answer:

A display of sleep stages achieved throughout the sleep period

Essentials of Polysomnography, Glossary

Question 69 Answer:

A tool or device on a polysomnograph which sets a limitation to the high-frequency signals that are allowed to pass through the amplifier

Essentials of Polysomnography, Glossary

Section 13: Terms and Definitions

Question 72

Hypercapnea

Section 13: Terms and Definitions

Question 74

Hypersomnia

Section 13: Terms and Definitions

Question 73

Hyperoxemia

Section 13: Terms and Definitions

Question 75

Hyperventilation

Question 74 Answer:

Excess lengths of levels of sleep or daytime sleepiness. The term is often used as a synonym for EDS.

Essentials of Polysomnography, Glossary

Question 72 Answer:

Excess levels of carbon dioxide (CO_2) in the blood

Essentials of Polysomnography, Glossary

Question 75 Answer:

A state of excessively fast breathing, resulting in decreased CO_2 levels and increased O_2 levels in the blood.

Essentials of Polysomnography, Glossary

Question 73 Answer:

The state of having too much oxygen in the blood

Essentials of Polysomnography, Glossary

Section 13: Terms and Definitions

Question 76

Hypnagogic foot tremor (HFT)

Section 13: Terms and Definitions

Question 78

Hypopnea

Section 13: Terms and Definitions

Question 77

Hypocapnea

Section 13: Terms and Definitions

Question 79

Hypoventilation

Question 78 Answer:
A 30% decrease in airflow for at least 10 seconds caused by a partial obstruction in the upper airway

Essentials of Polysomnography, Glossary

Question 76 Answer:
A sleep disorder characterized by rhythmic leg or foot movements at sleep onset

Essentials of Polysomnography, Glossary

Question 79 Answer:
Insufficient breathing which results in increased levels of CO_2 and decreased levels of O_2 in the blood

Essentials of Polysomnography, Glossary

Question 77 Answer:
Having too little carbon dioxide in the blood

Essentials of Polysomnography, Glossary

Section 13: Terms and Definitions

Question 80

Hypoxemia

Section 13: Terms and Definitions

Question 82

Impedance

Section 13: Terms and Definitions

Question 81

Hypoxia

Section 13: Terms and Definitions

Question 83

Inductive plethysmography

Question 82 Answer:

Resistance to the flow of electricity. In polysomnograph, EEG electrode impedances should be kept below 5,000 ohms.

Essentials of Polysomnography, Glossary

Question 80 Answer:

Having low oxygen levels in the blood

Essentials of Polysomnography, Glossary

Question 83 Answer:

A method of detecting respiratory effort by outputting changes in capacitance through an oscillator and to a calibrator unit

Essentials of Polysomnography, Glossary

Question 81 Answer:

The deficiency of oxygen supply to the bod

Essentials of Polysomnography, Glossary

Section 13: Terms and Definitions

Question 84

Inion

Section 13: Terms and Definitions

Question 86

Intercostal EMG

Section 13: Terms and Definitions

Question 85

Inspiratory phase

Section 13: Terms and Definitions

Question 87

Internodal pathways

Question 86 Answer:

An EMG channel used to measure respiratory effort by detecting activity in the intercostal muscles

Essentials of Polysomnography, Glossary

Question 84 Answer:

An anatomical landmark on the back of the head where the occipital bone protrudes from the skull. This landmark is used in the international 10/20 system of electrode placement to locate electrode sites.

Essentials of Polysomnography, Glossary

Question 87 Answer:

The pathways which the electrical impulses of the heart follow, from the SA node to the AV node

Essentials of Polysomnography, Glossar

Question 85 Answer:

Referring to the portion of the respiratory cycle in which inhalation occurs or during which time air is inhaled into the lungs

Essentials of Polysomnography, Glossary

Section 13: Terms and Definitions

Question 88

IPAP

Section 13: Terms and Definitions

Question 90

Klein-Levin syndrome

Section 13: Terms and Definitions

Question 89

Isomorphism

Section 13: Terms and Definitions

Question 91

Light therapy

Question 90 Answer:

A disorder that has recurrent hypersomnia as one of its symptoms

Question 88 Answer:

Inspiratory positive airway pressure. Positive airway pressure during the inhalation or inspiratory phase of respiration. EPAP and IPAP are identical during CPAP and dissimilar during bi-level PAP.

Question 91 Answer:

A treatment commonly used for insomnia and certain circadian rhythm disorders that includes exposing the eyes to additional levels of light in the morning hours to boost the circadian rhythm

Question 89 Answer:

Acting out dreams

Section 13: Terms and Definitions

Question 92

Low-frequency filter (LFF)

Section 13: Terms and Definitions

Question 94

Major body movement

Section 13: Terms and Definitions

Question 93

Maintenance of wakefulness test (MWT)

Section 13: Terms and Definitions

Question 95

Masseter

Question 94 Answer:

An epoch in which the patient's body movements obscure the tracings to the point that the sleep stage cannot be determined

Question 92 Answer:

A tool or device on a polysomnograph that sets a limitation to the low-frequency signals that are allowed to pass through the amplifier

Question 95 Answer:

A muscle in the chin and jaw area

Question 93 Answer:

A sleep study in which the patient is given several opportunities to remain awake while in a relaxed, darkened environment

Section 13: Terms and Definitions

Question 96

Mastoid

Section 13: Terms and Definitions

Question 98

Mechanical baseline

Section 13: Terms and Definitions

Question 97

Material Safety Data Sheet (MSDS)

Section 13: Terms and Definitions

Question 99

Melatonin

Question 98 Answer:

The vertical placement of a pen when the power to the amplifier is turned off

Question 96 Answer:

The lower part of the bone behind the ears. In polysomnography, the mastoid is used as a location for the reference electrodes M1 and M2.

Question 99 Answer:

A hormone secreted by the pineal gland that affects wakefulness

Question 97 Answer:

Information provided by the manufacturer of a potentially hazardous product that discloses proper uses and potential dangers

Section 13: Terms and Definitions

Question 100

Mercury strain gauge

Section 13: Terms and Definitions

Question 102

Montage

Section 13: Terms and Definitions

Question 101

Microarousal

Section 13: Terms and Definitions

Question 103

Movement arousal

Question 102 Answer:

The defined arrangement of channels and signal derivations on a polysomnogram

Question 100 Answer:

A device to detect respiratory effort by amplifying the change in resistance caused by circuit elongation and narrowing with a Wheatstone bridge box

Question 103 Answer:

An EEG arousal during which the patient moves

Question 101 Answer:

A brief EEG arousal or a partial awakening from sleep

Section 13: Terms and Definitions

Question 104

Multiple sleep latency test (MSLT)

Section 13: Terms and Definitions

Question 106

Narcolepsy tetrad

Section 13: Terms and Definitions

Question 105

Myoclonus

Section 13: Terms and Definitions

Question 107

Nasion

Question 106 Answer:

A group of symptoms commonly associated with narcolepsy, including EDS, hypnagogic hallucinations, sleep paralysis, and cataplexy. Few narcoleptics have all of these symptoms.

Question 104 Answer:

A daytime study consisting of five short nap opportunities of approximately 20 minutes each. Sleep latency is measured, and REM periods are considered abnormal. The study is commonly used to diagnose narcolepsy.

Question 107 Answer:

An anatomical landmark on the top or bridge of the nose where the forehead and nose meet. This landmark is used in the international 10/20 system of electrode placement to locate electrode sites.

Question 105 Answer:

A term referring to extremely brief muscle contractions or twitches

Section 13: Terms and Definitions

Question 108

Neurotransmitters

Section 13: Terms and Definitions

Question 110

Nocturnal confusion

Section 13: Terms and Definitions

Question 109

Nocturia

Section 13: Terms and Definitions

Question 111

Noradrenaline

Question 110 Answer:

A state of disorientation during, immediately before, or immediately after nighttime sleep

Question 108 Answer:

Chemicals in the brain that allow for the exchange of impulses from one neuron to the next

Question 111 Answer:

A chemical in the brain that maintains and enhances the activation of the cerebral cortex

Question 109 Answer:

Excessive or frequent urination during the night

Section 13: Terms and Definitions

Question 112

Ohm

Section 13: Terms and Definitions

Question 114

Paper speed

Section 13: Terms and Definitions

Question 113

Oxygen saturation

Section 13: Terms and Definitions

Question 115

Paradoxical sleep

Question 114 Answer:

In analogue polysomnography, the speed at which the paper is fed into the polysomnograph

Essentials of Polysomnography, Glossary

Question 112 Answer:

Unit of measurement for electrical impedances

Essentials of Polysomnography, Glossary

Question 115 Answer:

A term used for REM sleep. REM is considered paradoxical because the EEGs during REM are similar to the EEGs during wake, but the body is paralyzed.

Essentials of Polysomnography, Glossary

Question 113 Answer:

A measure of oxygen carried by the hemoglobin in the blood

Essentials of Polysomnography, Glossary

Section 13: Terms and Definitions

Question 116

Parkinson's disease

Section 13: Terms and Definitions

Question 118

Periodic breathing

Section 13: Terms and Definitions

Question 117

Perceptual disengagement

Section 13: Terms and Definitions

Question 119

Persistent insomnia

Question 118 Answer:

Episodes of repetitive central apneas

Essentials of Polysomnography, Glossary

Question 116 Answer:

A disease that often causes chronic pain and tremor and results in disruptions to normal sleep

Essentials of Polysomnography, Glossary

Question 119 Answer:

Insomnia that continues despite attempted treatment

Essentials of Polysomnography, Glossary

Question 117 Answer:

A change in consciousness that occurs at sleep onset in which the senses become partially or fully blocked

Essentials of Polysomnography, Glossary

Section 13: Terms and Definitions

Question 120

Phase advance

Section 13: Terms and Definitions

Question 122

Phasic

Section 13: Terms and Definitions

Question 121

Phase delay

Section 13: Terms and Definitions

Question 123

Physiologic calibrations

Question 122 Answer:

In polysomnography, an extremely brief event in sleep

Question 120 Answer:

A change in sleep to an earlier period in the 24-hour sleep–wake cycle

Question 123 Answer:

A series of simple tasks performed by the patient that serve as a baseline for scoring or the sleep study and ensure tracing reliability on the sleep study. These are also known as *biologic calibrations*.

Question 121 Answer:

A change in sleep to a later period in the 24-hour sleep–wake cycle

Section 13: Terms and Definitions

Question 124

Pickwickian syndrome

Section 13: Terms and Definitions

Question 126

Pineal gland

Section 13: Terms and Definitions

Question 125

Piezoelectric crystal

Section 13: Terms and Definitions

Question 127

Pittsburgh Sleep Quality Index (PSQI)

Question 126 Answer:

A gland in the brain that secretes melatonin

Question 124 Answer:

The former name for a sleep disorder characterized by obesity with somnolence, chronic hypoventilation, hypoxia, and secondary polycythemia

Question 127 Answer:

A series of questions in which a patient provides a subjective assessment of his or her sleep quality

Question 125 Answer:

A monitoring device that uses dielectric crystals under mechanical stress to generate a waveform showing respiratory effort

Section 13: Terms and Definitions

Question 128

Pneumatic respiration transducer

Section 13: Terms and Definitions

Question 130

Preauricular point

Section 13: Terms and Definitions

Question 129

Polarity convention

Section 13: Terms and Definitions

Question 131

Pressure transducer

Question 130 Answer:

An anatomical landmark used as a measuring point in the international 10/20 electrode placement system. This is located in front of the small notch at the midpoint of the ear.

Question 128 Answer:

A device for detecting respiratory effort that uses a cuff and bladder

Question 131 Answer:

A monitoring device that uses pressure from expired air to detect airflow

Question 129 Answer:

A standard used in EEG and polysomnography that specifies that a positive output signal is displayed as a downward pen deflection and a negative output signal is displayed as an upward pen deflection

Section 13: Terms and Definitions

Question 132

Pulmonary function test (PFT)

Section 13: Terms and Definitions

Question 134

Rebound sleep

Section 13: Terms and Definitions

Question 133

Purkinje fibers

Section 13: Terms and Definitions

Question 135

Referential derivation

Question 134 Answer:
Sleep after periods of deprivation, which usually consists of decreased sleep latency, increased stage R, and increased N3

Question 132 Answer:
A test designed to determine lung strength and volumes

Question 135 Answer:
A signal produced by comparing a signal transmitted through an exploring electrode to a signal transmitted through a reference electrode. This process is used in differential amplifiers.

Question 133 Answer:
Specialized myocardial fibers that conduct electrical impulses that enable the heart to contract

Section 13: Terms and Definitions

Question 136

Reference electrode

Section 13: Terms and Definitions

Question 138

Reticular activating system (RAS)

Section 13: Terms and Definitions

Question 137

REM extremity movement

Section 13: Terms and Definitions

Question 139

SaO_2

Question 138 Answer:

A system in the brain causing wakefulness and alertness

Essentials of Polysomnography, Glossary

Question 136 Answer:

An electrode or sensor used as a standard from which to compare potentials from an exploring electrode

Essentials of Polysomnography, Glossary

Question 139 Answer:

The amount of oxygen in the blood as read by an arterial blood gas

Essentials of Polysomnography, Glossary

Question 137 Answer:

A brief limb movement during REM sleep

Essentials of Polysomnography, Glossary

Section 13: Terms and Definitions

Question 140

Sampling rate

Section 13: Terms and Definitions

Question 142

Serotonin

Section 13: Terms and Definitions

Question 141

Sensitivity

Section 13: Terms and Definitions

Question 143

Sinoatrial (SA) node

Question 142 Answer:

A chemical in the brain that affects mood, appetite, aggression, body temperature, and sleep

Question 140 Answer:

The designated number of bits recorded per second in a channel

Question 143 Answer:

The point of the heart at which the electrical impulse begins. This is the pacemaker of the heart.

Question 141 Answer:

The ratio of signal input to the resulting wave. Sensitivity is usually measured in μV/mm.

Section 13: Terms and Definitions

Question 144

Sixty-Hertz filter

Section 13: Terms and Definitions

Question 146

Sleep debt

Section 13: Terms and Definitions

Question 145

Sleep architecture

Section 13: Terms and Definitions

Question 147

Sleep fragmentation

Question 146 Answer:

The amount of sleep an individual did not receive over a period of time but should have. This increases with sleep deprivation and can lead to excessive daytime sleepiness.

Question 144 Answer:

A unique filter pointed specifically at electrical activity in the 59-Hz to 61-Hz range to eliminate or attenuate 60-Hz activity

Question 147 Answer:

Brief EEG arousals or awakenings occurring during the night that reduce the amount of time spent asleep or in restorative stages of sleep

Question 145 Answer:

The pattern and percentage of REM and NREM stages of sleep achieved throughout the night

Section 13: Terms and Definitions

Question 148

Sleep hygiene

Section 13: Terms and Definitions

Question 150

Sleep inertia

Section 13: Terms and Definitions

Question 149

Sleep hyperhydrosis

Section 13: Terms and Definitions

Question 151

Sleep log

Question 150 Answer:

Feelings of tiredness that last longer than 10 minutes to 20 minutes after waking up

Question 148 Answer:

Practices that aid in initiating or maintaining sleep. These include going to bed at consistent times, using the bed only for sleeping, and avoiding heavy exercise just before retiring.

Question 151 Answer:

A diary of an individual's time in bed, estimated total sleep time, lights out time, lights on time, and daily activities. Sleep logs can help clinicians determine circadian rhythm disorders and causes of insomnia.

Question 149 Answer:

Profuse or excessive sweating during sleep

Section 13: Terms and Definitions

Question 152

Sleep mentation

Section 13: Terms and Definitions

Question 154

Sleep-onset REM period (SOREMP)

Section 13: Terms and Definitions

Question 153

Sleep-onset imagery

Section 13: Terms and Definitions

Question 155

Sleep paralysis

Question 154 Answer:

A REM period occurring at or just after sleep onset. This is considered abnormal and is often associated with narcolepsy and excessive daytime sleepiness.

Question 152 Answer:

Thoughts and feelings that take place during sleep

Question 155 Answer:

An event characterized by awakening and not being able to move for a period of time

Question 153 Answer:

The presence of mental images and experiences during the transition from wake to sleep

Section 13: Terms and Definitions

Question 156

Sleep restriction

Section 13: Terms and Definitions

Question 158

Snore sensor

Section 13: Terms and Definitions

Question 157

Snore microphone

Section 13: Terms and Definitions

Question 159

Soporific

Question 158 Answer:

A monitoring device that reads vibrations from the upper airway and delivers them to the polysomnograph to record

Essentials of Polysomnography, Glossary

Question 156 Answer:

The practice of limiting the amount of time spent in bed in an effort to treat insomnia

Essentials of Polysomnography, Glossary

Question 159 Answer:

A term describing something that causes sleep

Essentials of Polysomnography, Glossary

Question 157 Answer:

A monitoring device that detects noises and converts them to an electrical signal for the polysomnograph to record

Essentials of Polysomnography, Glossary

Section 13: Terms and Definitions

Question 160

SpO$_2$

Section 13: Terms and Definitions

Question 162

Strain gauge

Section 13: Terms and Definitions

Question 161

Stanford Sleepiness Scale

Section 13: Terms and Definitions

Question 163

Suprachiasmatic nucleus

Question 162 Answer:

A device to monitor expansion and contraction levels

Essentials of Polysomnography, Glossary

Question 160 Answer:

The percentage of oxygen in the blood as read by a pulse oximeter

Essentials of Polysomnography, Glossary

Question 163 Answer:

A structure in the brain responsible for the 24-hour circadian rhythm

Essentials of Polysomnography, Glossary

Question 161 Answer:

A scale consisting of seven statements describing subjective levels of sleepiness or alertness

Essentials of Polysomnography, Glossary

Section 13: Terms and Definitions

Question 164

Thalamus

Section 13: Terms and Definitions

Question 166

Thermocouple

Section 13: Terms and Definitions

Question 165

Thermistor

Section 13: Terms and Definitions

Question 167

Thermoregulation

Question 166 Answer:

A sensor placed in front of the nose and mouth that detects airflow by sensing temperature changes

Essentials of Polysomnography, Glossary

Question 164 Answer:

A structure in the brain responsible for relaying certain sensory information from the body to different parts of the brain

Essentials of Polysomnography, Glossary

Question 167 Answer:

Inherent regulation of body temperature in mammals

Essentials of Polysomnography, Glossary

Question 165 Answer:

A sensor that measures changes in temperature resulting from a patient's inhalations and exhalations

Essentials of Polysomnography, Glossary

Section 13: Terms and Definitions

Question 168

Tidal volume

Section 13: Terms and Definitions

Question 170

Time constant

Section 13: Terms and Definitions

Question 169

Time axis

Section 13: Terms and Definitions

Question 171

Tonic REM

Question 170 Answer:

The fall time of a calibration wave to 37% of its amplitude. This is synonymous with the low-frequency filter. The low-frequency filter is used to control slow-frequency waves.

Essentials of Polysomnography, Glossary

Question 168 Answer:

The estimated volume of air passed in and out of the lungs in a breath, usually measured in liters

Essentials of Polysomnography, Glossary

Question 171 Answer:

Periods of stage R in which no eye movements occur

Essentials of Polysomnography, Glossary

Question 169 Answer:

The horizontal time line of the polysomnogram that ensures the temporal relationship between signals being displayed

Essentials of Polysomnography, Glossary

Section 13: Terms and Definitions

Question 172

Transcutaneous CO_2

Section 13: Terms and Definitions

Question 174

Tricyclic antidepressants

Section 13: Terms and Definitions

Question 173

Transmembrane potential

Section 13: Terms and Definitions

Question 175

V waves

Question 174 Answer:

A group of medications designed to treat depression. Most of these also reduce REM sleep and are sometimes used to treat certain disorders associated with REM sleep.

Question 172 Answer:

A reading of carbon dioxide levels in the blood as measured by a heated sensor placed on the skin

Question 175 Answer:

Sharp negative deflections seen in an EEG channel. V waves are characteristic of the latter part of stage N1. V waves were formerly called *vertex waves* or *vertex sharp waves*.

Question 173 Answer:

Electrical activity across the cell surfaces

Section 13: Terms and Definitions

Question 176

Volt

Section 13: Terms and Definitions

Question 178

Zeitgeber

Section 13: Terms and Definitions

Question 177

Water-filled catheter

Question 178 Answer:

External stimuli such as light, melatonin, and physical activity that entrain biological rhythms to certain levels of wakefulness or sleep

Essentials of Polysomnography, Glossar

Question 176 Answer:

A measurement of electrical force

Essentials of Polysomnography, Glossary

Question 177 Answer:

A device used to detect respiratory effort

Essentials of Polysomnography, Glossary